Tools and Techniques in Computational Medicine

Tools and Techniques in Computational Medicine

Edited by **Marcus Lewis**

hayle
medical

New York

Published by Hayle Medical,
30 West, 37th Street, Suite 612,
New York, NY 10018, USA
www.haylemedical.com

Tools and Techniques in Computational Medicine
Edited by Marcus Lewis

© 2016 Hayle Medical

International Standard Book Number: 978-1-63241-415-1 (Hardback)

The publisher's policy is to use permanent paper from mills that operate a sustainable forestry policy. Furthermore, the publisher ensures that the text paper and cover boards used have met acceptable environmental accreditation standards.

Trademark Notice: Registered trademark of products or corporate names are used only for explanation and identification without intent to infringe.

Printed in the United States of America.

Contents

Preface

This book aims to highlight the current researches and provides a platform to further the scope of innovations in this area. This book is a product of the combined efforts of many researchers and scientists from different parts of the world. The objective of this book is to provide the readers with the latest information in the field.

Computational medicine is a rapidly growing field of medical science. It refers to the practice of using computer systems and software to diagnose different fatal diseases and to find how they are caused and the effects they have on human beings. It helps to study chronic diseases like cancer, heart ailments, etc. The aim of computational medicine is to study the growth of diseases in the human body and how it slowly kills the cells, tissues and other organs of our body. This book will bring forth some of the most innovative concepts and elucidate the new advances made in this area. It presents the complex subject of computational medicine in the most comprehensible format. It will serve as a reference guide to a broad spectrum of readers like students, doctors, experts, physicians, scientists, etc.

I would like to express my sincere thanks to the authors for their dedicated efforts in the completion of this book. I acknowledge the efforts of the publisher for providing constant support. Lastly, I would like to thank my family for their support in all academic endeavors.

Editor

Use of SSA and MCSSA in the Analysis of Cardiac RR Time Series

R. A. Thuraisingham

1A, Russell Street, Eastwood, NSW 2122, Australia

Correspondence should be addressed to R. A. Thuraisingham; ranjit@optusnet.com.au

Academic Editor: Gabriela Mustata Wilson

A new preprocessing procedure in the analysis of cardiac RR interval time series is described. It uses the singular spectrum analysis (SSA) and the Monte Carlo SSA (MCSSA) test. A novel feature of this preprocessing procedure is the ability to identify the noise component present in the series with a given probability and to separate the time series into a trend, signal, and noise. The MCSSA test involves testing whether the modes obtained from SSA can be generated by a noise process leading to separation of the noise modes from the signal. The procedure described here does not discard or modify any sample in the record but merely separates the time series into a trend, signal, and noise, allowing for further analysis of these components. The procedure is not limited to the length of the record and could be applied to nonstationary data. The basis functions used in SSA are data adaptive in that they are not chosen a priori but instead are dependent on the data set used, increasing flexibility to the analysis. The procedure is illustrated using the RR interval time series of a healthy, congestive heart failure, and atrial fibrillation subject.

1. Introduction

Singular spectrum analysis (SSA) [1–4] is an analytical tool that is used in time series analysis. Although it has been used widely in the analysis of environmental data [1–6] its use in biomedical signals has not received much attention. Some of biomedical signals that have been used to illustrate SSA are electroencephalogram (EEG) signals collected during evoked potential studies [7], ultrasound [8], and the electrocardiogram signal (ECG) [9, 10]. In the latter it was used to separate the fetal ECG signal from the maternal signal and in the separation of the heart sound artifact from the respiratory signals. This paper is an attempt to illustrate its value in the analysis of the cardiac RR time series data. The main focus in this paper is on preprocessing the cardiac RR interval series. It proposes an alternate procedure to the use of wavelet analysis for trend removal and the use of impulse rejection filter to remove artifacts [11]. Measured cardiac data contains a large amount of noise and nonlinear trend which require separation before any statistical assessment on the signal can be carried out. The method proposed here uses SSA, followed by the Monte Carlo singular spectrum analysis test (MCSSA) [1, 12]. It is a novel technique not only to separate the signal into various SSA modes but also to identify the SSA modes which correspond to noise. The MCSSA test [1, 12] involves testing the SSA modes of the original data with a large number of surrogate noise time series generated from random data having similar statistical properties of variance and autocovariance of lag 1 as the original series. The test identifies with a certain probability that certain SSA modes could be associated with autocorrelated noise. The use of such a test helps in the separation of the raw time series into a signal and noise. Some of the components in the signal are then fitted to the raw time series to match the trend, separating the raw series further into a trend, signal, and noise. The procedure is not limited to stationary data. The ability to identify certain SSA modes with noise processes of a given probability is a novel feature of the proposed procedure. This provides a certain confidence in the identification of the signal. Further the basis functions used in SSA for the separation of the signal are not chosen a priori as in the wavelet procedure but instead are dependent on the data used.

The SSA method and the MCSSA are described in Section 2. Section 3 is the results of the application of this technique in the analysis of three RR interval time series one from a healthy subject (N), the other two from subjects having congestive heart failure (CHF) and atrial fibrillation (AF). The data was obtained from MIT-BIH Normal Sinus Rhythm database and BIDMC Congestive Heart Failure database and MIT-BIH Atrial Fibrillation database, posted on Physionet [13]. Section 4 is the conclusion.

2. Method

2.1. Singular Spectrum Analysis. The term singular spectrum analysis comes from the spectral (eigenvalue) decomposition of a matrix X into its set (spectrum) of eigenvalues. These eigenvalues λ are the numbers that make the matrix $X - \lambda I$ singular where I is the unit matrix. The singular spectrum analysis (SSA) is the analysis of the time series using the singular spectrum. It was first introduced by Fraedrich [2] and Broomhead and King [3]. An excellent exposition of this technique is given by Elsner and Tsonis [1].

Time series are essential for describing and characterizing a physical system. This tool is a method to extract reliable information without relying on prior knowledge about the underlying physics or biology of the system. In SSA, the time series record is organized into a real symmetric matrix. This is done by making lagged or delayed copies of a segment of the time series. Suppose there are N_t values of a uniformly sampled time series x_i, $i = 1, 2, 3, \ldots, N_t$. An embedding dimension m is then chosen. The data is then arranged into an $(N \times m)$ matrix X with $N = N_t - m + 1$ as

$$X = 1/\sqrt{N} \begin{pmatrix} x_1 & x_2 & x_3 \cdots & x_m \\ x_2 & x_3 & x_4 \cdots & x_{m+1} \\ \cdots & \cdots & \cdots & \cdots \\ x_N & x_{N+1} & x_{N+2} \cdots & x_{N+m-1} \end{pmatrix}, \quad (1)$$

where $\sqrt{N}$ is a convenient normalization. The constructed matrix X is called the trajectory matrix, and it contains the complete record of patterns that have occurred within a window of size m. The elements of the matrix X are constructed as

$$X(i, j) = x_{i+j-1}, \quad 1 \le i \le N = N_t - m + 1; \ 1 \le j \le m. \quad (2)$$

The embedding dimension or also known as the window width determines the longest periodicity captured by SSA. A lagged covariance matrix S is then computed as the product of the trajectory matrix X and its transpose X^T given by

$$S = X^T X. \quad (3)$$

The matrix S is a real square symmetric ($m \times m$) matrix. Such a matrix can be made diagonal using a matrix E whose columns are orthonormal and a diagonal matrix Λ such that

$$S = E\Lambda E^T. \quad (4)$$

The square roots of the ordered real eigenvalues λ_k, $k = 1, \ldots, m$, of the matrix S are collectively called the singular spectrum. The corresponding eigenvectors $E(:, k)$ are referred to by different names such as basis functions, eigen vectors,

and empirical orthogonal Functions (EOF). E^T is the transpose of E.

The principal component a_k or sometimes referred to as the mode has N components where each component is obtained by projecting a time record each with m components onto to m components of the eigenvector k. The principal component matrix will therefore be an $m \times N$ matrix, where each row corresponds to an eigenvector with the N columns for the N time lags. The element $a(k, i)$ is given by

$$a(k, i) = \sum_{j=1}^{m} x_{i+j-1} E(j, k), \quad i = 1, 2, \ldots, N, \ k = 1, 2, \ldots, m. \quad (5)$$

The eigen values $\{\lambda_k\}$ correspond to the variance of each SSA mode $\{a(k)\}$.

As a result of orthogonality, each mode can be probed independently from the remainder of the time record. The entire time series can be reconstructed via reconstructed components (RC's) where each RC is associated with a mode and EOF. The component RC^k can be written as

$$RC^k_{i+j-1} = a(k, i) E(j, k), \quad i = 1, 2, \ldots, N, \ j = 1, 2, \ldots, m. \quad (6)$$

The original signal can be reconstructed from the RC's via

$$x_{i+j-1} = \sum_{k=1}^{m} RC^k_{i+j-1}, \quad i = 1, 2, \ldots, N, \ j = 1, 2, \ldots, m. \quad (7)$$

If filtering is carried out in the above summation k is restricted to values less than m.

Once the eigenvalues λ_k of the lagged covariance matrix S are determined, a plot of λ_k as a function of the mode k is carried out. If white noise is present there will be a clear break in the singular values, with the eigenvalues associated with the noise spreading out almost flat with low values. On the other hand if the noise is red there will be a gradual exponential decay which will make it difficult to separate the signal from noise. In the next section identifying the modes related to noise and signal will be carried out using MCSSA.

An oscillatory mode is characterized by a pair of nearly equal SSA eigenvalues and associated modes that are in approximate phase quadrature [1, 4]. Such a pair can represent efficiently a nonlinear, anharmonic oscillation. This allows an oscillatory mode to be detected. A single pair of data-adaptive SSA EOF's often will capture the basic periodicity of an oscillatory mode better than methods with fixed basis functions such as sines or cosines used in Fourier transform.

2.2. MCSSA. Monte Carlo SSA (MCSSA) [1, 12] is used to establish whether a given time series is distinguishable from a linear stochastic process which is normally considered as noise. Noise processes can be a described by a first order autoregressive process (AR(1)) where the value at a time $t(u_t)$ depends on the value at time $t - 1(u_{t-1})$ only

$$u_t = cu_{t-1} + e_t, \quad (8)$$

where c is a constant that represents the lag correlation between successive observations in the time series, referred to as the AR(1) coefficient, and e_t is a random error term with mean zero and variance σ^2. If $|c| < 1$, the series is stationary. If the noise is white, $c = 0$. For autocorrelated noise such as red noise where the power declines monotonically with increasing frequency, the range of c is within $1 > c > 0$.

For a series containing only white noise the eigen values of the lagged covariance matrix S are all equal. Further for a time series which contains a signal bearing component which is contaminated with white noise, the eigenvectors of the lagged covariance matrix S and S^{signal} are the same, and $\lambda_k = \lambda_k^{\text{signal}} + v^2$, where the noise variance is v^2 [1, page 71].

In order to determine whether the type of eigen spectrum obtained from the measured time series can be generated by an autocorrelated noise process, one estimates the AR(1) coefficient and the variance of the random error series e_t from the measured data, assuming it to be an AR(1) process. An estimate of the AR(1) is obtained from the normalized autocovariance coefficient (c) of the measured data at lag 1 and the variance of the error series $e_t (\sigma^2)$ from the variance of the data $(\text{var}(x))$ and $c, \sigma^2 = (1 - c^2)\text{var}(x)$ [14]. A number of different noise surrogate series $\{u_t\}$ are then generated to identify the auto correlated noise process as an AR(1) process of the type shown by (8). They are obtained with $u_0 = 0$, the AR(1) coefficient c and with different realizations of random data all having the same variance σ^2. For each realization of the surrogate noise series the lagged covariance matrix S^{noise} is evaluated and the eigenvalues $\{\lambda_k^{\text{noise}}\}$ are obtained from the diagonal elements of Λ^{noise} where $\Lambda^{\text{noise}} = E_X^T S^{\text{noise}} E_X$, E_X being the eigenvector matrix of the measured data [1, 12]. An identical transformation is applied to each surrogate S_{noise} to obtain the eigen values $\{\lambda_k^{\text{noise}}\}$, $k = 1, 2, \ldots, m$. There is no need to diagonalize each S_{noise}. The procedure measures the resemblance of a given surrogate with the measured data set. The ensemble of the sets of eigenvalues from the surrogate noise series is then used to test the hypothesis whether the eigen value of the measured time series can be attributed to an oscillatory mode. The 95 percentile of $\{\lambda_k^{\text{noise}}(j)\}$ $j = 1, 2, \ldots, ns$ where ns is the number of surrogates are then computed for each SSA mode k. If the eigen value λ_k of the measured time series is greater than the corresponding 95 percentile value for the eigenvalue of the surrogate data then the probability that the SSA mode is due to autocorrelated noise is less than 5%.

In this section the above procedure is illustrated for three RR data sets obtained from N, CHF, and AF subject [13], These three RR series have different characteristics and will provide a good example to understand this technique. The study in this report is limited to these three series and not to a bigger group since the focus of this study is to illustrate the technique instead of a statistical study on a group of RR series using this technique. In each of these cases 500 RR intervals were used. The embedding dimension m was chosen to have a value of 248. This choice was based on theoretical

TABLE 1: Significant SSA and oscillatory modes for N, CHF and AF data.

Date type	Signal—SSA modes						Oscillatory SSA modes
Healthy	1	2	10	11	14	15	10 11; 16 17; 22 23; 32 33; 65 66
	16	17	22	25	26		
	32	33	36	37	39		
	40	45	46	51	52		
	57	59	62	65	67		
	69	70	80	81	102		
CHF	1	2	3	4	5	6	7	7 8; 9 10; 15 16
	8	9	10	11	12	13	
	14	15	16	17	18	19	
	20	22	23	24	25		
	26	27	29	30	31	32	
AF	1	2	3	4	5	6	7	5 6; 10 11; 12 13; 16 17; 18 19; 25 26; 28 29; 30 31; 36 37; 43 44; 50 51; 52 53
	8	9	10	11	12	13	
	14	15	16	17	18	19	
	20	21	22	23	24		
	25	26	27	28	29		
	30	32	33	34	35		
	36	37	38	39	42		
	43	44	46	48	49		
	50	51	52	53	54		
	55	56	57	62			

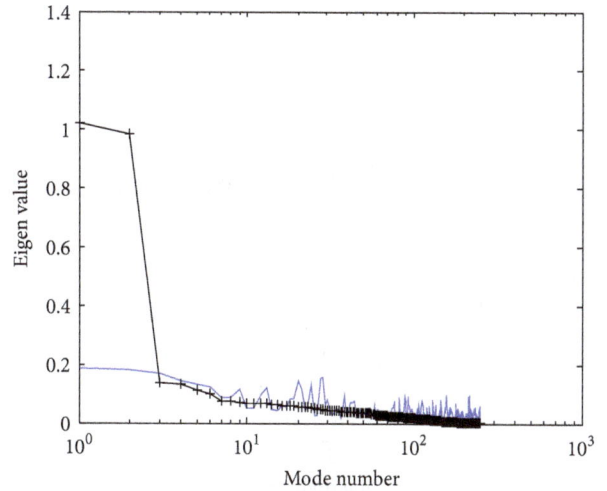

FIGURE 1: Eigen values of the SSA modes of the healthy data (red) along with the 95 percentile eigenvalues from an ensemble of 1000 surrogates generated by an AR(1) noisy process (blue).

results and studies based on a wide class of simulated and real data which indicate that the optimal choice of the embedding dimension or window length is close to one half of the time series length N [15, 16]. The number of noise surrogates used in MCSSA was 1000. That is, the surrogate list consists of 1000 different noise time series, with each time series containing 500 samples, the same number of samples as the time series that is being studied. This choice for the number of surrogates provided significance estimate to an accuracy of 1%, that is impossible to differentiate between 95% and 95.5% [1, page 97].

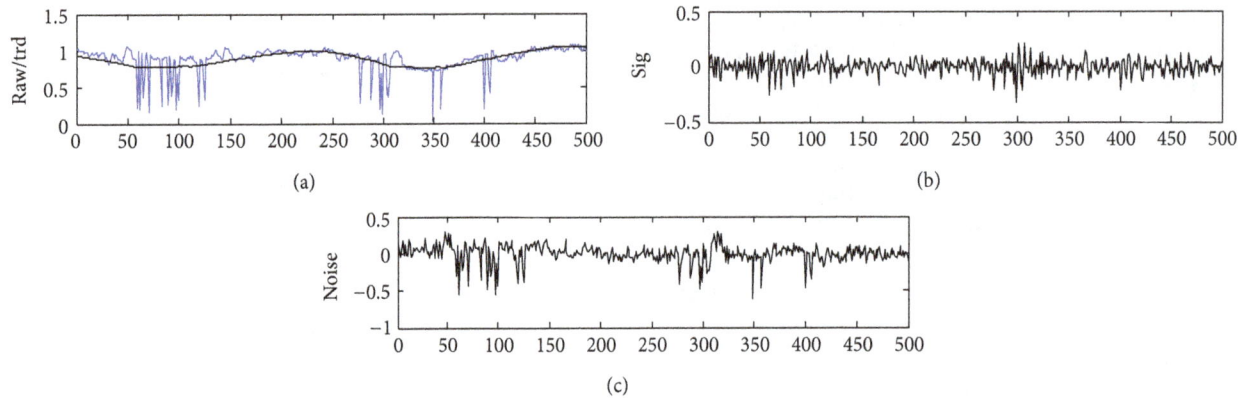

(a)

(b)

(c)

FIGURE 2: Healthy subject: (a) raw RR series (blue) and the trend (red); (b) the signal component of the raw series without the trend; (c) component of the raw series attributed to noise.

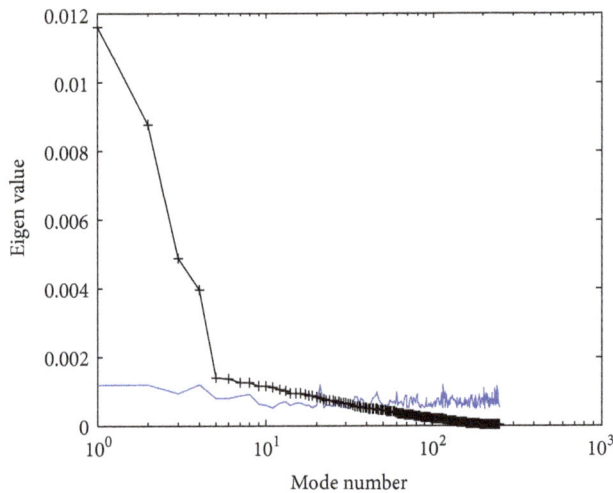

FIGURE 3: Eigen values of the SSA modes of the CHF data (red) along with the 95 percentile eigenvalues from an ensemble of 1000 surrogates generated by an AR(1) noisy process (blue).

Figure 1 shows the eigenvalues of the SSA modes of the data (red) along with the 95 percentile eigenvalues from an ensemble of 1000 surrogates generated by an AR(1) noisy process (blue). The information necessary to generate the noisy data is obtained from the measured data as described in Section 2.2. The SSA modes which are above the 95 percentile line are given in Table 1. These numbers total 31. That is, there are 31 eigenvalues associated with the signal and 217 with noise. Of this number, the modes where the consecutive eigen values are equal correspond to oscillatory modes having the same frequency but with phases offset by $\pi/2$. They are given in the second column of Table 1.

Before SSA is carried out the linear trend along with any residual mean is removed. The linear trend is removed by finding the best fit to a linear polynomial. The coarse nonlinear trend present in the series is then estimated from the first few signal modes with very high eigen values compared to the rest. In this case the first two SSA modes

contribute to this coarse nonlinear trend. The sum of the RC's that correspond to this nonlinear trend (SSA modes 1 and 2) is then added to the linear trend and mean to construct the observed trend of the raw RR series. This is shown as a red line superimposed on the raw RR series in Figure 2(a), where the healthy RR intervals are drawn. Figure 2(b) shows the sum of the RC's that constitute the signal SSA modes without the RC's of the trend. Figure 2(c) shows the part that is attributed to noise.

Figures 3 and 4 are similar plots for the CHF data while Figures 5 and 6 correspond to AF data. The numbers of the SSA modes that correspond to the signal and to the periodic signals are given in Table 1, both for the CHF and AF data.

The above results for the three different RR interval data sets illustrate the ability of the SSA technique to separate the raw series into a trend, signal, and noise. The trend seen in the raw time series is matched by the linear trend and a few low frequency RC's from the SSA. These RC's correspond to SSA modes having high eigen values, in comparison to the rest. Matching of the observed trend is carried out by successive inclusion of the RC's to the linear trend, beginning with the RC that corresponds to the highest eigen value, until a reasonable smooth reproduction of the trend is seen visually. The RC's that are used to construct the trend are a small subset of the RC's that are identified as the signal and obtained after filtering the noise components. For the examples chosen in this paper, the number of RC's that were used to construct the trend corresponded to the first two eigen values for N, first four for the CHF and the first eleven for the AF data. The eigen values corresponding to these RC's are quite separate from the rest. Although in this paper the RC's are chosen to visually match the trend observed, it is not limited to this procedure. Any other quantitative method could be chosen but it was found that the visual criterion was the safest procedure. What is identified is the coarse trend, and any procedure chosen must be verified visually to ensure that it is the coarse trend that is removed and not the signal.

The method adopted here to construct the trend and the signal is an alternate procedure to the use of wavelet analysis and the use of impulse rejection filter [11]. In the procedure mentioned in reference [11], the wavelet procedure

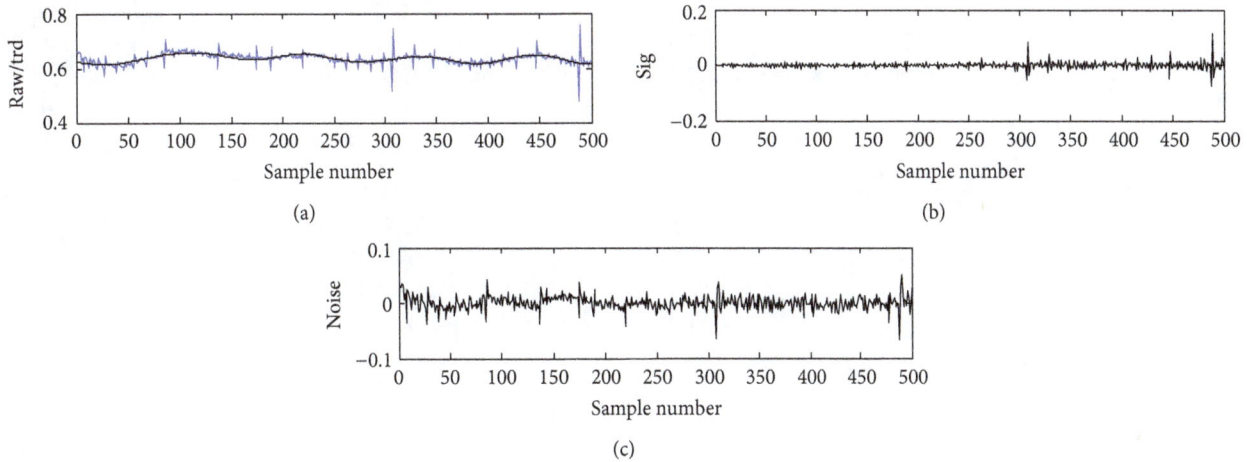

(a)

(b)

(c)

FIGURE 4: CHF subject: (a) raw RR series (blue) and the trend (red); (b) the signal component of the raw series without the trend; (c) component of the raw series attributed to noise.

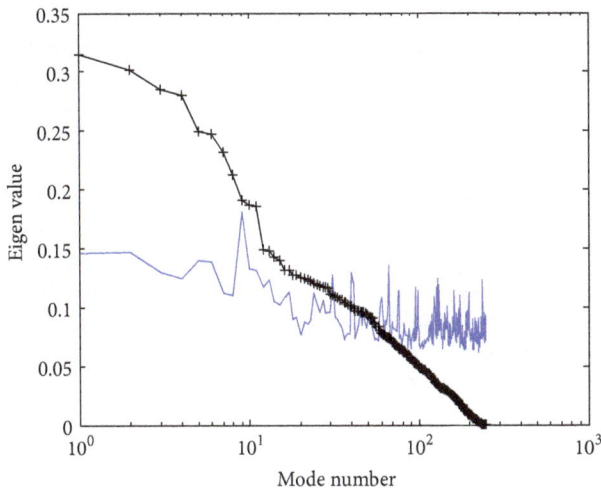

FIGURE 5: Eigen values of the SSA modes of the AF data (red) along with the 95 percentile eigenvalues from an ensemble of 1000 surrogates generated by an AR(1) noisy process (blue).

is used to remove the trend and the impulse rejection filter to remove the RR ectopic beats. The removed ectopic beats are replaced with the median RR value found in the adjacent sectors. Thus there is replacement of the original signal and no identification of the presence of colored or white noise. The present procedure is therefore different and superior. There is no replacement of any part of the signal but merely a separation of the signal into three categories: trend, signal, and noise. Further one of the main advantages of the present method is the filtering process for the noise which is verified by MCSSA.

The standard deviations of the signal for the N, CHF, and AF data are 0.067, 0.012, and 0.150 s, respectively. The depressed value for the standard deviation of the signal in CHF compared to N is in agreement with previous studies [11, 17]. Although the multiscale entropy (MSE) of a long AF record indicates that it can be approximated as white noise [18], the results on the SSA analysis done on a subset 500 samples from this same record indicate that such an approximation is invalid. If the AF record was white noise then the eigenvalues of SSA should all be equal [1, page 70]. This is not the case as can be seen from Figure 5 where the eigenvalues of AF are plotted. Further if the AF record is generated by a noise process, in MCSSA all the eigenvalues of the AF record should have been below the 95 percentile line, which is not evident. Also the visual presence of a nonlinear trend seen in the AF record is further evidence that there is correlation from neighboring samples. Such a result from a subset of a long record is not unexpected since the statistical properties of a finite sample from a large population will not always reflect the statistical properties of the larger group. This is the case when there are differing local time variations, which are averaged out when the sample number is increased. However the analysis of AF shows characteristics which indicate that it is more random than those of the CHF and N record. Let us examine this via the evaluation of the AR(1) coefficient which gives the correlation amongst neighboring samples.

Although the noise component is identified using the MC procedure, further separation of this noise as external or due to some internal cardiac process is not feasible at this stage. Assuming that all noise is internal, the AR(1) coefficient evaluated after removing only the linear trend from the data gives values of 0.493, 0.145, and −0.099 for the N, CHF and AF records, respectively. This shows that the correlation amongst the neighboring samples is the greatest for the N record with diminished correlations for the diseased subjects. Correlation is the least for the AF record indicating that it is more random. Since we do not expect all noise to be internal, another evaluation is carried out in the limit where all noise is external. In this case the linear trend and all noise are removed from the data sets and the AR(1) coefficient evaluated. The values for the AR(1) coefficient for the N, CHF, and AF records are 0.621, 0.231, and −0.101, respectively.

(a)

(b)

(c)

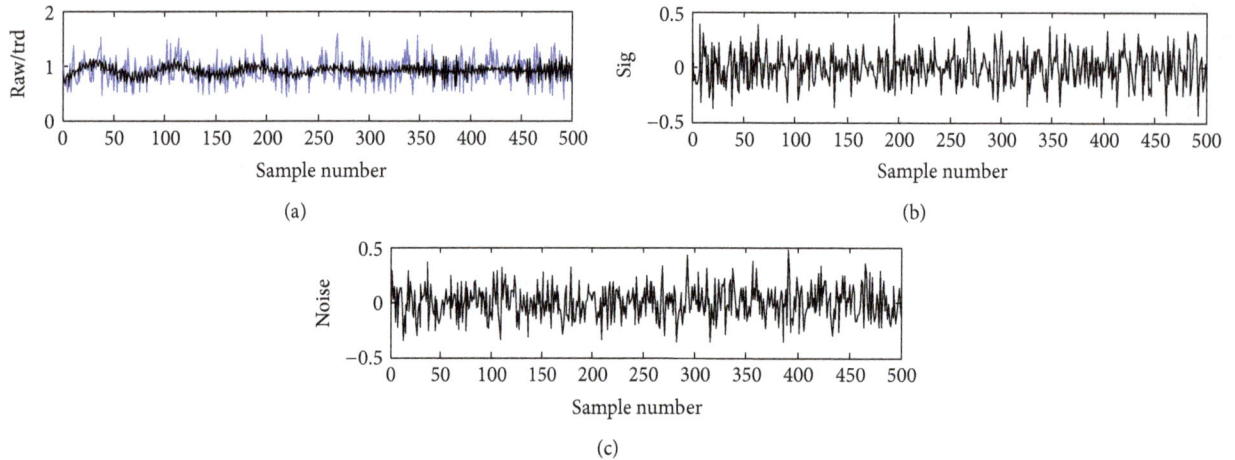

FIGURE 6: AF subject: (a) raw RR series (blue) and the trend (red); (b) the signal component of the raw series without the trend; (c) component of the raw series attributed to noise.

Again the neighboring correlations are in the order N > CHF > AF, with the AF record exhibiting the most random behavior. The presence of strong correlations in the healthy record and the diminished correlations amongst the diseased subjects is in agreement with the results of Costa et al. [18] showing that RR interval times of a healthy subject is more complex compared to those of a diseased subject.

The procedure outlined above using SSA does not discard or modify any samples in the record. It merely separates into different categories of nonlinear trend, signal, and noise. The nonlinear trend comprises a part the low frequency signal component which is added to the linear trend to fit the observed trend in to the measured data. The noise component is identified using a Monte Carlo procedure. Such an identification procedure for the noise component is an important feature of SSA. Since no part of the raw series is modified, with further available knowledge of external noise sources, it may be possible to separate noise components that are external from those that are heart related. This however is not carried here, since information about the external noise is unavailable. Although the example used in the illustration here has used a moderately small sample size, the method is not limited by such considerations. The choice of a moderate sample was made here merely from limitations to present details of such data in text. The division of a large sample into moderate subsets and performing SSA on them and then combining the results of the subsets is a computationally efficient procedure that can be adopted for large data sets.

4. Conclusion

A new preprocessing procedure in the analysis of cardiac RR interval time series using SSA is described. A Monte Carlo test is further carried to identify the noise component present in the time series. The latter procedure involves testing whether the SSA modes can be generated by a noise process, leading to a separation of the noise modes from the signal. Such an identification technique for the noise component is a novel feature of this preprocessing procedure. The procedure

does not discard or modify any sample in the record but merely separates the time series into a trend, signal, and noise, allowing further analysis of these components. The procedure is not limited to the length of the record and could be applied to nonstationary data. Another feature of this procedure is the basis functions used in the SSA analysis which are not chosen a priori as in wavelet analysis but instead are dependent on the data set used. The method adopted here to construct the trend and the signal is an alternate procedure to the use of wavelet analysis and the use of impulse rejection filter [11]. The method is illustrated using as an example RR interval time series of a healthy, congestive heart failure, and atrial fibrillation subject.

References

[1] J. B. Elsner and A. A. Tsonis, *Singular Spectrum Analysis: A New Tool in Time Series Analysis*, Plenum Press, New York, NY, USA, 1996.

[2] K. Fraedrich, "Estimating the dimensions of weather and climate attractors," *Journal of the Atmospheric Sciences*, vol. 43, pp. 419–432, 1986.

[3] D. S. Broomhead and G. P. King, "Extracting qualitative dynamics from experimental data," *Physica D*, vol. 20, no. 2-3, pp. 217–236, 1986.

[4] M. Ghil, M. R. Allen, M. D. Dettinger et al., "Advanced spectral methods for climatic time series," *Reviews of Geophysics*, vol. 40, no. 1, pp. 3-1–3-41, 2002.

[5] R. Vautard and M. Ghil, "Singular spectrum analysis in non-linear dynamics, with applications to paleoclimatic time series," *Physica D*, vol. 35, no. 3, pp. 395–424, 1989.

[6] H. N. Southgate, K. M. Wijnberg, M. Larson, M. Capobianco, and H. Jansen, "Analysis of field data of coastal morphological evolution over yearly and decadal timescales. Part 2: non-linear techniques," *Journal of Coastal Research*, vol. 19, no. 4, pp. 776–789, 2003.

[7] A. M. Tome, A. R. Teixeira, N. Figueiredo, I. M. Santos, P. Georgieva, and E. W. Lang, "SSA of biomedical signals: a linear invariant systems approach," *Statistics and Its Interface*, vol. 3, no. 3, pp. 345–355, 2010.

[8] W. C. A. Pereira, S. L. Bridal, A. Coron, and P. Laugier, "Singular spectrum analysis applied to backscattered ultrasound signals from in vitro human cancellous bone specimens," *IEEE Transactions on Ultrasonics, Ferroelectrics, and Frequency Control*, vol. 51, no. 3, pp. 302–312, 2004.

[9] M. Ghodsi, H. Hassani, and S. Sanei, "Extracting fetal heart signal from noisy maternal ECG by multivariate singular spectrum analysis," *Statistics and Its Interface*, vol. 3, no. 3, pp. 399–411, 2010.

[10] S. Sebastian and S. Rathnakara, "Separation of heart sound artifact from respiratory signals using singular spectrum based advanced line enhancer," *International Journal on Advanced Computer Theory and Engineering*, vol. 2, no. 4, pp. 107–112, 2013.

[11] R. A. Thuraisingham, "Preprocessing RR interval time series for heart rate variability analysis and estimates of standard deviation of RR intervals," *Computer Methods and Programs in Biomedicine*, vol. 83, no. 1, pp. 78–82, 2006.

[12] M. R. Allen and L. A. Smith, "Investigating the origins and significance of low-frequency modes of climate variability," *Geophysical Research Letters*, vol. 21, no. 10, pp. 883–886, 1994.

[13] A. L. Goldberger, L. A. Amaral, L. Glass et al., "PhysioBank, PhysioToolkit, and PhysioNet: components of a new research resource for complex physiologic signals," *Circulation*, vol. 101, no. 23, pp. E215–E220, 2000.

[14] http://www.statlab.uni-heidelberg.de/people/eichler/timeseries/ts5.pdf.

[15] H. Hassani, R. Mahmoudvand, M. Zokaei, and M. Ghodsi, "On the separability between signal and noise in singular spectrum analysis," *Fluctuation and Noise Letters*, vol. 11, Article ID 1250014, 25 pages, 2012.

[16] N. Golyandina, "On the choice of parameters in singular spectrum analysis and related sub space-based methods," *Statistics and Its Interface*, vol. 3, no. 3, pp. 259–279, 2010.

[17] A. Musialik-Łydka, B. Sredniawa, and S. Pasyk, "Heart rate variability in heart failure," *Polish Heart Journal*, vol. 58, no. 1, pp. 10–16, 2003.

[18] M. Costa, A. L. Goldberger, and C.-K. Peng, "Multiscale entropy analysis of complex physiologic time series," *Physical Review Letters*, vol. 89, no. 6, Article ID 068102, 4 pages, 2002.

2

On the Role of Optimal Counseling and Antiviral Therapy on Controlling HCV among Intravenous Drug Misusers

Steady Mushayabasa

Department of Mathematics, University of Zimbabwe, P.O. Box MP 167, Harare, Zimbabwe

Correspondence should be addressed to Steady Mushayabasa; steadymushaya@gmail.com

Academic Editor: Hon Keung Tony Ng

Hepatitis C virus (HCV) remains a major health challenge despite the availability of highly effective antiviral drugs. Prior studies suggest that many physicians are reluctant to treat intravenous drug misusers due to low levels of treatment adherence associated with intravenous drug misusers. HCV treatment guidelines and recommendations stipulate that HCV patients in treatment should abstain from intravenous drug misuse activities in order to reduce the likelihood of treatment failure, drug resistance, reinfection, superinfection, or mixed infection. In this paper, a mathematical model for exploring the transmission dynamics of HCV among intravenous drug misusers is proposed. The model incorporates essential characteristics of intravenous drug misusers such as relapse and nonadherence to treatment guidelines. With the aid of optimal control theory we assess the effects of time dependent HCV screening and treatment. Results from this study provide a framework for designing the appropriate strategies on controlling the long-term dynamics of HCV among intravenous drug users.

1. Introduction

Intravenous drug misuse continues to claim a large proportion of new hepatitis C virus (HCV) infections worldwide [1]. Despite advancements in the management of HCV and suggestions that treatment of recently acquired HCV can lead to virological response rate of up to 98%, low rates of treatment among HCV patients continue to be observed [2]. Apart from low treatment rates, nonadherence to HCV treatment guidelines and recommendations has been observed as one of the major challenges on effective HCV control among intravenous drug misusers [2, 3]. Adherence in the context of HCV treatment includes the patient's adherence to both the medication regimen and the overall medical plan [3]. Nonadherence to HCV treatment may be associated with a number of reasons among the following: higher pill burden and lengthy treatment, limited provider experience, lack of social support, and presence of cirrhosis [4].

This study aims to evaluate the effects of time dependent HCV screening and treatment. The application of optimal control theory on gaining insights into the long-term dynamics of HCV has been an interesting topic for a couple of researchers (e.g., see [5–8] and the references therein). In

2011, Martin et al. [5] developed a mathematical model to assess the impact of time dependent control on HCV antiviral treatment. Their work revealed, among others, that, with a fixed annual budget, greater impact on HCV control (measured by infections averted or prevalence reductions) and cost-effectiveness will be achieved in lower prevalence areas. Although nonadherence to HCV treatment is a major challenge on effective HCV control, few mathematical models have been proposed to assess its impact on HCV prevalence among intravenous drug misusers. It is against this background that this study is proposed.

2. Model Framework

We consider the mathematical model for HCV transmission among intravenous drug misusers proposed in [9]. The model utilizes a four-compartment model, tracking susceptible population S, HCV patients not in treatment I, HCV patients in treatment and having completely abstained from drug misuse activities A, and HCV patients in treatment and having partially abstained drug misuse activities B. Thus, the total population at time t is given by $N = S + I + A + B$.

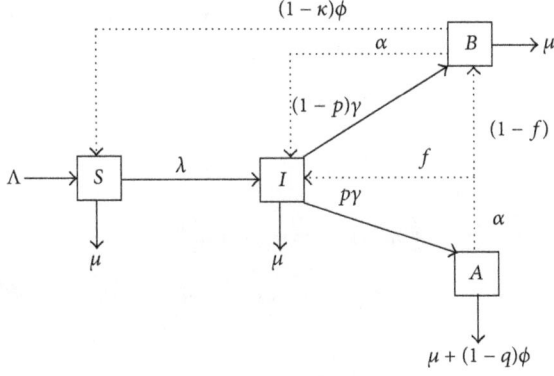

FIGURE 1: Flow diagram of the HCV transmission.

The dynamics of this model are governed by the following system of nonlinear differential equations:

$$\frac{dS}{dt} = \Lambda - (1 - \delta)\frac{\beta\left(cI + \theta\left(1 - \omega\right)B\right)S}{N} - \mu S + (1 - \kappa)\phi B,$$

$$\frac{dI}{dt} = (1 - \delta)\frac{\beta\left(cI + \theta\left(1 - \omega\right)B\right)S}{N} + \alpha\left(fA + B\right) - \left(\gamma + \mu\right)I,$$

$$\frac{dB}{dt} = (1 - p)\gamma I + (1 - f)\alpha A - \left(\alpha + (1 - \kappa)\phi + \mu\right)B,$$

$$\frac{dA}{dt} = p\gamma I - \left(\alpha + (1 - q)\phi + \mu\right)A.$$

(1)

The study assumes a homogeneous mixing population, with Λ denoting the entrance of new intravenous drug misusers; β is the probability of HCV transmission per needle sharing, c is the average number of needle sharing partners for individuals in class I per year, θ is the partner acquisition rate for individuals in class B per year, and θ is assumed to be less or equal to c due to the fact that individuals in treatment are assumed to have adopted a positive behavior towards the control of the epidemic. Hence, they are bound to reduce the number of partners compared to HCV patients unaware of their status; ω is a modification parameter accounting for the reduction in HCV infection by individuals in class B compared to those in class I (due to the fact that antiviral therapy reduces the viral load); the acute infection spontaneously clears in a proportion δ. Individuals in subgroup I seek treatment at rate γ. Upon commencing treatment, a fraction, p, of infectious individuals is assumed to fully abstain from drug misuse activities while the remainder $(1 - p)$ is assumed to partially abstain (i.e., they are assumed to continue participating in intravenous drug misuse activities with reduced partners); thus, they join class B. After successful treatment, a proportion $(1-\kappa)$ from class B recovers at rate ϕ and joins the susceptible class. A proportion $(1 - q)$ who successfully recovers from treatment in class A exits the model at rate ϕ. Natural mortality rate, μ, is assumed to be constant in all classes. Due to drug addiction, HCV patients in class A may relapse to drug misuse activities at rate α. Since class A constitutes HCV infected individuals who

would have fully abstained from drug misuse activities, we assume that a proportion f of those individuals who relapse join class I and the complementary proportion $(1 - f)$ moves to class B. All parameters in the model are strictly positive. The model flow diagram is depicted in Figure 1 with $\lambda = \beta(1 - \delta)[cI + \theta(1 - \omega)B]/N$.

3. The Optimal Control Problem

We introduce into the model system (1) time dependent control efforts $u_1(t)$ and $u_2(t)$ so that system (1) becomes

$$\frac{dS}{dt} = \Lambda - (1 - \delta)\frac{\beta\left[cI + \theta\left(1 - u_2\right)\left(1 - \omega\right)B\right]S}{N}$$
$$- \mu S + (1 - \kappa)\phi B,$$

$$\frac{dI}{dt} = (1 - \delta)\frac{\beta\left[cI + \theta\left(1 - u_2\right)\left(1 - \omega\right)B\right]S}{N}$$
$$+ \alpha\left(1 - u_2\right)\left(fA + B\right) - \left(u_1\gamma + \mu\right)I,$$

(2)

$$\frac{dB}{dt} = (1 - p)u_1\gamma I + (1 - u_2)\alpha A$$
$$- \left(\alpha\left(1 - u_2\right) + (1 - \kappa)\phi + \mu\right)B,$$

$$\frac{dA}{dt} = u_1\gamma pI - \left[(1 - u_2)\alpha + (1 - q)\phi + \mu\right]A.$$

The control functions u_1 and u_2 are bounded Lebesgue integrable functions. The control u_1 represents the efforts on screening and treatment of HCV patients unaware of their HCV status while control u_2 represents the efforts on monitoring and counseling of HCV patients in treatment. The problem is to maximize the objective functional as follows:

$$J\left(u_1, u_2\right)$$
$$= \int_0^{t_f}\left[(S + A) - \left(\pi_1 I + \pi_2 B\right) - \left(\pi_3 u_1^2 + \pi_4 u_2^2\right)\right]dt,$$

(3)

where t_f is the final time. The coefficients π_1 and π_2 represent the weight constants for infectious individuals in classes I and B, respectively. The parameters π_3 and π_4 are weights and benefit costs aimed at balancing the size of the terms u_1^2 and u_2^2, respectively. We seek to find an optimal control u_1^* or u_2^* such that

$$\mathcal{U} = \left\{\left(u_1\left(t\right), u_2\left(t\right)\right) \mid \left(u_1\left(t\right), u_2\left(t\right)\right) \text{ is measurable,}\right.$$
$$\left. 0 \le \left(u_1\left(t\right), u_2\left(t\right)\right) \le 1, \in \left[0, t_f\right]\right\},$$

(4)

where $\mathcal{U} = \{u_1(t), u_2(t) \mid u_1(t), u_2(t) \text{ is measurable}, 0 \le (u_1(t), u_2(t)) \le 1 \in [0, t_f]\}$ is the control set.

3.1. Existence of an Optimal Control Pair. The existence of optimal controls follows from standard results in optimal control theory [10, 11].

Theorem 1. *Consider the control problem with system (2). There exists an optimal control* $u^*(t) = (u_1^*, u_2^*) \in \mathcal{U}$ *such that*

$$J\left(u_1^*, u_2^*\right) = \max_{(u_1, u_2) \in \mathcal{U}} J\left(u_1, u_2\right). \tag{5}$$

Proof. The boundedness of solutions of system (2) for a finite time interval is used to prove the existence of an optimal control. To determine existence of an optimal control to our problem, we use a result from Fleming and Rishel (1975) (Theorem 4.1 pages 68-69) [10], where the following properties must be satisfied.

(1) The class of all initial conditions with an optimal control set u_1 or u_2 in the admissible control set along with each state equation being satisfied is not empty.

(2) The control set $\mathcal{U}$ is convex and closed.

(3) The right-hand side of the state is continuous, is bounded above by a sum of the bounded control and the state, and can be written as a linear function of each control in the optimal control sets u_1 and u_2, with coefficients depending on the time and the state variables.

(4) The integrand of the functional is concave on $\mathcal{U}$ and is bounded above by $c_2 - c_1 \left(|u_1|^2 + |u_2|^2\right)$, where $c_1, c_2 > 0$.

An existence result in Lukes (1982) (Theorem 9.2.1) [11] for the system (2) for bounded coefficients is used to give condition 1. The control set is closed and convex by definition. The right-hand side of the state system (2) satisfies condition 3 since the state solutions are a priori bounded. The integrand in the objective functional, $S + A - (\pi_1 I + \pi_2 B) - (\pi_3 u_1^2 + \pi_4 u_2^2)$, is Lebesgue integrable and concave on $\mathcal{U}$. Furthermore, $c_1, c_2 > 0$ and $\pi_1, \pi_2, \pi_3, \pi_4 > 1$, hence satisfying

$$S + A - \left(\pi_1 I + \pi_2 B\right) - \left(\pi_3 u_1^2 + \pi_4 u_2^2\right) \\ \leq c_2 - c_1 \left(|u_1|^2 + |u_2|^2\right), \tag{6}$$

where c_2 depends on the upper bound on S and $c_1 > 0$ since $\pi_3, \pi_4 > 0$. Therefore, the optimal control exists, since the states are bounded. $\square$

3.2. Characterization of the Optimality Control. Since there exists an optimal control for maximizing the functional (3) subject to system (2), we use Pontryagin's Maximum Principle

to derive the necessary conditions for this optimal control. The Lagrangian is defined as

$$L = S + A - \left(\pi_1 IX + \pi_2 B\right) - \left(\pi_3 u_1^2 + \pi_4 u_2^2\right)$$
$$+ \xi_1 \frac{dS}{dt} + \xi_2 \frac{dX}{dt} + \xi_3 \frac{dY}{dt} + \xi_4 \frac{dA}{dt}$$
$$= S - \left(\pi_1 X + \pi_2 Y\right) - \left(\pi_3 u_1^2 + \pi_4 u_2^2\right)$$
$$+ \xi_1 \left[\Lambda - (1 - \delta) \frac{\beta \left[cI + \theta (1 - u_2)(1 - \omega) B\right] S}{N}\right.$$
$$\left. - \mu S + (1 - \kappa) \phi B\right]$$
$$+ \xi_2 \left[(1 - \delta) \frac{\beta \left[cI + \theta (1 - u_2)(1 - \omega) B\right] S}{N}\right.$$
$$\left. + \alpha (1 - u_2)(fA + B) - (u_1 \gamma + \mu) I\right]$$
$$+ \xi_3 \left[(1 - p) u_1 \gamma I + (1 - u_2) \alpha A\right.$$
$$\left. - (\alpha (1 - u_2) + (1 - \kappa) \phi + \mu) B\right]$$
$$+ \xi_4 \left[u_1 \gamma p I - ((1 - u_2) \alpha + (1 - q) \phi + \mu) A\right]. \tag{7}$$

Theorem 2. *Given optimal controls u_1^* and u_2^* and solutions of the corresponding state system (2), there exist adjoint variables ξ_i, $i = 1, 2, \ldots, 4$, satisfying*

$$\frac{d\xi_1}{dt} = -\frac{\partial L}{\partial S}$$
$$= -1 + \mu \xi_1$$
$$+ \frac{\beta (1 - \delta) \left[cI + \theta (1 - u_2(t))(1 - \omega) B\right]}{N} (\xi_1 - \xi_2),$$

$$\frac{d\xi_2}{dt} = -\frac{\partial L}{\partial I}$$
$$= \pi_1 + \mu \xi_2 + u_1(t) \gamma (\xi_2 - (1 - p) \xi_3 - p \xi_4)$$
$$+ \frac{\beta c S (1 - \delta)}{N} (\xi_1 - \xi_2),$$

$$\frac{d\xi_3}{dt} = -\frac{\partial L}{\partial B}$$
$$= \pi_2 + \mu \xi_3 + (1 - \kappa) \phi (\xi_3 - \xi_1) + \alpha (1 - u_2(t))(\xi_3 - \xi_2)$$
$$+ \frac{\beta \theta S (1 - \delta)(1 - \omega)(1 - u_2(t))}{N} (\xi_1 - \xi_2),$$

$$\frac{d\xi_4}{dt} = -\frac{\partial L}{\partial A}$$
$$= -1 + (\mu + (1 - q) \phi) \xi_4 + \alpha (1 - u_2(t))$$
$$\times (\xi_4 - (1 - f) \xi_3 - f \xi_2), \tag{8}$$

with transversality conditions $\xi_i(t_f) = 0$ for $i = 1, 2, \ldots, 4$.

Proof. The form of the adjoint equation and transversality conditions are standard results from Pontryagin's Maximum Principle [10]; therefore, solutions to the adjoint system exist and are bounded. To determine the interior maximum of our Lagrangian, we take the partial derivate of L with respect to u_1 and u_2 and set it to zero. Thus,

$$u_1^* = \frac{\gamma\left(p\xi_4 + (1-p)\xi_3 - \xi_2\right)I}{2\pi_3},$$

$$u_2^* = \frac{\beta\theta cS(1-\delta)(1-\omega)(\xi_1 - \xi_2)B}{2\pi_4 N} \qquad (9)$$

$$+ \frac{\alpha\left[(B+fA)(\xi_3 - \xi_2) + (\xi_4 - \xi_3)A\right]}{2\pi_4}.$$

In compact form we have

$$u_1^* = \min\left\{\max\left\{0, \frac{\gamma\left(p\xi_4 + (1-p)\xi_3 - \xi_2\right)I}{2\pi_3}\right\}, 1\right\},$$

$$u_2^*$$

$$= \min\left\{\max\left\{0, \frac{\beta\theta cS(1-\delta)(1-\omega)(\xi_1 - \xi_2)B}{2\pi_4 N}\right.\right.$$

$$\left.\left. + \frac{\alpha\left[(B+fA)(\xi_3 - \xi_2) + (\xi_4 - \xi_3)A\right]}{2\pi_4}\right\}, 1\right\}.$$

$$(10)$$

The optimality system consists of the state system coupled with the adjoint system with the initial conditions, the transversality conditions, and the characterization of the optimal control. Substituting $u_1^*(t)$ and $u_2^*(t)$ for $u_1(t)$ and $u_2(t)$ in system (8) gives the optimality system. The state system and adjoint system have finite upper bounds. These bounds are needed in the uniqueness proof of the optimality system. Due to a priori boundedness of the state and adjoint functions and the resulting Lipschitz structure of the ordinary differential equations, we obtain the uniqueness of the optimal control for small t_f. The uniqueness of the optimal control follows from the uniqueness of the optimality system. $\square$

4. Numerical Results and Discussion

In this section, we numerically illustrate the optimal scenarios of the two controls $u_1(t)$ and $u_2(t)$. The optimal screening and treatment strategy is obtained by solving the optimality system (2) from the state and adjoint equations. An iterative method is used for solving the optimality system. We start to solve the state equations with a guess for the controls over the simulated time using a forward fourth-order Runge-Kutta scheme. Because of the transversality conditions (3), the adjoint equations are solved by a backward fourth-order Runge-Kutta scheme using the current iteration solution of the state equations. Then, the controls are updated by using a convex combination of the previous controls and the value from characterizations (10). This process is repeated and iteration is stopped if the values of unknowns at the previous iteration are very close to the ones at the present iteration [12].

4.1. Discussion of Parameter and Initial Population Estimates. Increasing the weights π_1 and π_2 leads to reduction in the population of subgroups I and B, respectively. In real world, parameter π_1 is greater than π_2 since HCV screening and treatment require a couple of procedures and a large population compared to counseling and monitoring of HCV patients in treatment. Similarly, $\pi_3 \geq \pi_4$. It follows that $\pi_1 = 1.1$, $\pi_2 = 1.5$, $\pi_3 = 0.3$, and $\pi_4 = 0.2$. We assume the following initial population sizes in our numerical simulations: $S(0) = 1500$, $I(0) = 500$, and $B(0) = A(0) = 0$.

4.2. Stopping Criteria. The implementation of the stopping criteria for the numerical scheme in this study uses the relative errors on controls, state variables, and adjoint variables. Thus, the optimal control iterations are performed until convergence in the relative update between all the state variables, the adjoint functions, and the control functions is less than a defined tolerance (TOL) value; that is,

$$\min_i \frac{\left|x_i^k - x_i^{k-1}\right|}{\left|x_i^k\right|} < \text{TOL}, \qquad (11)$$

where x_i is either the state variable, the adjoint function, or the control. The value TOL = 0.0001 is used in this study. Parameter values are defined in Table 1.

The effects of absence and presence of time dependent HCV screening and treatment are illustrated in Figure 2. Results from Figure 2 reveal that time dependent controls will have a remarkable impact on controlling new HCV infections among intravenous drug misusers. In Figures 2(c) and 2(d), one can observe that, in the interval 0–8 years, there is a higher population of HCV patients in treatment when there are time dependent controls compared to when there are no time dependent controls. However, the usefulness of time dependent controls is observed when $t > 8$; in this region, the population of HCV patients in treatment in the presence of time dependent controls is lower than the population of HCV patients in treatment in the absence of time dependent controls. Thus, the presence of time dependent control leads to low levels of HCV patients who will fail to adhere to HCV treatment, consequently leading to low treatment failure and high level of cessation in intravenous drug misuse activities.

Figure 3 illustrates the control profiles for the controls $u_1(t)$ and $u_2(t)$. In Figures 3(a) and 3(c), the control profile for control u_1 is at the upper bound from the start till the end. In Figure 3(b), the control profile for control u_2 is at the upper bound from the start till the end while in Figure 3(d) the control profile for control u_2 is at the upper bound from the start till when t is slightly above 15 years; thereafter, it drops sharply to the origin. The results here (Figure 3) suggest that, for effective HCV control among intravenous drug users, a slightly higher effort should be devoted to HCV screening and treatment than to counseling and monitoring.

5. Concluding Remarks

Intravenous drug misusers account for a disproportionately large burden of hepatitis C infection. Despite the availability of effective hepatitis C virus (HCV) antiviral therapy which

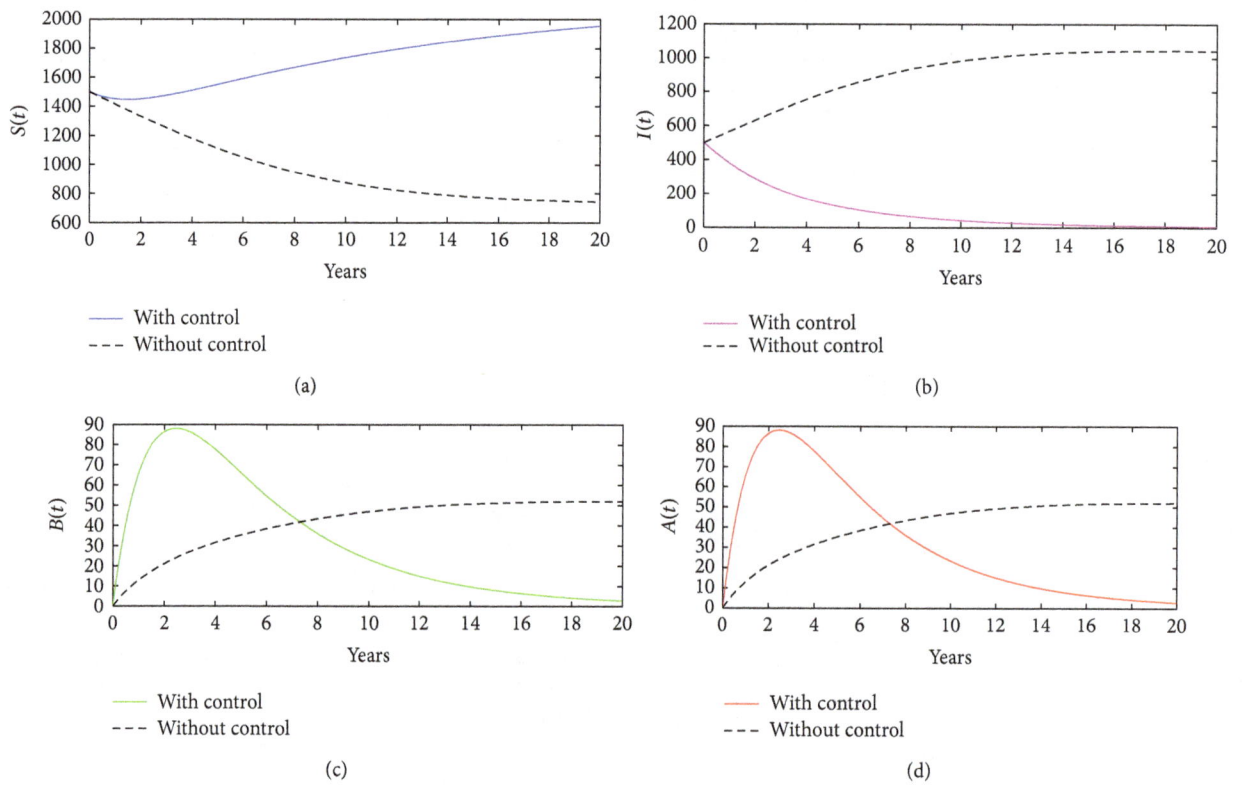

FIGURE 2: Simulations of model system (2) showing effects of presence and absence of time dependent controls on the long-term dynamics of HCV.

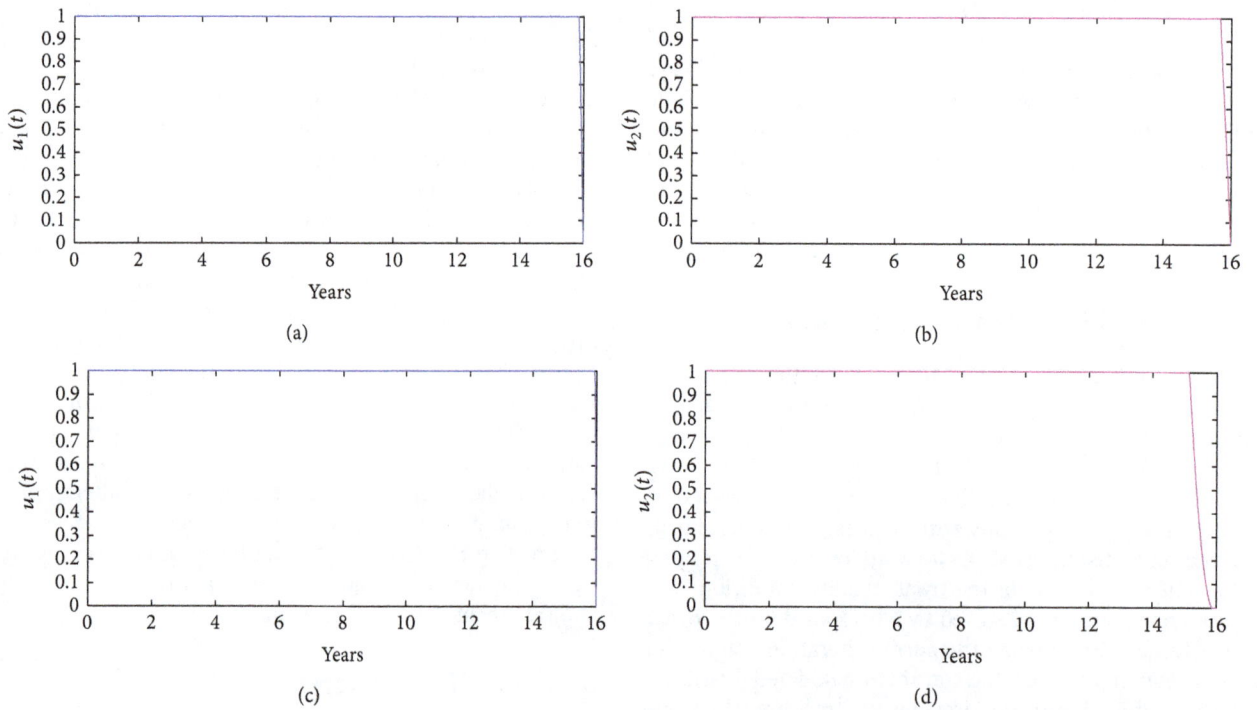

FIGURE 3: Simulations for the controls $u_1(t)$ and $u_2(t)$. In (a) $\pi_1 = 1.1, \pi_2 = 1.5$, and in (b) $\pi_1 = 1.5, \pi_2 = 1.1$.

TABLE 1: Model parameters and their baseline values.

Parameter description	Symbol	Units	Value (range)	Source
Relapse rate	α	Per year	0.1 (0.01–0.3)	[9]
Infection rate	β	Per year	0.1 (0.1834–0.2334)	[5]
Treatment rate	γ	Per year	0.02 (0.01–0.4)	[1]
Abstinence ratio	p	—	0.5 (0.01–0.6)	[9]
Modification factor	ω	—	0.5 (0.1–1.0)	[9]
1/treatment duration	ϕ	Per year	1.5 (0.9–1.992)	[9]
Natural mortality rate	μ	Per year	0.0142 (0.01–0.02)	[9]
New injector entrance rate	Λ	IDUs per year	250	Estimated
Average number of needle sharing partners for individuals in class I	c	IDUs per year	5.0 (1–10)	[9]
Partner acquisition for individuals in class B	θ	IDUs per year	3.0 (1–10)	[9]
Proportion of infections spontaneously clear	δ	—	0.26 (0.01–0.26)	[9]
Proportion of infections cured by treatment for class A	$1-q$	—	0.6 (0.5–0.625)	[9]
Proportion of infections cured by treatment for class B	$1-\kappa$	—	0.5 (0.5–0.625)	[9]
Proportion of relapse into class I	f	—	0.3 (0–0.3)	[9]

leads to a sustained virological response (SVR) rate of up to 98%, there continues to be a low rate of treatment uptake among intravenous drug misusers. In this paper, a mathematical model is proposed to assess the effects of time dependent HCV screening and treatment. The model incorporates counseling and monitoring of HCV patients in treatment. Monitoring and counseling may lead to a reduction in cases of treatment failure which arise due to nonadherence to HCV treatment guidelines and recommendations. The study reveals, among others, that more effort on HCV screening and treatment coupled with counseling may be effective on controlling HCV prevalence among intravenous drug misusers. Further analysis of the results suggests that effective time dependent HCV screening and treatment may be useful in combating new HCV infections even if <50% of HCV patients fail to completely quit drug misuse activities during the course of treatment. Although counseling and monitoring of a patient in treatment is never a bad idea, results in this study emphasize that a slightly higher effort should be devoted to HCV screening and treatment than to counseling and monitoring of HCV patients in treatment. Optimal control theory applied to an HCV model discussed in this paper provides a starting point for more elaborate models which can include drug resistance, superinfection, or mixed infection.

Conflict of Interests

The author declares that there is no conflict of interests regarding the publication of this paper.

Acknowledgments

The author is grateful to the Editor and the anonymous referees for their helpful comments which greatly improved the paper.

References

[1] S. Mushayabasa and C. P. Bhunu, "Hepatitis C and intravenous drug misuse: a modeling approach," *International Journal of Biomathematics*, vol. 7, no. 1, 2014.

[2] M. Hellard, R. Sacks-Davis, and J. Gold, "Hepatitis c treatment for injection drug users: a review of the available evidence," *Clinical Infectious Diseases*, vol. 49, no. 4, pp. 561–573, 2009.

[3] P. Higgs, R. Sacks-Davis, J. Gold, and M. Hellard, "Barriers to receiving hepatitis c treatment for people who inject drugs myths and evidence," *Hepatitis Monthly*, vol. 11, no. 7, pp. 513–518, 2011.

[4] Centers for Disease Control and Prevention, *Viral Hepatitis Surveillance*, Centers for Disease Control and Prevention, Atlanta, Ga, USA, 2009.

[5] N. K. Martin, A. B. Pitcher, P. Vickerman, A. Vassall, and M. Hickman, "Optimal control of hepatitis C antiviral treatment programme delivery for prevention amongst a population of injecting drug users," *PLoS ONE*, vol. 6, no. 8, Article ID e22309, 2011.

[6] A. Khan, S. Sial, and M. Imran, "Transmission dynamics of hepatitis C with control strategies," *Journal of Computational Medicine*, vol. 2014, Article ID 654050, 18 pages, 2014.

[7] S. Mushayabasa, C. P. Bhunu, G. Magombedze, and A. G. R. Stewart, "On the role of screening and educational campaigns on controlling HCV in correctional institutions," *Journal of Biological Systems*, vol. 21, no. 1, Article ID 1350007, 2013.

[8] S. Mushayabasa, C. P. Bhunu, and R. J. Smith, "Assessing the impact of educational campaigns on controlling HCV among women in prison settings," *Communications in Nonlinear Science and Numerical Simulation*, vol. 17, no. 4, pp. 1714–1724, 2012.

[9] S. Mushayabasa and C. P. Bhunu, "Mathematical analysis of hepatitis C model for intravenous drug misusers: impact of antiviral therapy, abstinence and relapse," *Simulation: Transactions of the Society of Modeling and Simulation International*, vol. 90, no. 5, pp. 487–500, 2014.

[10] W. H. Fleming and R. W. Rishel, *Deterministic and Stochastic Optimal Control*, Springer, 1975.

[11] D. L. Lukes, *Differential Equations: Classical to Controlled*, Mathematics in Science and Engineering, Academic Press, New York, NY, USA, 1982.

[12] E. Jung, S. Lenhart, and Z. Feng, "Optimal control of treatments in a two-strain tuberculosis model," *Discrete and Continuous Dynamical Systems B*, vol. 2, no. 4, pp. 473–482, 2002.

3

LASSO-ing Potential Nuclear Receptor Agonists and Antagonists: A New Computational Method for Database Screening

Sean Ekins,[1] Michael-R. Goldsmith,[2] Aniko Simon,[3] Zsolt Zsoldos,[3] Orr Ravitz,[3] and Antony J. Williams[4]

[1] *Collaborations in Chemistry, 5616 Hilltop Needmore Road, Fuquay-Varina, NC 27526, USA*
[2] *National Exposure Research Laboratory, US-Environmental Protection Agency, 109 TW Alexander Drive, Research Triangle Park, NC 27711, USA*
[3] *SimBioSys, Inc., 135 Queen's Plate Drive, Suite 520, Toronto, ON, Canada M9W 6V1*
[4] *Royal Society of Chemistry, 904 Tamaras Circle, Wake Forest, NC 27587, USA*

Correspondence should be addressed to Sean Ekins; ekinssean@yahoo.com and Michael-R. Goldsmith; goldsmith.rocky@epa.gov

Academic Editor: Gabriela Mustata Wilson

Nuclear receptors (NRs) are important biological macromolecular transcription factors that are implicated in multiple biological pathways and may interact with other xenobiotics that are endocrine disruptors present in the environment. Examples of important NRs include the androgen receptor (AR), estrogen receptors (ER), and the pregnane X receptor (PXR). In this study we have utilized the Ligand Activity by Surface Similarity Order (LASSO) method, a ligand-based virtual screening strategy to derive structural (surface/shape) molecular features used to generate predictive models of biomolecular activity for AR, ER, and PXR. For PXR, twenty-five models were built using between 8 to 128 agonists and tested using 3000, 8000, and 24,000 drug-like decoys including PXR inactive compounds (N = 228). Preliminary studies with AR and ER using LASSO suggested the utility of this approach with 2-fold enrichment factors at 20%. We found that models with 64–128 PXR actives provided enrichment factors of 10-fold (10% actives in the top 1% of compounds screened). The LASSO models for AR and ER have been deployed and are freely available online, and they represent a ligand-based prediction method for putative NR activity of compounds in this database.

1. Introduction

The nuclear receptor (NRs) family of transcription factors are important targets for therapeutic interventions for multiple diseases [1] and also may interact with other xenobiotics that are endocrine disruptors present in the environment [2]. It is therefore important to identify compounds that may specifically bind NRs and act as endocrine disruptors and develop synthetic compounds that can selectively (in a cell-type and/or tissue-selective manner) modulate NR pharmacology (reviewed in [3–9]). NRs including the androgen receptor

(AR; NR3C4), estrogen receptors α and β, (ERα and ERβ; NR3A1 and NR3A2) and pregnane X receptor (PXR; NR1I2) are particularly important as both therapeutic targets and for xenobiotics to mediate off-target effects.

The ERs are activated by 17β-estradiol while the AR is activated by testosterone and dihydrotestosterone and these receptors are transcriptional regulators of many genes [10] with important physiological functions [11–16]. The human PXR [17–19] similarly transcriptionally regulates genes involved in xenobiotic metabolism and excretion, as well as other cellular processes, including apoptosis [20–24]. Human

PXR is a broad specificity NR, binding a wide variety of molecules [25] and the activation of this NR can cause drug-drug interactions [23].

Multiple QSAR and machine learning models have been described for these NRs, to address endocrine disruptor risk assessment [26–28] and toxicological screening [29]. For example, a recent QSAR analysis of 74 natural or synthetic estrogens provided information on structural features for the activation of ERα and ERβ [30]. Nonlinear statistical machine learning methods have been applied to separate NR activators from nonactivators [31]. A virtual screening protocol identified ERβ specific ligands from a plant product-based database [32]; from 12 candidates evaluated by a fluorescence polarization binding assay, 3 had >100-fold selectivity to ERβ over ERα. The same approach has also been used to find compounds with good selectivity for ERα over ERβ [32, 33]. Bisson et al. have used computational methods that led to a nonsteroidal antiandrogen with improved AR antagonistic activity based on an initial screening of FDA approved new drugs [33]. Several groups have published datasets or performed modeling on ER and AR and these data are readily available for further evaluation with new modeling methods [34–38].

While the crystal structures of human PXR [39–43] have led to a greater understanding of the ligand binding domain (LBD) and ligand-receptor interactions [39–45], ligand-based computational models possess the key features for predicting binding [46–49]. PXR pharmacophores have been used to predict interactions for antibiotics [50] verified *in vitro*, and machine learning methods have also been evaluated [25, 38, 51–53]. Several protein-based docking studies have also been used to predict PXR agonists [25, 54–56], although machine learning methods appear to be advantageous to date.

We have recently described troubleshooting various computational methods [57] and specifically compared different methods for PXR [25]. There is a continuous search for new methods that might offer advantages for computational modeling to overcome some of these limitations and specifically for NRs [58]. A ligand-based software called LASSO (Ligand Activity by Surface Similarity Order) has been described that is focused on similarities in biomolecular activity rather than structural similarity [59]. The key components describing LASSO are the 23 kinds of Interacting Surface Point Type (ISPT) molecular descriptors (see Supplemental Table 1 available online at http://dx.doi.org/10.1155/2013/513537), which capture the essence of the surface point information in a feature vector containing the counts of each surface point type and create the feature vector for that ligand. This vector serves as the descriptor of that molecule with the assumption that ligands with similar feature vectors will have similar activity. A key property of the LASSO descriptor is its conformation independence which is due to the fact that it is defined by the number and type of Interacting Surface Points and not by their relative spacial distribution. LASSO has been shown to be able to readily screen over 1 million structures/minute, identify active molecules by enriching screened databases, and provide a means for scaffold hopping [59]. The current study applies LASSO to various NR datasets to generate models, validate them, and make the models available on a public website to illustrate how the method can be used. This work can be considered an extension of our previous troubleshooting studies [25, 57].

2. Materials and Methods

2.1. Training and Test Set Molecular Dataset Selection. One of the goals of this study was to determine what level of enrichment for binders (at weak or strong binding threshold) can be afforded using the ChemSpider LASSO descriptors (ligand-based approach) and compared with enrichment from a structure-based docking approach (eHiTS). For AR, the dataset consisting of 203 molecules with relative binding affinities and activity threshold classes of (a) strong, (b) moderate, (c) weak, and (d) inactive/nonbinding ligands, we evaluated the ability of LASSO to differentiate both (a) strong and (a + b) strong and moderate binders (all others were considered to be nonbinding). The training set for AR, derived with the LASSO descriptors, was obtained from the DUD set [60] and differ considerably from the test set. To evaluate the LASSO descriptors for the ER dataset consisting of 50 molecules with 15 "hits" (i.e., considerably weak binders) and 35 "nonhits" for the estrogen binding that differs considerably from the training set obtained again, we used the DUD ER (default or agonist and antagonist) as a training set [60].

In addition to the ChemSpider LASSO approach for the AR test set we used the eHiTS structure-based (molecular docking) screening strategy on two conformations of the AR (using PDB structures 2AMA and 1XNN) and reported the minimum score across the two conformations examined (this approach was used to add flexibility to the receptor). Similarly, for the ER dataset we docked against two functionally distinct conformations of the estrogen receptor (3ERT and 1GWR).

2.2. Datasets for LASSO Modeling: Structure File Preparation. The rat ER binding dataset (K_i values for 50 compounds of environmental relevance [35]) was obtained from EPA's DSSTox database (http://epa.gov/ncct/dsstox/ [34]). This dataset contains 15 industrial chemical "binders" (i.e., non-therapeutic) with significantly weaker binding affinities than what would be desired for drug lead candidates (i.e., 3–5-fold weaker binding affinity than the natural ligand 17β-estradiol). Similarly, the NCTR's rat AR activity dataset (competitive inhibition assays), also used in this study, contains 146 AR binders and 56 nonbinders (http://www.fda.gov/nctr/science/centers/toxicoinformatics/edkb/index.htm [37, 38]). All structures were imported into MOE and geometry optimized using the MMFFx forcefield in MOE (Chemical Computing Group, Montreal, Canada).

Three human PXR datasets were used, namely, dataset 1 represented 80 actives $EC_{50} < 100 \mu M$ and 64 inactives $EC_{50} > 100 \mu M$ that were drug-like molecules. The SMILES string for each molecule named or CAS number provided was obtained by downloading from either PubChem (http://pubchem.ncbi.nlm.nih.gov/) or ChemSpider (http://www.chemspider.com/) or sketched using the BUILDER module of SYBYL [56]. Dataset 2 represented 93 actives and 75 inactives that were drug-like molecules from a previous study [61]. The molecular structures encoded as SMILES strings [62] were downloaded from the supplementary information tables in the original publication [61]. Dataset 3 represented 30 actives and 89 inactives from a dataset of steroidal compounds (namely, androstanes, estratrienes, pregnanes and bile salts) as well as the ligands used in the crystal structures with hPXR activation determined by a luciferase-based reporter assay [25]. Human PXR activation was determined by a luciferase-based reporter assay as has been previously described in these and other publications.

2.3. LASSO Models for ER and AR.

2.3. LASSO Models for ER and AR. The methodology of LASSO has already been previously described in detail, [59] and the method performance in terms of diversity of test set and % enrichment of a database has also already been evaluated for the DUD set in paper just mentioned and also for other targets published elsewhere (http://www .simbiosys.com/ehits_lasso/ehits_lasso_table.html) to examine the performance of eHiTS LASSO, with this endocrine panel subset of target proteins of the total ~48 nuclear receptors. We used the newly assembled directory of useful decoys (DUD) [60] dataset to augment both the KIERBL and NCTR AR datasets.

2.4. PXR Models: Method I. The previously mentioned three PXR datasets were received from three different sources described earlier. Set 1, called: "hpxr_test," contained 80 actives and 64 inactives or decoys; set 2, called: "hpxr_train," contained 93 actives and 75 inactives; and finally set 3, called: "PXRl19-class," contained 30 actives with 89 inactives. Out of these three data sets, 7 screening prediction models were built using only the actives (the inactives were automatically generated by the software).

The following models were developed. Model 1 was trained on the first dataset (hpxr_test, 80 ligands) and tested with the other two sets (123 ligands). Model 2 was trained on the second dataset (hpxr_train, 93 ligands) and tested with the other two sets (110 ligands). Model 3 was trained on the third dataset (PXRl19-class, 30 ligands) and tested with the other two sets (173 ligands). Models 4–6 were trained on sets 1 and 2, that is, 173 ligands, sets 1 and 3, that is, 110 ligands, and sets 2 and 3, that is, 123 ligands and tested with the remaining one set of actives (i.e., 30, 93, and 80 ligands, resp.). Model 7 was trained on all actives (1, 2, and 3) and tested on the same. This was done as an extreme case to see the maximum potential training effect.

2.5. PXR Models: Method II. A second method for creating LASSO prediction models for the PXR test case was also investigated. Actives from the 3 datasets were all merged, resulting in an SDF file with 203 ligands with relative binding affinities and activity threshold classes (a) strong, (b) moderate, (c) weak, and (d) inactive/nonbinding ligands. To determine how many actives are needed to be selected for a good LASSO prediction model and also to see if the source of the actives is important, 25 LASSO models were developed

(Supplementary Table 2). Prediction models were built by selecting 8, 16, 32, 64, and 128 actives, starting from positions first, ninth, seventeenth, thirty-third, and sixty-fourth in the merged actives file.

The above 25 models were then tested for enrichment factor using the actives from the total active set and leaving out the ones used for training (this was 8, 16, 32, 64 or 128 ligands, resp.) mixed with drug-like decoys, that were obtained from another recent screening study [63]. To assess the effect of the size of the decoy set upon the prediction model, random 3000 (3 k), 8000 (8 k), and the whole 24,000 (24 k) decoy sets were used. In each case the decoys from all three sets received (228 structures in total) were added into the decoy test set.

3. Results

The enrichment plots shown for AR (Figure 1) and ER (Figure 2) with the percent actives recovered versus percent of dataset reveal an enrichment of ~2-fold at 20% of the dataset coverage regardless of whether a ligand or structure-based approach was used. For the AR dataset if the interaction threshold is specified as strong or strong + moderate, different levels of enrichment are incurred by either ChemSpider LASSO or eHiTS results. This translates into an improved performance of either ligand or structure-based screening approaches to bin molecules with stronger interactions (cyan and purple) than those substantially altered through the addition of weaker binding classes (magenta and yellow). Interestingly, in terms of the early-recognition problem, eHiTS is more sensitive (4-fold at 20%) than LASSO (1.5-fold at 20%); however, all 15 actives are captured by the LASSO descriptor within the first 37% of the dataset (with a minimum value of LASSO = 0.07) at considerably lower computational cost. A means of incorporating this into a real scenario would be to screen ChemSpider for AR with a descriptor above a threshold (in this case 0.07) from a specific dataset on ChemSpider and follow up these "hits" only with a more costly structure-based approach.

For the ER dataset where all 15 binders are in fact weak binders (i.e., 3 to 5 orders of magnitude weaker binders than the natural ligand 17β-estradiol) the default LASSO descriptors outperform (3-fold enrichment) the structure-based approach (2-fold enrichment) and the agonist-trained LASSO method outperforms the antagonist LASSO method (most likely due to a large diversity among antagonists than agonists). Here we can see that even for weakly interacting partners (i.e., low affinity binders for ER) we can still obtain enrichment that is substantially better than random.

These tandem virtual screening approaches combine computationally efficient ligand-based ChemSpider LASSO descriptors (since ChemSpider is at its core a rich and diverse collection of chemical structures, these were used in order to produce LASSO predictions for over 14 million compounds against a series of 40 targets including AR and ER. A LASSO search feature was added to ChemSpider to allow users to search the database by LASSO value (see Figure 3(a)). Scientists can readily search for the top 1000 compounds (or

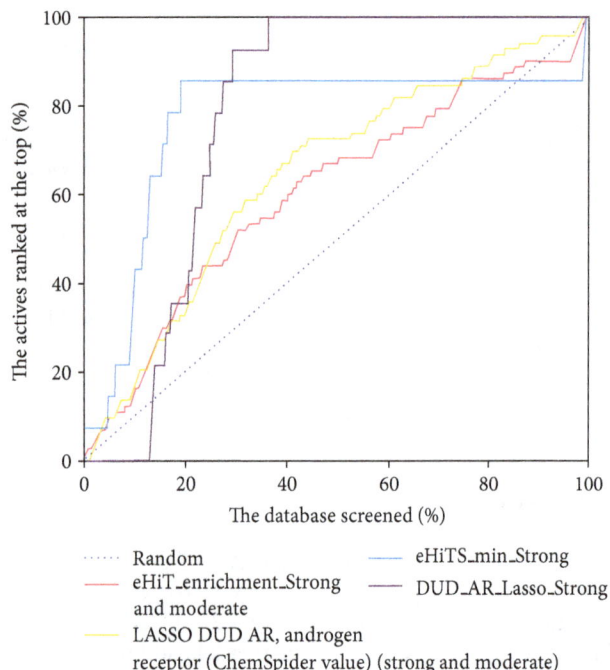

FIGURE 1: Enrichment plot for AR. Legend: blue dotted line: random hit rate, pink line: eHiTS docking score-based enrichment for strong and moderate binders (i.e., strong $Log_{IC_{50}}$ mean = −7.7, stdev = 0.7, moderate $Log_{IC_{50}}$ mean = −5.1, stdev = 0.6, probe DHT) from two crystal structures (1XNN and 2AMA), yellow line: LASSO DUD AR androgen receptor trained ligands (ChemSpider value with strong and moderate binding ligands as "hit" criteria), light blue: eHiTS minimum energy docking score from two crystal structures using strong binder hit criteria only (crystal structures 1XNN and 2AMA), purple: DUD LASSO using strong binders hit criteria only.

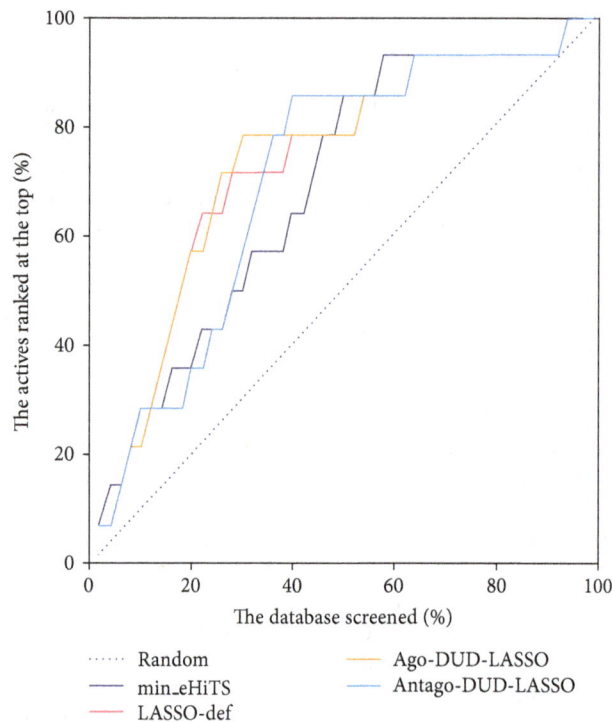

FIGURE 2: Enrichment plot for ER. Legend: purple dotted line: random hit rate, blue line: the minimum eHiTS docking score reported for two different crystal structures (Min_eHiTS, crystal structure = 3ERT and 1GWR), pink: using the default LASSO descriptors (LASSO-def), yellow: using the DUD AR agonist-trained descriptors as found on ChemSpider (agonist DUD LASSO), light blue: using the DUD AR antagonist trained descriptors as found on ChemSpider (antagonist DUD LASSO).

less) with the highest LASSO value for a particular target of interest. An advanced search in ChemSpider can combine LASSO value searches with other parameters such as molecular weight, rule of 5 values, and specific data sources (e.g., selecting molecules from commercial data sources only)) prior to more costly structure-based virtual screening strategies, dramatically improving virtual screening and "early-recognition problem" workflow efficiency.

Piggy-backing more costly structure-based virtual screening strategies on top of an initial screen dramatically assists in virtual screening endeavors and the early-recognition problem.

We have also shown an example of a molecule, mibolerone, a strong AR and ER binder based on LASSO (Figure 3(b)) which is known as a potent AR binder [64]. The LASSO surface point type values are shown in Supplemental Table 3 and more visually in Supplemental Figure 2.

When we used LASSO models with hPXR in method I (Figure 4) we found the best results with Model 1 which suggested 40% of the ligands can be pushed into the top 10% of the screened database resulting with an enrichment factor 4-fold better than random (Figure 5). In Method II we found the same enrichment factor using 64 actives in a 24 thousand compound decoy set (Figure 6). Another way to evaluate

the models is to present the statistics for using dataset 1 to predict dataset 2 (N = 168) for which we obtained sensitivity 12%, specificity 99%, accuracy 51%, and Matthews correlation 0.2. Using dataset 2 to predict dataset 1 gives similar results. These results suggest that the models could identify potential human PXR agonists in databases similar to other target proteins [59].

4. Discussion

For both the AR and ER ligands the main objective was to see how ligand-based screening tools, such as LASSO's ChemSpider implementation, perform such that they could be used for prioritizing chemicals for testing. The AR dataset contained a mixture of drug-like and environmental receptor modulators, whereas the ER dataset contained primarily environmental chemicals. Even in light of the relatively weak binding affinity of the "actives," that is, K_i of 10^{-4}–10^{-6}, while these would be poor candidates for lead optimization into drugs, they still pose an interaction potential with biological systems such as NRs if they bioaccumulate. Using these leads from LASSO screening with other methods such as molecular docking or free-energy perturbation simulations may also be useful. The validation of the approaches outlined above was pursued by

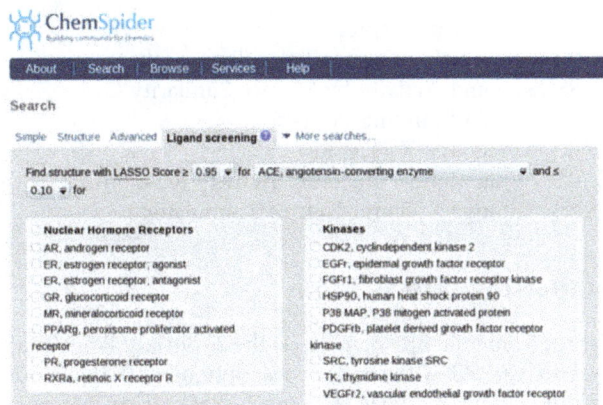

(a)

(b)

FIGURE 3: (a) LASSO models implemented in ChemSpider. (b) LASSO scores for Mibolerone, a strong AR and ER binder found with a LASSO search on ChemSpider. The LASSO score is significant only for 4 targets: MR, AR, ER and PR while the rest of the 40 targets are all 0.10 or below for this molecule.

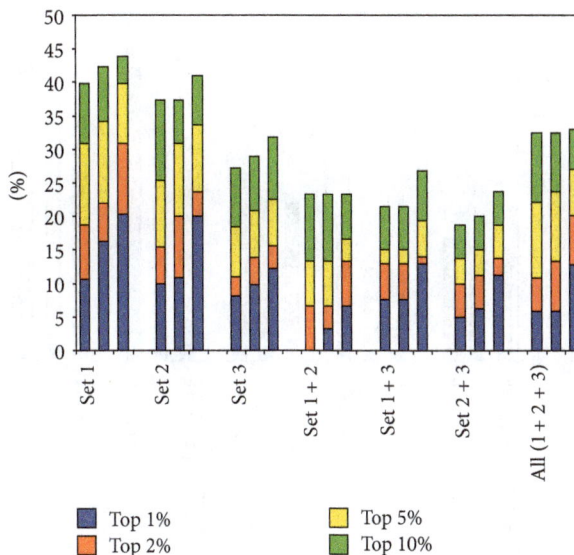

FIGURE 4: PXR LASSO 7 models derived in training method I.

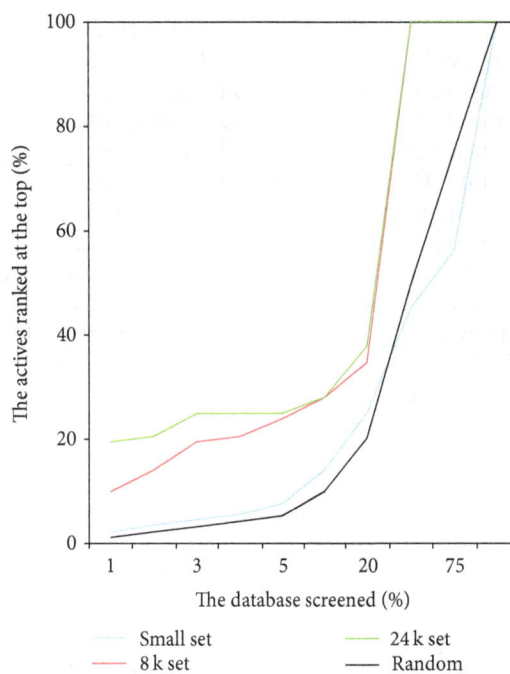

FIGURE 5: PXR LASSO enrichment for model from set 1.

examining two real datasets. These were the FDA's NCTR AR [38] and 50 environmental molecules evaluated for ER binding affinity [35]. In addition we have used multiple sets of PXR agonists described previously. Our results show enrichments of between 2-fold and 4-fold depending on the NR. For PXR there have been numerous recent studies using different machine learning methods and descriptors [25, 54, 56], and while the Matthews correlation coefficient in this study is lower than those in previous studies, the level of enrichment from between 4 fold (40% of actives in the top 10% of compounds screened) and 10-fold (10% actives in the top 1% of compounds screened) was very encouraging.

The molecular descriptors used in eHiTS LASSO are independent of ligand conformation and have been shown to successfully enrich screened databases across a wide range of target families [59]. Lying somewhere between a 2D and a 3D descriptor the ISPT descriptor does not contain any shape or 2D connectivity information. There may however be some molecular size information implicit in the descriptor due to capturing the counts of surface points and larger molecules will have more surface points than smaller molecules (and eHiTS LASSO may be somewhat sensitive to this).

The relatively high speed of eHiTS LASSO on a single CPU [59] makes it an ideal tool to be used as a predocking screen. From a troubleshooting perspective, eHiTS LASSO will return a high percentage of false positives, due to not considering 3D relationships of surface properties. Because of this, it will also return a higher percentage of different scaffolds, enabling scaffold hopping. It is also important to note that LASSO would not be able to differentiate stereo-isomerism apart from, perhaps, diastereomeric pairs which have structurally (configurationally) different features rather than conformationally different features, for which this method is conformation invariant.

Taking the results of eHiTS LASSO and feeding the top N% into a docking program would allow the docking program to weed out many of the false positives binders. For this

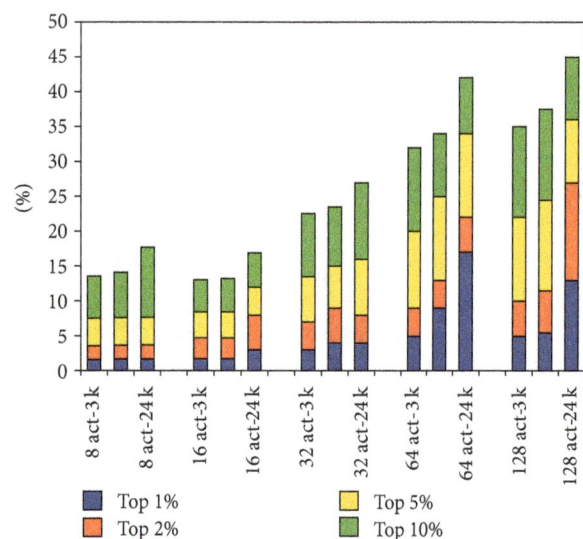

FIGURE 6: PXR LASSO average of 5 models over 5 runs derived in training method II.

reason, eHiTS LASSO is currently integrated with the commercially available eHiTS docking tool and can be readily used as a predocking screening tool for large virtual screens.

From the current study we have shown significant enrichments when testing computational models for AR, ER, and PXR. While AR and ER predictions are currently already implemented in ChemSpider, it is clear that adding predicted values for PXR and other NRs as they become available would be beneficial to the community in terms of accessing an open source of chemical structures with pregenerated descriptors. It should be noted however that the generation of model data for a database as large as that hosted by ChemSpider (now well over 25 million compounds) is not a small undertaking and consumes a significant amount of compute time, data preparation, and handling in order to deliver the models to the community for consumption.

The use of such ligand-based computational methods as exemplified by LASSO in this study could also be useful for the design and selection of chemical products that are less hazardous to human health and the environment. This may make them useful in green chemistry [65] (http://www.epa.gov/gcc/pubs/about_gc.html) as well as in biomedical research. The ready accessibility of such NR binding predictions from computational models like LASSO will be key in future for both pharmaceutical and environmental applications, and databases like ChemSpider can have an important role in providing them to the public as a predocking criteria, as we have demonstrated in this study. This study used published rat ER, AR and human PXR data. LASSO could also be applied to build models for the same NRs across multiple species, such that they could be used to estimate interspecies variation in ligand binding.

Abbreviations

AR: Androgen receptor
DUD: Directory of useful decoys
ER: Estrogen receptor
ISPT: Interacting Surface Point Type
LASSO: Ligand Activity by Surface Similarity Order
LBD: Ligand binding domain
PXR: Pregnane X receptor
QSAR: Quantitative Structure Activity Relationship
SNNS: Stuttgart Neural Network Simulator.

Supporting Information

The supplemental files contain (I) the 23 Surface Point Types used in LASSO with related descriptions, (II) the model building details for PXR (III) the LASSO 6.1 surface point types for Mibolerone, (IV) a visualization of the generalized surface-point types from LASSO for a histidine-like fragment as visualized in CheVi and (V) Mibolerone displayed in SimBioSys' CheVi 3D desktop visualization tool, showing the 3D structure, color-coded interaction surface of the molecule, and the surface point representation.

Disclaimer

This document has been subjected to review by the US Environmental Protection Agency and approved for publication.

Conflict of Interests

A. J. Williams is employed by the Royal Society of Chemistry which owns ChemSpider and associated technologies. S. Ekins and M. R. Goldsmith were on the advisory board for ChemSpider from June 2007 until May 2011. A. Simon, Z. Zsoldos, and O. Ravitz are employed by SimBioSys Inc. which owns LASSO and eHiTS.

References

[1] A. G. Smith and G. E. O. Muscat, "Skeletal muscle and nuclear hormone receptors: implications for cardiovascular and metabolic disease," *International Journal of Biochemistry and Cell Biology*, vol. 37, no. 10, pp. 2047–2063, 2005.

[2] A. K. Hotchkiss, C. V. Rider, C. R. Blystone et al., "Fifteen years after "wingspread"—environmental endocrine disrupters and human and wildlife health: where we are today and where we need to go," *Toxicological Sciences*, vol. 105, no. 2, pp. 235–259, 2008.

[3] S. Tenbaum and A. Baniahmad, "Nuclear receptors: structure, function and involvement in disease," *International Journal of Biochemistry and Cell Biology*, vol. 29, no. 12, pp. 1325–1341, 1997.

[4] A. Zimber and C. Gespach, "Bile acids and derivatives, their nuclear receptors FXR, PXR and ligands: role in health and disease and their therapeutic potential," *Anti-Cancer Agents in Medicinal Chemistry*, vol. 8, no. 5, pp. 540–563, 2008.

[5] P. L. Feldman, M. H. Lambert, and B. R. Henke, "PPAR modulators and PPAR pan agonists for metabolic diseases: the next generation of drugs targeting peroxisome proliferator-activated receptors?" *Current Topics in Medicinal Chemistry*, vol. 8, no. 9, pp. 728–749, 2008.

[6] X. Ma, J. R. Idle, and F. J. Gonzalez, "The pregnane X receptor: from bench to bedside," *Expert Opinion on Drug Metabolism and Toxicology*, vol. 4, no. 7, pp. 895–908, 2008.

[7] M. Bertolotti, C. Gabbi, C. Anzivino, L. Carulli, P. Loria, and N. Carulli, "Nuclear receptors as potential molecular targets in cholesterol accumulation conditions: insights from evidence on hepatic cholesterol degradation and gallstone disease in humans," *Current Medicinal Chemistry*, vol. 15, no. 22, pp. 2271–2284, 2008.

[8] E. E. Baulieu, M. Atger, and M. Best Belpomme, "Steroid hormone receptors," *Vitamins and Hormones*, vol. 33, pp. 649–736, 1975.

[9] D. V. Henley and K. S. Korach, "Endocrine-disrupting chemicals use distinct mechanisms of action to modulate endocrine system function," *Endocrinology*, vol. 147, no. 6, pp. S25–S32, 2006.

[10] M. D. Krasowski, E. J. Reschly, and S. Ekins, "Intrinsic disorder in nuclear hormone receptors," *Journal of Proteome Research*, vol. 7, no. 10, pp. 4359–4372, 2008.

[11] A. C. W. Pike, A. M. Brzozowski, R. E. Hubbard et al., "Structure of the ligand-binding domain of oestrogen receptor beta in the presence of a partial agonist and a full antagonist," *EMBO Journal*, vol. 18, no. 17, pp. 4608–4618, 1999.

[12] A. M. Brzozowski, A. C. W. Pike, Z. Dauter et al., "Molecular basis of agonism and antagonism in the oestrogen receptor," *Nature*, vol. 389, no. 6652, pp. 753–758, 1997.

[13] J. W. R. Schwabe, L. Chapman, J. T. Finch, D. Rhodes, and D. Neuhaus, "DNA recognition by the oestrogen receptor: from solution to the crystal," *Structure*, vol. 1, no. 3, pp. 187–204, 1993.

[14] J. S. Sack, K. F. Kish, C. Wang et al., "Crystallographic structures of the ligand-binding domains of the androgen receptor and its T877A mutant complexed with the natural agonist dihydrotestosterone," *Proceedings of the National Academy of Sciences of the United States of America*, vol. 98, no. 9, pp. 4904–4909, 2001.

[15] C. E. Bohl, C. Chang, M. L. Mohler et al., "A ligand-based approach to identify quantitative structure-activity relationships for the androgen receptor," *Journal of Medicinal Chemistry*, vol. 47, no. 15, pp. 3765–3776, 2004.

[16] P. L. Shaffer, A. Jivan, D. E. Dollins, F. Claessens, and D. T. Gewirth, "Structural basis of androgen receptor binding to selective androgen response elements," *Proceedings of the National Academy of Sciences of the United States of America*, vol. 101, no. 14, pp. 4758–4763, 2004.

[17] G. Bertilsson, J. Heidrich, K. Svensson et al., "Identification of a human nuclear receptor defines a new signaling pathway for CYP3A induction," *Proceedings of the National Academy of Sciences of the United States of America*, vol. 95, no. 21, pp. 12208–12213, 1998.

[18] B. Blumberg, W. Sabbagh Jr., H. Juguilon et al., "SXR, a novel steroid and xenobiotic-sensing nuclear receptor," *Genes and Development*, vol. 12, no. 20, pp. 3195–3205, 1998.

[19] S. A. Kliewer, J. T. Moore, L. Wade et al., "An orphan nuclear receptor activated by pregnanes defines a novel steroid signaling pathway," *Cell*, vol. 92, no. 1, pp. 73–82, 1998.

[20] S. Verma, M. M. Tabb, and B. Blumberg, "Activation of the steroid and xenobiotic receptor, SXR, induces apoptosis in breast cancer cells," *BMC Cancer*, vol. 9, article 3, 2009.

[21] D. Gupta, M. Venkatesh, H. Wang et al., "Expanding the roles for pregnane X receptor in cancer: proliferation and drug resistance in ovarian cancer," *Clinical Cancer Research*, vol. 14, no. 17, pp. 5332–5340, 2008.

[22] J. Zhou, M. Liu, Y. Zhai, and W. Xie, "The antiapoptotic role of pregnane X receptor in human colon cancer cells," *Molecular Endocrinology*, vol. 22, no. 4, pp. 868–880, 2008.

[23] A. Biswas, S. Mani, M. R. Redinbo et al., "Elucidating the 'Jekyll and Hyde' nature of PXR: the case for discovering antagonists," *Pharmaceutical Research*, vol. 26, no. 8, pp. 1807–1815, 2009.

[24] B. L. Urquhart, R. G. Tirona, and R. B. Kim, "Nuclear receptors and the regulation of drug-metabolizing enzymes and drug transporters: implications for interindividual variability in response to drugs," *Journal of Clinical Pharmacology*, vol. 47, no. 5, pp. 566–578, 2007.

[25] S. Ekins, S. Kortagere, M. Iyer et al., "Challenges predicting ligand-receptor interactions of promiscuous proteins: the nuclear receptor PXR," *PLoS Computational Biology*, vol. 5, no. 12, Article ID e1000594, 2009.

[26] N. Ai, R. K. DeLisle, S. J. Yu, and W. J. Welsh, "Computational models for predicting the binding affinities of ligands for the wild-type androgen receptor and a mutated variant associated with human prostate cancer," *Chemical Research in Toxicology*, vol. 16, no. 12, pp. 1652–1660, 2003.

[27] M. N. Jacobs, "In silico tools to aid risk assessment of endocrine disrupting chemicals," *Toxicology*, vol. 205, no. 1-2, pp. 43–53, 2004.

[28] W. Tong, R. Perkins, L. Xing, W. J. Welsh, and D. M. Sheehan, "QSAR models for binding of estrogenic compounds to estrogen receptor α and β subtypes," *Endocrinology*, vol. 138, no. 9, pp. 4022–4025, 1997.

[29] S. Ekins, L. Mirny, and E. G. Schuetz, "A ligand-based approach to understanding selectivity of nuclear hormone receptors PXR, CAR, FXR, LXRα, and LXRβ," *Pharmaceutical Research*, vol. 19, no. 12, pp. 1788–1800, 2002.

[30] T. Z. Bao, G.-Z. Han, J.-Y. Shim, Y. Wen, and X.-R. Jiang, "Quantitative structure-activity relationship of various endogenous estrogen metabolites for human estrogen receptor α and β subtypes: insights into the structural determinants favoring a differential subtype binding," *Endocrinology*, vol. 147, no. 9, pp. 4132–4150, 2006.

[31] D. Plewczynski, M. Von Grotthuss, S. A. H. Spieser et al., "Target specific compound identification using a support vector machine," *Combinatorial Chemistry and High Throughput Screening*, vol. 10, no. 3, pp. 189–196, 2007.

[32] L. Zhao and R. D. Brinton, "Structure-based virtual screening for plant-based EBβ-selective ligands as potential preventative therapy against age-related neurodegenerative diseases," *Journal of Medicinal Chemistry*, vol. 48, no. 10, pp. 3463–3466, 2005.

[33] W. H. Bisson, A. V. Cheltsov, N. Bruey-Sedano et al., "Discovery of antiandrogen activity of nonsteroidal scaffolds of marketed drugs," *Proceedings of the National Academy of Sciences of the United States of America*, vol. 104, no. 29, pp. 11927–11932, 2007.

[34] S. Laws et al., DSSTox EPA Estrogen Receptor Ki Binding Study (Laws et al.) Database—(KIERBL): SDF file and documentation. 2009 http://www.epa.gov/ncct/dsstox/sdf_kierbl.html.

[35] S. C. Laws, S. Yavanhxay, R. L. Cooper, and J. C. Eldridge, "Nature of the binding interaction for 50 structurally diverse chemicals with rat estrogen receptors," *Toxicological Sciences*, vol. 94, no. 1, pp. 46–56, 2006.

[36] J. R. Rabinowitz, S. B. Little, S. C. Laws, and M.-R. Goldsmith, "Molecular modeling for screening environmental chemicals for estrogenicity: use of the toxicant-target approach," *Chemical Research in Toxicology*, vol. 22, no. 9, pp. 1594–1602, 2009.

[37] H. Fang, W. Tong, W. S. Branham et al., "Study of 202 natural, synthetic, and environmental chemicals for binding to

the androgen receptor," *Chemical Research in Toxicology*, vol. 16, no. 10, pp. 1338–1358, 2003.

[38] D. Ding, L. Xu, H. Fang et al., "The EDKB: an established knowledge base for endocrine disrupting chemicals," *BMC Bioinformatics*, vol. 11, no. 6, article 5, 2010.

[39] R. E. Watkins, P. R. Davis-Searles, M. H. Lambert, and M. R. Redinbo, "Coactivator binding promotes the specific interaction between ligand and the pregnane X receptor," *Journal of Molecular Biology*, vol. 331, no. 4, pp. 815–828, 2003.

[40] R. E. Watkins, J. M. Maglich, L. B. Moore et al., "2.1 Å crystal structure of human PXR in complex with the St. John's wort compound hyperforin," *Biochemistry*, vol. 42, no. 6, pp. 1430–1438, 2003.

[41] Y. Xue, E. Chao, W. J. Zuercher, T. M. Willson, J. L. Collins, and M. R. Redinbo, "Crystal structure of the PXR-T1317 complex provides a scaffold to examine the potential for receptor antagonism," *Bioorganic and Medicinal Chemistry*, vol. 15, no. 5, pp. 2156–2166, 2007.

[42] J. E. Chrencik, J. Orans, L. B. Moore et al., "Structural disorder in the complex of human pregnane X receptor and the macrolide antibiotic rifampicin," *Molecular Endocrinology*, vol. 19, no. 5, pp. 1125–1134, 2005.

[43] D. G. Teotico, J. J. Bischof, L. Peng, S. A. Kliewer, and M. R. Redinbo, "Structural basis of human pregnane X receptor activation by the hops constituent colupulone," *Molecular Pharmacology*, vol. 74, no. 6, pp. 1512–1520, 2008.

[44] R. E. Watkins, G. B. Wisely, L. B. Moore et al., "The human nuclear xenobiotic receptor PXR: structural determinants of directed promiscuity," *Science*, vol. 292, no. 5525, pp. 2329–2333, 2001.

[45] Y. Xue, L. B. Moore, J. Orans et al., "Crystal structure of the pregnane X receptor-estradiol complex provides insights into endobiotic recognition," *Molecular Endocrinology*, vol. 21, no. 5, pp. 1028–1038, 2007.

[46] K. Bachmann, H. Patel, Z. Batayneh et al., "PXR and the regulation of apoA1 and HDL-cholesterol in rodents," *Pharmacological Research*, vol. 50, no. 3, pp. 237–246, 2004.

[47] S. Ekins, C. Chang, S. Mani et al., "Human pregnane X receptor antagonists and agonists define molecular requirements for different binding sites," *Molecular Pharmacology*, vol. 72, no. 3, pp. 592–603, 2007.

[48] S. Ekins and J. A. Erickson, "A pharmacophore for human pregnane X receptor ligands," *Drug Metabolism and Disposition*, vol. 30, no. 1, pp. 96–99, 2002.

[49] D. Schuster and T. Langer, "The identification of ligand features essential for PXR activation by pharmacophore modeling," *Journal of Chemical Information and Modeling*, vol. 45, no. 2, pp. 431–439, 2005.

[50] K. Yasuda, A. Ranade, R. Venkataramanan et al., "A comprehensive in vitro and in silico analysis of antibiotics that activate pregnane X receptor and induce CYP3A4 in liver and intestine," *Drug Metabolism and Disposition*, vol. 36, no. 8, pp. 1689–1697, 2008.

[51] A. Khandelwal, M. D. Krasowski, E. J. Reschly, M. W. Sinz, P. W. Swaan, and S. Ekins, "Machine learning methods and docking for predicting human pregnane X receptor activation," *Chemical Research in Toxicology*, vol. 21, no. 7, pp. 1457–1467, 2008.

[52] S. Kortagere, D. Chekmarev, W. J. Welsh, and S. Ekins, "Hybrid scoring and classification approaches to predict human pregnane X receptor activators," *Pharmaceutical Research*, vol. 26, no. 4, pp. 1001–1011, 2009.

[53] S. Ekins, E. J. Reschly, L. R. Hagey, and M. D. Krasowski, "Evolution of pharmacologic specificity in the pregnane X receptor," *BMC Evolutionary Biology*, vol. 8, no. 1, article 103, 2008.

[54] S. Kortagere, D. Chekmarev, W. J. Welsh, and S. Ekins, "Hybrid scoring and classification approaches to predict human pregnane X receptor activators," *Pharmaceutical Research*, vol. 26, no. 4, pp. 1001–1011, 2009.

[55] S. Kortagere, M. D. Krasowski, E. J. Reschly, M. Venkatesh, S. Mani, and S. Ekins, "Evaluation of computational docking to identify pregnane X receptor agonists in the toxcast database," *Environmental Health Perspectives*, vol. 118, no. 10, pp. 1412–1417, 2010.

[56] A. Khandelwal, M. D. Krasowski, E. J. Reschly, M. W. Sinz, P. W. Swaan, and S. Ekins, "Machine learning methods and docking for predicting human pregnane X receptor activation," *Chemical Research in Toxicology*, vol. 21, no. 7, pp. 1457–1467, 2008.

[57] S. Kortagere and S. Ekins, "Troubleshooting computational methods in drug discovery," *Journal of Pharmacological and Toxicological Methods*, vol. 61, no. 2, pp. 67–75, 2010.

[58] N. Ai, M. D. Krasowski, W. J. Welsh, and S. Ekins, "Understanding nuclear receptors using computational methods," *Drug Discovery Today*, vol. 14, no. 9-10, pp. 486–494, 2009.

[59] D. Reid, B. S. Sadjad, Z. Zsoldos, and A. Simon, "LASSO—ligand activity by surface similarity order: a new tool for ligand based virtual screening," *Journal of Computer-Aided Molecular Design*, vol. 22, no. 6-7, pp. 479–487, 2008.

[60] N. Huang, B. K. Shoichet, and J. J. Irwin, "Benchmarking sets for molecular docking," *Journal of Medicinal Chemistry*, vol. 49, no. 23, pp. 6789–6801, 2006.

[61] C. Y. Ung, H. Li, C. W. Yap, and Y. Z. Chen, "In silico prediction of pregnane X receptor activators by machine learning approaches," *Molecular Pharmacology*, vol. 71, no. 1, pp. 158–168, 2007.

[62] D. Weininger, "SMILES, a chemical language and information system. 1. Introduction to methodology and encoding rules," *Journal of Chemical Information and Computer Sciences*, vol. 28, pp. 31–36, 1988.

[63] G. B. McGaughey, R. P. Sheridan, C. I. Bayly et al., "Comparison of topological, shape, and docking methods in virtual screening," *Journal of Chemical Information and Modeling*, vol. 47, no. 4, pp. 1504–1519, 2007.

[64] L. R. Murthy, M. P. Johnson, and D. R. Rowley, "Characterization of steroid receptors in human prostate using mibolerone," *Prostate*, vol. 8, no. 3, pp. 241–253, 1986.

[65] A. M. Voutchkova, T. G. Osimitz, and P. T. Anastas, "Toward a comprehensive molecular design framework for reduced hazard," *Chemical Reviews*, vol. 110, no. 10, pp. 5845–5882, 2010.

4

QSAR Investigation on Quinolizidinyl Derivatives in Alzheimer's Disease

Ghasem Ghasemi,[1] Sattar Arshadi,[2] Alireza Nemati Rashtehroodi,[3] Mahyar Nirouei,[4] Shahab Shariati,[1] and Zinab Rastgoo[1]

[1] Department of Chemistry, Rasht Branch, Islamic Azad University, Rasht, Iran
[2] Department of Chemistry, Payame Noor University, Behshahr Branch, Behshahr, Iran
[3] Department of Chemistry, Payame Noor University, Sari Branch, Sari, Iran
[4] Department of Electrical Engineering, Lahijan Branch, Islamic Azad University, Lahijan, Iran

Correspondence should be addressed to Ghasem Ghasemi; ghasemi@iaurasht.ac.ir

Academic Editor: Hon Keung Tony Ng

Sets of quinolizidinyl derivatives of bi- and tri-cyclic (hetero) aromatic systems were studied as selective inhibitors. On the pattern, quantitative structure-activity relationship (QSAR) study has been done on quinolizidinyl derivatives as potent inhibitors of acetylcholinesterase in alzheimer's disease (AD). Multiple linear regression (MLR), partial least squares (PLSs), principal component regression (PCR), and least absolute shrinkage and selection operator (LASSO) were used to create QSAR models. Geometry optimization of compounds was carried out by B3LYP method employing 6–31 G basis set. HyperChem, Gaussian 98 W, and Dragon software programs were used for geometry optimization of the molecules and calculation of the quantum chemical descriptors. Finally, Unscrambler program was used for the analysis of data. In the present study, the root mean square error of the calibration and R^2 using MLR method were obtained as 0.1434 and 0.95, respectively. Also, the R and R^2 values were obtained as 0.79, 0.62 from stepwise MLR model. The R^2 and mean square values using LASSO method were obtained as 0.766 and 3.226, respectively. The root mean square error of the calibration and R^2 using PLS method were obtained as 0.3726 and 0.62, respectively. According to the obtained results, it was found that MLR model is the most favorable method in comparison with other statistical methods and is suitable for use in QSAR models.

1. Introduction

Alzheimer's disease (AD) is a debilitating illness with unmet medical needs [1]. The number of people afflicted with the disease worldwide is expected to be triple up to the year 2050 [2]. The multifactorial pathogenesis of AD includes accumulation of aggregates of β-amyloid (Aβ) and tau protein and loss of cholinergic neurons with consequent deficit of the neurotransmitter acetylcholine (ACh) [3, 4]. In advancing AD, AChE levels in the brain are declining [5].

The well-known theory of the quantitative structure-activity relationships (QSARs) [6–8] is based on the hypothesis that the biological activity of a chemical compound is mainly determined by its molecular structure [6]. QSAR attempts to find consistent relationship between biological activity and molecular properties, so that these "rules" can be used to predict the activity of new compounds from their structures.

Today, QSARs are being applied in many disciplines with much emphasis on drug design. Over the years of development, many methods, algorithms, and techniques have been discovered and applied in QSAR studies [9, 10]. To date, QSARs are among the important applications of chemometric tools with the objective of development of predictive models which can be used in different areas of chemistry including medicinal, agricultural, environmental, and materials [11–13].

Drug discovery often involves the use of QSAR to identify chemical structures that could have good inhibitory effects on specific targets [15]. The aim of QSAR analysis is to investigate

TABLE 1: Structures of quinolizidinyl derivatives of bi- and tricyclic systems used for QSAR model building [14].

General structure	X	Y	R	R□	Nr
(phenothiazine-type general structure with substituents X, Y, R, R')	S	N	$-CH_2-CH(CH_3)-N(Et)_2$	H	1
	S	N	$-(H_2C)_3-N(Et)_2$	CF_3	2
	S	N	$-(H_2C)_3-N$(piperidinyl)$-OH$	CN	3
	S	N	quinolizidinyl–CH$_2$–	H	4
	S	N	quinolizidinyl–CH$_2$–	CF_3	5
	O	N	quinolizidinyl–CH$_2$–	H	6
	CH_2	N	quinolizidinyl–CH$_2$–	H	7
	H_2C-CH_2	N	quinolizidinyl–CH$_2$–	H	8
	HC=CH	N	quinolizidinyl–CH$_2$–	H	9
	S	CH	H_2C–(piperidinyl)–N–CH_3	H	10
	S	CH	quinolizidinyl–CH$_2$–	H	11
	S	C-OH	quinolizidinyl–CH$_2$–	H	12
	S	C	quinolizidinyl–CH=	H	13
	H_2C-CH_2	C	quinolizidinyl–CH=	H	14

TABLE 1: Continued.

General structure	X	Y	R	R□	Nr
	HC=CH	C	quinolizidinyl–CH= (=CH$_2$), H	H	15
(fluorene, Y–R)		N	quinolizidinyl–CH$_2$, H		16
		CH	quinolizidinyl–CH$_2$, H		17
		CH	quinolizidinyl–CH$_2$, H		18
(diphenyl, Y–R)		N	quinolizidinyl–CH$_2$, H		19
		CH	quinolizidinyl–CH$_2$, H		20
		C	quinolizidinyl–CH= (=CH$_2$), H		21
		CH	quinolizidinyl–S–, H		22
(phenothiazine, X, Y, N–CO–R, R′)	S	CH	CH$_3$–CH–N(Et)$_2$	H	23
	S	CH	quinolizidinyl–CH$_2$, H	H	24
	S	CH	quinolizidinyl–CH$_2$, H	H	25
	S	CH	quinolizidinyl–S–CH$_2$, H	H	26
	S	CH	quinolizidinyl–S–CH$_2$, H	OCH$_3$	27

TABLE 1: Continued.

General structure	X	Y	R	R□	Nr
	S	CH	(S–CH(CH₃))	H	28
	S	CH	(S–(CH₂)₂)	H	29
	S	CH	(S–(CH₂)₃)	H	30
	S	CH	(S–(CH₂)₄)	H	31
	H₂C–CH₂	CH	(S–CH₂)	H	32
	HN–CO	N	(CH₂)	H	33
	HN–CO	N	(S–CH₂)	H	34
	NH		CH₃–CH–(CH₂)₃–N(Et)₂		35
	NH		(CH₂)		36
	NH		(S–(CH₂)₂)		37
	NH		(S–(CH₂)₃)		38
	S		(CH₂)		39

TABLE 1: Continued.

General structure	X	Y	R	R□	Nr
O=coumarin with O–R substituent			quinolizidinyl, NH–$(CH_2)_3$–		40
			quinolizidinyl, S–$(CH_2)_3$–		41
			quinolizidinyl, S–$(CH_2)_4$–		42

TABLE 2: The mean of selected descriptors.

Descriptor symbol	Descriptor group	Meaning
G (N⋯O)	Geometrical descriptors	Sum of geometrical distances between N⋯O
ARR	Constitutional descriptors	Aromatic ratio
Te	WHIM descriptors	T total size index/weighted by atomic Sanderson electronegativities
MATS6e	2D autocorrelations	Moran autocorrelation—lag 6/weighted by atomic Sanderson electronegativities
Mor31m	3D-MoRSE descriptors	3D-MoRSE— signal 31/weighted by atomic masses
Mor18m	3D-MoRSE descriptors	3D-MoRSE—signal 18/weighted by atomic masses

TABLE 3: The statistical parameters of different constructed QSAR models.

Method	RMSE		R^2	
	Calibration	Prediction	Calibration	Prediction
PLS	0.372616	0.466533	0.624241	0.426009
PCR	0.372537	0.484057	0.624401	0.407646
LASSO	—	—	0.766	

the correlation between activity, generally, biological activity, and the physicochemical properties of a set of molecules [16].

PLS regression technique is especially useful in quite common case where the number of descriptors (independent variables) is comparable to or greater than the number of compounds (data points), and/or there exist other factors leading to correlations between variables. In this case, the solution of classical least squares problem does not exist or is unstable and unreliable. On the other hand, PLS approach leads to stable, correct, and highly predictive models even for correlated descriptors [17].

PCR is a combination of principal component analysis (PCA) and MLR. The first step in PCR is to decompose a spectral data matrix using PCA. Generally, there are two types of decomposition techniques. The first technique is by computing eigenvectors and eigenvalues. We used singular value decomposition (SVD) to decompose the spectral data matrix. This is because SVD is generally accepted as the most stable and numerically accurate technique [18, 19].

LASSO translates each coefficient by a constant factor truncating at zero. This is called soft thresholding. Best subset selection drops all variables with coefficients smaller than the M_{th} largest. This is a form of hard thresholding.

2. Computational Details

The 3D structures of the molecules were drawn using the built optimum option of Hyperchem software (version 8.0). Then, the structures were fully optimized based on the ab initio method, using DFT level of theory. Hyperchem (version 3.0) and Dragon (version 3.0) programs were employed to calculate the molecular descriptors. All calculations were performed using Gaussian 98 W program series. Geometry optimization of compounds was carried out by B3LYP method employing 6–31 G basis set [20].

In this study, the independent variables were molecular descriptors, and the dependent variables were the actual half maximal inhibitory concentration (IC_{50}) values. More than 1498 theoretical descriptors were selected and calculated. These descriptors can be classified into several groups including: (i) constitutional, (ii) topological, (iii) molecular walk counts, (iv) BCUT, (v) Galvez topological charge indices, (vi) autocorrelations, (vii) charge, (viii) aromaticity indices, (ix) randic molecular profiles, (x) geometrical, (xi) RDF, (xii) MoRSE, (xiii) WHIM, (xiv) GETAWAY, (xv) functional groups, (xvi) atom-centred, (xvii) empirical, and (xviii) properties descriptors. Finally, Unscrambler (version 9.7) program was used for analysis of data and statistical calculation.

TABLE 4: Descriptors values for stepwise MLR model.

Molecule	G (N⋯O)	ARR	Te	MATS6e	Mor31m	Mor18m
1	0.000	0.500	13.546	0.045	−0.099	0.381
2	0.000	0.429	17.814	0.106	0.018	1.122
3	20.250	0.448	18.480	0.007	−0.294	1.186
4	0.000	0.414	15.923	0.007	−0.181	1.383
5	0.000	0.364	17.411	0.090	0.014	1.615
6	9.600	0.414	15.799	0.011	−0.113	0.104
7	0.000	0.414	16.071	0.022	−0.084	0.469
8	0.000	0.400	16.312	0.034	0.002	1.199
9	0.000	0.400	16.108	0.019	−0.191	1.233
10	0.000	0.480	14.345	0.088	0.225	1.547
11	0.000	0.414	15.271	0.119	0.106	2.132
12	4.490	0.400	15.838	−0.029	0.055	1.896
13	0.000	0.414	16.287	0.090	0.085	2.410
14	0.000	0.400	16.628	0.107	0.291	1.618
15	0.000	0.400	16.514	0.098	0.091	1.494
16	0.000	0.464	15.920	0.012	−0.039	0.330
17	0.000	0.429	14.869	0.129	0.083	1.143
18	0.000	0.429	14.841	0.129	0.083	0.946
19	0.000	0.444	13.992	0.003	−0.167	1.393
20	0.000	0.444	15.531	0.110	0.085	0.358
21	0.000	0.444	15.794	0.086	0.151	0.396
22	0.000	0.429	16.962	−0.002	0.004	0.488
23	2.850	0.480	14.983	−0.219	−0.126	1.175
24	3.590	0.387	14.711	−0.111	0.050	1.531
25	4.490	0.387	15.677	−0.111	0.210	1.747
26	6.090	0.364	19.718	−0.059	0.174	1.143
27	19.660	0.343	22.226	0.086	0.082	1.374
28	5.930	0.353	20.024	−0.050	−0.035	1.639
29	6.420	0.353	25.383	−0.101	0.140	1.918
30	7.620	0.343	28.305	−0.041	−0.007	1.792
31	9.500	0.333	36.586	−0.050	0.071	2.232
32	6.150	0.353	20.780	−0.113	−0.036	0.525
33	25.410	0.364	14.812	−0.051	−0.164	0.240
34	34.830	0.343	25.376	0.009	−0.292	0.729
35	19.340	0.400	24.194	0.080	−0.158	0.643
36	17.760	0.394	17.479	0.071	−0.267	1.192
37	19.490	0.333	26.550	0.079	−0.329	1.476
38	19.170	0.324	29.353	0.066	−0.033	1.304
39	12.740	0.333	19.215	0.087	0.048	1.531
40	43.630	0.200	17.259	−0.009	0.062	0.817
41	29.170	0.200	23.440	0.002	0.058	0.737
42	24.170	0.194	20.222	0.024	−0.122	0.665

For each compound in the training sets, the correlation equation was derived with the same descriptors. Then, the obtained equation was used to predict $\log (1/IC_{50})$ values for the compounds from the corresponding test sets. In the present work, the method of stepwise multiple linear regression (stepwise MLR) was used in order to select the most appropriate descriptor of all descriptors. Totally, 1498 descriptors were generated. In this study, two programs including SPSS (version 19) and Unscrambler were used for MLR, PLS, PCR, and LASSO.

3. Results and Discussions

The structures of the quinolizidinyl derivatives used in this study were shown in Table 1. Since, the variation in

TABLE 5: Experimental and predicted values of log $(1/IC_{50})$ using PCR and PLS methods.

Observed log (1/IC50)	Predicted PCR	Predicted PLS
1.531	1.534	1.426
1.653	1.656	1.656
0.854	1.340	1.327
1.591	1.679	1.675
1.771	1.713	1.893
1.568	1.647	1.661
1.699	1.657	1.660
1.74	1.482	1.401
0.919	1.429	1.351
1.634	1.572	1.489
0.845	1.684	1.677
1.623	2.260	2.324
1.763	1.630	1.625
1.663	1.423	1.341
0.919	1.282	1.203
1.613	1.560	1.602
1.653	1.574	1.614
1.681	1.574	1.614
0.949	1.047	1.080
0.826	1.042	1.073
1.544	1.068	1.100
1.653	0.919	0.956
1.653	1.767	1.701
1.69	1.693	1.726
1.477	1.689	1.722
1.505	1.358	1.370
1.672	1.212	1.275
1.602	1.467	1.503
1.672	1.160	1.153
0.833	0.962	0.919
0.756	0.733	0.630
1.532	1.161	1.076
1.623	1.579	1.584
1.462	1.193	1.171
1.69	1.491	1.387
0.863	0.521	0.581
−0.076	0.275	0.276
−0.658	0.022	−0.026
1.756	1.010	1.062
0.82	0.417	0.497
−0.456	0.431	0.495
0.079	0.273	0.337

the chemical structure of the considered compounds is low, the selection of chemical descriptors, which can encode small variations between structures of molecules in data set, is very important. In this way, GETAWAY descriptors are very informative 3D descriptors that can encode structural features of molecules. The four most significant descriptors which were selected are as follows [14, 20]:

G (N $\cdots$ O), ARR, Te, MATS6e, Mor31m, and Mor-18m.

The mean values of selected descriptors are shown in Table 2. As can be seen from this table, atomic masses and electronegativities were important descriptors in our study.

The selected descriptors through these methods were used to construct some linear models using PCR and PLS methods. Statistical parameters of different constructed QSAR models are shown in Table 3. R^2 and RMSE values for calibration in MLR method are better than the two other methods. In the present study, the root mean square error of the calibration and R^2 using MLR method were obtained as 0.1434 and 0.95, respectively.

Considering the experimental error, the overall prediction of the log $(1/IC_{50})$ values was quite satisfactory. The results of MLR method were much better than the two other methods.

In the present study, linear variable selection methods were used to select the most significant descriptors (stepwise MLR) (Table 4).

The performance of the QSAR model to predict log (IC_{50}) value was also estimated using the internal cross-validation method. The resulted predictions of the log $(1/IC_{50})$ using PLS and PCR methods in gas phase were given in Table 5.

4. Conclusion

In our study, the linear methods were used to select the most significant descriptors. The stepwise MLR, MLR, PLS, and PCR were used to construct a quantitative relation between the activities of quinolizidinyl derivatives and their calculated descriptors. MLR has been successfully used for finding a QSAR model for quinolizidinyl derivatives. It provides the best results in comparison with other studied methods. Our present attempt to correlate the log $(1/IC_{50})$ with theoretically calculated molecular descriptors has led to a relatively successful QSAR model that relates these derivatives. The results obtained from stepwise MLR method were suitable for drug design and classification.

Conflict of Interests

The authors declare that they have no conflict of interests.

Acknowledgment

The authors thank the Research vice Presidency of Islamic Azad University, Rasht Branch, for their encouragement, permission, and financial support.

References

[1] D. Selkoe, "Alzheimer's disease: genes, proteins, and therapy," *Physiological Reviews*, vol. 81, pp. 741–766, 2001.

[2] H. H. Griffiths, I. J. Morten, and N. M. Hooper, "Emerging and potential therapies for Alzheimer's disease," *Expert Opinion on Therapeutic Targets*, vol. 12, no. 6, pp. 693–704, 2008.

[3] J. R. Roland and H. Jacobsen, "Alzheimer's disease: from pathology to therapeutic approaches," *Angewandte Chemie*, vol. 48, no. 17, pp. 3030–3059, 2009.

[4] A. Gella and N. Durany, "Oxidative stress in Alzheimer disease," *Cell Adhesion and Migration*, vol. 3, no. 1, pp. 88–93, 2009.

[5] M. Mesulam, A. Guillozet, P. Shaw, and B. Quinn, "Widely spread butyrylcholinesterase can hydrolyze acetylcholine in the normal and Alzheimer brain," *Neurobiology of Disease*, vol. 9, no. 1, pp. 88–93, 2002.

[6] C. Hansch and A. Leo, *Exploring QSAR. Fundamentals and Applications in Chemistry and Biology*, American Chemical Society, Washington, DC, USA, 1995.

[7] H. Kubinyi, *QSAR: Hansch Analysis and Related Approaches*, Wiley-Interscience, New York, NY, USA, 2008.

[8] T. Puzyn, J. Leszczynski, and M. T. Cronin, *Recent Advances in QSAR Studies: Methods and Applications*, Springer, New York, NY, USA, 1st edition, 2009.

[9] L. He and P. C. Jurs, "Assessing the reliability of a QSAR model's predictions," *Journal of Molecular Graphics and Modelling*, vol. 23, no. 6, pp. 503–523, 2005.

[10] D. V. Eldred, C. L. Weikel, P. C. Jurs, and K. L. E. Kaiser, "Prediction of fathead minnow acute toxicity of organic compounds from molecular structure," *Chemical Research in Toxicology*, vol. 12, no. 7, pp. 670–678, 1999.

[11] Q. S. Du, P. G. Mezey, and K. C. Chou, "Heuristic molecular lipophilicity potential (HMLP): a 2D-QSAR study to LADH of molecular family pyrazole and derivatives," *Journal of Computational Chemistry*, vol. 26, no. 5, pp. 461–470, 2005.

[12] Q. S. Du, R. B. Huang, Y. T. Wei, L. Q. Du, and K. C. Chou, "Multiple field three dimensional quantitative structure-activity relationship (MF-3D-QSAR)," *Journal of Computational Chemistry*, vol. 29, no. 2, pp. 211–219, 2008.

[13] Q. S. Du, R. B. Huang, and K. C. Chou, "Recent advances in QSAR and their applications in predicting the activities of chemical molecules, peptides and proteins for drug design," *Current Protein & Peptide Science*, vol. 9, no. 3, pp. 248–259, 2008.

[14] B. Tasso, M. Catto, O. Nicolotti et al., "Quinolizidinyl derivatives of bi- and tricyclic systems as potent inhibitors of acetyl- and butyrylcholinesterase with potential in Alzheimer's disease," *European Journal of Medicinal Chemistry*, vol. 46, no. 6, pp. 2170–2184, 2011.

[15] E. K. Freyhult, K. Andersson, and M. G. Gustafsson, "Structural modeling extends QSAR analysis of antibody-lysozyme interactions to 3D-QSAR," *Biophysical Journal*, vol. 84, pp. 2264–2272, 2003.

[16] C. Karthikeyan, N. S. H. Moorthy N, and P. Trivedi, "QSAR study of substituted 2-pyridinyl guanidines as selective urokinase-type plasminogen activator (uPA) inhibitors," *Journal of Enzyme Inhibition and Medicinal Chemistry*, vol. 24, pp. 6–13, 2009.

[17] A. Höskuldsson, "PLS regression methods," *Journal of Chemometrics*, vol. 2, no. 3, pp. 211–228, 1988.

[18] P. J. Gemperline, "Principal component analysis," in *Practical Guide to Chemometrics*, pp. 69–104, CRC Press, 2nd edition, 2006.

[19] D. J. Livingstone and D. W. Salt, "Variable Selection—Spoilt for Choice?" *Reviews in Computational Chemistry*, vol. 21, pp. 287–348, 2005.

[20] G. Ghasemi, M. Nirouei, S. Shariati, P. Abdolmaleki, and Z. Rastgoo, *Arabian Journal of Chemistry*. In press.

5

Modeling Requirements for Computer Simulation of Cerebral Aneurysm

S. R. Ghodsi,[1] V. Esfahanian,[2] and S. M. Ghodsi[3]

[1] VFE Research Institute, University of Tehran (Campus 2), College of Engineering, 4th Floor of Institute of Petroleum Engineering Building, North Kargar Avenue, Tehran 14399-56191, Iran
[2] School of Mechanical Engineering, University of Tehran, Tehran 14399-56191, Iran
[3] Sina Trauma Research Center, Tehran University of Medical Science, Tehran 14399-56191, Iran

Correspondence should be addressed to S. R. Ghodsi; dr.sr.ghodsi@ut.ac.ir

Academic Editor: Michele Migliore

Background. In order to reduce the mortality risk of aneurysm rupture, a timely diagnosis and treatment are vital. There are different reasons for aneurysm, such as hypertension, arteriosclerosis, and heredity. An efficient and cost-effective method to study the generation, development, and rupture of aneurysm and also analysis of treatment methods can accelerate progress. The Computational Fluid Dynamics is a well-known tool to simulate various phenomena. A reliable virtual modeling in biology depends on our knowledge about variety of characteristics, that is, biological features, structural properties, and flow conditions. *Objective.* Because of the vast research about the related subjects, an organized review is required. The aim of current review article is classification of the required foundations for a reliable virtual modeling of cerebral aneurysm, especially in the Circle of Willis.

1. Introduction

Up to 50% cases of Subarachnoid Hemorrhage (SAH) result in fatality and 10%–15% lead to death before reaching a hospital [1]. Rupture of cerebral aneurysm is a well-known cause of SAH. The most prevalent location of cerebral aneurysm is Circle of Willis (CoW). Different factors can increase the risk of aneurysm generation and development, for instance aging, arteriosclerosis, and heredity. In addition, the characteristics of blood flow can exacerbate the problem. Thus it is required to gather various clinical and engineering aspects to reach an actual understanding of the nature of aneurysm.

An efficient and cost-effective way to modeling natural phenomena is numerical simulation. Increasing power of computing causes numerical simulation that plays a key role in recognition of various problems in engineering and medicine. The important point is the reliability of obtained results and the meaningful results of a numerical simulation that depend on variety of aspects.

The classification of related subjects to numerical simulation is a valuable step. Because of the complexity of blood supply system in the brain and also long-time history of

related research, it is necessary to review these studies. Two main groups are considered here: (1) fluid and structure and (2) flow and simulation. The tree of this classification is shown in Figure 1.

In fluid and structure section, there are three subcategories: blood properties, vessel properties, and cerebrovascular features. On the other side, the flow and simulation is divided to three subcategories: geometry and computational domain, numerical approaches, and flow regime features. The CoW is a collection of major vessels connected together and located at the bottom of the cerebral cavity and it is a common place for aneurysm [2]. The CoW combines the blood flow from the incoming afferent vessels and also transfers from a hemisphere to another [3]. The responsibility of CoW is compensating reduction of cerebral perfusion pressure, for example, when complete occlusion occurs in the internal carotid artery [4]. Some important physiological properties of CoW's vessels are presented in Table 1.

It was evident that the risk of transient ischemic attack is lower in the patients with healthy collateral circulations [5]. Approximately, at least 40%–50% of the people are confronted with the CoW's anomalies. The anomalies can be

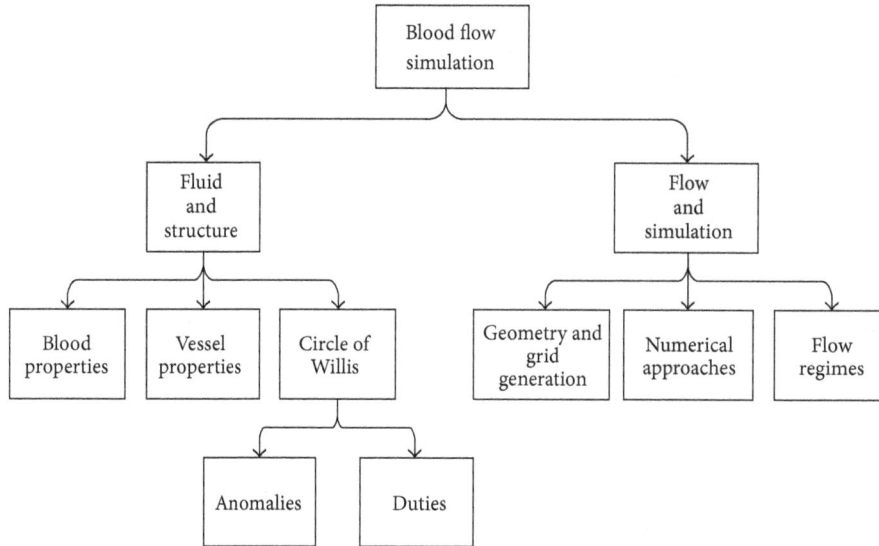

FIGURE 1: Classification of related subjects to the numerical simulation of blood flow in CoW.

classified in three cases: lack of some vessels, asymmetric, and different diameter of similar vessels.

The variations of CoW usually affect more than one segment. Papantchev et al. studied six types of common variations and their effects [6]. In order to know the condition of abnormality in Iranian population, 102 Iranian males were examined and classified in to the 22 common types of anomalies [7]. Because of the importance of CoW's anomalies, similar studies were performed in different countries. The data of 250 Egyptian patients showed that 68.3% and 38.3% of CoW consisted of complete anterior and complete posterior parts, respectively [8].

2. Required Data for Computation

The vessels of human are classified in three groups by size: arteries, veins, and capillaries. The artery and vein consist of three and two layers, respectively. The three layers are Tunica media, Tunica intima, and Tunica adventitia. Furthermore, the muscle layer in vein is considerably thinner than the artery's muscle layer [9].

Entire circulatory system is coated by endothelial cells. Low wall shear stress (less than 0.4 Pa) causes the proliferation of endothelial cells and also atherosclerosis. On the other side, high wall shear stress (more than 1.5 Pa) causes the reorientation of endothelial cells in the flow direction [10]. Some characteristics of vessels within the adult body are shown in Table 2. These data are important in computational domain generation. The complete data about other vessels and the variations are collected in the anatomy atlas [11]. The arterial bifurcation and atherosclerotic plaque can increase an abnormal shear stress on endothelium. The local arterial aggregate Young's Modulus of Elasticity decreases and subsequently causes an initial ballooning [12].

Obviously, the blood properties are required to simulate flow in arteries. The average adult has about 4 to 5 liters of blood. The red blood cells constitute about 45% of the volume

of blood, and the remaining cells (white blood cells and platelets) less than 1%. The fluid part of blood is called plasma and is about 55% [13].

The Reynolds number is an important flow criterion to identify the flow regime, that is, laminar or turbulent. Generally, the Reynolds number is the ratio of inertial forces to viscous forces. The Reynolds number is a dimensionless parameter

$$\mathrm{Re} = \frac{\rho u L_{\mathrm{ref}}}{\mu}, \tag{1}$$

where ρ, u, L_{ref}, and μ are density, velocity, reference length, and viscosity, respectively. The reference length is a characteristic of geometry, for example, the vessel's diameter. The Reynolds number in most of the vessels is lower than 500, just in Aorta and Vena cave it is about 3400. Thus, the blood flow is considered as laminar flow. However, under some conditions, for example, stenosis, the blood flow becomes turbulent in large diameter vessels, such as aorta [14].

If the Reynolds number is lower than the critical Reynolds, the flow is simulated as a laminar flow. The problem is finding the critical Reynolds number. In some cases the flow condition is on the border of turbulence and proper turbulent model is required [15]. The energy of blood flow decreases as a result of turbulence. Then the heart should add more energy to the blood flow. In addition, turbulence increases the perfusion pressure and also the required energy to overcome the additional resistance. In the microcirculation, including the arterioles, the linear relation between perfusion pressure and flow is

$$P_A - P_v = q R_p, \tag{2}$$

where P_A, P_v, q, and R_p are arterial pressure, venous pressure, flow rate, and peripheral resistance. The elasticity of the arterial network maintains high levels of perfusion pressure without overloading the heart, which is called the windkessel

TABLE 1: Physiological properties of CoW's vessels, such as length, radius, thickness, and elastic modulus [25].

	Arteries	Length (cm)	Initial diameter (cm)	Thickness (cm)	Elastic modulus (Pa) $\times 10^6$
1	Ascending aorta	4	2.4	0.163	0.4
2	Aortic arch I	2	2.24	0.126	0.4
3	Brachiocephalic	3.4	1.24	0.08	0.4
4	Aortic arch II	3.9	2.14	0.115	0.4
5	L. common carotid	20.8	0.5	0.063	0.4
6	R. common carotid	17.7	0.5	0.063	0.4
7	R. subclavian	3.4	0.846	0.067	0.4
8	Thoracic aorta	15.6	2	0.11	0.4
9	L. subclavian	3.4	0.846	0.067	0.4
10	L. ext. carotid	17.7	0.3	0.038	0.8
11	L. int. carotid I	17.7	0.4	0.05	0.8
12	R. int. carotid I	17.7	0.4	0.05	0.8
13	R. ext. carotid	17.7	0.3	0.038	0.8
14	R. vertebral	14.8	0.272	0.034	0.8
15	R. brachial	42.2	0.806	0.067	0.4
16	L. brachial	42.2	0.806	0.067	0.4
17	L. vertebral	14.8	0.272	0.034	0.8
18	L. int. carotid II	0.5	0.4	0.05	1.6
19	L. PCoA	1.5	0.146	0.018	1.6
20	R. PCoA	1.5	0.146	0.018	1.6
21	R. int. carotid II	0.5	0.4	0.05	1.6
22	Basilar	2.9	0.324	0.04	1.6
23	L. MCA	11.9	0.286	0.036	1.6
24	R. MCA	11.9	0.286	0.036	1.6
25	L. ACA, A1	1.2	0.234	0.029	1.6
26	R. ACA, A1	1.2	0.234	0.029	1.6
27	L. PCA, P1	0.5	0.214	0.027	1.6
28	R. PCA, P1	0.5	0.214	0.027	1.6
29	L. ACA, A2	10.3	0.24	0.030	1.6
30	R. ACA, A2	10.3	0.24	0.030	1.6
31	ACoA	0.3	0.148	0.019	1.6
32	L. PCA, P2	8.6	0.21	0.026	1.6
33	R. PCA, P2	8.6	0.21	0.026	1.6

TABLE 2: The properties of blood vessels.

Vessel	Number	Diameter (cm)	$Re_{average}$
Aorta	1	2.5	3400
Arteries	159	0.4	500
Arterioles	400	0.005	0.7
Capillaries	4500	0.0008	0.002
Venules	4000	0.002	0.01
Veins	40	0.5	140
Vena cava	18	3	3300

effect. The elastic function helps perfusion during diastole and generates the wave propagation [16].

The other main feature of fluid is viscosity. In the non-Newtonian fluid, there is a nonlinear relation between shear stress and shear rate. The non-Newtonian fluids are classified into the shear thinning and shear thickening. In shear thinning, increasing shear rate reduces the viscosity, and in shear thickening it is vice versa.

The human blood is considered as Newtonian fluid for all rates of shear when hematocrits are up to 12 percent. When the size of particles is significantly large in comparison with the channel's dimension, the fluid behaves like non-Newtonian fluid [9].

Consequently, in the large vessels such as arteries the blood is Newtonian, but in small vessels such as capillary, it is considered as non-Newtonian fluid. The effect of vessel's diameter on the viscosity is called Fahraeus-Lindqvist. As the diameter decreases (between 10 and 300 micrometers), the blood viscosity is reduced, because of the motion of erythrocytes in the center of the vessel and leaving plasma near the wall. A comprehensive study on different viscosity models of blood was performed by Yilmaz and Gundogdu. The models are classified into two groups including time independent and time dependent flow behavior models [17]. The impact of viscosity models on the simulation of aneurysm is studied by Evju et al. [18]. It has been shown that the nonlinear viscosity model can be important in some cases of aneurysm.

The shear forces due to the viscosity rises the pressure drop in network of vessels. Generally, the Hagen-Poiseuille equation is used to compute pressure drop of a laminar and incompressible flow in long cylindrical pipe:

$$\Delta p = \frac{8\mu L Q}{\pi r^4}, \tag{3}$$

where L, Q, and r are pipe's length, volumetric flow rate, and pipe's radius, respectively. The Hagen-Poiseuille equation is just used for a Newtonian fluid. In capillary vessel, the cross-section can be divided into two regions including a core and a cell-free plasma region near the wall. So, if the plasma layer thickness is δ, then

Core Region $\left(0 \leq r \leq r_{\text{cap}} - \delta\right)$

$$-\frac{\Delta p}{L} = \frac{1}{r}\frac{d}{dr}\left(\mu_c r \frac{du_c}{dr}\right)$$

$$\tag{4}$$

Cell-free plasma $\left(r_{\text{cap}} - \delta \leq r \leq r_{\text{cap}}\right)$

$$-\frac{\Delta p}{L} = \frac{1}{r}\frac{d}{dr}\left(\mu_p r \frac{du_p}{dr}\right),$$

where u_c, μ_c, u_p, and μ_p are velocity and viscosity in core and cell-free regions, respectively. Some assumptions are required to use these equations including no slip condition, zero-gradient in the center of vessel, and continuous velocity and shear stress at the regions' interface.

If an oscillating pressure gradient exists in the flow field, the velocity profile is a parabolic and proportional to the instantaneous flow rate and also the flow field is unsteady. Actually, in in vivo blood, the flow is affected by a pulsatile source. The inertia of the fluid in the central core prevents the core from following the applied gradient of pressure [19]. A dimensionless number, which is called Womersley, relates the frequency of unsteady pulsatile flow to viscous effect, in order to keep dynamic similarity in experimental scaling. The Womersley number implies how much of the vessel is affected by boundary layer, as follows:

$$\alpha \propto \frac{\text{unsteady inertial force}}{\text{viscous force}} \longrightarrow \alpha = r_{\text{ves}}\sqrt{\frac{\omega\rho}{\mu}}, \tag{5}$$

where ω is the angular frequency of the oscillation, that is, the frequency of the heart rate [19]. Small Womersley number ($\alpha \leq 1$) means the low frequency of pulsation. Therefore, parabolic profile of velocity is generated in each cycle and also Poiseuille's law is a good approximation [20]. On the other side, large number ($10 \leq \alpha$) means flat velocity profile, and the mean flow delays the pressure gradient by $90°$ [21].

Another important property of blood is density. Same as viscosity, not only the amount of density is not fixed for all cases, but also it is function of different variables, such as

species, gender, and body posture. The density of human blood is approximately 1056~1060 (kg/m^3). The density of blood plasma is approximately 1025 and 1125 (kg/m^3) [22].

The pressure gradient affording blood flow to the brain is called the Cerebral Perfusion Pressure (CPP). The variation of CPP is limited, because it can cause brain tissue to become ischemic, or rising Intracranial Pressure (ICP) [23]. The CPP is related to the cerebral blood flow (CBF) by the CerebroVascular Resistance (CVR) as follows:

$$\text{CBF} = \frac{\text{CPP}}{\text{CVR}}. \tag{6}$$

The autoregulation is a significant ability of human body to regulate the proper perfusion pressure for sensitive and vital organs. The brain arteries can respond to the perfusion pressure change by vasodilate or vasoconstrict, which is called autoregulation.

The autoregulation mechanism consists of two features, the autoregulation curve and the autoregulation dynamics [24]. In the autoregulation curve, the autoregulated range of pressure is approximately 75–175 mmHg and the overall steady-state blood flow rate is a function of mean arterial blood pressure:

$$Q_{ss} = \frac{1}{1 + A[O_2]_A}\left(MA + \frac{p_A - p_v}{R_0}\right), \tag{7}$$

where Q_{ss}, $[O_2]_A$, M, p_A, and p_v are the steady-state blood flow rate, arterial oxygen concentration, metabolic rate, arterial pressure, and venous pressure, respectively. The A and R_0 are two parameters to fit the autoregulation curve.

The upper and lower limits of the permeability are related to the arterial pressures limits of the autoregulated range. Therefore, the autoregulation dynamics are modeled using permeability (k) as follows:

$$\tau\frac{dk}{dx} = K_p\frac{Q_{ss} - Q}{Q_{ss}} + K_i\int_0^t \frac{Q_{ss} - Q}{Q_{ss}}dt, \tag{8}$$

where Q is time-varying flow rate and τ, K_p, and K_i are time constant, proportional, and integral gains, which are considered as 3, 70, and 0.1, respectively [24].

3. Simulation and Modeling Methods

The cerebral blood flow is a complex system, and CoW is just one of the important parts. Therefore, the systematic analysis is necessary for recognizing the functionality of CoW in this dynamic system. From the numerical modeling view point, there are three models of arterial blood flow [16].

3.1. Zero-Dimensional (0D) Models. The lumped element model describes the behavior of a distributed system into discrete entities under certain assumptions. The Windkesselmodel of the arterial network reveals a relation between pressure and flow at a specific arterial condition, without wave propagation consideration.

3.2. One-Dimensional (1D) Models.
The simplified equations of fluid motion are used to study the flow field. The wave-transmission characteristics are formulated by Womersley's oscillatory flow theory because of the hyperbolic feature of equations. A comprehensive literature review on the 1D models was performed by Reymond et al. [26].

3.3. Three-Dimensional (3D) Models.
In order to simulate accurately a segment of arterial tree, more comprehensive 3D model is required. Computational Fluid Dynamic (CFD) is a powerful tool to simulate complex flow field. The 0D and 1D modeling can reveal some useful and practical aspects about a real complex system. In order to investigate a phenomenon in detail, more accurate and applicable methods are required. If whole system of cerebral vessels is simulated by an accurate three-dimensional approach, the computational cost is beyond the power of current computing devices. The studies based on CFD are classified into three: the development, progression, and rupture of cerebral aneurysms [27]. The experiences show that image-based CFD is a capable facility to study interaction between hemodynamic loading and mechanobiological wall responses.

Combination of above methods can help improve prediction of complex problems. Quarteroni and Veneziani coupled 3D modeling of blood flow with a systemic, zero-dimensional, lumped model of circulation [28]. Beulen et al. derived boundary conditions in the first period from a one-dimensional wave propagation model and the initial pressure distribution [29].

One of the earliest studies about the mathematical model of saccular aneurysm in CoW was performed by Austin in 1971 [30]. The intracranial aneurysm was simulated using electrical circuit and also Duffing equation. He studied on the modeling of the effect of flow frequencies range on the flow condition in saccular aneurysm. This study was extended by Cronin to show the importance of pulsatile pressure in the danger of aneurysm rupture [31].

Cassot et al. developed a mathematical model to simulate the CoW flow and predict the effectiveness of anterior and posterior communicating arteries on the brain blood pressure [32]. This model was based on a linear function of the mean blood flow in 10 bifurcations in CoW and the difference of the pressures at the extremities of these nodes. After a decade, Lorthois et al. presented the modified and advanced 1D non-linear model using complex rheological properties of blood flow (such as and hematocrit distributions) in microcirculation [33, 34].

The equations of 1D models are based on the governing equations of flow motion. The laminar flow in arteries is same as steady and fully developed Poiseuille flow, therefore, the axial pressure gradient is computed as [35]

$$\frac{\partial p}{\partial z} = -\frac{8\pi\mu u}{A}. \tag{9}$$

In order to make conservation form, the equations are coupled in a system of equations as

$$\frac{\partial}{\partial t}\begin{bmatrix} A \\ u \end{bmatrix} + \frac{\partial}{\partial z}\begin{bmatrix} uA \\ \dfrac{u^2}{2} + \dfrac{p}{\rho} \end{bmatrix} = \begin{bmatrix} 0 \\ -\dfrac{8\pi\mu}{\rho}\dfrac{u}{A} \end{bmatrix}. \tag{10}$$

There are three variables in this system of equations, and an additional equation is needed to solve them. The third equation describes the relation between variation of artery's area and pressure (i.e., fluid-structure interaction). Therefore, the Laplace law for thin and homogenous elastic artery's wall is used to make this equation as follows:

$$p - p_0 = \beta\left(\sqrt{A} - \sqrt{A_0}\right), \qquad \beta = \frac{Eh_0\sqrt{\pi}}{A_0\left(1 - \sigma^2\right)}, \tag{11}$$

where A_0 and h_0 are the artery's area and wall thickness at the reference state. In addition, σ and E are Poisson's ratio and Young's Modulus.

The one-dimensional model can be deduced from the wave propagation relation. The average speed of blood in vessels is 0.5 m/s, but the wave speed is 5 m/s. The blood pressure and flow pulsations are considered as the wave propagation in the arterial network, which consist of information about the cardiovascular system [16].

An important factor in the instantaneous vessel's area is pressure difference between two sides of a vessel's wall, which is called transmural pressure (p_{tr}). There is a nonlinear and frequency relation between the transmural pressure and the area of the vessel, which is caused by complex nonlinearity and viscoelasticity of the arterial wall. The wave propagation speed of blood was introduced by Young as

$$c = \sqrt{\frac{A}{\rho C}} = \sqrt{\frac{Eh}{2\rho a}}, \tag{12}$$

where C is local area compliance. This equation is derived from simplified Newton's second law of motion and it is called Moens-Korteweg equation model.

Generally, the characteristic lines are defined in hyperbolic equations and they determine the behavior of solutions using invariant quantities along certain trajectories. The conservative form of hyperbolic system of equations appears as [35]

$$\frac{\partial U}{\partial t} + H\frac{\partial U}{\partial x} = C$$

$$U = \begin{bmatrix} A \\ u \end{bmatrix}, \qquad H = \begin{bmatrix} u & A \\ \dfrac{\beta}{2\rho\sqrt{A}} & u \end{bmatrix},$$

$$C = \begin{bmatrix} 0 \\ -\dfrac{1}{\rho}\left(\dfrac{8\pi\mu u}{A} + \dfrac{\partial p_0}{\partial x} - \dfrac{\beta}{2\sqrt{A_0}}\dfrac{\partial A_0}{\partial x} + \left(\sqrt{A} - \sqrt{A_0}\right)\dfrac{\partial \beta}{\partial x}\right) \end{bmatrix}. \tag{13}$$

The speed of waves from the heart (forward) is $u + c$ and also towards the heart (backward) is $u - c$. The forward-running wave is generated by the contraction of the heart and moves through the arterial network. When there is a variation in vessel properties, such as branch, the wave is reflected and moves back towards the heart. Therefore, there is a combination of forward- and backward-running waves.

In order to solve this system, the boundary conditions are required. The boundary conditions are reflecting and nonreflecting. In nonreflecting boundary conditions, the forward and backward waves are used at the inlet and outlet boundaries, respectively. Thus, the information from inside and outside of the domain are combined.

It should be noted that there are some difficulties in solution, such as discontinuity. A discontinuity is considered as a sudden jump; for example, stent or in a more prevalent case it is a vessel branching.

In the brain, aneurysms are often located at the lateral sides of curved vessels and at the bifurcations. The ruptured aneurysm is a common reason of death and also the surgery of aneurysm is high risk. Therefore, the recognition of different related subjects can improve the prediction of its behaviors. Different scientists studied the subjects, such as the reasons of aneurysm, the growth trend, and the effective factors. The effect of hemodynamic factors on the initiation, growth, and rupture of aneurysms is shown in different studies [36–39]. Furthermore, it is observed that the CFD-based prediction of aneurysm rupture is gradually becoming more confident and reliable [40].

Furthermore, the interaction between blood and vessel's wall play crucial role to simulate semireal pattern of fluid flow. The pressure and also blood velocity in large arteries are affected by the vessel deformability. The fluid-solid interaction (FSI) methods are used to predict this interaction. In simulation of a real situation, if the wall tension exceeds the wall tissue strength, the rupture of tissue should occur [41]. Furthermore, accuracy of modeling the arterial endothelial dysfunction plays an important role in prediction of long term vessel deformation [42].

Generally, there are some common points in FSI methods:

 (1) generated loads on the structure by fluid,

 (2) response of structure and impacts on the flow field,

 (3) computational domain and grid adaptation according to new conditions.

Based on significant development in computational fluid approaches and FSI methods and also advanced software to generate complex computational domain from in vivo medical imaging, the prediction of aneurysm behavior become more accurate and reliable [15, 43, 44]. Figueroa et al. developed a method in order to simulate blood flow in deformable models of arteries. They coupled the equations of the deformation of the vessel wall as a boundary condition for the fluid zone [45].

One of the first successful attempts to use FSI in predicting the abdominal aortic aneurysm was performed by Di Martino et al. [46]. The risk of rupture is a function of transversal diameter, that is, the maximum safe cross-sectional area of aneurysm. The aneurysm is usually asymmetric; therefore, the simple method, such as Laplace law

is not an appropriate solution of this question. An accurate 3D FSI simulation can predict correct relation between the growth rate of aneurysm and flow conditions. Li and Kleinstreuer used FSI simulation to investigate the geometry variations of abdominal aortic aneurysm, such as degree of asymmetry, neck angle, and bifurcation angle [47].

The functionalities and anomalies of CoW are studied using CFD tools [48–51]. Alnæs et al. developed a 3D simulation of CoW to study the impact of variations in vessel radii and bifurcation angles on wall shear stress and pressure on vessel walls [52]. It is shown that the rigid vascular wall is a good assumption for smaller vessels but not for larger arteries. In the CoW, this approximation could overestimate wall shear stress but probably not influence its spatial distribution.

Kim simulated the flow condition of CoW in two cases, including absence of left PCoA and absence of ACoA. It was shown that the autoregulation mechanism is strongly affected by the communicating arteries, PCoA and ACoA [53]. Long et al. studied on the CoW functionalities and abilities to supply blood in patients with unilateral carotid arterial stenosis. They selected four CoW configurations with an axisymmetric stenosis in an internal carotid artery (ICA) and also different boundary conditions [51].

In spite of these significant abilities, there are some difficulties to reach accurate and applicable predictions:

 (1) geometry generation according to the real situation,

 (2) generation of proper and efficient computational grid,

 (3) appropriate and efficient solver selection,

 (4) accurate initial and boundary conditions,

 (5) trace the result during the run carefully to improve the simulation,

 (6) present the final results in a user-friendly and inferable manner.

The most important subject in geometry generation is similarity with the physical domain. The simplest numerical form of aneurysm is a spherical and symmetric sac. But the actual geometry of aneurysms is irregular. Some software can generate real geometry from X-ray scans. For example, the mimiced software can produce actual geometry of organs from MRI of CT-scan files [54]. These tools can help reduce significantly the time of preprocessing and also improve the final results.

After the geometry and grid generation, the initial and boundary conditions are required. Generally, the boundary value problem is a differential equation with boundary conditions. The boundary conditions cause unique solution for problem, which is called well-posed problem. In addition, the relation between computational domain and outer regions is established with boundary condition. The boundary condition types are inlet, outlet, wall, symmetry, and periodic. Another important factor is initial condition, which specifies the condition of domain at the beginning.

The main step is selecting an appropriate numerical solver. As mentioned before, there are two regimes of flow, that is, laminar and turbulent. In laminar flow, the layers are parallel without any disruption, lateral mixing, and eddies [55]. Therefore, the discretized governing equation, that is, continuity, momentum, and energy, can be computed in coarse grid.

On the other hand, the turbulent flow is completely a complex regime with disruption, lateral mixing, and eddies. The implementation of discretized governing equation in turbulent flow needs very fine grid, and so unacceptable computational cost. This method is called Direct Numerical Simulation (DNS). DNS is not an applicable method in real situation. Alternatively, some simplified methods were developed in order to model the turbulent flow and reduce considerably the computational cost, such as Reynolds-Averaged Navier-Stokes (RANS). The comprehensive description of different methods of turbulent flow simulation is presented by Andersson et al. [56].

4. Discussion

The critical point in virtual simulation is the accuracy of prediction and consistency with the reality. The accuracy depends on the variety of factors. In the current paper, the important related subjects are reviewed in a classified manner. Although, different 1D and 3D simulations of CoW and cerebral aneurysm were carried out, many questions have been left. Some of important objectives of future studies are listed here.

(1) The cerebral perfusion is a vital subject and it is a function of flow rate and pressure. The amount of flow rate is known in normal condition and also the effect of some anomalies on flow rate was studied by 1D simulation [25]. However, the effect of anomalies and also 3D complexity is not completely obvious.

(2) The 0D or 1D modeling can help generate boundary conditions for 3D simulation. In addition, the 3D simulation can help improve the 1D modeling. As a result, 0D or 1D models and 3D simulation can have an effect on each other, simultaneously. It means that the local 3D simulation, that is, CoW, and global modeling, that is, cerebral blood system, should perform in a coupled condition. Regarding anomalies influence on the functionalities of CoW and also whole cerebral blood supply system, what is the relation between anomalies and cerebral blood supply?

Disclosure

There is no financial interest related to the material in the paper.

Conflict of Interests

The authors declare that there is no conflict of interests regarding the publication of this paper.

Authors' Contribution

Study concept and design was made by S. R. Ghodsi, V. Esfahanian, and S. M. Ghodsi. Drafting of the paper was made by S. R. Ghodsi. The sponsor had no role in the design and conduct of the study; collection, management, and analysis of the data; or preparation, review, and approval of the paper.

Acknowledgments

This study was carried out in VFE Research Institute in University of Tehran and based on a Project entitled as "3D Numerical Simulation of Flow in the Circle of Willis in Normal and Common Anomalies." In addition, many thanks to Sina Trauma Research Center, because of spiritual and financial sponsorship of the project.

References

[1] R. G. Whitmore, R. A. Grant, P. LeRoux, O. El-Falaki, and S. C. Stein, "How large is the typical subarachnoid hemorrhage? A review of current neurosurgical knowledge," *World Neurosurgery*, vol. 77, pp. 686–697, 2012.

[2] A. W. J. Hoksbergen, B. Fülesdi, D. A. Legemate, and L. Csiba, "Collateral configuration of the circle of Willis: transcranial color-coded duplex ultrasonography and comparison with postmortem anatomy," *Stroke*, vol. 31, no. 6, pp. 1346–1351, 2000.

[3] M. A. Neimark, A.-A. Konstas, A. F. Laine, and J. Pile-Spellman, "Integration of jugular venous return and circle of Willis in a theoretical human model of selective brain cooling," *Journal of Applied Physiology*, vol. 103, no. 5, pp. 1837–1847, 2007.

[4] X.-Q. Cheng, J.-M. Tian, C.-J. Zuo, J. Liu, Q. Zhang, and G.-M. Lu, "Quantitative perfusion computed tomography measurements of cerebral hemodynamics: correlation with digital subtraction angiography identified primary and secondary cerebral collaterals in internal carotid artery occlusive disease," *European Journal of Radiology*, vol. 81, pp. 1224–1230, 2012.

[5] K. R. D. De Silva, R. Silva, D. Amaratunga, W. Gunasekera, and R. W. Jayesekera, "Types of the cerebral arterial circle (circle of Willis) in a Sri Lankan population," *BMC Neurology*, vol. 11, article 5, 2011.

[6] V. Papantchev, S. Hristov, D. Todorova et al., "Some variations of the circle of Willis, important for cerebral protection in aortic surgery—a study in Eastern Europeans," *European Journal of Cardio-thoracic Surgery*, vol. 31, no. 6, pp. 982–989, 2007.

[7] B. Eftekhar, M. Dadmehr, S. Ansari, M. Ghodsi, B. Nazparvar, and E. Ketabchi, "Are the distributions of variations of circle of Willis different in different populations?—results of an anatomical study and review of literature," *BMC Neurology*, vol. 6, article 22, 2006.

[8] M. A. Maaly and A. A. Ismail, "Three dimensional magnetic resonance angiography of the circle of Willis: anatomical variations in general Egyptian population," *Egyptian Journal of Radiology and Nuclear Medicine*, vol. 42, no. 3-4, pp. 405–412, 2011.

[9] J. Ottesen, M. Olufsen, and J. Larsen, *Applied Mathematical Models in Human Physiology*, Department of Mathematics and Physics, Roskilde University, 2006.

[10] J. Janzen, "Ageing of the conduit arteries," *Journal of Pathology*, vol. 211, pp. 157–172, 2007.

[11] R. Uflacker and C. J. Feldman, *Atlas of Vascular Anatomy*, Williams & Wilkins, 1997.

[12] I. Chatziprodromou, A. Tricoli, D. Poulikakos, and Y. Ventikos, "Haemodynamics and wall remodelling of a growing cerebral aneurysm: a computational model," *Journal of Biomechanics*, vol. 40, no. 2, pp. 412–426, 2007.

[13] K. Rogers, *Blood: Physiology and Circulation*, Britannica Educational Publishing, 2012.

[14] http://www.cvphysiology.com/Hemodynamics/H007.htm.

[15] K. Valen-Sendstad, K.-A. Mardal, M. Mortensen, B. A. P. Reif, and H. P. Langtangen, "Direct numerical simulation of transitional flow in a patient-specific intracranial aneurysm," *Journal of Biomechanics*, vol. 44, no. 16, pp. 2826–2832, 2011.

[16] F. N. van De Vosse and N. Stergiopulos, "Pulse wave propagation in the arterial tree," *Annual Review of Fluid Mechanics*, vol. 43, pp. 467–499, 2011.

[17] F. Yilmaz and M. Y. Gundogdu, "A critical review on blood flow in large arteries; relevance to blood rheology, viscosity models, and physiologic conditions," *Korea Australia Rheology Journal*, vol. 20, no. 4, pp. 197–211, 2008.

[18] Ø. Evju, K. Valen-Sendstad, and K. A. Mardal, "A study of wall shear stress in 12 aneurysms with respect to different viscosity models and flow conditions," *Journal of Biomechanics*, vol. 46, pp. 2802–2808, 2013.

[19] C. Caro, *The Mechanics of the Circulation*, Cambridge University Press, 2012.

[20] Y. Huo and G. S. Kassab, "Pulsatile blood flow in the entire coronary arterial tree: theory and experiment," *The American Journal of Physiology—Heart and Circulatory Physiology*, vol. 291, no. 3, pp. H1074–H1087, 2006.

[21] Y. Fung, *Biomechanics: Circulation*, Springer, 1996.

[22] http://hypertextbook.com/facts/2004/MichaelShmukler.shtml.

[23] H. White and B. Venkatesh, "Cerebral perfusion pressure in neurotrauma: a review," *Anesthesia and Analgesia*, vol. 107, no. 3, pp. 979–988, 2008.

[24] S. Moore, T. David, J. G. Chase, J. Arnold, and J. Fink, "3D models of blood flow in the cerebral vasculature," *Journal of Biomechanics*, vol. 39, no. 8, pp. 1454–1463, 2006.

[25] J. Alastruey, K. H. Parker, J. Peiró, S. M. Byrd, and S. J. Sherwin, "Modelling the circle of Willis to assess the effects of anatomical variations and occlusions on cerebral flows," *Journal of Biomechanics*, vol. 40, no. 8, pp. 1794–1805, 2007.

[26] P. Reymond, Y. Bohraus, F. Perren, F. Lazeyras, and N. Stergiopulos, "Validation of a patient-specific one-dimensional model of the systemic arterial tree," *The American Journal of Physiology—Heart and Circulatory Physiology*, vol. 301, no. 3, pp. H1173–H1182, 2011.

[27] D. M. Sforza, C. M. Putman, and J. R. Cebral, "Computational fluid dynamics in brain aneurysms," *International Journal for Numerical Methods in Biomedical Engineering*, vol. 28, pp. 801–808, 2012.

[28] A. Quarteroni and A. Veneziani, "Analysis of a geometrical multiscale model based on the coupling of ODE and PDE for blood flow simulations," *Multiscale Modeling & Simulation*, vol. 1, pp. 173–195, 2003.

[29] B. W. A. M. M. Beulen, M. C. M. Rutten, and F. N. van de Vosse, "A time-periodic approach for fluid-structure interaction in distensible vessels," *Journal of Fluids and Structures*, vol. 25, no. 5, pp. 954–966, 2009.

[30] G. Austin, "Biomathematical model of aneurysm of the circle of willis, I: the duffing equation and some approximate solutions," *Mathematical Biosciences*, vol. 11, no. 1-2, pp. 163–172, 1971.

[31] J. Cronin, "Mathematical model of aneurysm of the circle of Willis: II. A qualitative analysis of the equation of Austin," *Mathematical Biosciences*, vol. 22, pp. 237–275, 1974.

[32] F. Cassot, M. Zagzoule, and J.-P. Marc-Vergnes, "Hemodynamic role of the circle of Willis in stenoses of internal carotid arteries. An analytical solution of a linear model," *Journal of Biomechanics*, vol. 33, no. 4, pp. 395–405, 2000.

[33] S. Lorthois, F. Cassot, and F. Lauwers, "Simulation study of brain blood flow regulation by intra-cortical arterioles in an anatomically accurate large human vascular network. Part II: flow variations induced by global or localized modifications of arteriolar diameters," *NeuroImage*, vol. 54, no. 4, pp. 2840–2853, 2011.

[34] S. Lorthois, F. Cassot, and F. Lauwers, "Simulation study of brain blood flow regulation by intra-cortical arterioles in an anatomically accurate large human vascular network: part I: methodology and baseline flow," *NeuroImage*, vol. 54, no. 2, pp. 1031–1042, 2011.

[35] J. P. Mynard and P. Nithiarasu, "A 1D arterial blood flow model incorporating ventricular pressure, aortic vaive ana regional coronary flow using the locally conservative Galerkin (LCG) method," *Communications in Numerical Methods in Engineering*, vol. 24, no. 5, pp. 367–417, 2008.

[36] J. R. Cebral, F. Mut, J. Weir, and C. M. Putman, "Association of hemodynamic characteristics and cerebral aneurysm rupture," *American Journal of Neuroradiology*, vol. 32, no. 2, pp. 264–270, 2011.

[37] J. Xiang, S. K. Natarajan, M. Tremmel et al., "Hemodynamic-morphologic discriminants for intracranial aneurysm rupture," *Stroke*, vol. 42, no. 1, pp. 144–152, 2011.

[38] Y. Qian, H. Takao, M. Umezu, and Y. Murayama, "Risk analysis of unruptured aneurysms using computational fluid dynamics technology: preliminary results," *American Journal of Neuroradiology*, vol. 32, no. 10, pp. 1948–1955, 2011.

[39] Y. Miura, F. Ishida, Y. Umeda et al., "Low wall shear stress is independently associated with the rupture status of middle cerebral artery aneurysms," *Stroke*, vol. 44, pp. 519–521, 2013.

[40] H. Takao, Y. Murayama, S. Otsuka et al., "Hemodynamic differences between unruptured and ruptured intracranial aneurysms during observation," *Stroke*, vol. 43, no. 5, pp. 1436–1439, 2012.

[41] J. G. Isaksen, Y. Bazilevs, T. Kvamsdal et al., "Determination of wall tension in cerebral artery aneurysms by numerical simulation," *Stroke*, vol. 39, no. 12, pp. 3172–3178, 2008.

[42] A. I. Barakat, "Blood flow and arterial endothelial dysfunction: mechanisms and implications," *Comptes Rendus Physique*, vol. 14, no. 6, pp. 479–496, 2013.

[43] R. Torii, M. Oshima, T. Kobayashi, K. Takagi, and T. E. Tezduyar, "Fluid-structure interaction modeling of blood flow and cerebral aneurysm: significance of artery and aneurysm shapes," *Computer Methods in Applied Mechanics and Engineering*, vol. 198, no. 45-46, pp. 3613–3621, 2009.

[44] K. Yokoi, F. Xiao, H. Liu, and K. Fukasaku, "Three-dimensional numerical simulation of flows with complex geometries in a regular Cartesian grid and its application to blood flow in cerebral artery with multiple aneurysms," *Journal of Computational Physics*, vol. 202, no. 1, pp. 1–19, 2005.

[45] C. A. Figueroa, I. E. Vignon-Clementel, K. E. Jansen, T. J. R. Hughes, and C. A. Taylor, "A coupled momentum method for modeling blood flow in three-dimensional deformable arteries," *Computer Methods in Applied Mechanics and Engineering*, vol. 195, no. 41-43, pp. 5685–5706, 2006.

[46] E. S. Di Martino, G. Guadagni, A. Fumero et al., "Fluid-structure interaction within realistic three-dimensional models of the aneurysmatic aorta as a guidance to assess the risk of rupture of the aneurysm," *Medical Engineering and Physics*, vol. 23, no. 9, pp. 647–655, 2001.

[47] Z. Li and C. Kleinstreuer, "A comparison between different asymmetric abdominal aortic aneurysm morphologies employing computational fluid-structure interaction analysis," *European Journal of Mechanics B*, vol. 26, no. 5, pp. 615–631, 2007.

[48] D. I. Zuleger, D. Poulikakos, A. Valavanis, and S. S. Kollias, "Combining magnetic resonance measurements with numerical simulations—extracting blood flow physiology information relevant to the investigation of intracranial aneurysms in the circle of Willis," *International Journal of Heat and Fluid Flow*, vol. 31, no. 6, pp. 1032–1039, 2010.

[49] T. David and S. Moore, "Modeling perfusion in the cerebral vasculature," *Medical Engineering and Physics*, vol. 30, no. 10, pp. 1227–1245, 2008.

[50] L. Grinberg, T. Anor, E. Cheever, J. R. Madsen, and G. E. Karniadakis, "Simulation of the human intracranial arterial tree," *Philosophical Transactions of the Royal Society A*, vol. 367, no. 1896, pp. 2371–2386, 2009.

[51] Q. Long, L. Luppi, C. S. König, V. Rinaldo, and S. K. Das, "Study of the collateral capacity of the circle of Willis of patients with severe carotid artery stenosis by 3D computational modeling," *Journal of Biomechanics*, vol. 41, no. 12, pp. 2735–2742, 2008.

[52] M. S. Alnæs, J. Isaksen, K.-A. Mardal, B. Romner, M. K. Morgan, and T. Ingebrigtsen, "Computation of hemodynamics in the circle of Willis," *Stroke*, vol. 38, no. 9, pp. 2500–2505, 2007.

[53] C. S. Kim, "Numerical simulation of auto-regulation and collateral circulation in the human brain," *Journal of Mechanical Science and Technology*, vol. 21, no. 3, pp. 525–535, 2007.

[54] http://www.materialise.com/.

[55] G. Batchelor, *An Introduction to Fluid Dynamics*, Cambridge University Press, 2000.

[56] B. Andersson, R. Andersson, L. Håkansso, M. Mortensen, R. Sudiyo, and B. van Wachem, *Computational Fluid Dynamics for Engineers*, Cambridge University Press, 2012.

6

Combined 3D QSAR Based Virtual Screening and Molecular Docking Study of Some Selected PDK-1 Kinase Inhibitors

Shalini Singh and Pradeep Srivastava

School of Biochemical Engineering, Indian Institute of Technology (Banaras Hindu University), Varanasi 221005, India

Correspondence should be addressed to Pradeep Srivastava; drpradeep19@gmail.com

Academic Editor: Jeon-Hor Chen

Phosphoinositide-dependent kinase-1 (PDK-1) is an important therapeutic target for the treatment of cancer. In order to identify the important chemical features of PDK-1 inhibitors, a 3D QSAR pharmacophore model was developed based on 21 available PDK-1 inhibitors. The best pharmacophore model (Hypo1) exhibits all the important chemical features required for PDK-1 inhibitors. The correlation coefficient, root mean square deviation (RMSD), and cost difference were 0.96906, 1.0719, and 168.13, respectively, suggesting a good predictive ability of the model (Hypo1) among all the ten pharmacophore models that were analyzed. The best pharmacophore model (Hypo1) was further validated by Fisher's randomization method (95%), test set method ($r = 0.87$), and the decoy set with the goodness of fit (0.73). Further, this validated pharmacophore model Hypo1 was used as a 3D query to screen the molecules from databases like NCI database and Maybridge. The resultant hit compounds were subsequently subjected to filtration by Lipinski's rule of five as well as the ADMET study. Docking study was done to refine the retrieved hits and as a result to reduce the rate of false positive. Best hits will further be subjected to in vitro study in future.

1. Introduction

Protein kinases are critical components of cellular signal transduction cascades [1]. Over 500 protein kinases in the human genome have been reported till date and they are considered as the second largest group of drug targets [2, 3]. Phosphoinositide-dependent kinase-1 (PDK-1), a 63 kDa serine/threonine kinase, is a major player in the PI3-kinase signaling pathway that regulates gene expression, cell cycle, growth, and proliferation [4–11]. PDK-1 is also termed as the "master kinase" because it phosphorylates highly conserved serine or threonine residues in the T-loop (or activation loop) of numerous AGC kinases, including PKB/AKT, PKC, p70S6K, SGK, and PDK-1 itself [12]. Although precise regulatory mechanisms vary, in the case of PKB/AKT, activation by PDK-1 is critically dependent on prior PI3 kinase activation and the presence of phosphatidylinositol-(3,4,5)-triphosphate (PIP3). A significant proportion (40–50%) of all tumors involve mutations in PIP3-3-phosphatase (PTEN) [13–15], which result in elevated levels of PIP3 and enhanced activation of PKB/AKT, p70S6K, and SGK. The inhibitors of

PDK-1 could potentially provide valuable therapeutic agents for the treatment of cancer.

Recognition process between ligand and model is based on spatial distribution of certain structural features of active site being complimentary to those of the interacting ligands, and the features common to the ligands would provide the information about the active site. A pharmacophore mapping is the essential step towards understanding of receptor-ligand recognition process and is established as one of the successful computational tools in rational drug design [16, 17]. This involves the identification of a three-dimensional arrangement of functional groups which a molecule must possess to be recognized by the receptor. Further, a model is generated by finding chemically important functional groups that are common to the molecules that bind. Pharmacophore can be derived by direct analysis of the structure of known ligand either in the most stable conformer or in the form observed when complexed with the target protein.

In the present study, a three-dimensional pharmacophore model for PDK-1 kinase inhibitors has been developed. The generated model is further utilized for screening of potentially active candidates from NCI and Maybridge database. The efficacy of these compounds is further validated by molecular docking.

2. Material and Methods

2.1. General Methodology. All pharmacophore models generation and Hypo1 based virtual screening were performed using the following tools.

HypoGen. It was implemented in Catalyst (Catalyst 4.1, Molecular Simulations Inc., San Diego, CA).

Fisher Randomization Test. It was done by CatScamble program implemented in Catalyst.

Lipinski Filtration. It was performed using Pipeline Pilot Studio (SciTegic Inc., San Diego, CA).

Ligandfit. Docking studies were achieved using Discovery Studio 2.5 (Accelrys Inc., San Diego, CA).

2.2. Data Set for Pharmacophore Analysis. A set of 83 different compounds were collected from different references [18–21], which have been identified and reported to be inhibitors of PDK-1 kinase. The inhibitory activity of these compounds, expressed as IC_{50} (i.e., concentration of compound required to inhibit 50% of PDK-1 kinase activity), was studied for all compounds. The IC_{50} values spanned across a wide range from 3.0 to 65,000 nM. Amongst 83 compounds, 21 compounds were selected as training set compounds and the rest of compounds were taken as a test set compounds. The chemical structures of all training set compounds are shown in Figure 1. The selection of the training set and test set were according to the following rules: (i) there is structural diversity among molecules, (ii) both training set and test set cover a wide range of activity, and (iii) the highest active compounds were included in the training set because they provide critical information for pharmacophore generation. The geometry of all compounds was built by using Accelrys Discovery Studio 2.5 [22]. All the compounds were minimized using the steepest descent algorithm with a convergence gradient value of 0.001 kcal/mol and a family of representative conformations was generated by fast conformational analysis methods using poling minimize algorithm [23] and CHARMM force field parameters [24]. A large number of confirmations of each compound were generated within an energy threshold of 20.0 kcal/mol above the global energy minimum.

2.3. Pharmacophore Modeling. Based on the conformations for each compound, HypoGen module of Discovery Studio 2.5 was used to construct the possible pharmacophore models [25]. Instead of using the lowest energy conformation of each compound, all the conformational models of each compound in the training set were used in Discovery Studio 2.5 for pharmacophore hypothesis generations. The training set compounds (21 in number) associated with their conformations were submitted to Discovery Studio 2.5

for 3D QSAR pharmacophore Generation (HypoGen). The HypoGen module generated hypothesis with features common in active molecule and missing from inactive molecule.

2.4. Model Validation. The statistical parameters, such as the cost value, determine the significance of the model. The best model was selected on the basis of significant statistical parameters, like high correlation (r), predicted the lowest total cost, and lower value of RMSD, and the value of the total cost should be closer to the fixed cost and far away from null cost. Another parameter, configuration cost, is also important for the determination of significance of the model, and it should be <17. The best hypothesis Hypo1 was also validated by test set validation method, Fischer's randomization validation, and decoy set method. Ligand pharmacophore mapping protocol was used for estimating the activity of all 62 test set compounds.

2.5. Decoy Set Validation. Results of test set validation method could only indicate that the generated pharmacophore model (Hypo1) has high efficiency in picking the active molecules but is not conformity as it also picked the inactive molecules. To further evaluate this, decoy set validation method was used to evaluate the efficiency of Hypo1 by calculating the GH (goodness of hit list) and EF (enrichment factor). A data set of small molecules was generated by decoy set finder 1.1 which included 1980 molecules with unknown activity and 20 active molecules were making a decoy set of 2,000 molecules. GH (goodness of hit list) and EF (enrichment factor) were calculated by the following equations:

$$EF = \frac{(Ha/Ht)}{(A/D)},$$

$$GH = \left\{ \frac{[Ha * (3A + Ht)]}{4HtA} \right\} * \left[1 - \frac{(Ht - Ha)}{(D - A)} \right], \tag{1}$$

where Ht = total number of molecules in hit list, Ha = total active molecules present in the hit list, A = total active molecules present in database, and D = total molecules present in decoy set.

The range of GH score varies from 0 to 1. GH score 0 means a null model, while the GH score 1 means generation of an ideal model.

Although when the GH score is higher than 0.7, it reflect the generation of a very good model. The EF and GH were found to be 69.23 and 0.73 (shown in Table 1) indicating that the generated pharmacophore model had a rationale for virtual screening.

2.6. Virtual Screening and ADMET Analysis. The final validated hypothesis (Hypo1) was used as a 3D structural query for retrieving potent compounds from NCI database and Maybridge database having 23,8819 molecules and 2,000 molecules, respectively. A systematic diagram of virtual screening protocol is shown in Figure 2.

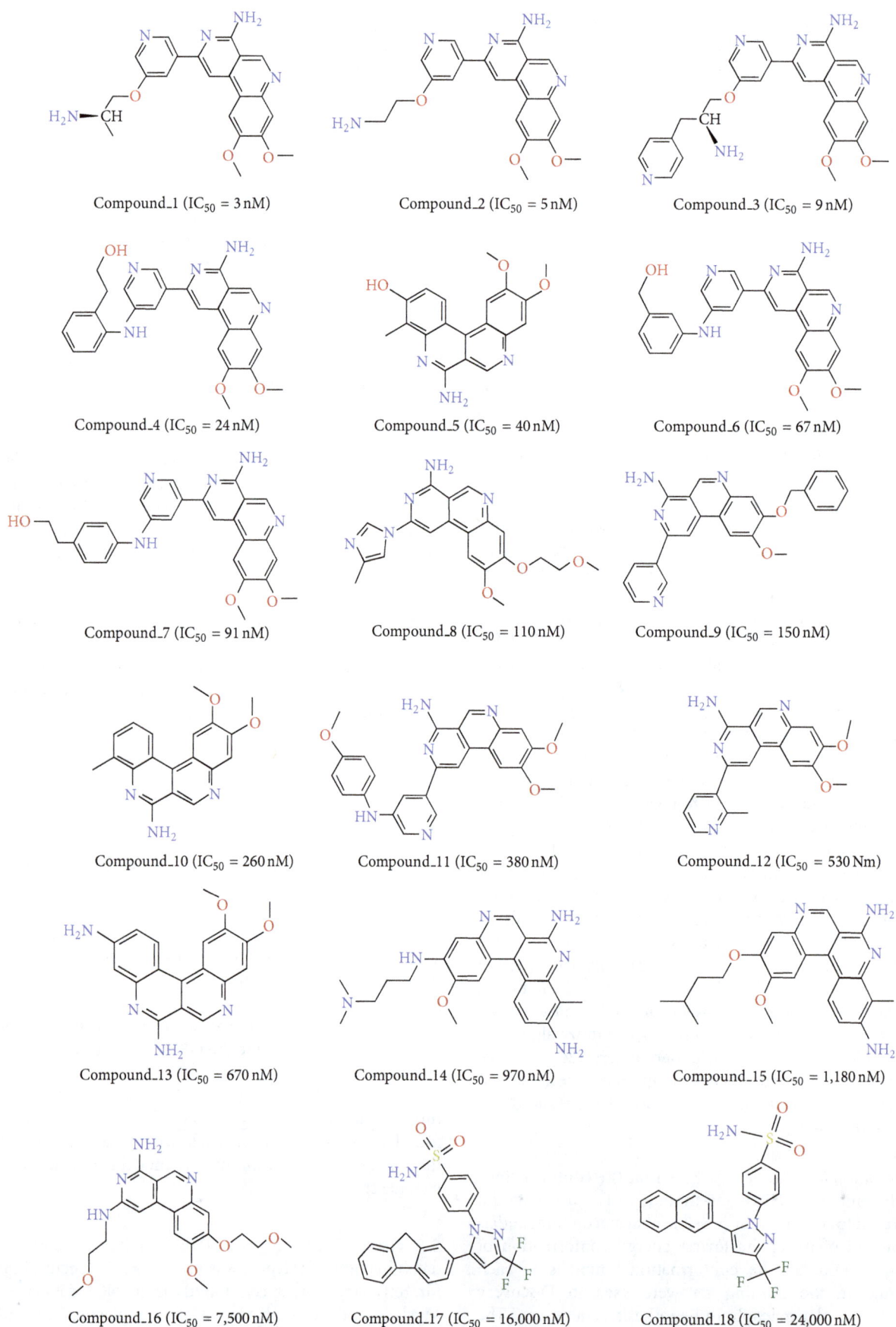

Compound_1 (IC$_{50}$ = 3 nM)

Compound_2 (IC$_{50}$ = 5 nM)

Compound_3 (IC$_{50}$ = 9 nM)

Compound_4 (IC$_{50}$ = 24 nM)

Compound_5 (IC$_{50}$ = 40 nM)

Compound_6 (IC$_{50}$ = 67 nM)

Compound_7 (IC$_{50}$ = 91 nM)

Compound_8 (IC$_{50}$ = 110 nM)

Compound_9 (IC$_{50}$ = 150 nM)

Compound_10 (IC$_{50}$ = 260 nM)

Compound_11 (IC$_{50}$ = 380 nM)

Compound_12 (IC$_{50}$ = 530 Nm)

Compound_13 (IC$_{50}$ = 670 nM)

Compound_14 (IC$_{50}$ = 970 nM)

Compound_15 (IC$_{50}$ = 1,180 nM)

Compound_16 (IC$_{50}$ = 7,500 nM)

Compound_17 (IC$_{50}$ = 16,000 nM)

Compound_18 (IC$_{50}$ = 24,000 nM)

(a)

FIGURE 1: Continued.

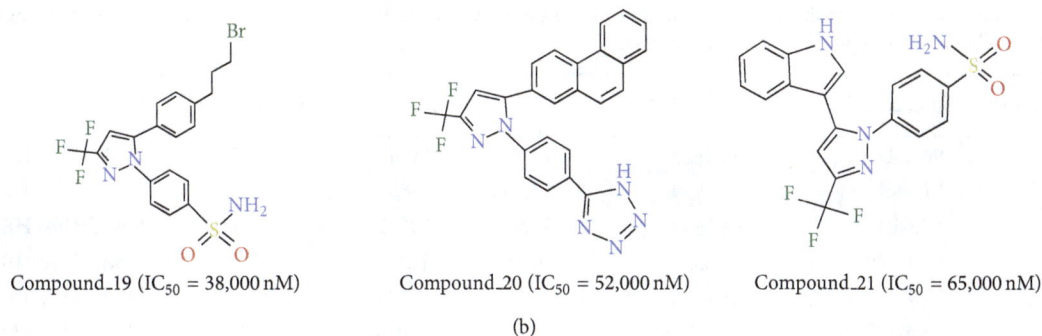

Compound_19 (IC_{50} = 38,000 nM)   Compound_20 (IC_{50} = 52,000 nM)   Compound_21 (IC_{50} = 65,000 nM)

(b)

FIGURE 1: Chemical structures of and activity data (IC_{50} values, nM) of 21 training set molecules applied for HypoGen pharmacophore generation.

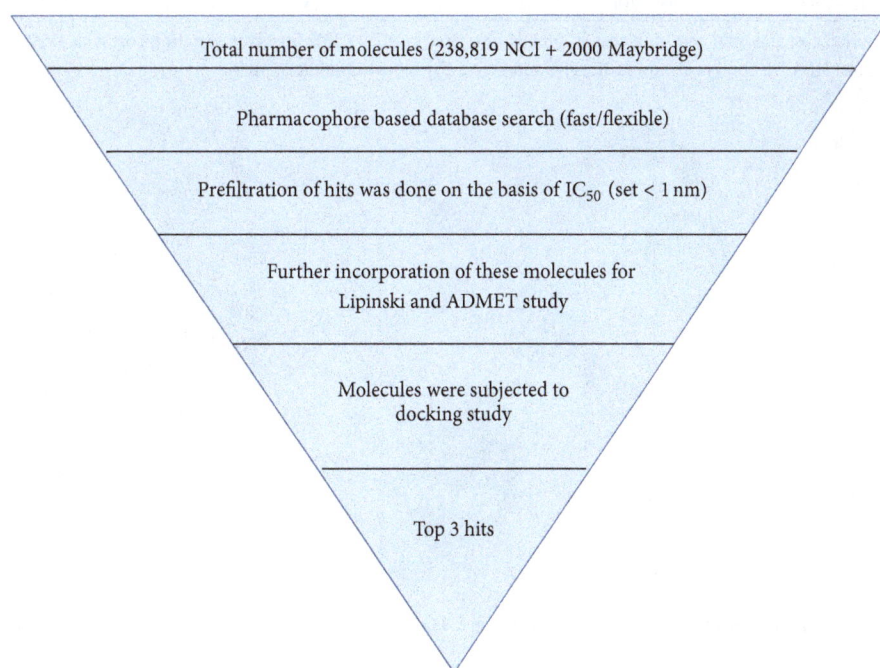

FIGURE 2: Diagrammatic representation of virtual screening protocol.

TABLE 1: Statistical parameters from the validation of the pharmacophore model by mean of decoy set.

Number	Parameters	Values
1	Total number of molecules in database (D)	2,000
2	Total number of active molecules in database (A)	20
3	Total number of hit molecules from database (Ht)	26
4	Total number of active molecules in hit list (Ha)	18
5	% yield of actives [(Ha/A) 100]	69.23
6	% ratio of actives in the hit list [(Ha/A) × 100]	90
7	Enrichment factor (EF) [(Ha × D)/(Ht × A)]	69.23
8	False negatives [A − Ha]	2
9	False positives [Ht − Ha]	8
10	GH score[a] (goodness of hit list)	0.73

[a][(Ha/4HtA)(3A + Ht) × [1 − (Ht − Ha)/(D − A)]].

3. Results and Discussion

3.1. Pharmacophore Modeling. Ten hypotheses were produced by 3D QSAR pharmacophore generation module of Accerlys Discovery Studio 2.5 through 21 training sets compounds (Table 2). Hypo1 was the most significant hypothesis characterized by high cost difference (168.48433), the lowest root mean square deviation (RMSD = 1.0719), and the best correlation coefficient (r = 0.96906). The fixed cost and the null cost values were 77.5618 and 258.686, respectively, with total cost value 90.2017 for Hypo1. This observation was much lower than null cost and closer to the fixed cost.

The best hypothesis (Hypo1) consists of four features, that is, two hydrogen bonds acceptor (HBA), one hydrogen bond donor (HBD), and one hydrophobic aliphatic feature (HyA). Figures 3(a) and 3(b) represent features of the best pharmacophore (Hypo1) and the distance and angular

TABLE 2: Information of statistical significance and predictive power presented in cost values measured in bits for top 10 hypotheses as a result of automated HypoGen pharmacophore generation process.

Hypothesis number	Total cost	Cost difference[a] (total cost-null cost)	Error	RMS	Correlation (r)	Features[b]
1	90.2017	168.4843	73.0296	1.0719	0.96906	HBA, HBA, HBD, and HyA
2	91.6361	167.0499	74.8623	1.1505	0.96423	HBA, HBA, HyA, and HyA
3	92.4311	166.2549	74.9287	1.1532	0.96414	HBA, HBA, HBD, and HyA
4	93.3537	165.3323	76.4684	1.2151	0.96002	HBA, HBA, HBD, and HyA
5	93.5794	165.1066	76.5881	1.2198	0.95971	HBA, HBA, HyA, and HyA
6	95.5213	163.1647	78.8279	1.3043	0.95376	HBA, HBA, HyA, and HyA
7	96.8603	161.8257	79.8688	1.34181	0.951035	HBA, HBD, HyA, and HyA
8	99.4115	159.4565	79.8688	1.34181	0.951035	HBA, HBD, HyA, and HyA
9	99.7217	158.9643	83.011	1.44906	0.942609	HBA, HBD, HyA, and HyA
10	99.7794	158.9066	83.1717	1.45431	0.942169	HBA, HBA, HBD, and HyA

[a]The cost difference between null cost and total cost; null cost is 258.686 bits; fixed cost is 77.5618 bits; configuration cost is 15.4729 bits.
[b]Abbreviation used for features: HBA: H-bond acceptor; HBD: H-bond donor; HyA: hydrophobic aliphatic.

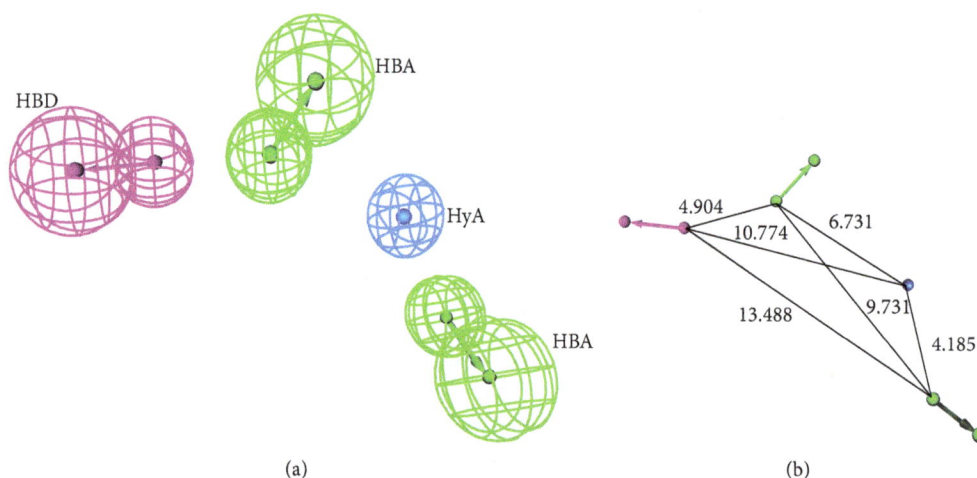

FIGURE 3: (a) Hypo1 (best pharmacophore) generated by HypoGen (3D QSAR pharmacophore protocol); (b) pharmacophore model with distance between chemical features.

constraints in the best pharmacophore (Hypo1). The experimental and estimated activities of the best pharmacophore hypothesis (Hypo1) for 21 training set compounds are shown in (Table 3). Figure 4(a) represents the top scoring hypothesis Hypo1, mapped on the most active compound 1 (IC_{50} = 3 nM) and Figure 4(b) represents the mapping of least active compound_21 (IC_{50} = 65,000 nM) of the training set.

3.2. Cost Analysis.
In addition to generating a hypothesis, HypoGen also provides two theoretical costs (represented in bit units) to help assess the validity of the hypothesis. The first is fixed cost (cost of an ideal hypothesis), which represents the simplest model that fits all data perfectly, and the second is the null cost (cost of null hypothesis), which represents the highest cost of a pharmacophore with no features and which estimates activity to be the average of the activity data of the training set molecules. They represent the upper and lower limits for the hypothesis that

are generated. A meaningful pharmacophore hypothesis may be generated when the difference between null hypothesis and the fixed hypothesis is large; a value of 40–60 bits may indicate that it has 75–90% probability of correlating the data. Other two parameters that also determine the quality of any pharmacophore are configuration cost or entropy cost and error cost. The configuration cost depends on the complexity of the pharmacophore and should have value <17 whereas the error cost is dependent on the root mean square difference between the estimated and the actual activity of the training set. The difference between total fixed cost and the null cost of the Hypo1 was observed to be 168.4843, which is more than 40–60, which depicts more than 90% probability of data correlation. Noticeably, the total cost of Hypo1 was much closer to the fixed cost than to the null cost. Furthermore, a high correlation coefficient of 0.96906 was observed with RMS value of 1.0719 and the configuration cost of 15.4729, demonstrating the development of a reliable pharmacophore model with high predictivity.

TABLE 3: Experimental biological data and estimated IC_{50} of training set molecules based on pharmacophore model Hypo1.

Compound no	IC_{50} value (nM)		Error	Uncertainty	Fit value
	Experimental	Expected			
1	3	2.4	−1.3	2	8.60
2	5	4.9	−1.0	2	8.29
3	9	14	+1.6	2	7.83
4	24	20	−1.2	2	7.67
5	40	130	+3.3	2	6.86
6	67	39	−1.8	2	7.40
7	91	110	+1.2	2	6.94
8	110	290	+2.6	2	6.52
9	150	230	+1.6	2	6.61
10	260	1000	+4.0	2	5.97
11	380	160	−2.4	2	6.71
12	530	1100	+2.0	2	5.94
13	670	1000	+1.5	2	5.97
14	690	420	−2.3	2	6.36
15	1200	390	−3.1	2	6.39
16	7500	27000	+2.7	2	5.55
17	16000	21000	+1.6	2	4.65
18	24000	21000	−1.1	2	4.65
19	38000	21000	−1.8	2	4.65
20	52000	93000	+1.8	2	4.01
21	65000	21000	−3.0	2	4.05

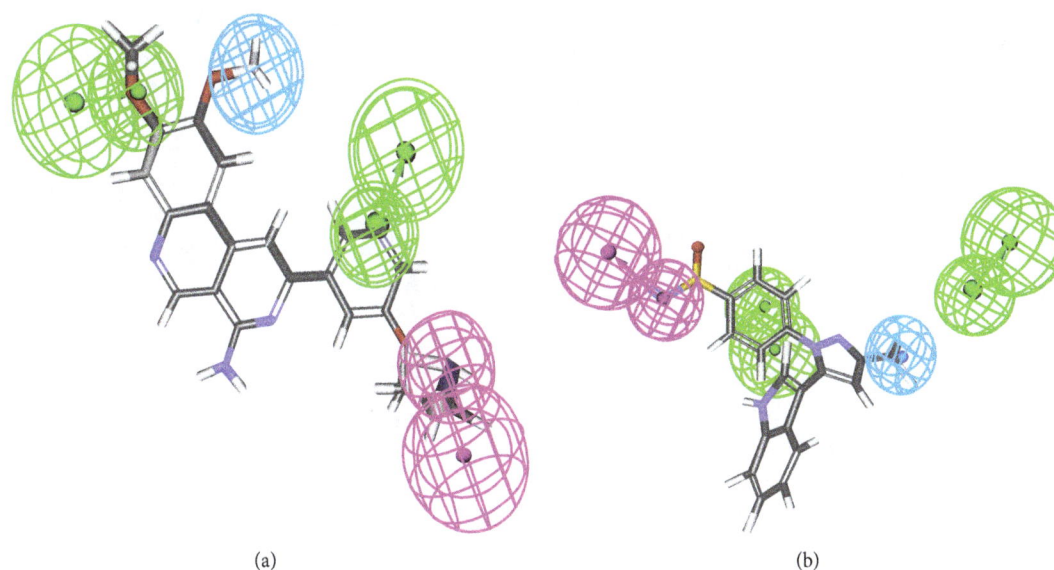

(a)   (b)

FIGURE 4: (a) The highest active compound (compound_1, IC_{50} = 3.0 nM) mapped on the best pharmacophore model; (b) the least active compound (Compound_21, IC_{50} = 65,000 nM) mapped on the best pharmacophore model (Hypo1). The most active compound exhibits a good fit with all features of the pharmacophore hypothesis, Hypo1, whereas in the least active compound it had hydrogen bond acceptor feature missing. Based on this, it may be concluded that two HBA features are important for PDK-1 kinase inhibitory activity.

3.3. Validation of Pharmacophore Model

3.3.1. Test Set Validation.
The test set method is for examining whether the pharmacophore model is capable of predicting the activities of external compounds of the test set series. The test set contains 62 compounds structurally different from the training set molecules. All the test set molecules were prepared in the same way as that for the training set molecules. Test set validation was done using ligand pharmacophore mapping protocol. The test set of 62 compounds were mapped on the Hypo1. It was observed that pharmacophore model performed well in estimation of activity of test set

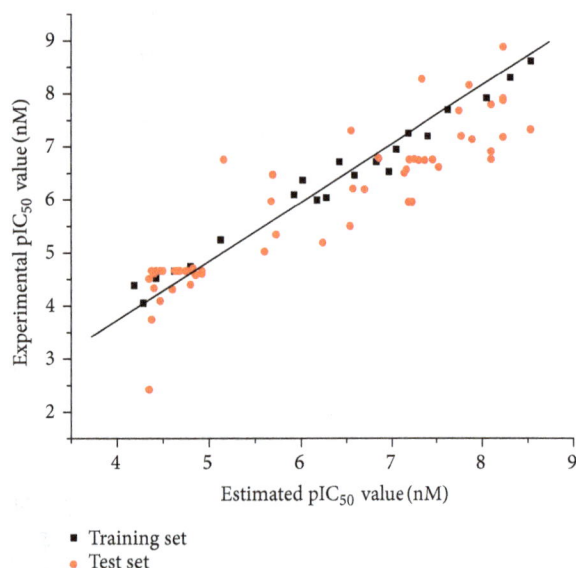

FIGURE 5: Regression plot of 62 test set molecules against Hypo1.

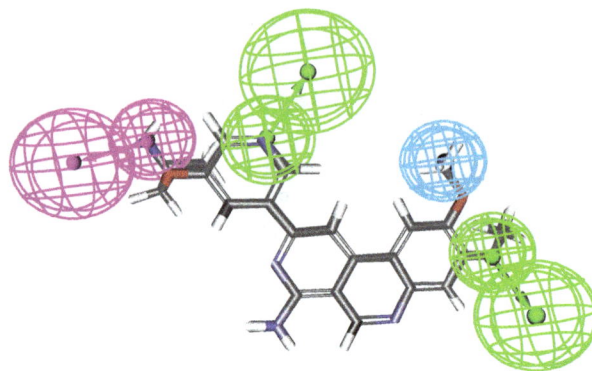

FIGURE 6: Most active test set compound (compound_22) mapped on the best pharmacophore model (Hypo1).

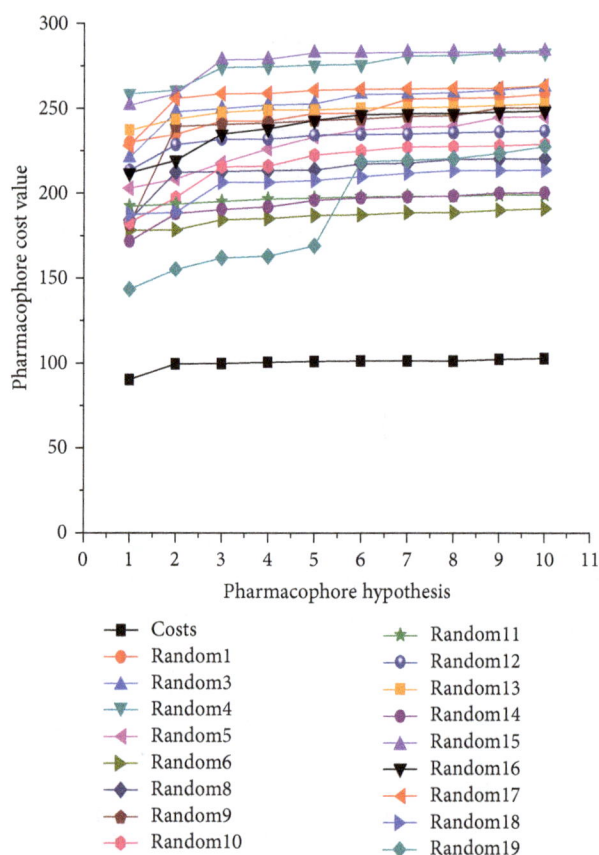

FIGURE 7: The difference in costs between the HypoGen runs and scrambled runs. The 95% confidence level was selected.

compounds, with a significant predictive correlation value ($r = 0.87$) between experimental and estimated activities (shown in Figure 5). The experimental and estimated activities of test set compounds mapped on the best hypothesis (Hypo1) were shown in (Table 4).

Further, another validation method was used to characterize the quality of the hypothesis using error ratio, which is the difference between estimated activity and experimental activity. Also an error ratio ≤10 depicts that there is no more than one order difference between estimated and experimental activity values, not more than one order. The best hypothesis (Hypo1) exhibited an error value ≤10 for 53 compounds out of 62 compounds. Only 9 compounds (compound_29, compound_32, compound_34, compound_38, compound_40, compound_51, compound_52, compound_53, and compound_55) with values > 10 were considered as outliers and rejected. The most potent compound_22 of the test set (IC_{50} = 6 nM) was mapped with Hypo1 (Figure 6). The best hypothesis (Hypo1) mapped very well, also all the chemical features of this compound matched and the estimated activity of this compound had an IC_{50} value of 1.3 nM. Based on these results, it was confirmed that one HBD, two HBA, and one HyA (hydrophobic aliphatic) features are essential for PDK-1 inhibitory activity.

3.3.2. Fisher's Validation. Fischer's randomization test method was used to evaluate the statistical relevance of Hypo1 by using the CatScramble program. The confidence level was fixed at 95%. The CatScramble program generated 19 random spreadsheets to construct hypothesis using exactly the same conditions as used in generating the original pharmacophore hypothesis. Total cost of 19 pharmacophore hypothesis generated randomly and the original pharmacophore hypothesis are also presented in Figure 7. It is observed that an original hypothesis (Hypo1) was far more superior to the 19 random hypotheses,

suggesting that Hypo1 is not generated by any chance event. These results have provided 95% confidence of the proposed hypothesis.

3.4. Pharmacophore Based Virtual Screening. The validated 3D QSAR pharmacophore model Hypo1 was used as a 3D structural query for retrieving potent compounds from NCI database and Maybridge database having 23,8819 molecules and 2,000 molecules, respectively. A total of 8,833 compounds

TABLE 4: Experimental biological data and estimated IC$_{50}$ of test set molecules based on pharmacophore model Hypo1.

Compound no	IC$_{50}$ (nM)		Error	Uncertainty	Fit value
	Experimental	Expected			
Compound_22	6	1.3	−4.6	2	8.87
Compound_23	47	5.2	−9.0	2	8.26
Compound_24	14	6.8	−2.0	2	8.14
Compound_25	6	11.9	+1.8	2	7.89
Compound_26	6	13.3	+2.2	2	7.85
Compound_27	8	15.9	+1.9	2	7.78
Compound_28	18	20.6	+1.4	2	7.66
Compound_29	3	46.8	+15.6	2	7.30
Compound_30	283	49.0	−5.8	2	7.29
Compound_31	17	62.2	+3.6	2	7.18
Compound_32	6	63.9	+10.5	2	7.17
Compound_33	13	71.0	+5.5	2	7.13
Compound_34	8	121.3	+15.2	2	6.89
Compound_35	144	159.2	+1.1	2	6.79
Compound_36	142	163.7	+1.1	2	6.76
Compound_37	57	166.9	+2.9	2	6.75
Compound_38	8	169.0	+21.1	2	6.75
Compound_39	65	173.1	+2.7	2	6.74
Compound_40	6,923	173.4	−39.9	2	6.74
Compound_41	35	173.7	+4.9	2	6.74
Compound_42	51	174.9	+3.4	2	6.73
Compound_43	43	176.8	+4.1	2	6.73
Compound_44	30	238.0	+7.9	2	6.60
Compound_45	70	264.1	+3.8	2	6.56
Compound_46	74	308.3	+4.2	2	6.49
Compound_47	2,033	332.1	+6.1	2	6.46
Compound_48	270	604.6	+2.2	2	6.20
Compound_49	200	604.6	+3.0	2	6.19
Compound_50	2,120	1,063.9	−1.9	2	5.95
Compound_51	60	1,070.4	+17.8	2	5.95
Compound_52	66	1,084.5	+16.4	2	5.94
Compound_53	290	3,107.8	+10.7	2	5.48
Compound_54	1,864	4,488.0	+2.4	2	5.33
Compound_55	580	6,336.0	+10.9	2	5.18
Compound_56	2,490	9,421.4	+3.8	2	5.00
Compound_57	15,000	19,013.5	+1.3	2	4.70
Compound_58	32,000	21,429.9	−1.5	2	4.65
Compound_59	38,000	21,429.8	−1.8	2	4.65
Compound_60	18,000	21,429.7	−1.2	2	4.65
Compound_61	32,000	21,430.2	−1.5	2	4.65
Compound_62	42,000	21,430.7	−1.9	2	4.65
Compound_63	32,000	21,430.9	−1.5	2	4.65
Compound_64	23,000	21,433.3	−1.1	2	4.65
Compound_65	15,000	21,434.2	−1.4	2	4.65
Compound_66	18,000	21,435.1	+1.2	2	4.65
Compound_67	22,000	21,436.7	−1.0	2	4.65
Compound_68	24,000	21,444.1	−1.1	2	4.65
Compound_69	21,000	21,446.6	+1.0	2	4.65

Table 4: Continued.

Compound no	IC$_{50}$ (nM)		Error	Uncertainty	Fit value
	Experimental	Expected			
Compound_70	12,000	21,449.9	+1.8	2	4.65
Compound_71	42,000	21,453.4	+1.3	2	4.65
Compound_72	17,000	21,454.8	+1.3	2	4.65
Compound_73	16,000	21,493.5	+1.3	2	4.64
Compound_74	34,000	21,538.8	+1.6	2	4.64
Compound_75	18,000	21,619.6	+1.2	2	4.64
Compound_76	12,000	24,152.4	+2.0	2	4.59
Compound_77	40,000	24,273.3	−1.6	2	4.59
Compound_78	14,000	25,463.7	+1.8	2	4.57
Compound_79	45,000	30,669.3	−1.5	2	4.49
Compound_80	16,000	39,286.2	+2.4	2	4.38
Compound_81	40,000	46,181.3	+1.1	2	4.31
Compound_82	25,000	48,798.6	+1.9	2	4.29
Compound_83	34,000	80,163.1	+2.3	2	4.07

exhibited good mapping with Hypo1 using fast and flexible search method. Out of total 8,833 compounds, 8,530 compounds were from NCI and 333 compounds were from Maybridge database. Out of these 8,833 molecules, 2033 molecules having their IC$_{50}$ < 1 μM were selected for further studies. Further sorting of these hits has been done by Lipinski's rule of five, to evaluate their drug similarity. Total 1,613 molecules passed this evaluative process. These 1,613 molecules were further evaluated for the ADMET studies. Only 842 molecules passed the ADMET filtration process. Those molecules were selected for further molecular docking studies, which exhibited estimated activity ≤0.5 μM. It was observed that only 43 molecules satisfied these conditions and further molecular docking study was prepared for these molecules.

3.5. Molecular Docking Studies. Further studies were conducted for selected compounds (retrieved hits) and evaluated the binding mode between compounds and protein. All the compounds and compound_1 were docked into the binding site of PDK-1 [26] (PDB entry: 1UU7) [27] by using LigandFit [28] docking method implemented in Discovery Studio 2.5 program package. Before docking all molecules, compound_1 (most active compound of the training set) was docked into the active site of PDK-1.

(a) Compound_1 Docking Description. Compound_1 has shown the docking energy of 64.5 kcal/mol and RMSD value of 0.841. This depicts that LigandFit docking method reproduced the original binding mode. Hence, for further docking of the LigandFit, docking method was used. It showed hydrogen bond interactions with important residues of amino acids, Lys111, Asp 230, Ala162, and Tyr 161 as shown in Figure 8(a).

(b) Other Compounds Docking Description. All 43 molecules (selected) were docked to the active sites of PDK-1 kinase, and, furthermore, only top 7 molecules, having high

docking energy, better hydrogen bond interactions with active site residues, and lower estimated activity (≤0.19 μM) were selected. The estimated activity, interaction energy, and LignadFit scores of all seven compounds along with compounds_1 are listed in Table 5. Finally, the three compounds which were selected for further analysis are NSC_218341, NSC_24871, and NSC_21193. Compound NSC_211930, NSC_218341, and NSC_24871 mapped to all features of the Hypo1. Compound NSC_211930 formed the hydrogen bonding with Ala162 a hinge region amino acid. While the amide group formed the hydrogen bond with Asp223, Lys111 was involved in the cation-pi interaction. Compound NSC_24871 formed the hydrogen bond interaction with Lys111, Ser160, and Ala162. It was observed that the phenyl ring of compound was sandwiched between the phenyl rings of Tyr161 and Phe93 and they formed the pi-pi interaction. Tyr161 formed pi-pi interactions with phenyl ring of Compound_218342, while the carboxyl groups were involved in the formation of two hydrogen bonds with Lys111 and Phe94. Phenolic oxygen was involved in formation of hydrogen bond with Ser162 and Ala162 amino acids. In all the cases, Try 161 was involved in forming pi-pi interaction with the phenyl ring of the compounds. 2D representation of molecular docking results of all three compounds was shown in the Figures 8(b), 8(c), and 8(d). Lys111 formed two hydrogen bonds with the two different oxygen atoms of phenyl groups of the Compound NSC_24871. Also one phenolic oxygen atom formed the two hydrogen bonds with the two hinge regions in amino acids, that is, Ser160 and Ala162. These three compounds retrieved from two databases (NCI & Maybridge), exhibited good interactions with important amino acids in the active sites. Among all three compounds, Compound NSC_218342 retrieved from the NCI database was observed to exhibit good estimated activity, fit values and docking score, and hydrogen bond interactions. Molecular docking results support that these molecules can be further taken as the potential leads for designing novel PDK-1 inhibitors in the future.

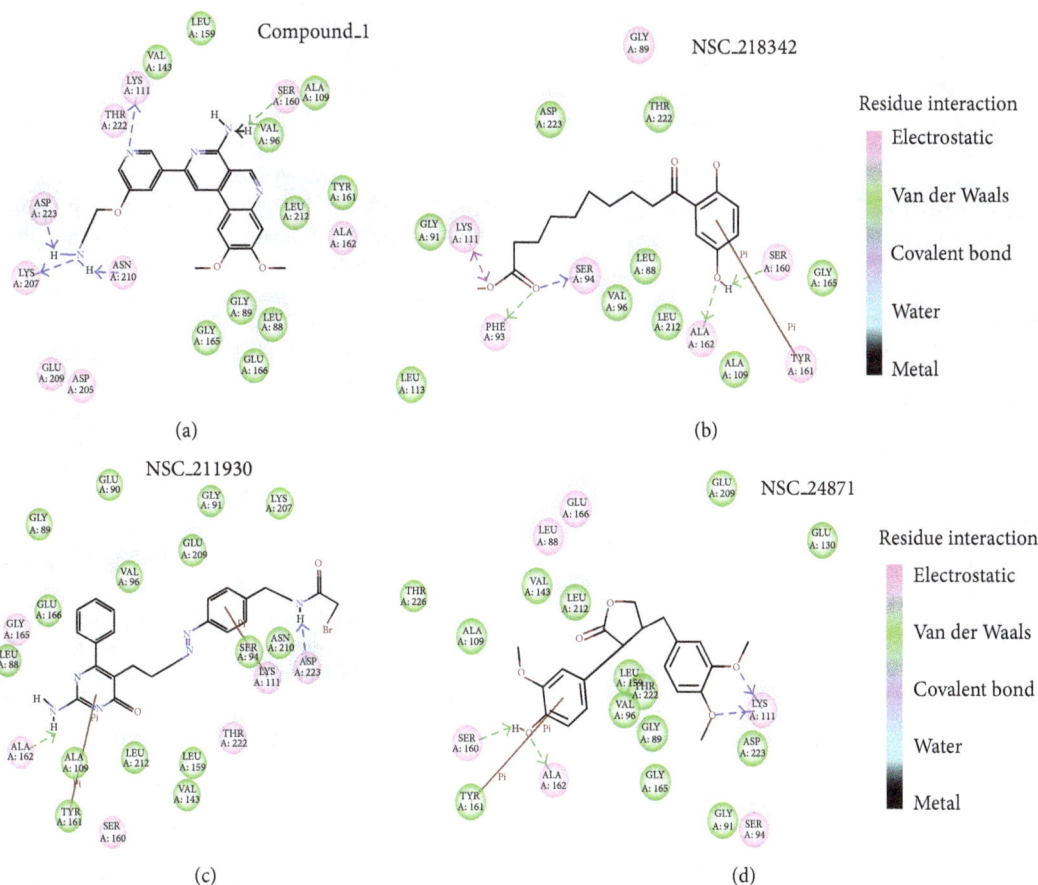

FIGURE 8: 2D representation of top docking hits retrieved from database and most active compound (Compound_1).

TABLE 5: The estimated activity, interaction energy, and LigandFit scoring results of top ranked four compounds obtained from the combination of Hypo1 based virtual screening and molecular docking studies.

Name	Est. (nM)	Interaction energy (kcal/mol)	LigScore1	LigScore2	-PLP1	-PLP2	-PMF
Compound_1	3.00	64.40	4.23	4.98	73.60	68.90	103.10
NSC_218342	31.40	65.39	4.93	4.25	61.42	59.79	83.91
NSC_24871	74.10	51.18	5.03	5.77	65.14	67.09	95.66
NSC_211930	82.00	57.30	6.17	6.23	79.00	71.43	75.76
NSC_84044	87.70	51.11	4.23	5.31	65.40	55.20	92.87
NSC_325657	93.80	55.47	5.84	6.16	75.72	73.50	106.54
NSC_343659	94.50	59.16	4.41	4.47	51.82	53.26	82.51
SB_01794	160.00	46.36	3.67	4.04	53.22	56.12	107.10

4. Conclusions

A ligand based computational method was used to identify molecular structural features required for effective PDK-1 inhibitors for discovery of drugs to prevent and cure wide variety of cancers. A data set of 83 compounds of selective PDK-1 inhibitors with their respective activities ranging over a wide range of magnitude has been used to generate pharmacophore hypothesis and to predict the activity successfully and accurately. A highly predictive pharmacophore model was generated based on 21 training set molecules, which had hydrogen bond acceptor, hydrogen bond donor, and hydrophobic aliphatic groups as chemical features which described their activities towards PDK-1 kinase. The validation of the model was based on 62 test set molecules, which finally showed that the model was able to differentiate various classes of PDK-1 inhibitors with a high correlation coefficient of 0.87 between experimental and predicted activities accurately. Further validation of Hypo1 was done by a decoy set method. The decoy set method exhibited GH score of 0.73 which depicts that designed model has very high efficiency in screening the molecules from database. Hypo1 was used as a 3D query to screen the potential molecules from the NCI database as well as Maybridge database. The hit compounds were filtered subsequently by Lipinski's rule of five and ADMET filtration. Further, molecule selection was refined by docking study. After the docking studies, it was observed that the 3 molecules (NSC_218342, NSC_24871, and NSC_211930) with different scaffolds exhibited better docking energy as well as better interaction. To conclude, the defined drug candidate is further evolved using in vitro and in vivo studies as anticancer molecule.

Conflict of Interests

The authors declare that there is no conflict of interests regarding the publication of this paper.

Acknowledgments

The authors thank Dr. J. A. R. P. Sarma, Senior Vice President, and Dr. K. V. Radhakishan, Ex-Director of GVK Biosciences Pvt., Ltd., for their cooperation and providing software facilities.

References

[1] M. A. Fabian, W. H. Biggs III, D. K. Treiber et al., "A small molecule-kinase interaction map for clinical kinase inhibitors," *Nature Biotechnology*, vol. 23, no. 3, pp. 329–336, 2005.

[2] G. Manning, D. B. Whyte, R. Martinez, T. Hunter, and S. Sudarsanam, "The protein kinase complement of the human genome," *Science*, vol. 298, no. 5600, pp. 1912–1934, 2002.

[3] I. Akritopoulou-Zanze and P. J. Hajduk, "Kinase-targeted libraries: the design and synthesis of novel, potent, and selective kinase inhibitors," *Drug Discovery Today*, vol. 14, no. 5-6, pp. 291–297, 2009.

[4] S. L. Anderson, D. Stokoe, H. Erdjument-Bromage et al., "Prohtein kinase B kinases that mediate phosphatidylinositol 3,4,5-trisphosphate-dependent activation of protein kinase B," *Science*, vol. 279, no. 5351, pp. 710–714, 1998.

[5] D. R. Alessi, M. Deak, A. Casamayor et al., "3-Phosphoinositide-dependent protein kinase-1 (PDK-1): structural and functional homology with the *Drosophila* DSTPK61 kinase," *Current Biology*, vol. 7, pp. 776–789, 1997.

[6] R. A. Currie, K. S. Walker, A. Gray et al., "Role of phosphatidylinositol 3,4,5-trisphosphate in regulating the activity and localization of 3-phosphoinositide-dependent protein kinase-1," *Biochemical Journal*, vol. 337, no. 2-3, pp. 575–583, 1999.

[7] T. Kobayashi and P. Cohen, "Activation of serum- and glucocorticoid-regulated protein kinase by agonists that activate phosphatidylinositide 3-kinase is mediated by 3-phosphoinositide-dependent protein kinase-1 (PDK-1) and PDK2," *Biochemical Journal*, vol. 339, no. 2, pp. 319–328, 1999.

[8] T. Kobayashi, M. Deak, N. Morrice, and P. Cohen, "Characterization of the structure and regulation of two novel isoforms of serum- and glucocorticoid-induced protein kinase," *Biochemical Journal*, vol. 344, no. 1, pp. 189–197, 1999.

[9] J. Park, M. L. Leong, P. Buse, A. C. Maiyar, G. L. Firestone, and B. A. Hemmings, "Serum and glucocorticoid-inducible kinase (SGK) is a target of the PI 3-kinase-stimulated signaling pathway," *The EMBO Journal*, vol. 18, no. 11, pp. 3024–3033, 1999.

[10] N. Pullen, P. B. Dennis, M. Andjelkovic et al., "Phosphorylation and activation of p70^{s6k} by PDK-1," *Science*, vol. 279, no. 5351, pp. 707–710, 1998.

[11] D. R. Alessi, M. T. Kozlowski, Q. P. Weng, N. Morrice, and J. Avruch, "3-phosphoinositide-dependent protein kinase 1 (PDK-1) phosphorylates and activates the p70 S6 kinase *in vivo* and *in vitro*," *Current Biology*, vol. 8, no. 2, pp. 69–81, 1998.

[12] A. Mora, D. Komander, D. M. F. van Aalten, and D. R. Alessi, "PDK-1, the master regulator of AGC kinase signal transduction," *Seminars in Cell and Developmental Biology*, vol. 15, no. 2, pp. 161–170, 2004.

[13] P. L. Dahia, "PTEN, a unique tumor suppressor gene," *Endocrine-Related Cancer*, vol. 7, no. 2, pp. 115–129, 2000.

[14] I. Sansal and W. R. Sellers, "The biology and clinical relevance of the *PTEN* tumor suppressor pathway," *Journal of Clinical Oncology*, vol. 22, no. 14, pp. 2954–2963, 2004.

[15] M. Cully, H. You, A. J. Levine, and T. W. Mak, "Beyond PTEN mutations: the PI3K pathway as an integrator of multiple inputs during tumorigenesis," *Nature Reviews Cancer*, vol. 6, no. 3, pp. 184–192, 2006.

[16] Y. Kurogi and O. F. Guner, "Pharmacophore modeling and three-dimensional database searching for drug design using catalyst," *Current Medicinal Chemistry*, vol. 8, no. 9, pp. 1035–1055, 2001.

[17] O. F. Guner, O. Clement, and Y. Kurogi, "Pharmacophore modeling and three dimensional database searching for drug design using catalyst: recent advances," *Current Medicinal Chemistry*, vol. 11, no. 22, pp. 2991–3005, 2004.

[18] H. K. Kyung, W. Allan, B. F. J. Middleton et al., "Benzo[c][2,7]naphthyridines as inhibitors of PDK-1," *Bioorganic and Medicinal Chemistry Letters*, vol. 19, no. 17, pp. 5225–5228, 2009.

[19] N. Thomas, G. D. Russell, I. Charles et al., "The identification of 8,9-dimethoxy-5-(2-aminoalkoxy-pyridin-3-yl)-benzo[c][2,7]naphthyridin-4-ylamines as potent inhibitors of 3-phosphoinositide-dependent kinase-1 (PDK-1)," *European Journal of Medicinal Chemistry*, vol. 45, no. 4, pp. 1379–1386, 2010.

[20] J. Zhu, J.-W. Huang, P.-H. Tseng et al., "From the cyclooxygenase-2 inhibitor celecoxib to a novel class of 3-phosphoinositide-dependent protein kinase-1 inhibitors," *Cancer Research*, vol. 64, no. 12, pp. 4309–4318, 2004.

[21] A. Gopalsamy, M. Shi, D. H. Boschelli et al., "Discovery of dibenzo[c,f][2,7]naphthyridines as potent and selective 3-phosphoinositide-dependent kinase-1 inhibitors," *Journal of Medicinal Chemistry*, vol. 50, no. 23, pp. 5547–5549, 2007.

[22] *Accelrys Discovery Studio 2. 5*, Accelrys, San Diego, Calif, USA, 2009, http://www.accelrys.com/.

[23] A. Smellie, S. Teig, and P. Towbin, "Poling: promoting conformational variation," *Journal of Computational Chemistry*, vol. 16, no. 2, pp. 171–187, 1995.

[24] B. R. Brooks, R. E. Brucolleri, B. D. Olafson, D. J. States, S. Swaminathan, and M. Karplus, "CHARMM: a program for macromolecular energy, minimization, and dynamics calculations," *Journal of Computational Chemistry*, vol. 4, no. 2, pp. 187–217, 1983.

[25] H. Li, J. Sutter, and R. Hoffmann, *Pharmacophore Perception and Development and Use in Drug Design*, International University Line, La Jolla, Calif, USA, edited by O. F. Guner, 2000.

[26] J. R. Medina, C. W. Blackledge, D. A. Heerding et al., "Aminoindazole PDK-1 inhibitors: a case study in fragment-based drug

discovery," *ACS Medicinal Chemistry Letters*, vol. 1, no. 8, pp. 439–442, 2010.

[27] D. Komander, G. S. Kular, A. W. Schüttelkopf et al., "Interactions of LY333531 and other bisindolyl maleimide inhibitors with PDK-1," *Structure*, vol. 12, no. 2, pp. 215–226, 2004.

[28] C. M. Venkatachalam, X. Jiang, T. Oldfield, and M. Waldman, "LigandFit: a novel method for the shape-directed rapid docking of ligands to protein active sites," *Journal of Molecular Graphics and Modelling*, vol. 21, no. 4, pp. 289–307, 2003.

7

Genetic Algorithm Based Approach in Attribute Weighting for a Medical Data Set

Kirsi Varpa, Kati Iltanen, and Martti Juhola

Computer Science, School of Information Sciences, University of Tampere, 33014 Tampere, Finland

Correspondence should be addressed to Martti Juhola; martti.juhola@sis.uta.fi

Academic Editor: Martin J. Murphy

Genetic algorithms have been utilized in many complex optimization and simulation tasks because of their powerful search method. In this research we studied whether the classification performance of the attribute weighted methods based on the nearest neighbour search can be improved when using the genetic algorithm in the evolution of attribute weighting. The attribute weights in the starting population were based on the weights set by the application area experts and machine learning methods instead of random weight setting. The genetic algorithm improved the total classification accuracy and the median true positive rate of the attribute weighted k-nearest neighbour method using neighbour's class-based attribute weighting. With other methods, the changes after genetic algorithm were moderate.

1. Introduction

One of the most commonly used simple classification methods is the nearest neighbour (NN) method that classifies a new case into the class of its nearest neighbour case [1]. The nearest neighbour method is an instance-based learning method that searches for the most similar case of the test case from the training data by some distance measure, usually with the Euclidean distance. A natural extension to NN is the k-nearest neighbour (k-NN) method that assigns the majority class of the k nearest training cases for the test case [2]. Different refinements and extensions have been proposed for k-NN in order to improve classification results and overcome classification problems, for example, distance-weighting of neighbours [2], extensions using properties of the data set [3], weighting of attributes [2, 4, 5], and attribute weight optimization with genetic algorithms (GA) [6–11].

Genetic algorithms [12, 13] and other evolution algorithms [14, 15] have been utilized in various complex optimization and simulation problems because of their powerful search and optimization capabilities. A search method of a genetic algorithm is a combination of directed and stochastic search and the search can be done multidirectionally because GA maintains a population of potential solutions from the search space [14]. The basics of the search method of GA

underlie in natural selection and genetic inheritance [12]; individuals of the population are used in the reproduction of new solutions by means of crossover and mutation. Genetic algorithms have been used with various machine learning methods to optimize weighting properties of the method. Since our research is based on the nearest neighbour search applying machine learning methods, we concentrate on related works where GAs have been applied only with the k-nearest neighbour method. Kelly and Davis [6] combined the GA with a weighted k-nearest neighbour (wk-NN) method in the algorithm called GA-WKNN in order to find a single attribute weight vector that would improve the classification results of the wk-NN. A similar kind of approach was used in [7] where GA was combined with the wk-NN and a parallel processing environment in order to optimize classification of large data sets. In both studies, a set of real-valued weights for attributes to discriminate all classes of data were achieved as a result after GA runs. The study of Hussein et al. [8] showed that GA can be applied successfully in setting a real-valued weight set for 1-NN classifier but the improvement of accuracy happened at the expense of increase in processing time. Results showed that GA methods combining the wk-NN outperformed the basic k-NN [6–8]. However, a single set of weights for all classes is not always the best solution because attributes have a different effect on classes [11]. Therefore, solutions for searching for a weight for each class and attribute have been developed. Lee et al. [9] combined the GA-based attribute weighting method with a modified k-NN, thus, forming an adaptive feature weighting method A3FW-MNN that used different sets of attribute weights for different classes. Also, Mateos-García et al. [10] assigned different weights to every attribute depending on each class in their evolutionary algorithm called Label Dependent Feature Weighting (LDFW) algorithm.

In this research we studied whether the classification performance of the attribute weighted machine learning methods based on the nearest neighbour search can be improved when using the genetic algorithm in the evolution of attribute weighting based on the experts and machine learning methods when runs were made with a medical data set. This medical data has been our test data in our previous researches [16, 17].

2. Material

In this research an otoneurological data set having 951 cases from seven different vertigo diseases (classes) (Table 1) was used. The data was collected over a decade starting from the 1990s in the Department of Otorhinolaryngology at Helsinki University Central Hospital, Finland, where experienced specialists confirmed all the diagnoses. The distribution of the disease classes is imbalanced; over one-third of the cases belong to the Menière's disease class (36.8%), whereas the smallest disease class benign recurrent vertigo has only 2.1% of the cases.

In total, the data includes 176 attributes concerning a patient's health status: occurring symptoms, medical history, and clinical findings in otoneurologic, audiologic, and imaging tests [18, 19]. Clinical testing has not been done to every patient and, therefore, there are several test results that have missing values of the attributes. Attributes with low frequencies of available values were left outside this research. After leaving out the attributes having over 35% missing values, 94 attributes remained to be used in this research: 17 quantitative (integer or real value) and 77 qualitative attributes (of which 54 were binary (yes/no), 20 were ordinal, and 3 were nominal). Genetic algorithm runs were done with the data including missing attribute values.

3. Genetic Algorithm

The basic idea of the genetic algorithm is the following: in the beginning, a population of individuals is formed either randomly or with information about the application domain. Traditionally, a binary representation of the individuals has been used but in multidimensional and numerical problems real-valued representation is nowadays used [14]. In each generation, the individuals of the population are evaluated with an objective evaluation function, thus, giving the individual its fitness rate. A selection method is used to find the fittest individuals for a new population. Some individuals of the new population undergo reproduction by means of crossover and mutation. In the crossover, the information of the individuals

TABLE 1: The frequency distribution of vertigo disease classes.

	Disease name	Abbreviation	Frequency	%
1	Acoustic neurinoma	ANE	131	13.8
2	Benign positional vertigo	BPV	173	18.2
3	Menière's disease	MEN	350	36.8
4	Sudden deafness	SUD	47	4.9
5	Traumatic vertigo	TRA	73	7.7
6	Vestibular neuritis	VNE	157	16.5
7	Benign recurrent vertigo	BRV	20	2.1
	Total		951	100

is swapped in their corresponding elements. Mutation alters one or more elements of the individual arbitrarily. Elitism is a commonly applied survivor selection method. It keeps the current fittest individual unchanged in the population so the high-performance individuals are not lost from one generation to the next [20]. The GA can be ended after a fixed number of iterations or if no further improvement is observed after some number of generations.

We utilized the genetic algorithm in the evolution of the attribute weight values. A pseudocode of the used genetic algorithm is given in Pseudocode 1. A population contained 21 individuals that used real-valued representation instead of binary presentation because the attribute weight values were described with real-valued numbers, not just with 0 and 1. Each individual consisted of seven different attribute weight sets for 94 attributes. The individuals of the starting population were based on the weights set by the experts and machine learning methods. The starting population is defined more accurately in Section 3.1. The genetic algorithm used a roulette-wheel selection in parent selection and a uniform crossover with discrete recombination in offspring creation. The crossover was done in 80.0% probability ($p_c = 0.8$) and the crossover points were selected randomly and independently for each gene (a field on an individual). Mutation was done in 1.0% probability ($p_m = 0.01$) for the gene and it was done also in a uniform manner: a random value was drawn from the range [0, 1] which was set as a new value in the current position. In addition, elitism was used in order to keep the best individual within the population during runs. We did not want to lose the best performing weight set during the evolution. If the number of the individuals was higher than 21 in the end of the generation, a survivor selection was used. The individuals were ordered by their classification performance and the individuals with the lowest accuracy were discarded from the population. The genetic algorithm ended after 20 generations or if the best classification accuracy maintained the same during 10 successive generations. Furthermore, if all the individuals were the same in the population, the evaluation ended. The parameters used in the GA runs are described in Table 2.

The genetic algorithm runs were done separately with three different machine learning methods used in the population evaluation: with the nearest pattern method of the otoneurological expert system (ONE), with the

$$\text{data } D = \begin{matrix} [Case_1 \\ \vdots \\ Case_{951}] \end{matrix} = \begin{matrix} [[c_{1,1},\dots,c_{1,94}] \\ \vdots \\ [c_{951,1},\dots,c_{951,94}]] \end{matrix}$$

$$\text{population } Weights = \begin{matrix} [Weight_1 \\ \vdots \\ Weight_{21}] \end{matrix} = \begin{matrix} [[w_{1,1,1},\dots,w_{1,1,94};\dots;w_{1,7,1},\dots,w_{1,7,94}] \\ \vdots \\ [w_{21,1,1},\dots,w_{21,1,94};\dots;w_{21,7,1},\dots,w_{21,7,94}]] \end{matrix}$$

```
population_size = 21
p_c = 0.8              //Crossover rate
p_m = 0.01            //Mutation rate
divide data D into 10 equally-sized subsets
for cv_round = 1 to 10 do
        divide training data D-d_cv_round into train (6 subsets) and test (3 subsets) data
        initialize methods with train data:
                cwk-NN and wk-NN OVA: HVDM initialization
                ONE: fitness value calculation for values of attributes
        evaluate starting population Weights with test data and ONE/cwk-NN/wk-NN OVA
        while ending terms of GA are not fulfilled do
                //Survivor selection: Elitism
                search for the individual with the highest fitness rate from the population
                //Parent selection: Roulette-wheel selection with fitness-proportionate selection
                for each individual in the population do
                        calculate individual's fitness proportionate rate = individual's fitness rate/sum of individuals'
                        fitness rates
                        calculate individual's cumulative fitness proportionate rate
                end for
                while nr of individuals in the mating pool is smaller than population_size do
                        generate a random number r from [0, 1]
                        search for the jth individual that has smaller cumulative fitness proportionate rate than r
                        add the jth individual in the mating pool
                end while
                //Crossover: Uniform crossover with discrete recombination
                for each individual in the mating pool do
                        generate a random number s from [0, 1]
                        if s is smaller than p_c then
                                add the individual in the parent pool
                        else
                                add the individual in the new population (offspring is a direct copy of its parent)
                        end if
                end for
                while two individuals can be taken from the parent pool do
                        if two individuals are exactly the same then
                                add the first individual into the new population
                                take new individual from the parent pool to use in the crossover
                        end if
                        for each disease class weight set do
                                select the crossover points randomly
                                swap information of two individuals in the corresponding crossover points (create children)
                        end for
                        add children in the new population
                end while
                //Mutation: Uniform mutation
                for each individual in the new population do
                        for each gene of individual do
                                generate a random number t from [0, 1]
                                if t is smaller than p_m then
                                        select a random value v from the range [0, 1]
                                        set the value v as a new value of the gene
                                end if
                        end for
                end for
```

PSEUDOCODE 1: Continued.

```
            evaluate children and mutated individuals in the new population with test data and
            ONE/cwk-NN/wk-NN OVA
            add the elite individual without changes into the new population
            //Survivor Selection
            if nr of individuals in the new population is larger than population_size then
                    sort cases descending by their fitness rate
                    discard the last cases in order to have correct nr of individuals in the population
            else if nr of individuals in the new population is smaller than population_size then
                    select randomly missing cases from the old population
            end if
        end while
        initialize methods with training data D-d_cv_round:
            cwk-NN and wk-NN OVA: HVDM initialization
            ONE: fitness value calculation for values of attributes
        evaluate the individual with the highest fitness rate after GA with testing data d_cv_round and
        ONE/cwk-NN/wk-NN OVA
    end for
```

PSEUDOCODE 1: Pseudocode of the genetic algorithm used in the evolution of the attribute weight values with 10-fold cross-validation.

TABLE 2: Parameters used with the genetic algorithm.

Genetic algorithm parameters	
Crossover rate	0.8
Mutation rate	0.01
Population size	21
Generation	20 (and 100 for ONE)
Elitism	Yes (1 individual)

attribute weighted k-nearest neighbour method using neighbour's class based attribute weighting (cwk-NN), and with the attribute weighted k-nearest neighbour method using one-versus-all the other (OVA) classifiers (wk-NN OVA). The evaluation methods are defined more accurately in Section 3.2. During the genetic algorithm runs, for each individual in the population its fitness rate was calculated with the method at hand; that is, the individual was evaluated against the method. Within the methods cwk-NN and ONE, the fitness rate for the individual was defined with a total classification accuracy (ACC) and within the wk-NN OVA with a true positive rate (TPR). The total classification accuracy was used with the ONE and the cwk-NN because all seven disease classes were classified at the same time whereas the wk-NN OVA concentrated on one disease class (and its weight set) at a time. During GA wk-NN OVA runs, it was more important to find the weight set that separated well the cases of the disease class at hand from the others than to classify the other cases also well.

The total classification accuracy showed the percentage of all correctly classified cases within the data set:

$$ACC = 100 \frac{t_{pos}}{n_{cases}} \%, \qquad (1)$$

where t_{pos} was the total number of cases correctly classified within classes and n_{cases} was the total number of cases used

in the classification. The true positive rate expressed the percentage of correctly inferred cases within the class as

$$TPR = 100 \frac{t_{pos_c}}{n_{cases_c}} \%, \qquad (2)$$

where t_{pos_c} was the number of correctly classified cases in class c and n_{cases_c} was the number of all cases in class c. With the cwk-NN and wk-NN OVA methods, the classification performance was calculated from the seven nearest neighbour method (7-NN) results and with the ONE from the first diagnosis suggestion (ONE1). However, for disease class benign recurrent vertigo (BRV) with the wk-NN OVA method it was necessary to use the TPR of three nearest neighbours (3-NN) as the fitness rate because of the small size of the disease class at hand. Otherwise the TPR for classifying BRV would have always been zero. Nonetheless, if there occurred a situation where TPR of 3-NN was zero with all individuals in the starting population, a new population was created randomly and evaluated. Random new population was created at most ten times and if the TPR did not change during 10 runs, GA run was ended.

A 10-fold cross-validation (CV) [2] was used in evaluating the classification performance of the genetic algorithm. The data was randomly divided into 10 subsets of approximately equal size. The division was made in a stratified manner to ensure that the class distribution of each subset resembled the skewed class distribution of the entire data set. In the beginning, one cross-validation partition (10% of the data) was left aside to test the performance of the found best individual after genetic algorithm run. The nine cross-validation partitions (90%) were used during the training process. In order to calculate the fitness rate for each individual in the population during genetic algorithm runs, the training data was further divided into two parts: six cross-validation parts were used for training and three cross-validation parts were used for testing the current machine learning method used in the fitness rate calculation. Thus, during the genetic algorithm run 60%–30% data division was used. After the genetic algorithm run, the individual having the highest fitness rate was declared as a result of weight combination and it was then tested with the left aside test data subset. The 10-fold cross-validation was repeated ten times. In total, there were 100 test runs per each evaluation method used in the genetic algorithm. The same cross-validation divisions were used with all the evaluation methods—that is, each method had the same training and testing sets used during the genetic algorithm runs.

3.1. Starting Population.
The starting population consisted of 21 individuals. Each individual included seven different attribute weight sets (weights for 94 attributes), one set for each disease class. Instead of selecting the starting individuals at random, we decided to use good "guesses" as a starting point. Therefore, the starting individuals were based on the attribute weights defined by the domain experts (three different weight set versions) and learnt by three machine learning methods (the Scatter method [21–23] and the weighting method of the instance-based learning algorithm IB4 [24] and its variant IB1w). Based on the weight sets defined by the experts and the machine learning methods, two different modifications were created from weight sets with 50% random mutation, thus having 18 weight sets in total. In addition to these, three totally random weight sets were created into the starting population.

The weight values were computed with the machine learning methods from the imputed data set, that is, from the data set where the missing values of attributes were substituted with the class-wise modes of the qualitative and the class-wise medians of the quantitative attributes. In total, 10.1% of the values of attributes were missing in the data set. The imputation was done class-wise on the basis of the whole data prior to data division into training and testing sets. The calculation of the weights was repeated 10 times for each CV training set in the Scatter, IB4, and IB1w methods and the mean weights of the 10 repetitions were used in the classification to handle the randomness in these methods. The weights defined by the application area experts were the same for each CV training set.

The experts' weights were based on three different combinations. The first weight set included the original attribute weights defined by a group of experienced otoneurological physicians for the decision support system ONE made in the 1990s [25]. The second and the third weight sets were defined by two domain specialists during the upgrade process of the decision support system in the 2000s [16].

The Scatter method is normally used for attribute importance evaluation [21–23]. It calculates a scatter value for an attribute that expresses the attributes' power to separate classes in the data set. For attribute weighting purposes, the scatter values were calculated for each attribute in different class versus other classes' situations. In order to use the scatter values as attribute weights, it was necessary to take inverses of scatter values.

The weight calculation method of the IB4 classification method computes attribute weights independently for each class with a simple performance feedback algorithm [24]. The attribute weights of IB4 reflect the relative relevancies of the attributes in the class. The difference between IB4 and its simpler version IB1w is that IB1w saves all processed cases in its class descriptions and does not discard any cases from the class descriptions during runs. Also, the cases with poor classification records are kept in class descriptions with IB1w whereas IB4 discards these cases based on their past performance during classification.

More detailed description of the machine learning methods Scatter, IB4, and IB1w and their use in weight formation will be given in the paper [17].

In order to have different weight sets comparable to each other during the genetic algorithm runs, the attribute weights were normalized into range [0, 1]. The values of each weight set were divided by the highest weight value occurring in the weight calculation method at issue.

3.2. Evaluation Methods

3.2.1. Nearest Pattern Method of ONE.
The first method used within the genetic algorithm to evaluate the performance of the individuals in the population was the inference mechanism of the otoneurological decision support system ONE [26]. Its inference mechanism resembles the nearest neighbour methods of pattern recognition. Instead of searching for the nearest case from the training set, it searches for the most fitting class for a new case from its knowledge base.

In the knowledge base of ONE, a pattern is given to each class that corresponds to one vertigo disease. The pattern can be considered a profile of a disease as it describes its related symptoms and signs. Each class in the knowledge base is described with a set of attributes with weight values expressing their significance for the class. In addition, a fitness value for each attribute value is given to describe how it fits the class. The fitness values for attribute values were computed on the basis of the 60% part of training data. Fitness values can have values between 0 and 100. The fitness value 0 means that the attribute value does not fit the class, whereas the fitness value 100 shows that the value fits the class perfectly. The weight values for attributes were given in the population in the GA; thus, the weight values varied from 0 to 1. The greater weight value is, the more important the attribute is for the class.

The inference mechanism calculates scores for the classes from the weight and fitness values of the attributes. The score $S(c)$ for a class c is calculated in the following way:

$$S(c) = \frac{\sum_{a=1}^{A(c)} x(a)\, w(c,a)\, f(c,a,j)}{\sum_{a=1}^{A(c)} x(a)\, w(c,a)}, \qquad (3)$$

where $A(c)$ is the number of the attributes associated with class c, $x(a)$ is 1 if the value of attribute a is known and otherwise 0, $w(c,a)$ is the weight of the attribute a for class c, and $f(c,a,j)$ is the fitness value for the value j of the attribute a for class c [26]. In the case of quantitative attributes, the fitness values are interpolated by using the attribute values in the knowledge base as interpolation points. The fitness values are altered to the range of 0 to 1 during the inference process.

In addition to the score, the minimum and maximum scores are calculated for the classes using the lowest and the highest fitness values for the attributes having missing values.

The classes are ordered primarily by the score and secondarily by the difference of the minimum and maximum score. If the classes have the same score but one class has a smaller difference between the minimum and maximum scores than the others, the class having the smallest difference is placed higher in order. If the classes have the same score and the minimum and maximum score difference, their order is selected randomly. The class having the highest score is referred to as the best diagnosis suggestion.

Some vertigo diseases resemble each other by having a similar kind of symptoms with other diseases during some phase of the disease and, in addition, some patients can actually have two (or more) vertigo diseases present concurrently [27]. Therefore, it is good to check the classification results of ONE with more than one disease suggestion. In the end, the final diagnostic choice must be made by the physician based on the information given on all alternative diseases [27].

3.2.2. Attribute Weighted k-Nearest Neighbour Method Using Neighbour's Class-Based Attribute Weighting.

The other method used in the population evaluation was the attribute weighted k-nearest neighbour method using neighbour's class-based attribute weighting (cwk-NN). The distance measure of the basic k-nearest neighbour method [1] was expanded to take the attribute weighting into account [6]. Lee et al. [9] used a similar class-dependent attribute weighting with their modified k-nearest neighbour method where different attribute weight sets for different classes were determined with the adaptive-3FW feature weighting method. With our cwk-NN the attribute weighting depends on the disease class of the neighbour case. Thus, there ought to be as many attribute weights sets available as there are classes.

The distance measure used with the cwk-NN was the Heterogeneous Value Difference Metric (HVDM) [28] expanded with the attribute weighting. HVDM was used because it can handle both qualitative and quantitative attributes in the data set. The attribute weighted HVDM is defined as

$$\text{weighted\_HVDM}\ (x, y) = \sqrt{\sum_{a=1}^{m} w_{ca} d_a(x_a, y_a)^2}, \quad (4)$$

where m is the number of attributes, c is the disease class of the case y, w_{ca} is the weight of the attribute a in class c, and $d_a(x_a, y_a)$ is the distance between the values x_a and y_a for attribute a. The distance function $d_a(x_a, y_a)$ is defined as

$$d_a(x_a, y_a)$$

$$= \begin{cases} 1, & \text{if } x \text{ or } y \text{ is unknown} \\ \text{normalized\_vdm}_a(x_a, y_a), & \text{if } a \text{ is qualitative} \\ \text{normalized\_diff}_a(x_a, y_a), & \text{otherwise.} \end{cases}$$

$$(5)$$

Because HVDM computes distances to qualitative and other attributes with different measurement ranges, it is necessary to scale their results into approximately the same range in order to give each attribute a similar influence on the overall distance [28]. The normalized distance to a quantitative attribute is calculated with (6):

$$\text{normalized\_diff}_a(x_a, y_a) = \frac{|x_a - y_a|}{4\sigma_a}, \quad (6)$$

where σ_a is the standard deviation of the numeric values of attribute a in the training set of the current classifier, and to a nominal attribute with (7):

$$\text{normalized\_vdm}_a(x_a, y_a) = \sqrt{\sum_{c=1}^{C} \left| \frac{N_{a,x,c}}{N_{a,x}} - \frac{N_{a,y,c}}{N_{a,y}} \right|^2}, \quad (7)$$

where C is the number of output classes in the problem domain (in this case $C = 7$), $N_{a,x(y),c}$ is the number of cases in T that have a value x (or a value y) for attribute a and the output class c, and $N_{a,x(y)}$ is the number of cases in T that have a value x (or a value y) for attribute a [28]. In other words, we are calculating the conditional probabilities to have the output class c when having attribute a with the value x (or the value y).

This approach allowed modifications of all the weights at the same time.

3.2.3. Attribute Weighted k-Nearest Neighbour Method Using One-versus-All Classifiers.

In addition to the neighbour's class-based attribute weighting the attribute weighted k-nearest neighbour method was tested with one-versus-all classifiers (wk-NN OVA). Within this method, the multiclass classification problem was converted into multiple binary classifiers—that is, the m class problem was divided into m binary problems [29]. Each binary OVA classifier was trained to separate a class from all the other classes by marking the cases of this one class as member cases and the cases of the other classes as nonmember cases in the training set.

The attribute weighted k-NN OVA is an instance-based learning method that searches for the k most similar cases (neighbours) of a new case from each classifier separately. There is one classifier per each class and each classifier gives a vote for the case being a member or nonmember of the class based on the majority class of the k neighbours. The final class of the new case is assigned from a classifier suggesting the case being a member of a class. There can occur a situation in which the new case gets more than one member of a class vote (a tie situation) or all of the classifiers vote for the other class (the case to be a nonmember of all the classes). In a tie situation the class of the new case is determined by searching for the most similar member case from the member voting classifiers. The case gets the class of the member case with the shortest distance to it. When all the classifiers vote for the case to be a nonmember, the basic 1-nearest neighbour classifier using the whole training data containing the original disease classes is employed to find the most similar case (and its class) for the new case.

The distance measure used in the wk-NN OVA was also the HVDM measure. The difference in the HVDM description in (4) is that the c is the class of the classifier at issue, not

TABLE 3: Example evaluation computation time of one population (21 individuals, one generation) in GA runs with different computers.

Computer	Example one population evaluation time			
	GA ONE	*GA cwk-NN*	*GA wk-NN OVA*	Specifications
C1	3 min 25 s	48 min 54 s	4 h 57 min 8 s	W7 Intel Core i7-3540M 3.00 GHz, 16 GB RAM
C2	—	49 min 53 s	6 h 59 min 16 s	I3-530 2.93 GHz, 12 GB RAM
C3	—	3 h 47 min 41 s	9 h 41 min 9 s	Q6600 2.4 GHz, 8 GB RAM
C4	—	3 h 12 min 41 s	21 h 14 min 0 s	HP ProLiant DL580 G7 server: 4^* Intel Xeon X7560 2.26 GHz, 1 TB RAM
C5	—	3 h 4 min 58 s	7 h 22 min 52 s	DL785 G5 server: 8^* AMD Opteron 8360 SE 2.5 GHz, 512 GB RAM
C6	—	—	10 h 34 min 55 s	Intel Core2 Duo E6750 2.66 GHz, 2 GB RAM

TABLE 4: The ending time of the genetic algorithm runs within different evaluation methods.

Genetic algorithm	*GA ONE*	*GA cwk-NN*	*GA wk-NN OVA*	*GA ONE100*
Ended before 20th generation [%]	75.0	18.0	82.9	39.0^*
Ended on 10th generation [%]	48.0	6.0	54.9	12.0^*
Ended on 20th generation [%]	25.0	82.0	17.1	61.0^*

* The ending generations of the *GA ONE100* runs was examined before 100th generation, on 50th generation and on 100th generation.

the class of the case y. In addition, in (7) *wk*-NN OVA has two output classes ($C = 2$). The data in the learning set T of the classifier is divided into the member and nonmember classes.

4. Results

The results of the GA runs with ONE and *cwk*-NN as an evaluation method were the averages of the 10 times repeated 10-fold cross-validation whereas the results with the *wk*-NN OVA were the averages of the 5 times repeated 10-fold cross-validation. The 10-fold cross-validation was repeated only five times with the *GA wk*-NN OVA due to its huge computation time. For example, the evaluation of a population (21 individuals in one generation in a GA run) in one cross-validation set with the *GA ONE* lasted 3 minutes and 25 seconds, with the *GA cwk*-NN 48 minutes and 54 seconds, and with the *GA wk*-NN OVA 4 hours, 57 minutes, and 8 seconds when running the GA with the computer C1 (Table 3). With the other computers, the computation was even slower. Thus, at worst, the computation time of one cross-validation set lasting 20 generations with the computer C1 and *GA wk*-NN OVA was over four days (over 12 days with C4) assuming that within each generation all individuals were evaluated. In practice, the number of evaluated individuals varied within generations due to the crossover and the mutation. Notice that computers C4 and C5 were servers having several other users simultaneously and, thus, we had only minor part of their CPU in use. During *GA cwk*-NN and *GA wk*-NN OVA runs, the GA was run parallel in five computers, thus, having at best 11 parallel GA runs in process. *GA ONE* was run only with the computer C1.

The number of generations in the GA runs with all used evaluation methods varied from 10 to 20. In total, 75.0%, 18.0%, and 82.9% of GA runs ended before the 20th generation due to having the same best accuracy (*GA ONE* and *GA cwk*-NN) or TPR (*GA wk*-NN OVA) in 10 consecutive GA runs with ONE method, *cwk*-NN, and *wk*-NN OVA, respectively (Table 4). With the *GA wk*-NN OVA, all the

GA runs with the disease classes sudden deafness, traumatic vertigo, and benign recurrent vertigo ended before the 20th generation and with the other classes from 58.0% to 88.0% of the runs. If the number of ending generation was 10, this meant that the best ACC or TPR in the population did not change at all during the GA run and, therefore, the run was ended. *GA cwk*-NN ended after 10 generations only in 6.0% of the GA runs whereas *GA ONE* and *GA wk*-NN OVA ended during the GA runs around half of runs (in 48.0% and 54.9% of runs, resp.). In the *GA wk*-NN OVA runs, this happened especially with disease class traumatic vertigo where all CV runs ended after 10 generations and with sudden deafness (96.0%) and benign recurrent vertigo (94.0%). The other disease classes ended during the *GA wk*-NN OVA runs after 10 generations from 12.0% (acoustic neurinoma) to 34.0% (vestibular neuritis) of the runs. Most of the *GA cwk*-NN runs lasted 20 generations (82.0%) whereas only a fourth of the *GA ONE* runs and 17.1% of the *GA wk*-NN OVA runs went through 20 generations.

Within the *GA wk*-NN OVA runs of the disease class benign recurrent vertigo occurred situations where the TPRs in the starting population were zero regardless of using the TPR of 3-NN instead in population evaluation. The TPR of 3-NN was used with BRV instead of 7-NN because of the small size of the disease class. The TPRs of starting individuals were zero in 30 out of 50 cross-validation sets within the *GA wk*-NN OVA run concentrating on the BRV. In this case, new starting individuals were created randomly. Random individual creation was repeated in different cross-validation sets from one to five and nine times. The *GA wk*-NN OVA run ended if the TPR of starting population stayed zero ten times. This happened in 14 (28.0%) cross-validation sets only with the disease class benign recurrent vertigo.

In order to see the effect of genetic algorithm on the population, we examined the worst and the best total classification accuracies of individuals (the attribute weight vectors) in the beginning and in the end of the genetic algorithm run. The mean worst and the mean best total accuracies and their standard deviations with GA runs using ONE and *cwk*-NN as

TABLE 5: The mean and its standard deviation of the best and worst total classification accuracies of individuals in the starting and ending populations occurring during different GA runs within 10 times (in *GA wk-NN OVA* 5 times) repeated 10-fold cross-validation.

Method	Population	Best accuracy [%]		Worst accuracy [%]	
		Mean	Std dev.	Mean	Std dev.
GA ONE (ONE1)	start	74.0	0.8	49.8	1.6
	end	73.8	0.7	61.4	2.8
	end 100	73.9	0.9	66.5	2.0
GA cwk-NN (7-NN)	start	63.6	1.6	27.9	2.2
	end	68.3	1.9	56.2	2.2
GA wk-NN OVA (7-NN)	start	79.2	0.5	75.3	0.5
	end	78.6	0.9	78.7	0.8

TABLE 6: The starting point of the genetic algorithm using ONE inference (*GA ONE*), the attribute weighted *k*-nearest neighbour method with neighbour's class-based attribute weighting (*GA cwk-NN*) and with OVA classifiers (*GA wk-NN OVA*) as evaluation method. The true positive rates (TPR) of seven disease classes and the total classification accuracies of the best individual from the starting population are given in percentages (%) from 10 times (five times with *GA wk-NN OVA*) repeated 10-fold cross-validation.

	Disease	ANE	BPV	MEN	SUD	TRA	VNE	BRV	Median TPR	Total accuracy
	Cases	131	173	350	47	73	157	20		951
GA ONE	ONE1	63.5	55.0	91.1	67.4	84.0	67.5	37.0	67.4	74.0
	ONE12	76.0	84.7	96.6	97.0	96.3	75.4	69.5	84.7	87.5
	ONE123	88.1	94.7	98.1	99.6	99.9	84.6	86.0	94.7	93.8
GA cwk-NN	1-NN	47.6	50.2	75.7	28.7	59.0	55.0	10.5	50.2	58.8
	3-NN	48.9	52.5	82.2	24.0	58.9	57.0	9.0	52.5	61.9
	5-NN	49.0	54.4	85.1	21.1	57.0	56.5	8.5	54.4	62.9
	7-NN	48.9	55.0	86.6	19.6	56.3	57.8	5.5	55.0	63.6
	9-NN	49.2	56.0	87.8	16.4	53.4	57.5	3.5	53.4	63.7
GA wk-NN OVA	1-NN	70.4	73.5	85.0	67.2	62.7	78.2	19.0	70.4	75.8
	3-NN	71.1	75.8	91.8	73.2	61.1	79.4	18.0	73.2	79.2
	5-NN	70.7	75.7	92.8	74.5	62.5	79.5	15.0	74.5	79.6
	7-NN	69.9	74.7	93.0	73.2	60.0	80.1	15.0	73.2	79.2
	9-NN	68.9	73.2	93.2	71.9	58.1	80.5	16.0	71.9	78.7

an evaluation method were calculated from 10 times repeated 10-fold cross-validation and with GA runs using *wk*-NN OVA from 5 times repeated 10-fold cross-validation (Table 5). The mean best accuracies stayed approximately the same with the *GA ONE*, whereas the mean best accuracy increased 4.7% with the *GA cwk-NN* and decreased 0.6% with the *GA wk-NN OVA*. The improvement can be seen from the mean worst classification accuracies: the worst accuracy occurring in the population increased during GA runs, especially with the *GA cwk-NN* (28.3%). With the *GA ONE*, the mean worst accuracy improved 11.6% when using at most 20 generations and 16.7% when using at most 100 generations. With the *GA wk-NN OVA*, the improvement was moderate (3.4%) but one must notice that its mean worst classification accuracy was already over 75% in the starting population, which was better than the mean best accuracies of the other methods.

The more detailed results of the *GA ONE*, the *GA cwk-NN*, and the *GA wk-NN OVA* runs in the beginning and in the end with the best individual occurring in the population are given in Tables 6 and 7. The true positive rates of the disease classes

are shown with *GA ONE* for the first (ONE1), the first and second (ONE12), and the first, second, and third (ONE123) diagnosis suggestions of ONE and with *GA cwk-NN* and *GA wk-NN OVA* for one, three, five, seven, and nine nearest neighbours (1-NN–9-NN). During cross-validation runs in GA, the individuals were evaluated by the total classification accuracy of the ONE1 with the *GA ONE* and of the 7-NN with the *GA cwk-NN* and by the true positive rate of the 7-NN with the *GA wk-NN OVA* (except with disease class BRV that used the TPR of 3-NN). The true positive rate was used as a fitness rate with the *GA wk-NN OVA* instead of the total accuracy because it concentrated on classifying one disease class at a time whereas *GA ONE* and *GA cwk-NN* classified all seven disease classes at the same time.

Within 20 generations lasting GA, the best improvement between the start population and the end population was yielded with the *GA cwk-NN* that improved the total classification accuracies and the mean true positive rates when using one to nine nearest neighbours in the classification. Total classification accuracy of the *GA cwk-NN* rose at best 5.1%

TABLE 7: The end result of the genetic algorithm using ONE inference (*GA ONE*), the attribute weighted *k*-nearest neighbour method with neighbour's class-based attribute weighting (*GA cwk-NN*) and with OVA classifiers (*GA wk-NN OVA*) as evaluation method in population evaluation after at most 20 generations. The true positive rates (TPR) of seven disease classes and the total classification accuracies of the best individual in the end population are given in percentages (%) from 10 times (five times with *GA wk-NN OVA*) repeated 10-fold cross-validation.

	Disease	ANE	BPV	MEN	SUD	TRA	VNE	BRV	Median TPR	Total accuracy
	Cases	131	173	350	47	73	157	20		951
GA ONE	ONE1	63.5	55.4	90.8	66.2	83.0	68.0	31.5	66.2	73.8
	ONE12	77.0	82.7	96.4	93.6	96.2	76.2	62.0	82.7	87.0
	ONE123	87.6	92.8	98.0	98.5	99.5	84.4	84.5	92.8	93.2
GA cwk-NN	1-NN	70.2	50.0	68.4	30.6	70.0	60.3	15.0	60.3	61.1
	3-NN	70.8	53.9	78.1	27.7	72.5	62.9	14.5	62.9	65.9
	5-NN	70.5	56.1	81.5	23.2	71.9	63.8	12.0	63.8	67.4
	7-NN	69.5	56.6	84.7	21.1	71.0	63.9	8.5	63.9	68.3
	9-NN	69.0	57.5	86.6	18.1	69.7	64.1	6.0	64.1	68.8
GA wk-NN OVA	1-NN	71.5	74.1	84.6	67.2	67.1	77.8	18.0	71.5	76.2
	3-NN	71.6	75.3	91.7	74.9	66.8	78.7	16.0	74.9	79.5
	5-NN	70.4	73.6	92.2	77.0	63.6	79.2	14.0	73.6	79.1
	7-NN	70.4	71.8	92.6	77.0	59.5	79.6	13.0	71.8	78.6
	9-NN	70.5	72.4	92.7	74.9	59.7	79.6	13.0	72.4	78.7

(in 9-NN) and median TPR 10.7% (in 9-NN). The GA had a smaller effect on the results of the *GA ONE* and the *GA wk-NN OVA*. The results in the start population and in the end population stayed quite near each other. Small improvement in the mean total classification accuracy and the mean TPR can be seen with the *GA wk-NN OVA* using one or three nearest neighbours in the classification. Otherwise, the total classification accuracies decreased a bit when using the *GA ONE* and with the *GA wk-NN OVA* using five or seven neighbours in the classification.

Changes within the true positive rates of disease classes compared to the start and end results varied between methods. The *GA cwk-NN* mainly increased the TPRs. During GA runs, it increased the most the TPR of acoustic neurinoma (22.6% in 1-NN) and traumatic vertigo (16.3% in 9-NN). Menière's disease was the only class where the TPR decreased (at worst −7.3% in 1-NN) during *GA cwk-NN* runs. With the *GA ONE*, the TPRs of classes mainly decreased. It decreased the most the TPR of benign recurrent vertigo (−7.5% in ONE12) and sudden deafness (−3.4% in ONE12). However, small increase in TPR can be seen with acoustic neurinoma (1.0% in ONE12) and with vestibular neuritis (0.8% with ONE12). With the *GA wk-NN OVA*, some TPRs increased and some decreased. The TPR increased the most with traumatic vertigo (5.8% in 3-NN) and sudden deafness (3.8% in 7-NN) and decreased the most with benign recurrent vertigo (−3.0% in 9-NN) and benign positional vertigo (−2.9% in 7-NN).

Because the computation time with the ONE method was so much faster than with the *k*-nearest neighbour methods, the evolution of the population with *GA ONE* runs was tested also with 100 generations in addition to the 20 generations. The ending condition was also changed: the GA run ended if the maximum accuracy stayed the same in 50 successive runs or 100 generations were run. In total, 39.0% of the *GA ONE100*

TABLE 8: The end result of the genetic algorithm using ONE inference in population evaluation after at most 100 generations. True positive rates and the total classification accuracies of the best individual in the end populationare given in percentages [%] from 10 times repeated 10-fold cross-validation.

Disease	Cases	*GA ONE 100*		
		ONE1	ONE12	ONE123
ANE	131	67.1	79.9	89.6
BPV	173	56.9	82.0	92.8
MEN	350	89.9	96.1	97.9
SUD	47	61.7	90.9	97.0
TRA	73	80.3	96.4	99.7
VNE	157	69.6	78.7	86.0
BRV	20	23.0	53.5	75.0
Median TPR		67.1	82.0	92.8
Total accuracy	951	73.9	87.3	93.5

runs ended before the 100th generation and within 12.0% of the runs there was no change in the best total classification accuracy during 50 generations (Table 4). The classification results of the *GA ONE100* runs are given in Table 8. The increase of generations from 20 to 100 did not affect much the mean total classification accuracy nor the mean median TPR. Within disease classes, benign recurrent vertigo suffered the most from the generation increase: its true positive rate decreased at worst −16.0% (ONE12) compared to the starting population and −9.5% (ONE123) compared to the 20th generation. The best TPR increase was achieved with acoustic neurinoma: 3.9% from the starting population and 3.6% from the 20th generation.

5. Discussion and Conclusion

Genetic algorithm runs were done with three different population evaluation methods in order to see whether the classification performance of the attribute weighted methods based on the nearest neighbour search can be improved when using the genetic algorithm in the evolution of attribute weighting. The attribute weighting in the starting population was based on the weights described by the application area experts and machine learning methods instead of random weight setting. The genetic algorithm runs were done separately with the nearest pattern method of ONE (*GA ONE*), with the attribute weighted k-nearest neighbour method using neighbour's class-based attribute weighting (*GA cwk-NN*), and with the attribute weighted k-nearest neighbour method using one-versus-all classifiers (*GA wk-NN OVA*). The 10-fold cross-validation was repeated 10 times with *GA ONE* and *GA cwk-NN* and 5 times with *GA cwk-NN OVA* due to its huge computation time.

The GA runs lasted at maximum 20 generations, 10 generations if there were no change in the best classification accuracy. Most of the GA runs with *GA ONE* and *GA wk-NN OVA* ended before the 20th generation (75.0% and 82.9%, resp.) and around half (!) of the GA runs ended without a change in the best classification (ended after 10 generations; 48.0% and 54.9%, resp.). Only 18.0% of the *GA cwk-NN* runs ended before the 20th round and 6.0% after 10 generations.

The total classification accuracies and the mean true positive rates were improved within *GA cwk-NN* runs whereas with *GA ONE* and *GA wk-NN OVA* the results in the beginning and in the end population stayed quite near each other. One reason why the GA did not improve much the total classification accuracies with the *GA ONE* and the *GA wk-NN OVA* might be that the attribute weights used in the starting population were already optimized for separate disease classes. In addition, also the fitness values for ONE method can be said to be the best occurring fitness values because they were computed from the otoneurological data with the machine learning method.

Hussein et al. [8] noticed that in some applications a strict cost-benefit analysis may rule out the use of genetic algorithm optimization because of its increase in processing time (e.g., 100–150% increase in counting time compared to the basic classifier with 200 train and test cases and over 400% when using 3824 train cases and 1797 test cases with k-NN leave-one-out). Also, Kelly and Davis [6] admit that it can take a tremendous amount of time to find high-performance weight vectors for variably weighted machine learning methods. The results in [3] showed that the extensions of the k-NN yielded generally better results at the cost of speed since all extensions required a training phase. In this research, the *GA wk-NN OVA* was really time-consuming compared to *GA cwk-NN* and *GA ONE*. However, if the weight calculation needs to be done only once or quite seldom, the time issue is not that crucial, especially if it improves the performance of the method.

In this study the weights set by the experts and learnt by machine learning methods were used as a starting point. This helped a lot the search of appropriate weights but there might be different attribute weight combinations with as good or even better classification results. Therefore it would be good to test genetic algorithm also with totally random starting population and with several different parameters in offspring creation and mutation.

Conflict of Interests

The authors declare that there is no conflict of interests regarding the publication of this paper.

Acknowledgments

The first author acknowledges the support of Onni and Hilja Tuovinen Foundation, Oskar Öflund's Foundation, and Finnish Cultural Foundation, Päijät-Häme Regional fund who granted scholarships for her postgraduate studies. The authors are grateful to Docent E. Kentala, M.D., and Professor I. Pyykkö, M.D., for their help in collecting the otoneurological data and medical advice.

References

[1] T. M. Cover and P. E. Hart, "Nearest neighbor pattern classification," *IEEE Transactions on Information Theory*, vol. 13, no. 1, pp. 21–27, 1967.

[2] T. Mitchell, *Machine Learning*, McGraw-Hill, New York, NY, USA, 1997.

[3] Z. Voulgaris and G. D. Magoulas, "Extensions of the k nearest neighbour methods for classification problems," in *Proceedings of the 26th IASTED International Conference on Artificial Intelligence and Applications (AIA '08)*, pp. 23–28, ACTA Press, Anaheim, Calif, USA, February 2008.

[4] J. M. Sotoca, J. S. Sánchez, and F. Pla, "Estimating feature weights for distance-based classification," in *Proceedings of the 3rd International Workshop on Pattern Recognition in Information Systems (PRIS '03)*, Angers, France, 2003.

[5] E. Marchiori, A. Ngom, E. Formenti, J.-K. Hao, X.-M. Zhao, and T. van Laarhoven, "Class dependent feature weighting and k-nearest neighbor classification," in *Proceedings of the 8th IAPR International Conference on Pattern Recognition in Bioinformatics (PRIB '13)*, vol. 7986 of *LNBI*, pp. 69–78, Springer, Berlin, Germany, 2013.

[6] J. D. Kelly and L. Davis, "A hybrid genetic algorithm for classification," in *Proceedings of the 12th International Joint Conference on Artificial Intelligence (IJCAI '91)*, vol. 2, pp. 645–650, Morgan Kaufmann, San Franciso, Calif, USA, 1991.

[7] W. F. Punch, E. D. Goodman, M. Pei, L. Chia-Shun, P. Hovland, and R. Enbody, "Further research on feature selection and classification using genetic algorithms," in *Proceedings of the 5th International Conference on Genetic Algorithms (ICGA '93)*, pp. 557–564, University of Illinois, Champaign, Ill, USA, 1993.

[8] F. Hussein, N. Kharma, and R. Ward, "Genetic algorithms for feature selection and weighting, a review and study," in *Proceedings of the 6th International Conference on Document Analysis and Recognition (ICDAR '01)*, pp. 1240–1244, Seattle, Wash, USA, 2001.

[9] H. Lee, E. Kim, and M. Park, "A genetic feature weighting scheme for pattern recognition," *Integrated Computer-Aided Engineering*, vol. 14, no. 2, pp. 161–171, 2007.

[10] D. Mateos-García, J. García-Gutiérrez, and J. C. Riquelme-Santos, "Label dependent evolutionary feature weighting for remote sensing data," in *Proceedings of the 5th International Conference on Hybrid Artificial Intelligence Systems*, pp. 272–279, Springer, 2010.

[11] D. Mateos-García, J. García-Gutiérrez, and J. C. Riquelme-Santos, "On the evolutionary optimization of k-NN by label-dependent feature weighting," *Pattern Recognition Letters*, vol. 33, no. 16, pp. 2232–2238, 2012.

[12] D. E. Goldberg, *Genetic Algorithms in Search, Optimization, and Machine Learning*, Addison-Wesley, Reading, Mass, USA, 1989.

[13] M. Mitchell, *An Introduction to Genetic Algorithms*, MIT Press, Cambridge, Mass, USA, 1996.

[14] Z. Michalewicz, *Genetic Algorithms + Data Structures = Evolution Programs*, Springer, Berlin, Germany, 1992.

[15] A. E. Eiben and J. E. Smith, *Introduction to Evolutionary Computing*, Springer, Berlin, Germany, 2003.

[16] K. Varpa, K. Iltanen, M. Juhola et al., "Refinement of the otoneurological decision support system and its knowledge acquisition process," in *Proceedings of the 20th International Congress of the European Federation for Medical Informatics (MIE '06)*, pp. 197–202, Maastricht, The Netherlands, 2006.

[17] K. Varpa, K. Iltanen, M. Siermala, and M. Juhola, "Attribute weighting with scatter and instance-based learning methods evaluated with otoneurological data," *International Journal of Computational Medicine and Healthcare*, 2013.

[18] E. Kentala, I. Pyykkö, Y. Auramo, and M. Juhola, "Database for vertigo," *Otolaryngology—Head and Neck Surgery*, vol. 112, no. 3, pp. 383–390, 1995.

[19] K. Viikki, *Machine learning on otoneurological data: decision trees for vertigo diseases [Ph.D. thesis]*, Department of Computer Sciences, University of Tampere, Tampere, Finland, 2002, http://urn.fi/urn:isbn:951-44-5390-5.

[20] K. A. De Jong, *Analysis of the behaviour of a class of genetic adaptive systems [Ph.D. thesis]*, Computer and Communication Sciences Department, The University of Michigan, Ann Arbor, Mich, USA, 1975, http://hdl.handle.net/2027.42/4507.

[21] M. Siermala, M. Juhola, J. Laurikkala, K. Iltanen, E. Kentala, and I. Pyykkö, "Evaluation and classification of otoneurological data with new data analysis methods based on machine learning," *Information Sciences*, vol. 177, no. 9, pp. 1963–1976, 2007.

[22] M. Juhola and M. Siermala, "A scatter method for data and variable importance evaluation," *Integrated Computer-Aided Engineering*, vol. 19, no. 2, pp. 137–139, 2012.

[23] M. Juhola and M. Siermala, "Scatter Counter program and its instructions," 2014, http://www.uta.fi/sis/cis/research_groups/darg/publications/scatterCounter_2_7_eng.pdf.

[24] D. W. Aha, "Tolerating noisy, irrelevant and novel attributes in instance-based learning algorithms," *International Journal of Man-Machine Studies*, vol. 36, no. 2, pp. 267–287, 1992.

[25] E. Kentala, Y. Auramo, M. Juhola, and I. Pyykkö, "Comparison between diagnoses of human experts and a neurotologic expert system," *Annals of Otology, Rhinology and Laryngology*, vol. 107, no. 2, pp. 135–140, 1998.

[26] Y. Auramo and M. Juhola, "Modifying an expert system construction to pattern recognition solution," *Artificial Intelligence in Medicine*, vol. 8, no. 1, pp. 15–21, 1996.

[27] E. Kentala, Y. Auramo, I. Pyykkö, and M. Juhola, "Otoneurological expert system," *Annals of Otology, Rhinology and Laryngology*, vol. 105, no. 8, pp. 654–658, 1996.

[28] R. D. Wilson and T. R. Martinez, "Improved heterogeneous distance functions," *Journal of Artificial Intelligence Research*, vol. 6, pp. 1–34, 1997.

[29] M. Galar, A. Fernández, E. Barrenechea, H. Bustince, and F. Herrera, "An overview of ensemble methods for binary classifiers in multi-class problems: experimental study on one-vs-one and one-vs-all schemes," *Pattern Recognition*, vol. 44, no. 8, pp. 1761–1776, 2011.

8

Mathematical Modeling of the Expert System Predicting the Severity of Acute Pancreatitis

Maria A. Ivanchuk,[1] **Vitalij V. Maksimyuk,**[2] **and Igor V. Malyk**[3]

[1] Department of Biological Physics and Medical Informatics, Bukovinian State Medical University, Kobyljanska Street 42, Chernivtsi 58000, Ukraine
[2] Department of Surgery, Bukovinian State Medical University, Golovna Street 137, Chernivtsi 58000, Ukraine
[3] Department of the System Analysis and Insurance and Financial Mathematics, Chernivtsi National University of Yuriy Fedkovich, Unversitetska Street 12, Chernivtsi 58012, Ukraine

Correspondence should be addressed to Maria A. Ivanchuk; mgracia@ukr.net

Academic Editor: Daniel Kendoff

The method of building the hyperplane which separates the convex hulls in the Euclidean space R^n is proposed. The algorithm of prediction of the presence of severity in patients based on this method is developed and applied in practice to predict the presence of severity in patients with acute pancreatitis.

1. Introduction

During the last decades, pronounced tendency to the relentless increase in morbidity in acute pancreatitis is observed. Thus, the depth of pathomorphological pancreatic parenchyma lesions can vary from the development of edematous pancreatitis up to pancreatic necrosis. However, accurate predicting of the probable nature of the lesion of the pancreas in the early stages of acute pancreatitis is one of the most difficult problems of modern pancreatology. Diagnostic and the predictive probability of existing laboratory and instrumental diagnostic markers and rating scales does not exceed 70–80% [1–3]. Such situation is a major difficulty in selecting the adequate treatment strategy in the initial stages of acute pancreatitis. Thus the search for new methods of accurate predicting of acute pancreatitis' severity becomes an urgent problem.

Development of mathematical approaches for prediction in medicine was developed by Fisher, the father of the linear discriminant analysis [4]. Currently, there are many approaches to solving this problem: cluster analysis, the construction of predictive tables, image recognition, and linear programming. Fundamentals of building the prognostic tables and Wald serial analysis are described in [5]. Cluster analysis is commonly used for solving the tasks of medical prediction.

In the paper [6], the procedure of cluster analysis with a study of the indices of the daily variability of cardiac rhythm in patients with the ischemic disease of heart is examined. In [7] using national data from the Scientific Registry of Transplant Recipients authors compare transplant and wait-list hospitalization rates. They suggest two marginal methods to analyze such clustered recurrent event data; the first model postulates a common baseline event rate, while the second features cluster-specific baseline rates. Results from the proposed models to those based on a frailty model were compared with the various methods compared and contrasted. Three major considerations in designing a cluster analysis are described in [8]. The first relates to selection of the individuals. The second consideration is selection of variables for measurement and the third consideration is how many variables to choose to enter into a cluster analysis. To classify clinical phenotypes of anti-neutrophil cytoplasmic antibody-associated vasculitis, cluster analysis was used in [9]. Researches on the general theory of diagnosis, classification, and application of optimization methods for pattern recognition, solving applied problems in medicine and biology, are conducted by Mangasarian et al. for many years [10].

But universal method for solving problems of recognition, identification, and diagnosis does not exist. Therefore, development of methods for predicting in medicine still remains relevant. One among the many challenges of recognition is the task of constructing hyperplanes which separate two convex sets. Many manuscripts [11–16] are devoted to the solution of this problem.

We propose a methodology for constructing convex hulls and their separation, which can be used for modeling expert medical prognostic systems (e.g., to separate groups of patients with different degrees of severity of the disease for prediction of severity in patients).

2. Methods

2.1. Separation of the Convex Hulls. Let us have two sets of points $A = \{a_i = (a_i^1, a_i^2, \ldots, a_i^n), i = \overline{1, m_A}\}$ and $B = \{b_i = (b_i^1, b_i^2, \ldots, b_i^n), i = \overline{1, m_B}\}$ in Euclidean space R^n. Let m be number of points in the set. We must find the separate hyperplane:

$$L_p = \{x \in R^n : \langle p, x \rangle = \gamma\}, \quad p \neq 0, \tag{1}$$

where $\langle p, x \rangle$ is the scalar product of the vectors p and x such that sets A and B can be placed in the different half-spaces:

$$L_p^+ = \{x \in R^n : \langle p, x \rangle > \gamma\},$$
$$L_p^- = \{x \in R^n : \langle p, x \rangle < \gamma\}. \tag{2}$$

To build the convex hull conv_A for the set A, for each of $C_{m_A}^n$ points' combinations from the set A, if it is possible, build the hyperplane

$$H_p = \{x \in R^n : \langle p, x \rangle = \beta\}, \quad p \neq 0. \tag{3}$$

Coordinates of the vector $p = (p^1, \ldots, p^n)$ are found as minors $(n-1)$ order for elements of the first row of the matrix:

$$\begin{pmatrix} x^1 - a_1^1 & x^2 - a_1^2 & \cdots & x^n - a_1^n \\ a_2^1 - a_1^1 & a_2^2 - a_1^2 & \cdots & a_2^n - a_1^n \\ \cdots & \cdots & \cdots & \cdots \\ a_n^1 - a_1^1 & a_n^2 - a_1^2 & \cdots & a_n^n - a_1^n \end{pmatrix}, \tag{4}$$

where $x \in R^n$, $a_i \in A$, $i = \overline{1, n}$. Coefficient β is determined from the following equation:

$$\beta = -\left(a_1^1 p^1 + a_1^2 p^2 + \cdots + a_1^n p^n\right). \tag{5}$$

If all points of the set A are in the one of half-spaces of hyperplane H_p, then polygon $a_1 a_2 \cdots a_n$ is one of the convex hull's hyperfaces. The complex of all hyperfaces is the convex hull conv_A.

Point $b_i \in B$ is called outlier if point b_i is internal for the conv_A. Point b_i is outlier if there is at least one hyperface $a_1 a_2 \cdots a_n \in \text{conv}_A$ that

$$\left|\overrightarrow{cf}\right| = \left|\overrightarrow{cb_i}\right| + \left|\overrightarrow{b_i f}\right|, \tag{6}$$

where point $c \in \text{int conv}_A$, point f is the intersection point of the hyperplane H_p ($a_1 a_2 \cdots a_n \in H_p$), and line

$$\frac{x^1 - c^1}{b^1 - c^1} = \frac{x^2 - c^2}{b^2 - c^2} = \cdots = \frac{x^n - c^n}{b^n - c^n}. \tag{7}$$

To find the point f let us write (3) in parametric form:

$$x^1 = c^1 + \left(b^1 - c^1\right) t$$
$$x^2 = c^2 + \left(b^2 - c^2\right) t$$
$$\cdots$$
$$x^n = c^n + \left(b^n - c^n\right) t. \tag{8}$$

Put (8) in the hyperplane equation (3) and find parameter t:

$$t^* = \frac{p^1 c^1 + p^2 c^2 + \cdots + p^n c^n + \beta}{p^1 \left(c^1 - b^1\right) + p^2 \left(c^2 - b^2\right) + \cdots + p^n \left(c^n - b^n\right)}. \tag{9}$$

To find coordinates of the point f let us put (9) in (8):

$$f^1 = c^1 + \left(b^1 - c^1\right) t^*$$
$$f^2 = c^2 + \left(b^2 - c^2\right) t^*$$
$$\vdots$$
$$f^n = c^n + \left(b^n - c^n\right) t^*. \tag{10}$$

After finding all outliers from the sets A and B eject outliers from the set, with less number of outliers. Build the new convex hulls and find the outliers. If there are outliers in the new convex hulls, eject them. If there are not any outliers, the convex hulls do not intersect. According to consequence of Hahn-Banach theorem there is a nonzero linear functional L_p that separates conv_A and conv_B [17].

Find the separating functional L_p as hyperplane parallel to one of convex hulls' hyperfaces. Choose hyperface so that convex hulls conv_A and conv_B are in different half-spaces formed by hyperplane parallel to this hyperface. Find points $a_{\min} \in \text{conv}_A$ and $b_{\min} \in \text{conv}_B$ so that $|\overrightarrow{a_{\min} b_{\min}}| = \min(|\overrightarrow{a_i b_j}| : a_i \in \text{conv}_A, b_j \in \text{conv}_B, i = \overline{1, m_A}, j = \overline{1, m_B})$. Let $d_{\min} \in \overrightarrow{a_{\min} b_{\min}}$. For each hyperface $\{H_{A_{\min}} : H_{A_{\min}} \subset \text{conv}_A; a_{\min} \in H_{A_{\min}}\}$ and $\{H_{B_{\min}} : H_{B_{\min}} \subset \text{conv}_B; b_{\min} \in H_{B_{\min}}\}$ build the parallel hyperplane $\{L_p : d_{\min} \in L_p; L_p \| H_{A_{\min}}$ or $L_p \| H_{B_{\min}}\}$. If $a_i \in L_p^+$, for all $a_i \in A$, $i = \overline{1, m_A}$, and $b_j \in L_p^-$, for all $b_j \in B$, $j = \overline{1, m_B}$, then L_p is separating hyperplane.

2.2. Modeling the Expert System of Predicting the Presence of Severity in Patients. Let us have two groups of patients: A, patients with severity, and B, patients without severity. There are n_0 parameters (factors which affect the severity) known for each patient.

During modelling we used the terms sensitivity (Se) and specificity (Sp):

$$Se = \frac{a}{a+c}, \qquad Sp = \frac{d}{b+d}, \qquad (11)$$

where a is the true positives, b is the false positives (overdiagnosis errors), c is the false negatives (underdiagnosis errors), and d is the true negatives. The sensitivity of a clinical test refers to the ability of the test to correctly identify those patients with the disease. The specificity of a clinical test refers to the ability of the test to correctly identify those patients without the disease [18].

We created an algorithm of modelling the expert system in a way that uses the least amount of features for the best result. Information of the parameters was found using Kulback's information measure [5]. We built convex hulls for the most informative factor. If convex hulls intersect, we found outliers—the points from the set A that are internal to $conv_B$ and the points from the set B that are internal to $conv_A$. The set A outliers are underdiagnosis errors. The set B outliers are overdiagnosis errors. We built the prognostic system to find the patients with severity, so we rejected the outliers from the set B. Let the set $O_B = \{o_i : o_i \in B \cap \text{int } conv_A, i = \overline{1, m_{O_B}}\}$ be the set of outliers from B. After rejecting, we get a new set $B' = B/O_B$.

If you build the expert system for differential diagnosis, you reject outliers out of the set where there are less of them.

If the percentage of rejected points is more than the significance level

$$\frac{m_{O_B}}{m_B} > \alpha, \qquad (12)$$

the next (the most informative) factor was added. The space dimension is increased by 1. In the new space convex hulls were built and the outliers were rejected. The space dimension was increased until preassigned significance level. If all available diagnostic information was used, but preassigned significance level was not reached, then decision of not sufficient information was taken. When preassigned significance level was reached, we found the separating hyperplanes. The algorithm for modelling the prognostic system is represented on the Figure 1. The results were checked in the control group and the hyperplane with maximal sensitivity was chosen.

The complexity of this algorithm is $O(m^{n+1})$ [19] if the convex hulls are built by search of all combinations of points. The complexity of this algorithm is $O(m^2)$ if the convex hulls are built by Jarvis march or "gift wrapping" algorithm [20].

3. Results

3.1. The Expert System of Predicting the Presence of Severity in Patients with Acute Pancreatitis. The research involved 60 persons with severe and 28 patients with nonsevere acute pancreatitis. Among them, there were 57 (64.8%) men and 31 (35.2%) women. The mean age was 48.54 years (±15.18) in males and 56.21 (±17.91) in females. The most common etiology was alcohol consumption (48.3%), followed by gallstones (34.2%). In 17.5% no identifiable cause was found.

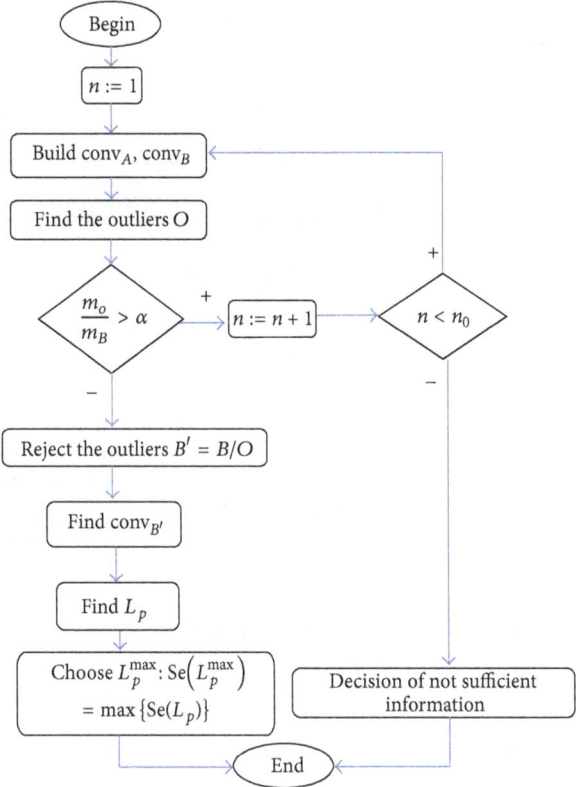

FIGURE 1: Algorithm for modelling the prognostic system.

The diagnostic criteria for acute pancreatitis were those defined by the 2006 AP Guidelines, as the presence of at least two of the following features: (1) characteristic abdominal pain, (2) elevation over 3 times the upper normal limit of serum amylase/lipase, and (3) characteristic features on computer tomography (CT) scan [21]. Severe acute pancreatitis was diagnosed according strictly to Atlanta criteria: Early Prognostic Scores, APACHE II ≥ 8, Ranson ≥ 3; Organ Failure, systolic pressure < 90 mmHg, creatinine > 2.0 mg/L after rehydration, PaO_2 ≤ 60 mmHg; Local Complications (on CT scan), Necrosis, Abscess, and Pseudocyst [22].

Patients were divided into two samples—training (50 patients with severity and 20 without them) and control (10 patients with severity and 8 without). The level of significance was $\alpha = 0,01$. The algorithm presented above was used for patients with training set.

For $n = 1$, the percentage of outliers was 29.5%.

For $n = 2$, the percentage of outliers was 3%.

For $n = 3$, the percentage of outliers was 1.4%.

For $n = 4$, the percentage of outliers was 0%.

We got 8 hyperplanes which separate the convex hulls of the training samples. Two of them had higher sensitivity and specificity (we got only 1 (6%) of underdiagnosis errors and there were no overdiagnosis errors for the control sample with these hyperplanes):

$$- 18937.5x^1 - 200.3x^2 + 5007.3x^3$$

$$+ 42348x^4 + 310958.6 = 0,$$

$$- 4802.5x^1 - 142.8x^2 + 5007.3x^3$$

$$+ 2158.1x^4 + 177176.4 = 0,$$

(13)

where x^1 is time before hospitalization, x^2 is blood lipase, x^3 is amylase urine, and x^4 is BMI.

So, we built the expert system with sensitivity Se = 94%.

Statistical errors are seen only in 1 patient in the control group, who were diagnosed with interstitial edematous pancreatitis development on the background severe diabetes mellitus. According to Expert System the acute pancreatitis without severity was predicted. This error, in our view, is associated with late ambulation of the patient for medical care as a result of atypical course of acute pancreatitis, increased blood and urine amylase, and increased BMI, which is the characteristic signs of diabetes mellitus. That is, in this case, some of the most important prognostic parameters of acute pancreatitis have been characterized by different diseases in particular of diabetes mellitus, which caused the error.

4. Conclusions

The method of separation of convex hulls in Euclidean space by constructing a separating hyperplane parallel to one of the convex hulls hyperfaces is proposed. On the basis of this method the algorithm for modelling the prognostic system is stated. The proposed algorithm is applied in practice to predict the presence of severity in patients with acute pancreatitis and gives 94% correct results for the control sample, while diagnostic and the predictive probability of existing laboratory and instrumental diagnostic markers and rating scales does not exceed 70–80%. Clinical application of the developed mathematical model predicting the severity of acute pancreatitis promotes proper choice of treatment tactics and allows improving final results of these patients' treatment.

Conflict of Interests

The authors declare that there is no conflict of interests regarding the publication of this paper.

References

[1] E. J. Balthazar, "Acute pancreatitis: assessment of severity with clinical and CT evaluation," *Radiology*, vol. 223, no. 3, pp. 603–613, 2002.

[2] G. Sathyanarayan, P. K. Garg, H. K. Prasad, and R. K. Tandon, "Elevated level of interleukin-6 predicts organ failure and severe disease in patients with acute pancreatitis," *Journal of Gastroenterology and Hepatology*, vol. 22, no. 4, pp. 550–554, 2007.

[3] A. K. Khanna, S. Meher, S. Prakash et al., "Comparison of ranson, Glasgow, MOSS, SIRS, BISAP, APACHE-II, CTSI scores,

IL-6, CRP, and procalcitonin in predicting severity, organ failure, pancreatic necrosis, and mortality in acute pancreatitis," *HPB Surgery*, vol. 2013, Article ID 367581, 10 pages, 2013.

[4] R. A. Fisher, *Contributions To Mathematical Statistics*, John Wiley & Sons, 1950.

[5] E. V. Gubler and A. A. Genkin, *Primenenie Neparametricheskih Kriteriev Statistiki v Medico-Biologicheskih Issledovanijah (Using the Nonparametric Statistic Criteria in Medical and Biological Researches)*, Leningrad, Russia, 1973.

[6] A. I. Borodulin, A. V. Sviridov, and O. V. Sudakov, "Using the cluster analysis in the in the diagnostic of ischemic heart disease," *Prikladnie Informacionnie Aspekti Medicini*, no. 2, pp. 28–32, 2008.

[7] D. E. Schaubel and J. Cai, "Analysis of clustered recurrent event data with application to hospitalization rates among renal failure patients," *Biostatistics*, vol. 6, no. 3, pp. 404–419, 2005.

[8] M. Weatherall, P. Shirtcliffe, J. Travers, and R. Beasley, "Use of cluster analysis to define COPD phenotypes," *European Respiratory Journal*, vol. 36, no. 3, pp. 472–474, 2010.

[9] A. Mahr, S. Katsahian, H. Varet et al., "Revisiting the classification of clinical phenotypes of anti-neutrophil cytoplasmic antibody-associated vasculitis: a cluster analysis," *Annals of the Rheumatic Diseases*, vol. 72, no. 6, pp. 1003–1010, 2013.

[10] O. L. Mangasarian, W. N. Street, and W. H. Wolberg, "Breast carter diagnosis and prognosis via linear programrnig," *Operation Research*, vol. 43, no. 4, 1995.

[11] A. I. Golikov, Y. G. Evtushenko, and S. Ketabchi, "On families of hyperplanes that separate polyhedra," *Computational Mathematics and Mathematical Physics*, vol. 45, no. 2, pp. 238–253, 2005.

[12] A. R. Alimov and V. Y. Protasov, "Separation of convex sets by extreme hyperplanes," *Fundamental and Applied Mathematics*, vol. 17, no. 4, pp. 3–12, 2012.

[13] I. I. Eremin, "Fejér methods for the strong separability of convex polyhedral sets," *Russian Mathematics*, no. 12, pp. 33–43, 2006.

[14] A. V. Ershova, "Algorithm of the disjoint convex polyhedral separating using Fejer mappings," *Sistemi Upravlenia I Informacionnie Tehnologii*, vol. 1, no. 35, pp. 53–56, 2009.

[15] C. Böhm and H.-P. Kriegel, "Determining the convex hull in large multidimensional databases," in *Data Warehousing and Knowledge Discovery*, vol. 2114 of *Lecture Notes in Computer Science*, pp. 294–306, Springer, 2001.

[16] G. Fung, R. Rosales, and B. Krishnapuram, "Learning rankings via convex hull separation," in *Proceedings of the Annual Conference on Neural Information Processing Systems (NIPS '05)*, pp. 395–402, December 2005.

[17] A. N. Kolmogorov and S. V. Fomin, *Elements of the Theory of Functions and Functional Analysis*, Courier Dover, 1999.

[18] D. G. Altman, *Practical Statistics for Medical Research*, Chapman & Hall/CRC, London, UK, 1991.

[19] S. A. Abramov, *Lectures at Algorithmic Complexity*, MTSNMO, Moscow, Russia, 2009.

[20] F. Preparata and M. Shamos, *Computational Geometry—An Introduction*, Springer, 1985.

[21] P. A. Banks and M. L. Freeman, "Practice guidelines in acute pancreatitis," *The American Journal of Gastroenterology*, vol. 101, no. 10, pp. 2379–2400, 2006.

[22] E. L. Bradley III and C. F. Frey, "A clinically based classification system for acute pancreatitis: summary of the International Symposium on Acute Pancreatitis, Atlanta, Ga, September 11 through 13, 1992," *Archives of Surgery*, vol. 128, no. 5, pp. 586–590, 1993.

9

Transmission Dynamics of Hepatitis C with Control Strategies

Adnan Khan, Sultan Sial, and Mudassar Imran

Department of Mathematics, Lahore University of Management Sciences, Lahore 54792, Pakistan

Correspondence should be addressed to Mudassar Imran; mudassar.imran@lums.edu.pk

Academic Editor: Darryl D. D'Lima

We present a rigorous mathematical analysis of a deterministic model, for the transmission dynamics of hepatitis C, using a standard incidence function. The infected population is divided into three distinct compartments featuring two distinct infection stages (acute and chronic) along with an isolation compartment. It is shown that for basic reproduction number $R_0 \leq 1$, the disease-free equilibrium is locally and globally asymptotically stable. The model also has an endemic equilibrium for $R_0 > 1$. Uncertainty and sensitivity analyses are carried out to identify and study the impact of critical parameters on R_0. In addition, we have presented the numerical simulations to investigate the influence of different important parameters on R_0. Since we have a locally stable endemic equilibrium, optimal control is applied to the deterministic model to reduce the total infected population. Two different optimal control strategies (vaccination and isolation) are designed to control the disease and reduce the infected population. *Pontryagin's Maximum Principle* is used to characterize the optimal controls in terms of an optimality system which is solved numerically. Numerical results for the optimal controls are compared against the constant controls and their effectiveness is discussed.

1. Introduction

Hepatitis C (HCV) is an important public health problem, as it is the common cause of liver diseases throughout the world [1]. The disease was first recognized in 1975 and its causative agent was identified in 1989. Hepatitis C is characterized by an acute (often asymptotic) stage, which, in most cases, is followed by a chronic stage that can result in cirrhosis and liver cancer. The hepatitis C virus (causative agent) is an enveloped RNA virus, which is further characterized to be a positive-sense single stranded virus belonging to the family Flaviviridae and is considerably small in size. Replication of the RNA-based virus involves the use of the enzyme RNA-dependent RNA polymerase (RdRP), which has a high error rate while going through this process. World Health Organization's report suggests that around 3% of the world population has been infected with HCV. The population infected with chronic HCV, who are at risk of developing liver cancer or cirrhosis, is estimated to be around 170 million. Furthermore, nearly 350,000 people die annually throughout the globe as a result of HCV-related liver diseases [2].

Hepatitis C can be characterized by two distinct stages: an acute stage and a chronic stage. Initially, infection by HCV causes an acute HCV which is usually asymptotic. Only about 15% of the cases show mild symptoms like decreased appetite, nausea, fatigue, joint or muscle pains, and weight loss. In 20% of the cases, the infection may resolve spontaneously. And the remaining 80% of the people exposed to HCV progress to the chronic stage of the infection by developing a chronic infection, which can last for decades. During the starting years of infection, most people experience minimal or no symptoms at all. However, HCV becomes the main cause of liver cancer and cirrhosis after several years of living with it. About 1%–5% of chronic HCV patients die from liver cancer or cirrhosis and nearly 5%–20% develop cirrhosis over 30 years. Patients with cirrhosis are 20 times more likely to develop hepatocellular carcinoma, at the rate of 13% each year. Moreover, 27% of cirrhosis cases and 25% of hepatocellular carcinoma cases worldwide are estimated to be caused by HCV [3–5].

Depending on the genotype of the HCV, the standard treatment of infected patients includes a combination of pegylated interferon (peg IFN-α) and the robust antiviral drug Ribavirin, for a period of 24 or 48 weeks [6]. The reaction to treatment also differs by genotype and lies between 70% and 80% for genotypes 2 and 3, while it is almost non existent for genotype 6. Recently, there have been promising treatment advances of genotype 1 using directly acting antiviral agents (DAAs). However, to prevent the infection, there is still a need to create effective vaccine strategy. Vaccines, which are used in preclinical and clinical trials, involve DNA-based proteins, recombinant proteins, synthetic peptide vaccines, and so forth. The future design of vaccines, along with the use and success of previously mentioned vaccines, has been discussed here [7]. However, no long-term immunity is granted in recovering from hepatitis C infection. So, this absence of acquired immunity must be shown in any model for hepatitis C. This is done by allowing recovered patients to become susceptible again.

Several studies have been carried out [8–13] and they are pertinent to our work. Most of these papers classify individuals in the population into different states and then formulate a system of ordinary differential equations (ODE) to analyze the time-evolution of each of these population states. Reade et al. [12] present an ODE model of infections with acute and chronic stages. Similarly, by Luo and Xiang, [10] a four state system was analyzed with exposed, acute and chronic states. Suna et al. [13] present a study on a SEIRS model where it was assumed that recovered individuals lose their infection-acquired immunity. Martcheva and Castillo-Chavez in [11] have formulated a model for hepatitis C lacking an exposed class and have discussed the stability of the equilibrium states.

We will formulate a five-state deterministic model with individuals in the population being classified as susceptible, acute, chronic, isolated, and recovered. Individuals suffering from acute and chronic stages of the infections are represented by acute and chronic states, respectively. The isolated state represents the chronically infected individuals getting isolated. The isolation of those with disease symptoms is probably the first infection control measure in recorded human history [14]. Over the decades, quarantine and isolation have been used to reduce the transmission of numerous emerging and reemerging human diseases such as leprosy, plague, cholera, typhus, yellow fever, smallpox, diphtheria, tuberculosis, measles, Ebola, pandemic influenza, and, more recently, SARS [15–20].

Previous models of HCV, particularly the models calculating the threshold quantity basic reproduction number R_0, have included the treatment and/or vaccination and have discussed the control of the disease by looking at the role of disease transmission parameters in the reduction of R_0 and the prevalence of the disease. However, these models did not account for time-dependent control strategies since their discussions are based on prevalence of the disease at equilibria. Optimal control theory has been employed to make decisions involving epidemic and biological models. The desired results and performance of the control functions depend on the different situations. Lenhart's HIV models [21, 22] used optimal control to design the treatment strategies. Jung et al. [23] provide a very good example of deciding how to divide the efforts between two treatment strategies (case holding and case finding) of the two-strain TB model. Yan et al. [24] used an optimal isolation campaign to fight the SARS epidemic. Study control strategies produce valuable theoretical results which can be used to suggest or design epidemic control programs. Depending on a chosen goal (or goals), various objective criteria may be adopted.

Our model extends previous work done on modeling the spread of hepatitis C in several key ways. First, we introduce an isolation class and qualitatively assess the effects of this isolation class on the transmission dynamics. Quarantine of individuals suspected of being exposed to a disease and the isolation of those with disease symptoms constitute what probably is the first infection control measure since the beginning of recorded human history [14]. However, almost no analysis of the effects of an isolation class on diseases with a chronic stage has been done and, therefore, our paper will be one of the first attempts to study the effect of isolation on the spread of a disease with a chronic stage. In addition, we will model the force of infection by a proportionate mixing, with the possibility of secondary infections due to contact with individuals who belong to the acute, chronic, or isolation class. Furthermore, we consider the disease-induced death rates for HCV in our model and will also take into account the possibility of recovery at every stage of the disease. These features add to the complexity of our model and make it considerably more insightful from an epidemiological perspective than previous models [11, 25].

In the paper, Section 2 presents a rigorous mathematical analysis of the deterministic model. It is shown that for basic reproduction number $R_0 \leq 1$, the disease-free equilibrium is locally and globally asymptotically stable. Further, the model has an endemic equilibrium, which exists if $R_0 > 1$ and persists in this case. The effect of using isolation on population is discussed using a threshold quantity. Sensitivity and uncertainty analyses are carried out to study the impact of crucial parameters on R_0. The existence of a locally stable endemic equilibrium, in case of $R_0 > 1$, encourages us to use a time-dependent optimal control strategy to prevent and control HCV. In Section 3, we designed two different optimal control strategies (vaccination and isolation) and performed numerical simulations to illustrate the effects of an optimal control strategy. Conclusion is presented in the last section.

2. Model Formulation and Steady State Analysis

2.1. Model Formulation. We formulate a five-state model with individuals classified as susceptible, acute, chronic, isolated and recovered. Hep C has an extremely slow progression that makes it difficult to characterize the natural history of the disease [3]. The following assumptions will therefore be made.

(1) All infected individuals develop the acute form of Hep C first.

(2) Individuals with either the acute or chronic form of Hep C are capable of transmitting the disease.

(3) Individuals with the acute form of the disease either progress to the chronic form or recover naturally. Since the acute form of the disease is largely asymptomatic, there is little chance of treatment at this stage.

(4) There is no permanent immunity against HCV after recovery; thus the recovered individuals move back to the susceptible.

In addition, the model will assume that the susceptible population S has a constant recruitment rate Π and natural death rate μ. Susceptible individuals who get infected suffer from the acute form of hepatitis C and move to the compartment A with the force of infection given by λ. Individuals in A, in addition to the natural death rate μ, die at a disease-induced death rate δ_a. They also have a natural recovery rate of κ. Individuals with the acute form of the infection progress to the chronic form of the disease at a rate ξ, in which case the individual is shifted to compartment C. Individuals in C, in addition to the natural death rate μ, also die at a disease-induced death rate δ_c. Furthermore, these individuals recover at a rate ψ and thus move to the recovered compartment S. Also, the individuals in compartment C are isolated and moved to compartment Q at a rate α. Individuals in Q, in addition to the natural death rate μ, also die at a disease-induced death rate δ_q. Isolated individuals can either recover at a rate γf or become acutely infected with HCV at a rate $\gamma(1 - f)$. The individuals in R are prone to the natural death rate μ, or they become susceptible again and enter the S compartment at a rate of ω. Recovery from HCV does not result in immunity.

Mathematically, the model is as follows:

$$\frac{dS}{dt} = \Pi + \omega R - \lambda S - \mu S,$$

$$\frac{dA}{dt} = \lambda S + \gamma(1 - f)Q - (\xi + \kappa + \mu + \delta_a)A,$$

$$\frac{dC}{dt} = \xi A - (\alpha + \psi + \mu + \delta_c)C, \qquad (1)$$

$$\frac{dQ}{dt} = \alpha C - (\gamma + \mu + \delta_q)Q,$$

$$\frac{dR}{dt} = \gamma f Q + \kappa A + \psi C - (\omega + \mu)R,$$

where

$$\lambda = \frac{\beta(\eta A + C + \zeta Q)}{N}. \qquad (2)$$

The descriptions of variables and parameters of model (1) are as follows.

Variable

$N(t)$: Total population
$S(t)$: Population of susceptible individuals
$A(t)$: Population of individuals with acute Hep C
$C(t)$: Population of individuals with chronic Hep C
$Q(t)$: Population of isolated individuals
$R(t)$: Population of recovered individuals.

Parameter

Π: Recruitment rate
μ: Natural death rate
δ_a: Disease-induced death rate for individuals with acute Hep C
δ_c: Disease-induced death rate for individuals with chronic Hep C
δ_q: Disease-induced death rate for isolated individuals
γ: Recovery rate of isolations
f: Fraction of isolated that becomes susceptible
ξ: Progression rate from acute to chronic
α: Isolation rate of chronic individuals
κ: Natural recovery rate for acute individuals
ψ: Recovery rate for chronic individuals
ω: Progression rate of recovered individuals to susceptible individuals
β: Effective contact rate
η: Modification parameter for reduction in infectiousness of acute individuals
ζ: Modification parameter for reduction in infectiousness of quarantined individuals.

Since (1) is a model for human populations, all the associated parameters are nonnegative. Furthermore, the following result holds and can be proved easily.

Lemma 1. *The variables of model (1) are nonnegative for all time $t > 0$. In other words, solutions of the system (1) with positive initial data will exist and remain positive for all $t > 0$. Moreover, the closed set*

$$D = \left\{(S, A, C, Q, R) \in R_+^5 : S + A + C + Q + R \leq \frac{\Pi}{\mu}\right\} \qquad (3)$$

is positively invariant and global attractor.

Since the region D is positively invariant and global attractor, it is sufficient to consider the dynamics of the flow generated by model (1) (Figure 1) in region D, where the model is considered to be epidemiologically and mathematically well posed.

2.2. Disease-Free Equilibrium (DFE). In this section, we discuss the existence and stability of the disease-free equilibrium (DFE).

2.2.1. Local Stability. Model (1) has a disease-free equilibrium DFE, obtained by setting the right-hand sides of the equations in (1) to zero, given by

$$\aleph_0 = (S^*, A^*, C^*, Q^*, R^*) = \left(\frac{\Pi}{\mu}, 0, 0, 0, 0\right). \qquad (4)$$

The local stability property of $\aleph_0$ will be determined using the next generation operator method described in [26].

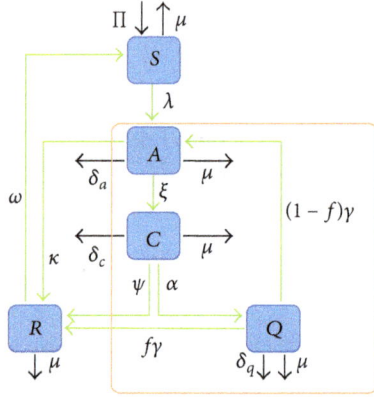

FIGURE 1: Schematic diagram of model (1).

The nonnegative matrix F, of the new infection terms, and the M-matrix, V, of the transition terms associated with model (1), are given by

$$F = \begin{pmatrix} \beta\eta & \beta & \beta\zeta \\ 0 & 0 & 0 \\ 0 & 0 & 0 \end{pmatrix},$$

$$V = \begin{pmatrix} \xi + \kappa + \mu + \delta_a & 0 & -\gamma(1-f) \\ -\xi & \alpha + \psi + \mu + \delta_c & 0 \\ 0 & -\alpha & \gamma + \mu + \delta_q \end{pmatrix}. \tag{5}$$

The eigenvalues of matrix FV^{-1} are

$$\left\{ 0, 0, \frac{\beta\left[\eta k_2 k_3 + \xi k_3 + \zeta\alpha\xi\right]}{k_1 k_2 k_3 - \alpha\xi k_4} \right\}. \tag{6}$$

It follows that the basic reproduction number $R_0 = \rho(FV^{-1})$ is given by

$$R_0 = \frac{\beta\left[\eta k_2 k_3 + \xi k_3 + \zeta\alpha\xi\right]}{k_1 k_2 k_3 - \alpha\xi k_4} > 0, \tag{7}$$

where

$$\begin{aligned} k_1 &= \left(\xi + \kappa + \mu + \delta_a\right), \\ k_2 &= \left(\alpha + \psi + \mu + \delta_c\right), \\ k_3 &= \left(\gamma + \mu + \delta_q\right), \\ k_4 &= \gamma(1-f). \end{aligned} \tag{8}$$

The basic reproduction number is interpreted as the average number of new infections that one infectious individual can produce if introduced into a population composed of susceptible individuals. Susceptible individuals acquire infection following contact with either an acute (A), chronic (C), or isolated (Q) individual. The number of infections produced by an acutely infected individual (near the DFE) is $\beta\eta/k_1$ given by the product of the infection rate of an acute individual ($\beta\eta$) and the average duration in the acute class ($1/k_1$). Furthermore, the number of infections

produced by a chronically infected individual (near the DFE) is $\beta\xi/k_1 k_2$ given by the product of the infection rate of a chronic individual (β), the average duration in the chronic C class ($1/k_2$), and the probability that an acute individual survives and progresses to the chronic stage ξ/k_1. Similarly, the number of infections produced by an isolated individual (near the DFE) is $\beta\zeta\xi\alpha/k_1 k_2 k_3$ given by the product of the infection rate of an isolated individual ($\beta\zeta$), the average duration in the isolated class ($1/k_3$), and the probability that an acute individual survives and progresses to the isolated stage $\xi\alpha/k_1 k_2$. Finally, we observe that a fraction $\xi\alpha\gamma(1-f)/k_1 k_2 k_3$ of newly infected individuals will reenter the acute class. Thus, the average number of new infections generated by a single infectious individual is given by

$$\left(\frac{\beta\eta}{k_1} + \frac{\beta\xi}{k_1 k_2} + \frac{\beta\zeta\xi\alpha}{k_1 k_2 k_3}\right)\sum_{n=0}^{\infty}\left[\frac{\xi\alpha\gamma(1-f)}{k_1 k_2 k_3}\right]^n$$

$$= \left(\frac{\beta\eta}{k_1} + \frac{\beta\xi}{k_1 k_2} + \frac{\beta\zeta\xi\alpha}{k_1 k_2 k_3}\right)\left[\frac{1}{1 - (\xi\alpha\gamma(1-f)/k_1 k_2 k_3)}\right]$$

$$= R_0. \tag{9}$$

The local stability of the DFE holds due to Theorem 2 of [26].

Lemma 2. *The DFE, $\aleph_0$, of model (1) is locally asymptotically stable if $R_0 < 1$ and unstable if $R_0 > 1$.*

Lemma 2.2 implies that with $R_0 < 1$, a small influx of infectious individuals will not lead to a large outbreak of the disease. To ensure that disease elimination is independent of the initial sizes of subpopulations, it is necessary to show that the DFE is globally asymptotically stable if $R_0 < 1$. This is explored below.

2.2.2. Global Stability

Theorem 3. *The DFE of model (1), given by (4), is globally asymptotically stable whenever $R_0 \leq 1$.*

Proof. Consider the following Lyapunov function:

$$L = aA + cC + qQ, \tag{10}$$

where

$$a = \frac{k_2 k_3}{k_1 k_2 k_3 - \alpha\xi k_4},$$

$$c = \frac{\beta k_3 + \alpha\left[\beta\zeta + k_4\right]}{k_1 k_2 k_3 - \alpha\xi k_4}, \tag{11}$$

$$q = \frac{k_2\left[\beta\zeta + k_4\right]}{k_1 k_2 k_3 - \alpha_\xi k_4}.$$

Clearly L is positive definite. We have

$$\dot{L} = a\,\dot{A} + c\,\dot{C} + q\,\dot{Q}$$

$$= a\lambda S + ak_4 Q - ak_1 A + c\xi A - qk_3 Q + q\alpha C - ck_2 C$$

$$= a\beta\frac{[\eta A + C + \zeta Q]}{N}S + [ak_4 - qk_3]Q$$

$$\quad + [c\xi - ak_1]A + [q\alpha - ck_2]C$$

$$\leq [a\beta\eta + c\xi - ak_1]A + [a\beta + q\alpha - ck_2]C$$

$$\quad + [a\beta\zeta + ak_4 - qk_3]Q$$

$$= \frac{[\beta\eta k_2 k_3 + \xi\beta k_3 + \xi\alpha\beta\zeta + \xi\alpha\beta k_4 - k_1 k_2 k_3]}{k_1 k_2 k_3 - \alpha\xi k_4}A$$

$$\quad + \frac{[k_2 k_3 \beta + \alpha k_2 \beta\zeta + \alpha k_2 k_4 - \beta k_3 k_2 - \alpha k_2 \beta\zeta - \alpha k_2 k_4]}{k_1 k_2 k_3 - \alpha\xi k_4}C$$

$$\quad + \frac{[k_2 k_3 \beta\zeta + k_2 k_3 k_4 - k_2 k_3 \beta\zeta - k_2 k_3 k_4]}{k_1 k_2 k_3 - \alpha\xi k_4}Q$$

$$= (R_0 - 1)A.$$

$$(12)$$

Thus,

$$\dot{L} \leq (R_0 - 1)A \leq 0, \quad \text{for } R_0 < 1. \tag{13}$$

It follows that $\dot{L} \leq 0$ for $R_0 < 1$ with $\dot{L} = 0$ if and only if $A = C = Q = 0$ or $R_0 = 1$. Hence, L is a Lyapunov function on D.

The largest invariant set in $\{(S, A, C, Q, R) \in D \mid \dot{L} = 0\}$ is the singleton $\{\aleph_0\}$. According to the LaSalle Invariance Principle, $\aleph_0$ is globally asymptotically stable in D if $R_0 < 1$. This means that, with $R_0 < 1$, every solution to the system (1) with initial conditions in D approaches $\aleph_0$ as $t \rightarrow \infty$:

$$(S, A, C, Q, R) \longrightarrow \aleph_0 = \left(\frac{\Pi}{\mu}, 0, 0, 0, 0\right) \quad \text{as } t \longrightarrow \infty.$$

$$(14)$$

$\square$

The epidemiological implication of the above result is that the disease can be eliminated from the population if the basic reproduction number R_0 can be brought down to and maintained at a value less than unity (i.e., the condition $R_0 < 1$ is sufficient and necessary for disease elimination). Figure 2 depicts numerical results by simulating model (1) using various initial conditions with $R_0 < 1$. It is evident from the simulation that all initial solutions converged to DFE, $\aleph_0$, in-line with Theorem 3.

2.3. Endemic Equilibrium. In this section the existence and stability of endemic equilibrium of model (1) will be discussed. We define endemic equilibrium to be those fixed points of the system (1) in which at least one of the infected compartments of the model is nonzero.

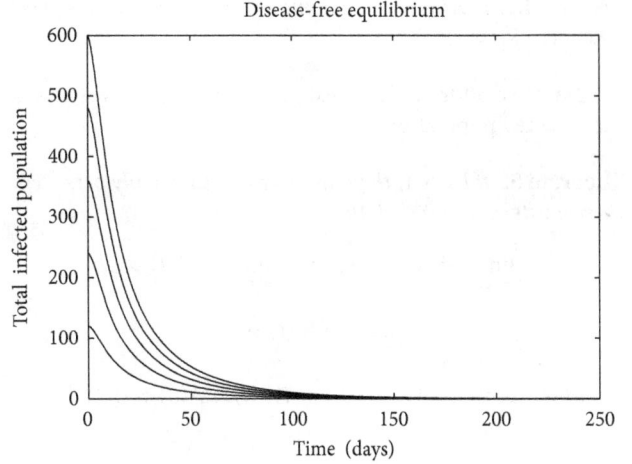

FIGURE 2: Disease-free equilibrium: $R_0 = 0.7994$. Simulation shows the total infected population with different initial infected population sizes. The parameter values are given in the appendix.

Let $\aleph_1 = (S^{**}, A^{**}, C^{**}, Q^{**}, R^{**})$ denote an arbitrary endemic equilibrium of model (1) so that $N^{**} = S^{**} + A^{**} + C^{**} + Q^{**} + R^{**}$. Solving the equations of model (1) at steady state gives

$$A^{**} = \frac{k_2}{\xi}C^{**},$$

$$Q^{**} = \frac{\alpha}{k_3}C^{**},$$

$$S^{**} = \frac{1}{\lambda^{**}}\left(\frac{k_1 k_2 k_3 - \alpha\xi k_4}{\xi k_3}\right)C^{**}, \tag{15}$$

$$R^{**} = \frac{1}{k_5}\left(\frac{f\gamma\alpha}{k_3} + \frac{\kappa k_2}{\xi} + \psi\right)C^{**},$$

where

$$\lambda^{**} = \beta\frac{[\eta A^{**} + C^{**} + \zeta Q^{**}]}{N^{**}}, \quad k_5 = (\omega + \mu). \tag{16}$$

Consider S^{**}. Then, using λ^{**} and (15) from above we have the following endemic states:

$$A^{**} = \frac{k_2}{\xi}\left[\frac{R_0 - 1}{Y}\right]S^{**},$$

$$C^{**} = \left[\frac{R_0 - 1}{Y}\right]S^{**},$$

$$Q^{**} = \frac{\alpha}{k_3}\left[\frac{R_0 - 1}{Y}\right]S^{**},$$

$$R^{**} = \frac{1}{k_5}\left[\frac{k_2 k_3 + k_3\kappa\xi + \gamma f\alpha k_2}{k_2 k_3}\right]\left[\frac{R_0 - 1}{Y}\right]S^{**},$$

$$(17)$$

where

$$Y = \left[\frac{k_2}{\xi} + 1 + \frac{\alpha}{k_3}\right]. \tag{18}$$

Hence, we have the following result.

Lemma 4. *Model* (1) *has endemic equilibria, given by* $\aleph_1$ (15), *whenever* $R_0 > 1$.

Now, we address the question of uniform persistence of the infected population.

Theorem 5. *If* $R_0 > 1$, *then the disease is uniformly persistent: there exists an* $\epsilon > 0$ *such that*

$$\lim_{t \to \infty} \inf A(t) > \epsilon, \qquad \lim_{t \to \infty} \inf C(t) > \epsilon,$$

$$\lim_{t \to \infty} \inf Q(t) > \epsilon, \tag{19}$$

for all solutions (S, A, C, Q, R) *of* (1) *with* $A(0) > 0$, $C(0) > 0$, *and* $Q(0) > 0$.

Proof. Let $X = \{(S, A, C, Q, R) \in R_+^5 : A = C = Q = 0\}$. Thus, X is the set of all disease-free states of (1) and it can be easily verified that X is positively invariant. Let $M = D \cap X$. Since both D and X are positively invariant, M is also positively invariant. Also note that $\aleph_0 \in M$ and $\aleph_0$ attracts all the solutions in X. So, $\Omega(M) = \{\aleph_0\}$. The equations for the infected components of (1) can be written as

$$x'(t) = Y(x) x(t), \tag{20}$$

where $x(t) = (A(t), C(t), Q(t))^T$, $Y(x) = [(S/N)F - V]$. It is clear that $Y(\aleph_0) = F - V$. Also it is easy to check that $Y(\aleph_0)$ is irreducible. We will apply Lemma A.4 in [27] to show that M is a uniform weak repeller. Since $\aleph_0$ is a steady state solution, we can consider it to be a periodic orbit of period $T = 1$. $P(t, x)$, the fundamental matrix of the solutions for (20), is e^{tY}. Since the spectral radius of $Y(\aleph_0) = R_0 > 1$, the spectral radius of $e^{Y(\aleph_0)} > 1$. So condition 2 of Lemma A.4 is satisfied. Taking $x = \aleph_0$, we get $P(T, \aleph_0) = e^{Y(\aleph_0)}$ which is a primitive matrix, because $Y(\aleph_0)$ is irreducible, as mentioned in Theorem A.12(i) [28]. This satisfies the condition 1 of Lemma A.4. Thus, M is a uniform weak repeller and disease is weakly persistent. M is trivially closed and bounded relative to D and hence, compact. Therefore, by Theorem 1.3 [29], we have that M is a uniform strong repeller and disease is uniformly persistent. $\square$

The epidemiological implication of Theorem 5 is that the disease will persist in the population whenever $R_0 > 1$. Numerical simulation results, depicted in Figure 3 using different initial conditions, shows convergence of solutions to the $\aleph_1$ in-line with Theorem 5.

2.4. Sensitivity Analysis. The asymptotic dynamics of the model are completely determined by the threshold quantity R_0, which determines the prevalence of the disease. Since we have a deterministic model, the only uncertainty is generated by the input variation and parameters. Therefore, we present parameter-related global uncertainty and sensitivity analyses on R_0. Parameter estimates can be uncertain because of many reasons including natural variation, error in measurements, or a lack of measuring techniques. Uncertainty analysis qualitatively decides which parameters are most influential in

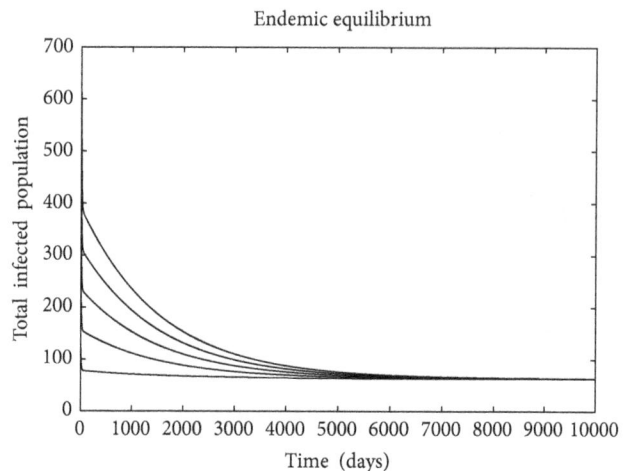

FIGURE 3: Endemic equilibrium: $R_0 = 1.5545$. Simulation shows the total infected population with different initial infected population sizes. The parameter values are given in the appendix.

the model output (R_0 in our case) and quantifies the degree of confidence in the existing data and parameter estimation. On the other hand, the sensitivity analysis identifies critical model parameters and quantifies the impact of each input parameter on the value of an output, in the presence of other input parameters.

Ideally, uncertainty and sensitivity analyses should be performed simultaneously. Here we use the Latin-hypercube sampling based method to quantify uncertainty and sensitivity of R_0 as a function of 12 model parameters (μ, γ, ξ, α, κ, ψ, β, η, ζ, δ_a, δ_c and δ_q). For the sensitivity analysis, partial rank correlation coefficient (PRCC) measures the impact of the parameters on the output variable. PRCC provides a measure of monotonicity after the removal of the linear effects of all but one variable. PRCC method uses the rank transformation of the data (i.e., replacing the values with their ranks) to reduce the effects of nonlinearity. The Rank Correlation Coefficient (RCC) indicates the degree of monotonicity between the input and output variables. The resultant data are considered partially in some sense, that is, partial rank correlation coefficients (PRCC) are computed that take into account the correlations among other input variables. The basic reproduction number R_0 is the output measure in the sensitivity and uncertainty analyses.

The assumed distributions of the model parameters used in the two analyses are mentioned in the appendix. Our estimate of R_0 for Hep C from uncertainty analysis is 1.33 with 95% CI (1.1, 1.95) as shown in Figure 4. The probability that $R_0 > 1$ is 90%. This suggests that Hep C will get endemic under the preset conditions. However, the time taken to reach that state could be large.

The sensitivity analysis suggests that the most significant (PRCC values above 0.5 or below −0.5 in Figure 5) sensitivity parameters to R_0 are α, κ, β, and ζ. This suggests that these parameters need to be estimated with precision to capture the transmission dynamics of the Hep C. The analyses further suggest that the isolation strategy aimed to reduce the infected population yields the desired result.

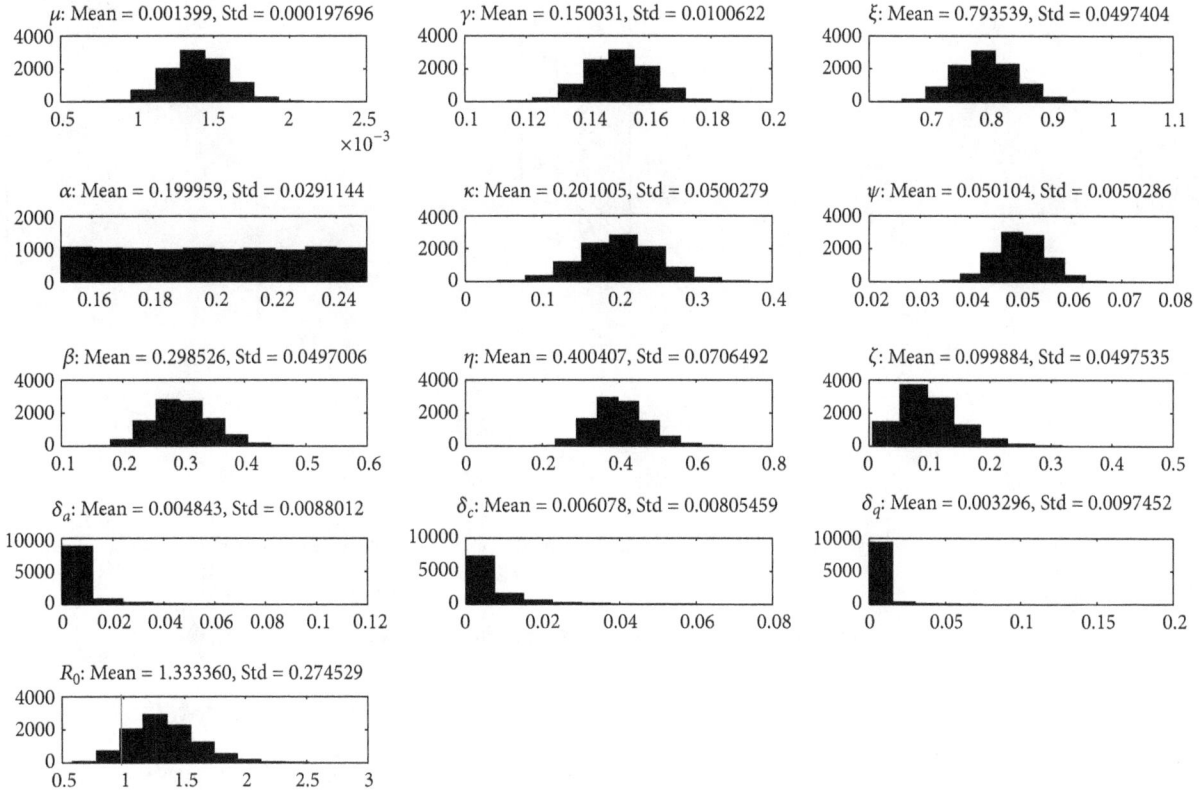

FIGURE 4: Uncertainty analysis: the probability that $R_0 > 1$ is 90% with 95% confidence interval (1.1, 1.95). This suggests that hepatitis C will get endemic under the present conditions. However, the time taken to reach that state could be large. 10000 values were generated for each parameter according to their distributions and mean values. Values of parameters given in Appendix were used to calculate R_0.

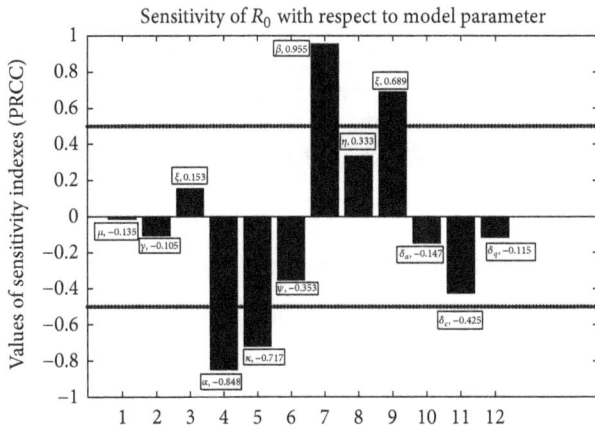

FIGURE 5: Sensitivity analysis: the proportion of chronically infected being quarantined α, proportion of acute infections recovering spontaneously κ_1, effective contact rate β, and modification parameter for infectiousness of quarantined ζ are the most significant parameters. This means that even a small error in the estimation of these parameters can greatly affect the value of R_0 and hence the analysis of our model. Partial rank correlation coefficients (PRCC) are calculated with respect to R_0. Parameters with modulus of PRCC values in excess of 0.5 are declared sensitive to R_0.

Since we are interested in the influence of critical model parameters on the basic reproductive number and hence the prevalence of chronic Hep C, we conduct numerical simulation to investigate it. In order to qualitatively measure the effect of isolation on the transmission dynamics of Hep C, a threshold analysis of the parameter associated with the isolation of chronically infected individuals is discussed (α). We computed the partial derivative of R_0 with respect to this parameter.

For the case of the isolation of chronically infected individuals, it is easy to see that

$$\frac{\partial R_0}{\partial \alpha} = ((\beta \eta k_1 + \beta \zeta \xi)(k_1 k_2 k_3 - \alpha \xi k_4)$$
$$- \beta (\eta k_1 k_2 + \xi k_3 + \zeta \alpha \xi)(k_1 k_3 - \xi k_4))$$
$$\times ((k_1 k_2 k_3 - \alpha \xi k_4)^2)^{-1}$$

(21)

which simplifies to

$$\frac{\partial R_0}{\partial \alpha} = \beta \xi k_1 k_3 \left[\zeta (k_2 - \alpha) + \frac{\eta k_4 (k_2 - \alpha)}{k_3} + \frac{\xi k_4}{k_1} - k_3 \right],$$

(22)

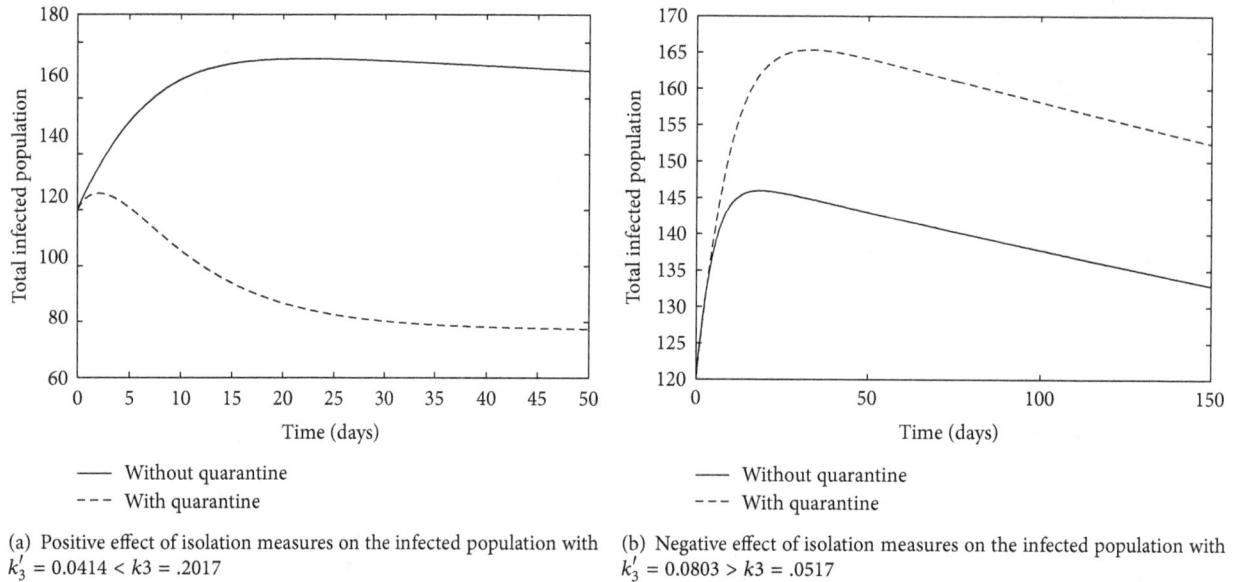

(a) Positive effect of isolation measures on the infected population with $k_3' = 0.0414 < k3 = .2017$

(b) Negative effect of isolation measures on the infected population with $k_3' = 0.0803 > k3 = .0517$

FIGURE 6: Effect of isolation on the infected population.

where

$$k_2 - \alpha = \psi + \mu + \delta_c > 0. \tag{23}$$

Now we have

$$\frac{\partial R_0}{\partial \alpha} < 0 (> 0) \quad \text{iff } k_3' < k_3 (> k_3), \tag{24}$$

where

$$k_3' = \zeta (k_2 - \alpha) + \frac{\eta k_4 (k_2 - \alpha)}{k_3} + \frac{\xi k_4}{k_1} > 0. \tag{25}$$

Thus, the isolation of chronically infected individuals will reduce R_0 and, therefore, reduce disease burden (new infections, mortality, etc.) if k_3' does not exceed the threshold k_3 (which is the rate of transfer of individuals out of the isolation state). This case is presented in Figure 6(a).

On the other hand, if $k_3' > k_3$, then the use of isolation (of chronically infected individuals) will increase R_0, and, consequently, increase disease burden (hence, the use of isolation is detrimental to the community in this case). This case is presented in Figure 6(b). This important result is summarized below.

Lemma 6. *The use of isolation of the chronically infected individuals will have positive (negative) population-level impact if $k_3' < (>)k_3$.*

Now we present the simulations of the critical parameters (as identified by sensitivity analysis) and R_0. Figure 7 presents the dependence of the basic reproductive number on the parameters α and ξ, where α denotes the isolation rate of chronic and ξ denotes the progression rate to chronic from acute. From the contour plot, we see that if ξ is larger, then R_0

is always greater than one, which implies that it is important to control the acute Hep C. Figure 7(b) shows that the basic reproductive number may be less than one if α and ξ can be restricted to a range, leading to the potential extinction of the disease.

The dependence of basic reproductive number R_0 on the recovery rate κ, isolation rate α, and effective contact rate is explored in Figure 8. From Figure 8(a), it is clear that high isolation rate with low effective contact will result in smaller value of R_0. Furthermore, R_0 is very sensitive to β and basic reproductive number increases sharply when β is slightly increased. Therefore, keeping the effective contact rate low will result in disease extinction. In Figure 8(b), larger recovery rate of chronic individuals κ results in smaller values of R_0. However, still the R_0 increases as β increases but smoothly and not sharply as seen in Figure 8(a).

3. Optimal Control Strategies

Pontryagin and Boltyanskii [30] formulated the optimal control theory for models with underlying dynamics defined by a system of ordinary differential equations. The theory, application areas, and the numerical methods have progressed considerably. Pontryagin's Maximum Principle allows us to adjust the control in a model to achieve the desired results. The control parameters are mostly functions of time appearing as coefficients in the model.

Optimal control theory has been employed to make decisions involving epidemic and biological models. The desired results and performance of the control functions depend on the different situations. Lenhart's HIV models [21, 22] used optimal control to design the treatment strategies. Jung et al.

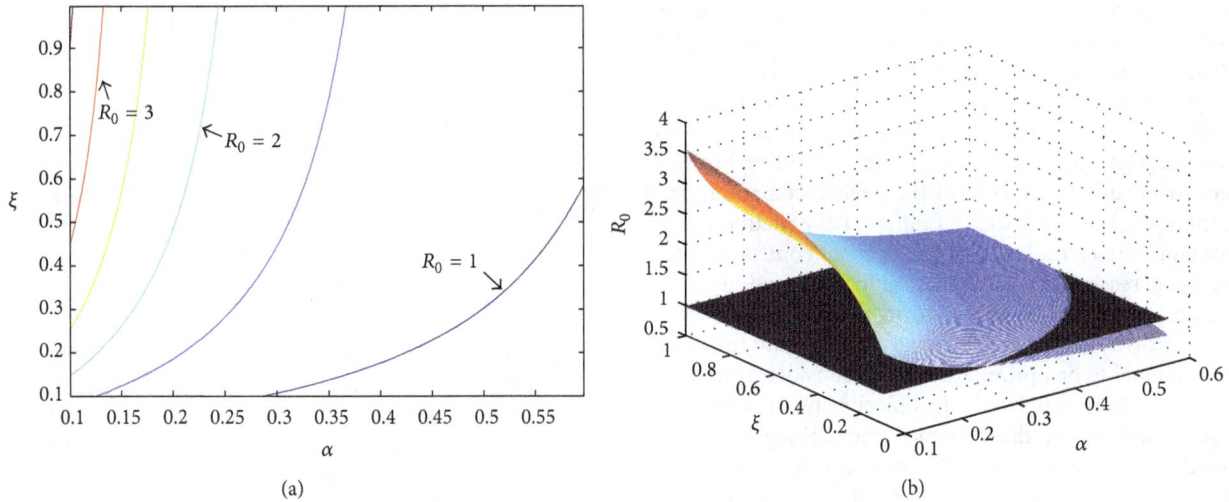

FIGURE 7: Plots of the basic reproductive number R_0 in terms of the parameters α and ξ, which show the estimated effects of α and ξ on R_0. (a) A contour plot of the surface R_0 for the values of $R_0 = 1, 2, 3$. (b) Two surfaces, R_0 and the constant 1, are plotted to show the curve on which $R_0 = 1$.

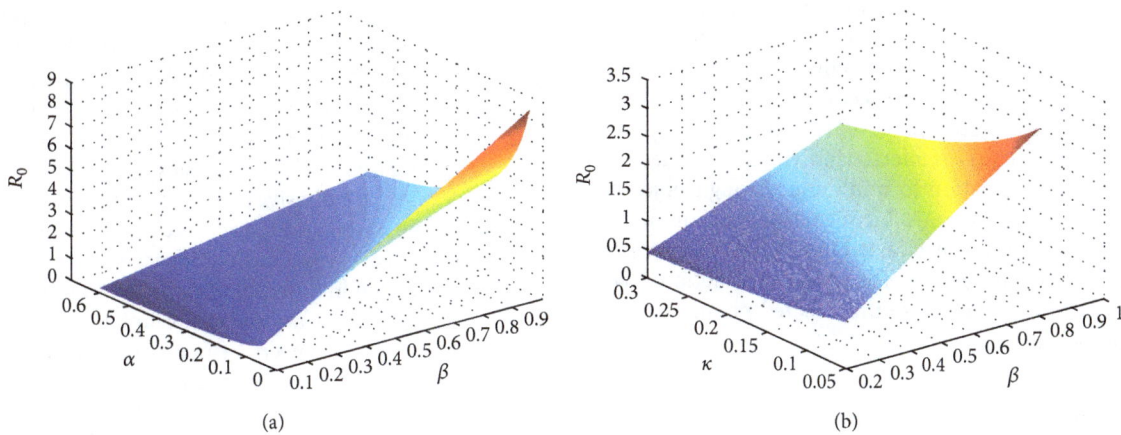

FIGURE 8: Plots of the basic reproductive number R_0 in terms of the parameters β, α, and κ, which show the effects of β, α, and κ on R_0. (a) Effect of isolation rate α and effective contact rate β on the R_0. (b) Effect of recovery rate of chronic κ and effective contact rate β on the R_0.

[23] provide a very good example of deciding how to divide the efforts between two treatment strategies (case holding and case finding) of the two-strain TB model. Yan et al. [24] used an optimal isolation strategy to fight the SARS epidemic. In [31] Joshi formulated two control functions as coefficients of the ODE system representing treatment effects in a two-drug regime in an HIV immunology model. The goal was to maximize the concentration of T cells while minimizing the toxic effects of the drug. The analytic and numerical results illustrated the level of two drugs to be used over the chosen time interval. The required balancing effect between two competing goals was well predicted by optimal control theory. Behncke [32] studied SIR models including vaccination, isolation, and health promotion campaign and obtained analytical results for optimal control. The optimal

control intervention policies for stochastic epidemic models were treated by Clancy [33].

Pontryagin's Maximum Principle appends an adjoint system of differential equations with terminal boundary conditions to the original model (state system) of differential equations, in the attempt to characterize an optimal control. The optimality system, which characterizes the optimal controls, consists of the differential equations of the original model (state system) along with the adjoint differential equations (adjoint system). The adjoint system has the same number of equations as in the state system. The adjoint functions behave very similar to the Lagrange multipliers (appending constraints to the function of several variables to be maximized or minimized). The adjoint variables maximize or minimize the state variables with respect to the desired objective functional. The details of the necessary conditions for the adjoint and optimal controls are presented here [30, 34, 35]. For the application of these results see [21].

Optimal control techniques are used to optimize the models given by system of differential equations. While formulating an optimal control problem, deciding how and where to introduce the control (through vaccination, drug treatment etc.) in the system of differential equation is very important. The formulation of the optimal control problem must be a reasonable and practical representation of the situation to be considered. The form of the optimal control depends heavily on the system being analyzed and the objective functional to be optimized. We will consider a quadratic dependence on the control in the objective functional.

The questions of the existence and uniqueness of the optimal control in an optimality system can be dealt with using the Lipschitz properties of the differential equations [30, 34]. For a detailed example, see the work of Fister et al. [21] and Fleming and Rishel [34]. After establishing the existence and the uniqueness results, we can confidently continue to numerically solve the optimality system to get the desired optimal control.

In this section, we consider two different time-dependent control strategies to prevent and control the spread of Hep C in the population. The first strategy is to introduce vaccination to our population and see the effects on the prevalence of the Hep C. We introduce a vaccination control, which is a function of time, in our model of differential equations to minimize the population of infected individual while keeping the cost of the vaccination to minimum through objective functional. Next strategy introduces control function for the isolation rate of chronically infected individuals to minimize the total infected population. The objective functional was designed carefully to minimize the infected population and the cost of the isolation facility.

3.1. Vaccination Control. The use of vaccination is an important disease control and prevention measure. Optimal vaccination control strategy for an SIR model has been devised using dynamic programming technique [36]. Also the optimal control strategies have been investigated for TB control [23, 37]. We have analyzed the dynamics of the model without vaccination in the last section which had a locally stable equilibrium. In this section we will explore the effects of a vaccination campaign on our deterministic model of Hep C by including vaccination. After including vaccination the model is given as follows:

$$\frac{dS}{dt} = \Pi + \omega R - \lambda (1 - v) S - (1 - \sigma) \lambda v S - \mu S - \sigma v S,$$

$$\frac{dA}{dt} = \lambda (1 - v) S + (1 - \sigma) \lambda v S$$
$$+ \gamma (1 - f) Q - (\xi + \kappa + \mu + \delta_a) A,$$

$$\frac{dC}{dt} = \xi A - (\alpha + \psi_1 + \mu + \delta_c) C,$$

$$\frac{dQ}{dt} = \alpha C - (\gamma + \mu + \delta_q) Q,$$

$$\frac{dR}{dt} = \gamma f Q + \psi C + \kappa A - (\omega + \mu) R,$$

(26)

where

$$\lambda = \frac{\beta (\eta A + C + \zeta Q)}{N}.$$ (27)

In addition to the dynamics of the original model (1), now the susceptible population is being vaccinated at per capita rate v (vaccine coverage rate). The vaccination rate v includes both the medical inoculation and the educational campaigns to prevent Hep C. We also have to consider the partial efficiency of the vaccine, due to which only σ ($0 \le \sigma \le 1$) fraction of the vaccinated susceptible individuals go to the recovered class (σ is the vaccine efficacy). The remaining $(1 - \sigma)$ fraction of the vaccinated susceptible individuals goes to the acute class as a result of their contact with the infected individuals. When $\sigma = 0$, it means that the vaccine has no effect at all and when $\sigma = 1$, the vaccine is perfectly effective.

It is well understood that in order to eradicate an epidemic we have to vaccinate a large fraction of the susceptible population. Take the example of smallpox, its eradication was achieved after an intensive worldwide vaccination campaign and a very high vaccination rate [38]. However, in some infectious diseases such as measles and TB, the disease persists despite the extensive usage of vaccine, mainly because of low vaccine efficacy [39] and vaccination campaigns that could not reach everyone. Different vaccination policies have been implemented in different parts of the world. Practically, the cost of vaccine is a very important factor influencing the policy. Hence, we need to find a balance between the rate of vaccinating susceptible individuals and the cost of the vaccination. Now we design an optimal vaccination strategy to minimize an objective functional that takes into account both the cost and the number of infectious individuals. Now let the vaccination rate be given as function of time $v(t)$ in model (26). The control set **V** is

$$\mathbf{V} = \{v(t) : 0 \le v(t) \le b, 0 \le t$$
$$\le T, v(t) \text{ is Lebesgue measurable}\}.$$
(28)

The goal is to minimize the cost function defined as

$$J[v] = \int_0^T P_1 C + P_2 A + P_3 Q + \frac{1}{2} W v^2 (t).$$ (29)

This performance specification involves the numbers of individuals of acute, chronic, and isolated, respectively, as well as the cost of applying vaccination control (v). This cost also includes the cost for organization and management of vaccine and so forth. Hence, the cost function should be nonlinear. In this paper, a quadratic function is implemented for measuring the control cost [21–24]. The coefficients P_1, P_2, P_3, and W are balancing cost factors due to scales and importance of the four parts of the objective function. We need to find an optimal control $v^*(t)$ such that

$$J\left[v^*\right] = \min_{v \in V} J\left[v\right]. \qquad (30)$$

The existence of a solution to the optimal control problem can be obtained by verifying sufficient conditions. We refer to the conditions in Theorem III.4.1 and its corresponding corollary in [34]. The boundedness of solutions to the system (26) for the finite time interval is needed to establish these conditions. Pontryagin's Maximum Principle [30] provides the necessary conditions to be satisfied by the optimal vaccination $v(t)$. This principle reduces (26), (28), and (29) into a problem of minimizing pointwise a Hamiltonian, H, with respect to v:

$$H = P_1 C + P_2 A + P_3 Q + \frac{1}{2} W v^2(t) + \sum_{i=1}^{i=5} \lambda_i k_i, \qquad (31)$$

where k_i represents the right hand side of model's (26) ith differential equation. Using Pontryagin's Maximum principle [30] and the optimal control existence result from [34], we have the following.

Theorem 7. *There exists a unique optimal $v^*(t)$ which minimizes J over* **V***. Also, there exists adjoint system of λ_i's such that*

$$\frac{d\lambda_1}{dt} = \left(\lambda\left(1 - v^*\right) + (1 - \sigma) v^* \lambda + \sigma v^* + \mu\right) \lambda_1$$
$$- \left(\left(1 - v^*\right) \lambda + (1 - \sigma) v^* \lambda\right) \lambda_2,$$
$$\frac{d\lambda_2}{dt} = \left(\frac{\beta\eta\left(1 - v^* + (1 - \sigma) v^*\right) S}{N}\right) \lambda_1$$
$$+ \left(k_1 - \frac{\beta\eta\left(1 - v^* + (1 - \sigma) v^*\right) S}{N}\right) \lambda_2$$
$$- \xi \lambda_3 \lambda_1 - \kappa \lambda_5 - P_2,$$
$$\frac{d\lambda_3}{dt} = \left(\frac{\beta\left(1 - v^* + (1 - \sigma) v^*\right) S}{N}\right) \lambda_1$$
$$- \frac{\beta\left(1 - v^* + (1 - \sigma) v^*\right) S}{N} \lambda_2$$
$$+ k_2 \lambda_3 - \alpha \lambda_4 - \psi \lambda_5 - P_1,$$
$$\frac{d\lambda_4}{dt} = \left(\frac{\beta\zeta\left(1 - v^* + (1 - \sigma) v^*\right) S}{N}\right) \lambda_1$$
$$- \left(k_4 + \frac{\beta\zeta\left(1 - v^* + (1 - \sigma) v^*\right) S}{N}\right) \lambda_2$$
$$+ k_3 \lambda_4 - \gamma f \lambda_5 - P_3, \qquad (32)$$

$$\frac{d\lambda_5}{dt} = \omega \lambda_1 + k_5 \lambda_5,$$
$$k_1 = \left(\xi + \kappa + \mu + \delta_a\right), \qquad k_2 = \left(\alpha + \psi_1 + \mu + \delta_c\right),$$
$$k_3 = \left(\gamma + \mu + \delta_q\right), \qquad k_4 = \gamma\left(1 - f\right),$$
$$k_5 = \left(\omega + \mu\right). \qquad (33)$$

The transversality condition gives

$$\lambda_i\left(T\right) = 0. \qquad (34)$$

The vaccination control is characterized as

$$v^*\left(t\right)$$
$$= \min\left[b, \max\left(0, \frac{S}{W}\left(\lambda\lambda_1\left(1 - \sigma\right) + \sigma\lambda_1 + \lambda\lambda_2\right.\right.\right. \qquad (35)$$
$$\left.\left.\left. - \lambda\lambda_1 - \lambda\lambda_2\left(1 - \sigma\right)\right)\right)\right].$$

Proof. Clearly the integrand of J is convex with respect to $v(t)$. Also the solutions of (26) are bounded as $N(t) \le \Pi/\mu$ for all time. Also it is easily verifiable that the state system (26) has the Lipschitz property with respect to the state variables. With these properties and using Corollary 4.1 of [34], we have the existence of the optimal control.

Since we have the existence of the optimal vaccination control, using Pontryagin's Maximum Principle, we obtain

$$\frac{d\lambda_1}{dt} = -\frac{\partial H}{\partial S}, \qquad \lambda_1\left(T\right) = 0,$$
$$\vdots \qquad (36)$$
$$\frac{d\lambda_5}{dt} = -\frac{\partial H}{\partial R}, \qquad \lambda_5\left(T\right) = 0$$

evaluated at the optimal control, which results in the stated adjoint system (32). The optimality condition is

$$\left.\frac{\partial H}{\partial v}\right|_{v^*} = 0. \qquad (37)$$

Therefore, on the set $\{t : 0 < v^*(t) < b\}$, we obtain

$$v^* = \frac{S}{W}\left(\lambda\lambda_1\left(1 - \sigma\right) + \sigma\lambda_1 + \lambda\lambda_2 - \lambda\lambda_1 - \lambda\lambda_2\left(1 - \sigma\right)\right). \qquad (38)$$

Considering the bounds on v^*, we have the characterizations of the optimal control as in (35). Clearly the state and the adjoint functions are bounded. Also it is easily verifiable that state system and adjoint system have Lipschitz structure with respect to the corresponding variables; we obtain the uniqueness of the optimal control for sufficiently small time T [30, 34]. The uniqueness of the optimal control pair follows from the uniqueness of the optimality system, which consists of (26) and (32), with characterizations (35). There is a restriction on the length of the time interval in order

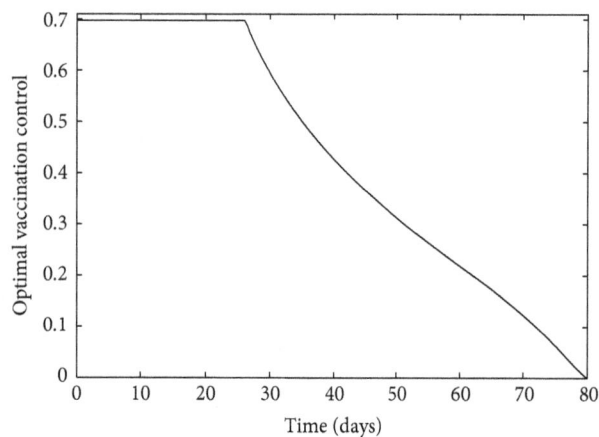

(a) Optimal vaccination control $v(t)$

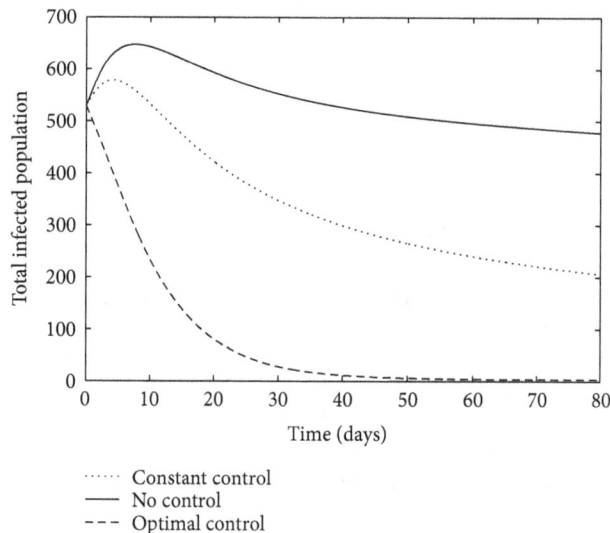

(b) Total infected population with different control strategies

FIGURE 9: Simulations show the optimal vaccination control and its effectiveness. The left simulation presents the vaccination strategy to be followed to prevent the epidemic and disease spread. The right simulation presents comparison of the total chronically infected individuals under optimal and constant control. Clearly optimal strategy prevents the epidemic and retains the infected population to a minimum.

to guarantee the uniqueness of the optimality system. This restriction on the length of the time interval is due to the opposite time orientations of (26) and (32); the state problem has initial values and the adjoint problem has final values. For example, see [21]. This restriction is very common in control problems [22]. ☐

The following optimality system, consisting of 10 equations, characterizes the optimal vaccination control as defined in above theorem. It consists of five equations of (26) with initial condition $\{S(0) = S_0, A(0) = A_0, C(0) = C_0, Q(0) = Q_0, R(0) = R_0\}$ and five equations of (32) with transversality condition $\{\lambda_1(T) = \lambda_2(T) = \lambda_3(T) = \lambda_4(T) = \lambda_5(T) = 0\}$.

Next, we discuss the numerical solutions of the optimality system and the corresponding optimal control pairs and the parameters. The optimal vaccination strategy is obtained by solving the optimality system (26) and (32), consisting of 10 ODEs from the state and adjoint equations. An iterative method is used for solving the optimality system. We start to solve the state equations with a guess for the control $v(t)$ over the simulated time using a forward fourth-order Runge-Kutta scheme. The adjoint functions have final time conditions. Because of this transversality condition on the adjoint functions (32), the adjoint equations are solved by a backward fourth-order Runge-Kutta scheme using the current iteration solution of the state equations. Then, the controls are updated by using a convex combination of the previous control and the value from the characterizations in (35). This process is repeated and iteration is stopped if the values of unknowns at the previous iteration are very close to the ones at the present iteration.

Numerical solutions to the optimal system (26) and (32) are carried out using MATLAB and are presented here. The parameter values and the initial conditions are given in the appendix. The parameter values used have $R_0 > 1$ when the model without control is considered. Thus, the disease is not expected to die out without intervention strategies.

Figure 9(a) represents the control strategy to be employed for the optimal results. This control strategy minimizes both the cost and the infected population ($A + C + Q$). It is well understood that in order to eradicate an epidemic, a large fraction of susceptible population needs to be vaccinated. Therefore, an upper bound of $b = 0.7$ was chosen for vaccination control $v(t)$. The optimal control v is at its upper bound during the first 60 days and then v is steadily decreasing to 0. In fact, at the beginning of simulated time, the optimal control is staying at its upper bound in order to vaccinate as many susceptible individuals as possible to prevent the individuals from getting infected. The steady decrease of the v is determined by the balance between the cost of the infected individuals and the cost of the controls. Figure 9(b) shows the total infected population for the optimal vaccination control, constant vaccination, and without control. It is easy to see that the optimal control is much more effective for reducing the number of infected individuals and decreasing the time-span of the epidemic. As normally expected, in the early phase of the epidemic breakouts, keeping the vaccination controls at their upper bound will directly lead to the decrease of the number of the infected people.

Figure 10 shows the cost associated with the optimal and constant control strategy. It is clear that the cost of optimal strategy is much less than the cost of constant strategy. In fact the costs differ by order of magnitude of ten. Figure 11 represents the population sizes of the distinct

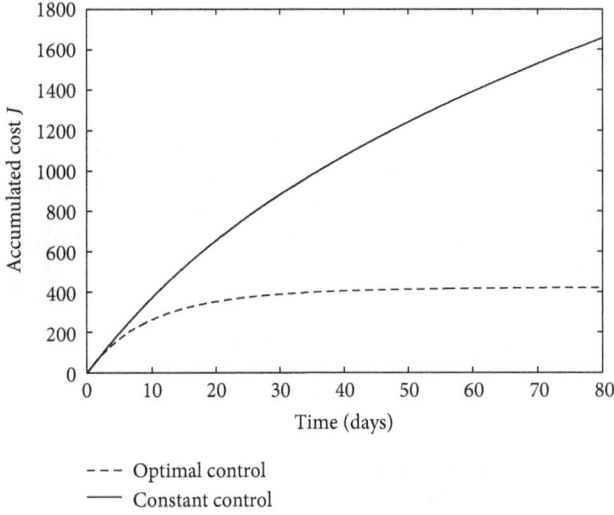

FIGURE 10: Simulation of accumulated cost of different control strategies.

--- Optimal control
— Constant control

infected states (acute, chronic, and isolated) and with optimal control strategy, population sizes go to minimum in short period of time.

3.2. Isolation Control. Several approaches to Hep C vaccine development have now been studied and include synthetic peptides, DNA [40], recombinant E1 and E2 proteins [41], and prime-boost strategies [42]. Success of these approaches has been limited for a number of reasons including: the delivery of a limited number of protective viral epitopes, the inclusion of incorrectly folded recombinant proteins, the limited humoral and cell mediated responses that are associated with DNA vaccines, and the use of adjuvants with relatively poor potency. It is also now apparent that vaccine inducing strong T cell responses alone may not be sufficient to prevent hepatitis C infection [40]. An effective preventive vaccine against Hep C will, therefore, need to induce strong neutralizing and cellular immune responses [7].

Since an effective vaccine is not available against all the genotypes of Hep C, we have to look for alternate strategies to control the spread of Hep C. The quarantine and isolation of those individuals with disease symptoms constitute what is probably the first infection control measure since the beginning of recorded human history [14]. In our model of Hep C, the isolation compartment was introduced to investigate the effect on the infected population size and results were discussed in the last section. Now we can attempt to control the isolation rate of the chronically infected individuals in order to control the Hep C. This section will explore the effects of isolation control rate, of chronically infected individuals, on the total size of the infected population. The model including the required control is as follows:

$$\frac{dS}{dt} = \Pi + \omega R - \lambda S - \mu S,$$

$$\frac{dA}{dt} = \lambda S + \gamma (1 - f) Q - (\xi + \kappa + \mu + \delta_a) A,$$

$$\frac{dC}{dt} = \xi A - (\psi + u_1 + \mu + \delta_c) C,$$

$$\frac{dQ}{dt} = u_1 C - (\gamma + \mu + \delta_q) Q,$$

$$\frac{dR}{dt} = \gamma f Q + \kappa A + \psi C - (\omega + \mu) R,$$

$$(39)$$

where

$$\lambda = \frac{\beta (\eta A + C + \zeta Q)}{N}. \qquad (40)$$

In addition to the dynamics of the original model (1), now we have a control parameter for the isolation rate of the chronically infected individuals labeled as u_1. The control u_1 represents the fraction of the chronically infected individuals that are being isolated in order to decrease the rate of the spread of infection.

Now we design an optimal control strategy to minimize an objective functional that takes into account both the cost and the number of infectious individuals. Now let the isolation rate be $u_1(t)$ for model (39). The control set $\mathbf{U}$ is

$$\mathbf{U} = \{u_1(t) : 0 \le u_1(t) \le b,$$

$$0 \le t \le T, u_1(t) \text{ are Lebesgue measurable}\}. \qquad (41)$$

The objective functional is defined as

$$J[u_1] = \int_0^T P_1 C + P_2 Q + \frac{1}{2} W u_1^2(t), \qquad (42)$$

where we want to minimize the infectious individuals, while also keeping the cost of the isolation facilities low. W_1, P_1, P_2, and P_3 are the weight parameters. We need to find an optimal control $u_1^*(t)$ such that

$$J[u_1^*] = \min_{u_1 \in U} J[u_1]. \qquad (43)$$

Pontryagin's Maximum Principle [30] provides the necessary conditions to be satisfied by the optimal vaccination $v(t)$. This principle reduces (39), (41), and (42) into a problem of minimizing pointwise a Hamiltonian H, with respect to u_1, defined as

$$H = P_1 C + P_2 Q + \frac{1}{2} W u_1^2(t) + \sum_{i=1}^{i=4} \lambda_i k_i, \qquad (44)$$

where k_i represents the right hand side of model's (39) ith differential equation. Using Pontryagin's Maximum Principle [30] and the optimal control existence result from [34], we have the following.

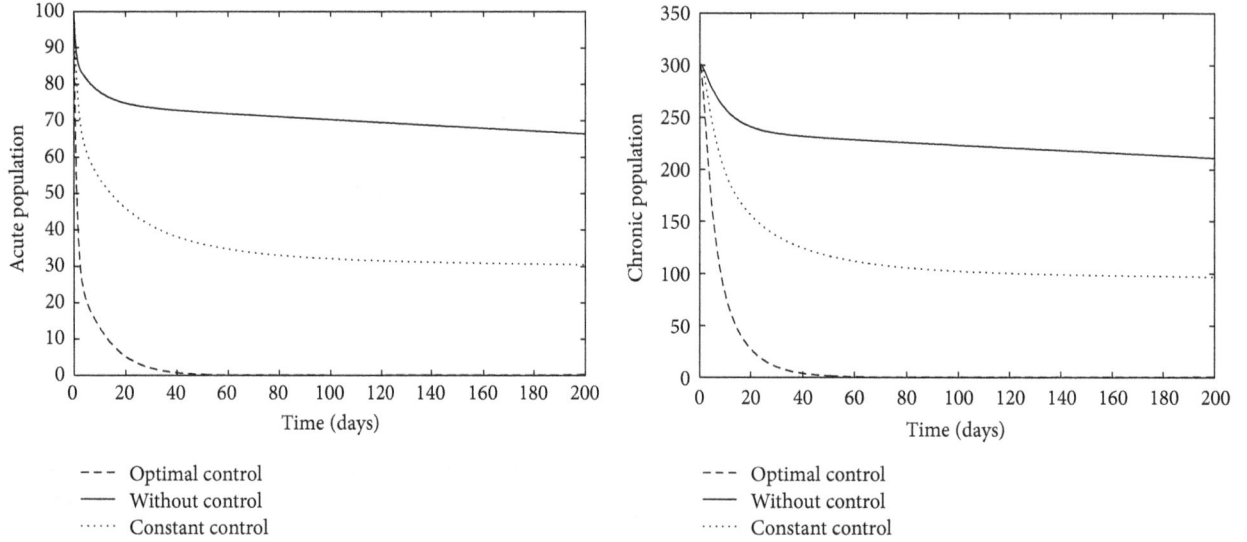

(a) Simulation of acute (Hep C) population with different control strategies

(b) Simulation of chronic (Hep C) population with different control strategies

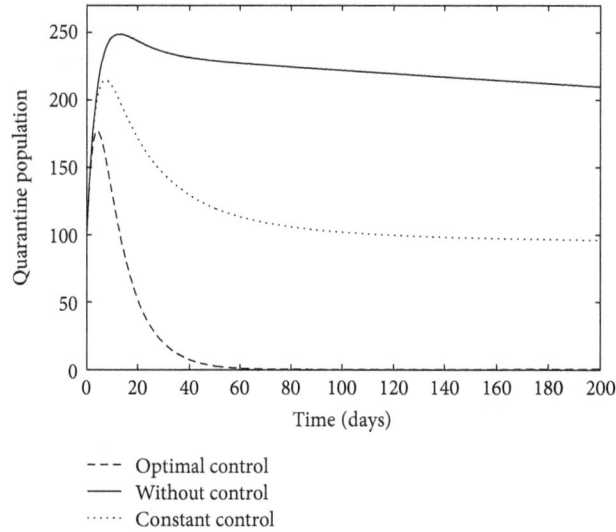

(c) Simulation of isolated population with different control strategies

FIGURE 11: Population sizes of different infected compartments under vaccination strategy. This simulation presents comparison of the total chronically infected, isolated, and acute individuals under optimal and constant control. Clearly optimal strategy prevents the epidemic and retains the infected population to a minimum.

Theorem 8. *There exists a unique optimal control $u_1^*(t)$ which minimizes J over $\mathbf{U}$. Also, there exists adjoint system of λ_i's such that*

$$\frac{d\lambda_1}{dt} = (\lambda + \mu)\lambda_1 - \lambda\lambda_2,$$

$$\frac{d\lambda_2}{dt} = \left(\frac{\beta\eta S}{N}\right)\lambda_1 + \left(k_1 - \frac{\beta\eta S}{N}\right)\lambda_2 - \xi\lambda_3 - \kappa\lambda_5,$$

$$\frac{d\lambda_3}{dt} = \left(\frac{\beta\eta S}{N}\right)\lambda_1 - \frac{\beta S}{N}\lambda_2 + k_2\lambda_3 - u_1^*\lambda_4 - \psi\lambda_5 - P_1,$$

$$\frac{d\lambda_4}{dt} = \left(\frac{\beta\zeta S}{N}\right)\lambda_1 - \left(k_4 + \frac{\beta\zeta S}{N}\right)\lambda_2 + k_3\lambda_4 - \gamma f\lambda_5 - P_2,$$

$$\frac{d\lambda_5}{dt} = \omega\lambda_1 + k_5\lambda_5,$$

(45)

where $k_2 = (u_1 + \psi + \mu + \delta_c)$ and all other k's are given above. The transversality condition is

$$\lambda_i(T) = 0.$$

(46)

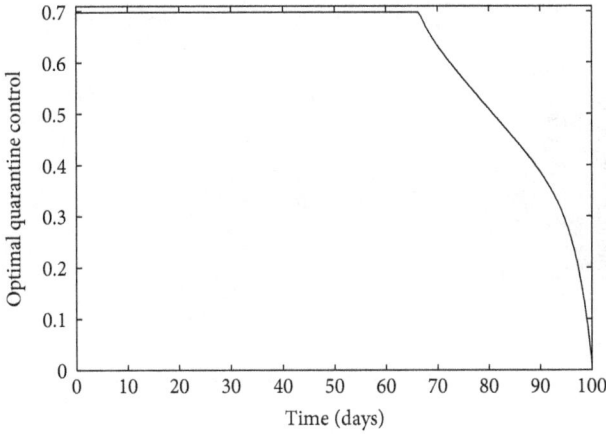

(a) Optimal isolation control $v(t)$

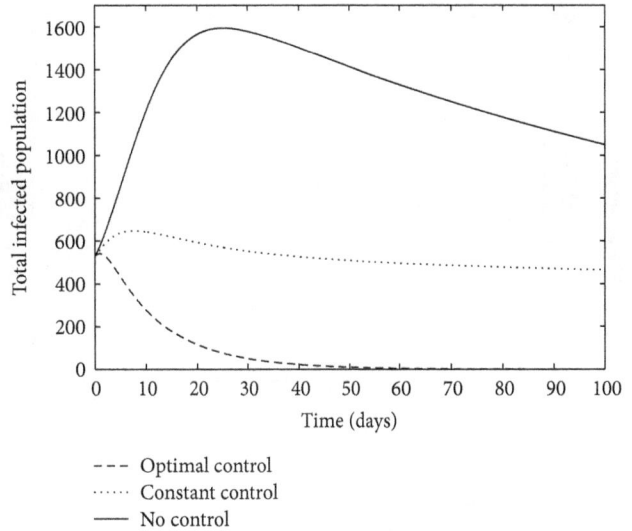

--- Optimal control
······ Constant control
— No control

(b) Total infected population with different control strategies

FIGURE 12: Simulations show the optimal isolation control and its effectiveness. The left simulation presents the isolation strategy to be followed to prevent the epidemic and disease spread. The right simulation presents comparison of the total chronically infected individuals under optimal and constant control. Clearly optimal strategy prevents the epidemic and retains the infected population to a minimum.

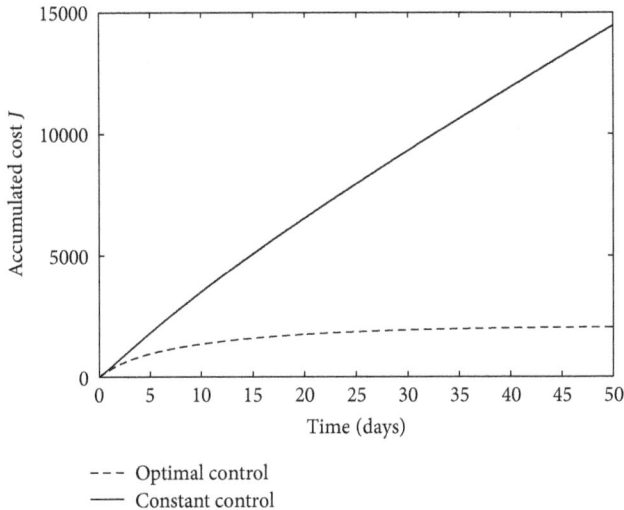

--- Optimal control
— Constant control

FIGURE 13: Accumulated cost of different control strategies: simulation presents comparison of the cost incurred to implement optimal and different constant control strategies to control hepatitis C.

The optimal treatment control pair is characterised as

$$u_1^*(t) = \min\left[b, \max\left(0, \frac{C(\lambda_3 - \lambda_4)}{W}\right)\right]. \quad (47)$$

The proof is identical to the proof of Theorem 7.

In this case the system of 10 differential equations, as stated above, characterizes the optimal treatment control pair, consisting of five equations of system (39) and five equations of system (45).

Now, we discuss the numerical solutions of the optimality system and the corresponding optimal control pair and the parameters. The optimal treatment strategy is obtained by solving the optimality system (39) and (45), consisting of 10 ODEs from the state and adjoint system. The method is discussed in the last section.

Figure 12(a) represents the optimal isolation strategy to be employed to minimize the cost and the infected population. Considering the practical constraints, an upper bound of $b = 0.7$ was chosen for the optimal isolation control $u_1(t)$. The optimal control u_1 is at its upper bound during the first 70 days and then u_1 is steadily decreasing to 0. In fact, at the beginning of simulated time, the optimal control is staying at its upper bound in order to isolate as many chronically infected individuals as possible to prevent the infected population from increasing. The steady decrease of u_1 is determined by the balance between the cost of the infected individuals and the cost of the controls. Figure 12(b) shows the total infected population for the optimal control, constant control, and without control. It is clear that with the use of an optimal control strategy the disease can be eradicated in a short period of time. Figure 13 shows the cost associated with the optimal and constant control strategy. It is clear that the cost of optimal strategy is much less than the cost of constant strategy and in fact differs by order of magnitude of tens. Figure 14 represents the population sizes of the distinct infected states (acute, chronics and isolated) and with optimal control strategy, population sizes go to minimum in short period of time.

4. Conclusions

This paper has discussed the transmission dynamics of the Hep C and eventually formulated an optimal control strategy to prevent disease spread. At first, a deterministic epidemic

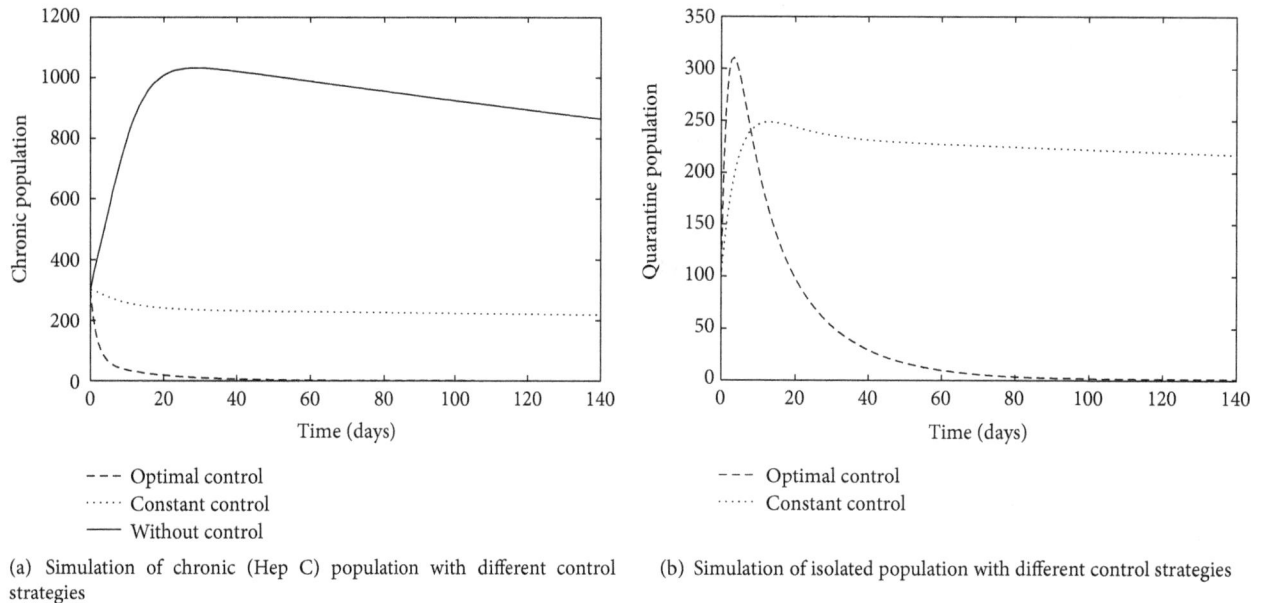

(a) Simulation of chronic (Hep C) population with different control strategies

(b) Simulation of isolated population with different control strategies

FIGURE 14: Population Sizes of different infected compartments under optimal Isolation strategy. Simulation presents comparison of the total chronically infected and isolated individuals under optimal and constant control. Clearly optimal strategy prevents the epidemic and retains the infected population to a minimum.

model for the spread of Hep C, which incorporates the possibility of an isolation state, is formulated. Global analysis of the equilibrium solution is performed. The existence of a disease-free equilibrium and an endemic equilibrium is shown. It is further demonstrated that the disease-free equilibrium is globally asymptotically stable for values of the basic reproduction number (R_0 < 1). The disease uniformly persists when R_0 > 1. In addition, it is shown that the endemic equilibrium is locally asymptotically stable for values of the basic reproduction number (R_0 > 1) assuming constant total population. It is also shown that numerical simulations of the deterministic model agree with the theoretical results. Finally, the sensitivity and uncertainty analyses were performed along with numerical simulations to study the influence of vital parameters on the disease spread.

The model is most sensitive to the control variables α (proportion of chronic population being isolated) and β (effective contact rate); given the nature of the disease, controlling the isolation parameter (i.e., devising an effective isolation strategy) seems to be the most workable solution.

Since we have a stable endemic equilibrium, we formulated (time-dependent) optimal control strategies to fight Hep C. We considered the two most effective strategies known to prevent disease spread, vaccination and isolation separately. Absence of an effective vaccine against all known genotypes of Hep C made us consider vaccination and isolation strategy separately. We assumed that the vaccination not only includes medical vaccination, but also the education and awareness schemes about Hep C.

The numerical results show that the proportion that is isolated optimally with respect to time has a higher favorable impact (as compared to implementing a high but

constant isolation rate) on keeping the cost of disease control low. However, it should be pointed out that the ideal time varying optimal strategy might not be applied easily. Still, it does provide a basis on which can be designed practical quasioptimal control strategies.

Next we consider the possibility of an effective vaccine becoming available for Hep C. We formulate a possible optimal time varying vaccination strategy; our analysis shows that it is not required to vaccinate a constant proportion of the susceptible population over time, but rather the optimal policy (being cost effective) is to start with vaccinating a constant proportion of the susceptibles and then progressively reducing the fraction of the susceptibles vaccinated.

Although the early diagnosis and treatment of Hep C virus infection are desirable to prevent spread of infection and to reduce the risk of progression of disease, the majority of acute individuals are asymptomatic and most infected persons are unaware of their exposure to the virus. More public awareness of Hep C may also increase the recovery from acute stage in the model. The goal of therapy is to prevent complications and death from the infection. Therapy along with an effective isolation strategy can greatly reduce the prevalence of Hep C.

Appendix

Parameter Values

Sensitivity analysis is shown in Table 1.

Disease-free equilibrium: $\Pi = 0.12, \gamma = 0.2, f = 0.8, \kappa = 0.2, \omega = 0.95, \mu = .00004566, \xi = 0.8, \delta_a = 0.000233, \delta_c = 0.00233, \delta_q = 0.001667, \eta = 0.4, \zeta = 0.1, \beta = 0.18$.

TABLE 1: Sensitivity analysis.

Parameter	Mean, standard (distribution)
μ	$1E^{-3}, 2E^{-4}$ (N)
δ_a	$6.3E^{-3}, E^{-4}$ (G)
δ_c	$9.3E^{-3}, E^{-4}$ (G)
δ_q	$3.3E^{-3}, E^{-4}$ (G)
γ	$0.15, 0.01$ (N)
ξ	$0.8, 0.05$ (N)
α	$0.2, 0.05$ (U)
κ	$0.2, -0.05$ (N)
ψ	$0.05, 5E^{-3}$ (N)
β	$0.3, 0.05$ (G)
η	$0.4, 0.05$ (G)
ζ	$0.1, 0.05$ (G)

The N, U, and G stand for normal, uniform, and gamma distribution, respectively.

Endemic equilibrium: $\beta = 0.35$; all other values are the same.

Optimal vaccination control: $\Pi = 1.2, \gamma = 0.2, f = 0.8, \kappa = 0.2, \omega = 0.95, \mu = .0004566, \xi = 0.8, \alpha = 0.2, \psi = 0.05, \delta_a = 0.000233, \delta_c = 0.00233, \delta_q = 0.001667, \eta = 0.4, \zeta = 0.1, \beta = 0.35, P_1 = .1, P_2 = 0.05, P_3 = 0.05, W = 1, \sigma = 0.9, a_1 = 0, b_1 = 0.9, v = .15$.

Optimal isolation control: $P_1 = 0.1$, $P_2 = 0.01$, $P_3 = 0.01$, $W_1 = 2$, $a_1 = 0$, $b_1 = 0.7$.

Conflict of Interests

The authors declare that there is no conflict of interests regarding the publication of this paper.

References

[1] A. M. Di Bisceglie, "Hep C," The Lancet, vol. 350, pp. 1209–1211, 1998.

[2] N. Jiwani and R. Gul, "A Silent Storm: Hep C in Pakistan," Journal of Pakistan Medical Students, vol. 1, pp. 89–91, 2011.

[3] A. M. Di Bisceglie, S. E. Order, J. L. Klein et al., "The role of chronic viral hepatitis in hepatocellular carcinoma in the United States," American Journal of Gastroenterology, vol. 86, no. 3, pp. 335–338, 1991.

[4] G. Fattovich, G. Giustina, F. Degos et al., "Morbidity and mortality in compensated cirrhosis type C: a retrospective follow-up study of 384 patients," Gastroenterology, vol. 112, no. 2, pp. 463–472, 1997.

[5] Y. Hutin, M. E. Kitler, G. J. Dore et al., "Global Burden of Disease (GBD) for Hep C," The Journal of Clinical Pharmacology, vol. 44, pp. 20–29, 2004.

[6] A. Jawaid and A. K. Khuwaja, "Treatment and vaccination for Hep C: present and future," Journal of Ayub Medical College, Abbottabad, vol. 20, pp. 129–133, 2008.

[7] J. Torresi, D. Johnson, and H. Wedemeyer, "Progress in the development of preventive and therapeutic vaccines for Hep C virus," Journal of Hepatology, vol. 54, pp. 1273–1285, 2011.

[8] S. Busenberg and P. van den Driessche, "Analysis of a disease transmission model in a population with varying size," Journal of Mathematical Biology, vol. 28, no. 3, pp. 257–270, 1990.

[9] I. K. Dontwi, N. K. Frempong, D. E. Bentil, I. Adetunde, and E. Owusu-Ansah, "Mathematical modeling of Hep C Virus transmission among injecting drug users and the impact of vaccination," American Journal of Scientific and Industrial Research, vol. 1, pp. 41–46, 2010.

[10] F. Luo and Z. Xiang, "Global analysis of an endemic model with acute and chronic stages," International Mathematical Forum, vol. 7, pp. 75–81, 2012.

[11] M. Martcheva and C. Castillo-Chavez, "Diseases with chronic stage in a population with varying size," Mathematical Biosciences, vol. 182, no. 1, pp. 1–25, 2003.

[12] B. Reade, R. G. Bowers, M. Begon, and R. Gaskell, "A model of disease and vaccination for infections with acute and chronic phases," Journal of Theoretical Biology, vol. 190, pp. 355–367, 1998.

[13] S. Suna, C. Guob, and C. Lia, "Global analysis of an SEIRS model with saturating contact rate," Applied Mathematical Sciences, vol. 6, pp. 3991–4003, 2012.

[14] H. W. Hethcote, "Mathematics of infectious diseases," SIAM Review, vol. 42, no. 4, pp. 599–653, 2000.

[15] G. Chowell, N. W. Hengartner, C. Castillo-Chavez, P. W. Fenimore, and J. M. Hyman, "The basic reproductive number of Ebola and the effects of public health measures: the cases of Congo and Uganda," Journal of Theoretical Biology, vol. 229, no. 1, pp. 119–126, 2004.

[16] M. Lipsitch, "Transmission dynamics and control of severe acute respiratory syndrome," Science, vol. 300, pp. 1966–1970, 2003.

[17] J. O. Lloyd-Smith, A. P. Galvani, and W. M. Getz, "Curtailing transmission of severe acute respiratory syndrome within a community and its hospital," Proceedings of the Royal Society B, vol. 170, pp. 1979–1989, 2003.

[18] R. G. McLeod, J. F. Brewster, A. B. Gumel, and D. A. Slonowsky, "Sensitivity and uncertainty analyses for a sars model with time-varying inputs and outputs," Mathematical Biosciences and Engineering, vol. 3, pp. 527–544, 2006.

[19] X. Yan and Y. Zou, "Optimal and sub-optimal quarantine and isolation control in SARS epidemics," Mathematical and Computer Modelling, vol. 47, pp. 235–245, 2008.

[20] X. Yan and Y. Zou, "Control of Epidemics by quarantine and isolation strategies in highly mobile populations," International Journal of Information and Systems Sciences, vol. 5, no. 3-4, pp. 271–286, 2009.

[21] K. R. Fister, S. Lenhart, and J. S. McNally, "Optimizing chemotherapy in an HIV model," Electronic Journal of Differential Equations, vol. 1998, no. 32, pp. 1–12, 1998.

[22] D. Kirschner, S. Lenhart, and S. Serbin, "Optimal control of the chemotherapy of HIV," Journal of Mathematical Biology, vol. 35, no. 7, pp. 775–792, 1997.

[23] E. Jung, S. Lenhart, and Z. Feng, "Optimal control of treatments in a two-strain tuberculosis model," Discrete and Continuous Dynamical Systems B, vol. 2, no. 4, pp. 473–482, 2002.

[24] X. Yan, Y. Zou, and J. Li, "Optimal quarantine and isolation strategies in epidemics control," World Journal of Modelling and Simulation, vol. 33, pp. 202–211, 2007.

[25] I. K. Dontwi, N. K. Frempong, D. E. Bentil, I. Adetunde, and E. Owusu-Ansah, "Mathematical modeling of Hepatitis C Virus transmission among injecting drug users and the impact

of vaccination," *American Journal of Scientific and Industrial Research*, vol. 1, pp. 41–46, 2010.

[26] P. van den Driessche and J. Watmough, "Reproduction numbers and sub-threshold endemic equilibria for compartmental models of disease transmission," *Mathematical Biosciences*, vol. 180, pp. 29–48, 2002.

[27] A. S. Ackleha, B. Maa, and P. L. Salceanua, "Persistence and global stability in a selectionmutation size-structured model," *Journal of Biological Dynamics* , vol. 5, no. 5, pp. 436–453, 2011.

[28] H. L. Smith and P. Waltman, *The Theory of the Chemostat*, Cambridge University Press, Cambridge, UK, 1995.

[29] H. R. Thieme, "Persistence under relaxed point-dissipativity," *SIAM Journal on Mathematical Analysis*, pp. 407–435, 1993.

[30] L. S. Pontryagin and V. G. Boltyanskii, *The Mathematical Theory of Optimal Processes*, Golden and Breach Science, 1986.

[31] H. R. Joshi, "Optimal control of an HIV immunology model," *Optimal Control Applications and Methods*, vol. 23, no. 4, pp. 199–213, 2002.

[32] H. Behncke, "Optimal control of deterministic epidemics," *Optimal Control Applications and Methods*, vol. 21, no. 6, pp. 269–285, 2000.

[33] D. Clancy, "Optimal intervention for epidemic models with general infection and removal rate functions," *Journal of Mathematical Biology*, vol. 39, no. 4, pp. 309–331, 1999.

[34] W. H. Fleming and R. W. Rishel, *Deterministic and Stochastic Optimal Control*, Springer, 1975.

[35] M. L. Kamien and N. L. Schwartz, *Dynamic Optmisation*, North Holland, Amsterdam, The Netherlands, 1991.

[36] H. W. Hethcote and P. Waltman, "Optimal vaccination schedules in deterministic epidemic model," *Mathematical Biosciences*, vol. 18, pp. 365–381, 1973.

[37] F. B. Agusto, "Optimal chemoprophylaxis and treatment control strategies of a tuberculosis transmission model," *World Journal of Modelling and Simulation*, vol. 5, no. 3, pp. 163–173, 2009.

[38] H. W. Hethcote, "An immunization model for a heterogeneous population," *Theoretical Population Biology*, vol. 14, no. 3, pp. 338–349, 1978.

[39] A. A. Saylers and D. D. Whitt, *Bacterial Paathogenesis A*, ASM Press, Washington, DC, USA, 2001.

[40] Q.-L. Choo, G. Kuo, R. Ralston et al., "Vaccination of chimpanzees against infection by the hepatitis C virus," *Proceedings of the National Academy of Sciences of the United States of America*, vol. 91, no. 4, pp. 1294–1298, 1994.

[41] W. Hackbusch, "A numerical method for solving parabolic equations with opposite orientations," *Computing*, vol. 20, no. 3, pp. 229–240, 1978.

[42] M. Puig, K. Mihalik, J. C. Tilton et al., "CD4+ immune escape and subsequent t-cell failure following chimpanzee immunization against hepatitis C virus," *Hepatology*, vol. 44, no. 3, pp. 736–745, 2006.

10

Structure-Based Virtual Screening and Molecular Dynamic Simulation Studies to Identify Novel Cytochrome *bc1* Inhibitors as Antimalarial Agents

**Rahul P. Gangwal, Gaurao V. Dhoke, Mangesh V. Damre,
Kanchan Khandelwal, and Abhay T. Sangamwar**

*Department of Pharmacoinformatics, National Institute of Pharmaceutical Education and Research (NIPER),
Sector 67, S.A.S. Nagar, Punjab 160 062, India*

Correspondence should be addressed to Abhay T. Sangamwar; abhays@niper.ac.in

Academic Editor: Said Audi

Cytochrome *bc1* (EC 1.10.2.2, *bc1*) is an essential component of the cellular respiratory chain, which catalyzes electron transfer from quinol to cytochrome c and concomitantly the translocation of protons across the membrane. It has been identified as a promising target in malaria parasites. The structure-based pharmacophore modelling and molecular dynamic simulation approach have been employed to identify novel inhibitors of cytochrome *bc1*. The best structure-based pharmacophore hypothesis (Hypo1) consists of one hydrogen bond acceptor (HBA), one general hydrophobic (HY), and two hydrophobic aromatic features (HYAr). Further, hydrogen interactions and hydrophobic interactions of known potent inhibitors with cytochrome *bc1* were compared with Hypo1, which showed that the Hypo1 has good predictive ability. The validated Hypo1 was used to screen the chemical databases. The hits obtained were subsequently subjected to the molecular docking analysis to identify false-positive hits. Moreover, the molecular docking results were further validated by molecular dynamics simulations. Binding-free energy analysis using MM-GBSA method reveals that the van der Waals interactions and the electrostatic energy provide the basis for favorable absolute free energy of the complex. The five virtual hits were identified as possible candidates for the designing of potent cytochrome *bc1* inhibitors.

1. Introduction

The cytochrome *bc1* complex (EC 1.10.2.2, *bc1*) is a vital component of the cellular respiratory chain and the photosynthetic apparatus in photosynthetic bacteria [1]. It is found on the plasma membrane of bacteria and in the inner mitochondrial membrane of eukaryotes [2]. It consists of two heme groups, cytochrome b, iron-sulfur protein (ISP), with a Rieske-type Fe2S2 cluster and cytochrome c1 that undergoes reduction and oxidation during turnover of the enzyme [3]. The role of cytochrome *bc1* complex is to catalyze the electron transfer from quinol to a soluble cytochrome c (cyt c), and this electron transfer couples to the translocation of protons across the membrane [4]. Due to its important role in the life cycle, inhibition of the *bc1* complex has become an important target in the discovery of new antimalarial agent [5].

Atovaquone is a competitive inhibitor of the quinol oxidation site of cytochrome bc1. It has also shown potential role against pneumocystis pneumonia and toxoplasmosis in immunocompromised individuals [6–8]. So far, two separate catalytic sites within the *bc1* complex have been identified and confirmed by X-ray crystallographic studies: the quinol oxidation site (Q_o site) and the quinone reduction site (Q_i site) [9]. Based on the specific binding interactions and conformational changes observed in both cyt b and the ISP domain into the *bc1* complex, Q_o inhibitors were further divided into two subgroups. subgroup I (Pf inhibitors) contains stigmatellin (SMA), famoxadone (FMX), and UHDBT, while subgroup II (Pm inhibitors) includes azoxystrobin (AZ) and methoxyacrylate-type inhibitors (MOA), KM, pyraclostrobin (PY), and many others [10]. The ISP domain is still mobile after binding of subgroup II inhibitors but becomes fixed after the binding of subgroup I inhibitors [11].

In the present study, we aim to identify the structural features essential for inhibition of cytochrome *bc1* and thereby design of potent Q_o site inhibitors. Structure-based virtual screening and molecular dynamic simulations approaches have been applied to achieve this goal. The best structure-based qualitative pharmacophore hypothesis (Hypo1) was generated, validated, and used as a 3D query to screen Specs, NCI, and ChemDiv databases. The hits were subsequently filtered by docking study. Further, the hits obtained were validated by molecular dynamics simulations. Finally, five novel compounds with diverse scaffolds were identified as possible candidates for the designing of potent cytochrome *bc1* inhibitors.

2. Materials and Methods

2.1. Data Sets. The most important step in the pharmacophore modeling is the selection of suitable training set, responsible for determining the quality of the generated pharmacophore [12]. In this study, structure-based pharmacophore hypothesis was generated using a potent inhibitor (FMX) and cytochrome *bc1* complex. The known cytochrome *bc1* inhibitors were collected from the literature and used as a test set for validation of developed pharmacophore hypotheses.

2.2. Pharmacophore Modelling. Pharmacophore modeling studies were carried out using LigandScout3.0 and Accelrys Discovery Studio2.5 (DS2.5) software package installed on IBM graphics workstation [13, 14]. From the available crystal structures of cytochrome *bc1*, one crystal structure was selected for generation of the structure-based pharmacophore models based on their IC_{50} values of cocrystallized ligand, resolution, and source organism. LigandScout3.0, an automated tool for pharmacophore generation, was used to study the interaction between the inhibitors and amino acids in the active site of cytochrome *bc1*. It identifies protein ligand interactions such as hydrogen bond, charge transfer, and hydrophobic regions and also define excluded volume spheres based on the side chain atoms to characterize the inaccessible areas for any potential ligand. Initially, pharmacophore hypothesis was generated by Create Simplified Pharmacophore (Catalyst) module of LigandScout. The generated pharmacophore hypothesis was exported in .hypoedit format and then converted into .chm format using the Hypoedit tool in DS2.5 and used as a 3D query for the screening process [15].

2.3. Validation of Pharmacophore Model. Validation of the developed pharmacophore model was done to determine its capability in differentiating active and the least active or inactive compounds and further performing virtual screening of databases. For the validation purpose two different methods, test set prediction and decoy test, were employed. In the test set predication, a set of 80 inhibitors of diverse chemical classes were prepared (see Supplementary Table 1 available online at http://dx.doi.org/10.1155/2013/637901) [11, 16–19].

The test compounds were classified into the most active (IC_{50} < 1000 nM) and the least active (IC_{50} > 1000 nM) inhibitors based on their inhibitory activity. The molecules were sketched and minimized in Catalyst, and conformational analysis was carried out. For each molecule a maximum of 255 conformers (with an energy threshold of 4 kcal/mol) were generated and considered for model validation. Flexible method was employed for fitting the molecule to the pharmacophore hypothesis. This method ensures an exhaustive conformational mapping even for most complex molecules. Default values were used for all other parameters in the conformational analysis. All the test set inhibitors were mapped on the developed pharmacophore hypothesis, and FitValue was predicted for each inhibitor. Further, for evaluation purpose, test set inhibitors were divided into active and the least active based on the predicted FitValues. The hit rate of pharmacophore hypothesis was calculated to analyse efficiency of developed pharmacophore hypothesis in differentiating between active and the least active.

For further validation of generated hypothesis, decoy set was generated using DecoyFinder1.1 [20]. Decoys are molecules that are supposed to be inactive against a target and used to validate the performance of the virtual screening workflow. To avoid bias in the enrichment factor calculation, decoys should resemble ligands physically, while still being chemically distinct from them. Decoys were selected if they are having similarity to that of the active ligands with respect to physical descriptors (molecular weight, number of rotational bonds, hydrogen bond donor count, hydrogen bond acceptor count, and the octanol-water partition coefficient) and deprived of the chemical descriptors to any of the active ligands [20]. 34 active cytochrome *bc1* inhibitors were included in the database to calculate various statistical parameters such as accuracy, precision, sensitivity, specificity, goodness of hit score (GH), and enrichment factor (*E* value). Out of these, GH and *E* value are the two major parameters, playing significant role in identifying capability of the generated pharmacophore hypothesis [21].

2.4. Virtual Screening. Virtual screening of chemical databases is a fast and accurate method, which helps to identify novel and potential leads suitable for further development. It has an advantage over any *de novo* design methods in which retrieved hits can be easily obtained for biological testing. Three commercially available databases of diverse chemical compounds were used in virtual screening. The databases were first screened for their drug-like properties using Lipinski's rule of five and subsequently submitted to DEREK for different toxicity filters. Fast/Flexible and Best/Flexible are the two databases searching options available in DS2.5. In our study, we performed virtual screening using Best/Flexible search option. The validated pharmacophore hypothesis Hypo1 was used as a 3D query in database screening. The hits obtained from pharmacophore based virtual screening were evaluated for drug-like properties using QED value. For calculation of QED value, physicochemical properties such as MW, ALOGP, number of HBDs, number of HBAs, molecular PSA, number of ROTBs, and the number of AROMs were calculated using the DS2.5. Finally, a substructure search was performed against each compound using a curate reference set of 94 functional moieties that are potentially mutagenic, are reactive, or have unfavorable pharmacokinetic properties. The number of matches for each compound was captured (ALERTS) [22]. The unweighted and weighted QED values were calculated based on the previously mentioned molecular properties by using following formulae:

$$\text{QED} = \exp\left(\frac{1}{n}\sum_{i=1}^{n}\ln d_i\right),$$

$$\text{QED}_w = \exp\left(\frac{\sum_{i=1}^{n} w_i \ln d_i}{\sum_{i=1}^{n} w_i}\right),$$

(1)

where d is the derived desirability function corresponding to different molecular properties; w is the weight applied to each function; n is the number of molecular properties [23]. Hit compounds that passed all of these tests were taken for molecular docking analysis using Glide5.5.

2.5. Molecular Docking. To investigate the detailed intermolecular interactions between the virtual hits and cytochrome *bc1*, an automated docking program Glide5.5 was used [24]. Three-dimensional structure information about the target protein was taken from the protein data bank (PDB ID: 1L0L). Cocrystallized ligand (Famoxadone) was docked into cytochrome *bc1* to validate the docking protocol. The protocol followed for docking studies of virtual hits included processing of the protein and ligand preparation. During protein preparation, ligand molecules were deleted, hydrogen atoms were added, solvent molecules were deleted; and bond orders for crystal protein were adjusted and minimized up to 0.30 Å RMSD [25, 26]. An active site of 10 Å was created around the cocrystallized ligand. The extraprecision (XP) mode and other default parameters of Glide software were used for the docking studies.

2.6. Molecular Dynamics Simulation. The screened virtual hits were further validated, for its binding affinity with the active site residue of cytochrome *bc1*, by performing the molecular dynamics (MD) simulations. MD studies of the cytochrome *bc1* complex with cocrystallized ligand (Famoxadone), and top two virtual hits were performed using AMBER11 [27]. The input files for the MD simulations were prepared in tleap module of AMBER, in which the system was hydrated by TIP3P water box of 10 Å and neutralized by counter ions. The minimization of the initial solvated system was performed in two steps; in the first step, only water was permitted to move employing 500 cycles of the steepest descent followed by 500 cycles of conjugate gradient method. In the second step, the entire system was subjected for minimization using 500 cycles of the steepest descent followed by 500 cycles of conjugated gradient method. The heating of the system was carried out at 310 K using Langevin thermostat. SHAKE algorithm was implemented for hydrogen constraints. The force of 2 kcal/mol/Å^2 on the heavy atoms of the complex was restrained during density equilibration. Whole system equilibration was performed

over a period of 1000 ps. Production phase of 5000 ps was carried out using NPT ensemble at 310 K and one atmospheric pressure. Nonbonded cutoff of 8 Å and step size of 2 fs was used for the simulations.

Furthermore, the binding affinity of the cocrystallized ligand and top two virtual hits were calculated by the molecular mechanics generalized Born surface area (MM-GBSA) method integrated into AMBER11 [28]. Binding-free energy (ΔG_{Bind}) of inhibitors at the binding site was calculated by using (2)

$$\Delta G_{\text{Bind}} = G_{\text{Complex}} - G_{\text{Protein}} - G_{\text{Ligand}},$$

(2)

where G_{Complex}, G_{Protein}, and G_{Ligand} represent the free energies of complex, protein, and the ligand, respectively. Free energy (G) of each state was calculated using the following equations:

$$G = E_{\text{MM}} + G_{\text{GB}} + G_{\text{SA}} - \text{TS},$$

(3)

$$E_{\text{MM}} = E_{\text{vdW}} + E_{\text{ele}} + E_{\text{int}},$$

(4)

where E_{MM} represents the molecular mechanical energy; G_{GB} and G_{SA} are the contributions from polar and nonpolar terms of the free energy of the solvent continuum, and TS represents the entropic contribution of the solute. E_{MM} was obtained using (4), in which E_{ele} is electrostatic energy, E_{vdW} is van der Waals energy, and E_{int} is internal energy. G_{GB} was calculated based on the generalized Born model. G_{SA} was computed by the molsurf module of AMBER according to (5), which is proportional to the solvent accessible surface area (SASA):

$$G_{\text{SA}} = \gamma \times \text{SASA} + b.$$

(5)

3. Results and Discussion

3.1. Generation of Pharmacophore Model. The overall workflow followed during identification of novel cytochrome *bc1* inhibitors is as shown in Figure 1. The reported crystal structures of cytochrome *bc1* from the protein data bank were analyzed for organism source, conformations, bound inhibitors, and their activity. Finally, one cocrystallized structure of cytochrome *bc1* was selected for development of structure-based pharmacophore hypothesis. The binding site analysis was performed for better understanding of the specificity and pharmacophore requirement of inhibitors. The binding site was characterized by several direct interactions such as hydrogen bond interactions, π-π interaction, and lipophilic side chains complement, which reflects the hydrophobic nature of an active site.

For structure-based pharmacophore studies, we have used LigandScout3.0, which provides the interactions between protein and ligand as well as some excluded volume spheres corresponding to their 3D structures of protein. In this study, the coordinates of cytochrome *bc1* complex (PDB ID: 1L0L) and insight from molecular docking analysis of known cytochrome bc1 inhibitors were used for generation of structure-based pharmacophore hypothesis. In developed structure-based pharmacophore hypothesis, one HBA was pointed towards Glu271. Also, molecular docking analysis

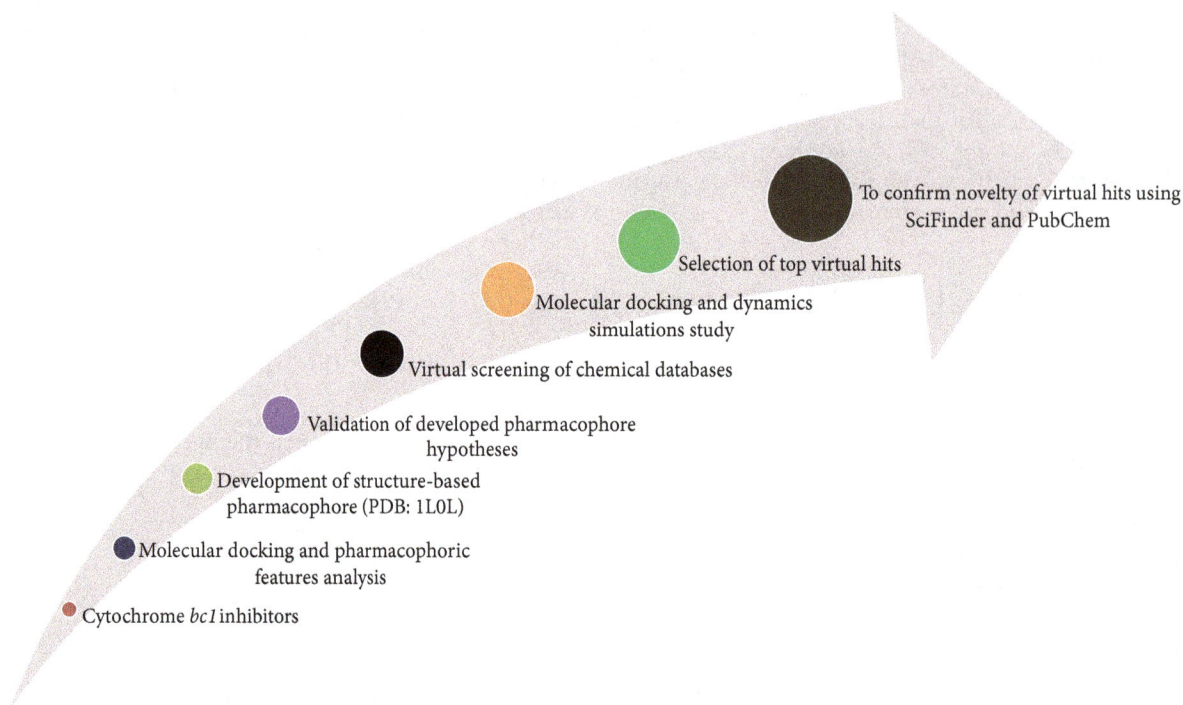

FIGURE 1: The overall work flow followed during identification of novel cytochrome *bc1* inhibitors.

reveals that the oxygen atom of most potent inhibitors (IC_{50} value < 100 nM) was accepting an H-bond from NH of Glu271. Hence, HBA was considered as an important chemical feature to identify novel cytochrome *bc1* inhibitors. Finally, four-feature structure-based hypothesis (Hypo1) was generated, which consists of one HBA, one general hydrophobic (HY), and two hydrophobic aromatic features (HYAr).

3.2. Pharmacophore Model Validation. Figure 2 shows the chemical features of a pharmacophore hypothesis (Hypo1) with their interfeature distance constraints. The test set prediction was performed to validate the developed pharmacophore hypothesis. The Hypo1 pharmacophore hypothesis was used to estimate the FitValue of test set compounds. The inhibitors showing FitValue higher than 2.38 considered as active and the rest were considered as the least active. The hit rate of pharmacophore hypothesis suggested that the developed pharmacophore hypothesis can differentiate between active and the least active. In detail, 50 of 57 highly active and 18 of 23 the least active compounds were predicted correctly by the Hypo1. Seven active compounds were underestimated as the least active, whereas five compounds are overestimated as active by Hypo1. Figure 3 shows the mapping of the most active and the least active compound from the test set over Hypo1. The highly active compound was mapped accurately to all features of Hypo1. While, in case of the least active compounds, one HBA was missing and two HYAr features were mapped partially.

Finally, DecoyFinder1.1 was employed to generate small database (*D*) containing 1258 compounds, which includes 34

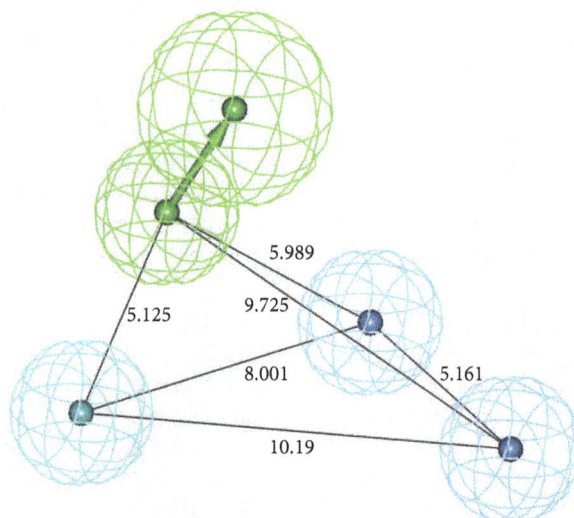

FIGURE 2: Chemical features of the structure-based pharmacophore hypothesis with interfeature distance constraints.

actives and 1224 decoys. This database was used to validate the generated hypothesis (Hypo1), whether it is capable of distinguishing the actives from decoys or not. The hypothesis Hypo1 was used as a 3D structural query to perform screening of decoy database and then accuracy, precision, sensitivity, and specificity were calculated. The hits were selected based on the FitValue. Furthermore, for the analysis of results,

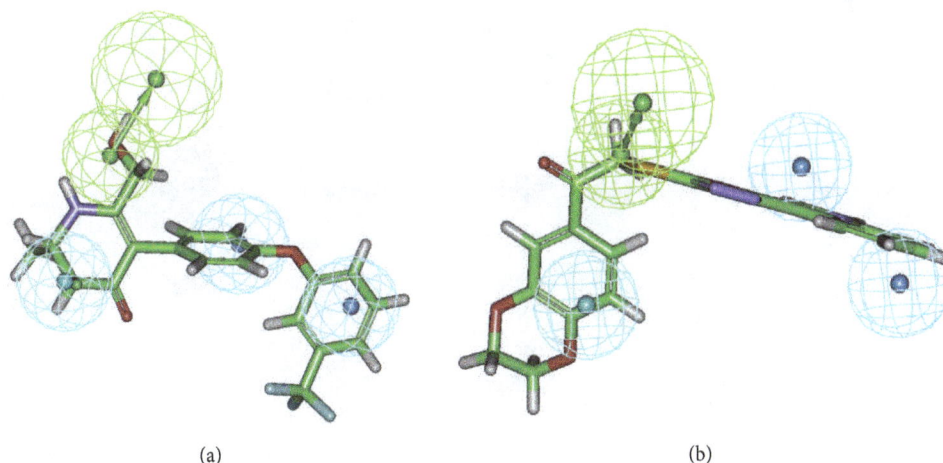

(a)   (b)

FIGURE 3: The most active and the least active compound from the test set aligned with pharmacophore hypotheses.

TABLE 1: The statistical parameters obtained from decoy test.

Sr. no.	Parameter	Hypo1
1	Total compounds in database (D)	1258
2	Total number of actives in database (A)	34
3	Total hits (H_t)	42
4	Active hits (TP)	30
5	True negative (TN)	1216
6	Enrichment factor or enhancement (E)	26.42
7	False negatives (FN = A− TP)	4
8	False positives (FP = H_t− TP)	8
9	GH score (goodness of hit list)	0.748
10	Accuracy = (TP + TN)/(TP + TN + FP + FN)	0.990
11	Precision = TP/(TP + FP)	0.789
12	Sensitivity = TP/(TP + FN)	0.882
13	Specificity = TN/(TN + FP)	0.993

the enrichment factor (E value) and goodness of hit score (GH) were calculated using the following formulae:

$$E = \frac{(\text{TP} \times D)}{(\text{Ht} \times A)},$$

$$\text{GH} = \left(\frac{\text{TP}}{4\text{Ht}A}\right)(3A + \text{Ht}) \times \left(1 - \left(\frac{\text{Ht} - \text{TP}}{D - A}\right)\right), \quad (6)$$

where D, A, Ht, and TP represent the total number of compounds of the database, total number of actives, total number of compounds screened by a pharmacophore model, and total number of active compounds screened, respectively [29]. Hypo1 has shown an E value of 26.42. The calculated GH score was greater than 0.5, specifies that the quality of developed pharmacophore was significant (Table 1). From the overall validation results, we assure that the Hypo1 hypothesis could discriminate between the active and the least active compounds. Hence, we have used Hypo1 hypothesis for virtual screening to select or discriminate the suitable cytochrome *bc1* inhibitors.

3.3. Sequential Virtual Screening. Sequential virtual screening was performed as depicted in the flowchart (Figure 4). The NCI, ChemDiv, and Specs databases were screened using Lipinski's rule of five, which comprised 87374, 843113, and 276807 compounds, respectively. Further, the hits obtained were screened for several toxicity filters, such as carcinogenicity, chromosome damage, genotoxicity, hERG channel inhibition, hepatotoxicity, mutagenicity, and thyroid toxicity using DEREK. After applying toxicity filter 622196 compounds were obtained and subsequently screened by the validated pharmacophore hypothesis (Hypo1). 381734 compounds were mapped to the Hypo1 pharmacophore hypothesis, which included some structurally similar compounds to that of existing cytochrome *bc1* inhibitors, and some novel scaffolds were also identified. A set of 340 hit compounds from Hypo1 screening were selected based on the estimated FitValue > 2.50. Out of these, 236 compounds having QED value > 0.50 were selected and subjected to further analysis by molecular docking to avoid the false-positive hits from virtual screening.

3.4. Molecular Docking Studies. Recently in molecular dynamic study, Zhao et al. have reported that the side chains of hydrophobic residues of the active site showed the conformational stability, except the phenyl group of Phe274, which exhibited the significant conformational flexibility in different complexes [1]. The conformational flexibility of phenyl group of Phe274 allows optimizing the corresponding π-π interactions. The phenyl ring of the cyanophenoyl group is almost vertical to the pyrimidyl ring due to the presence of the linear cyano group in AZ. As a result, the pyrimidyl ring is not able to form ideal π-π interaction parallel with the phenyl ring of Phe274. On the contrary, myxothiazol is more potent than AZ because its thiazole ring parallels well with the phenyl group of Phe274 and from the ideal π-π interaction [1]. These facts suggested that the π-π interaction between inhibitors and the phenyl of Phe274 is essential for inhibitory activity. Thus π-π interaction with Phe274 is considered as essential during molecular docking analysis.

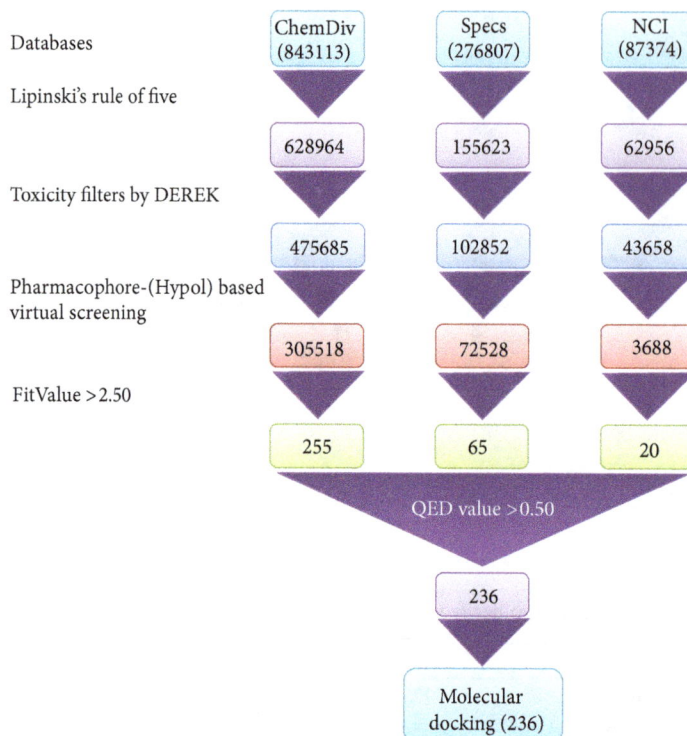

FIGURE 4: The sequential virtual screening followed during identification of novel cytochrome *bc1* inhibitors.

Docking studies were carried out to identify false-positive hits from virtual screening process and to explore the interaction between the virtual hits and cytochrome *bc1*. All the test set compounds along with virtual hits were docked into the active site of cytochrome *bc1* (PDB ID: 1L0L) using Glide program. Glide score, which differentiates compounds based on their interacting pattern, is calculated for all molecules. The cocrystallized ligand famoxadone (FMX) was docked into the active site of cytochrome *bc1* to validate the docking protocol with RMSD of 0.320 Å. FMX contains three aromatic rings, the central five-membered oxazolidinedione ring carries a phenyl amino group and a phenoxyphenyl group. In detail, it forms one strong hydrogen bond with an amide group of the conserved Glu271. The hydrophobic environment is formed by the Phe274, Tyr131, Tyr273, Phe91, and Tyr278 allowing formation of a network of π-π interactions with the two phenyl groups of famoxadone. Top virtual hits were showing similar interaction pattern to that of FMX along with some additional hydrogen bonds and hydrophobic interactions. The binding interaction pattern observed during docking studies was complementary with that of the hydrogen bond acceptor and hydrophobic features of pharmacophore hypotheses. On the basis of molecular docking analysis five virtual hits (Figure 5) with diverse scaffolds were identified as potential cytochrome *bc1* inhibitors. Figure 6 shows 2D interaction pose of FMX and top virtual hit at the active site of cytochrome *bc1*. The Glide score, FitValue, and QED value of top five virtual hits are shown in Table 2.

Further, these five hit compounds were confirmed by the PubChem [30] and SciFinder [31] scholar search tools, as

TABLE 2: The Glide Score, FitValue, and QED values of top five virtual hits.

Compound name	Glide score	FitValue	QED weighted
ZINC17170092	−10.891	2.997	0.532
ZINC09153263	−10.744	2.999	0.605
ZINC09833402	−10.545	3.903	0.500
ZINC24611274	−10.437	2.999	0.691
ZINC01061443	−10.407	2.998	0.529

unreported for cytochrome *bc1* inhibition. Hence, we suggest that these virtual hits with diverse scaffolds are novel as cytochrome *bc1* inhibitors.

3.5. Molecular Dynamic Simulation. In order to verify whether the results obtained by the molecular docking analysis were robust or a fortuitous, we have carried out molecular dynamics simulations with cocrystallized ligand (FMX) and top two virtual hits. The atomic RMSDs of the Cα, C, and N atoms of the protein and the ligands obtained during the trajectories and the initial structures were monitored during the simulations. The sharp rise was observed up to first 50 ps, and the function remained stable for the rest of the simulation. The system reached a constant temperature. The total energy was fluctuating around an average energy with the system stabilization at a given temperature of 310 K and 1 atmospheric pressure. The RMSD of the molecular dynamics simulation was stable after 1 ns of the equilibrium. Both protein-ligand trajectories

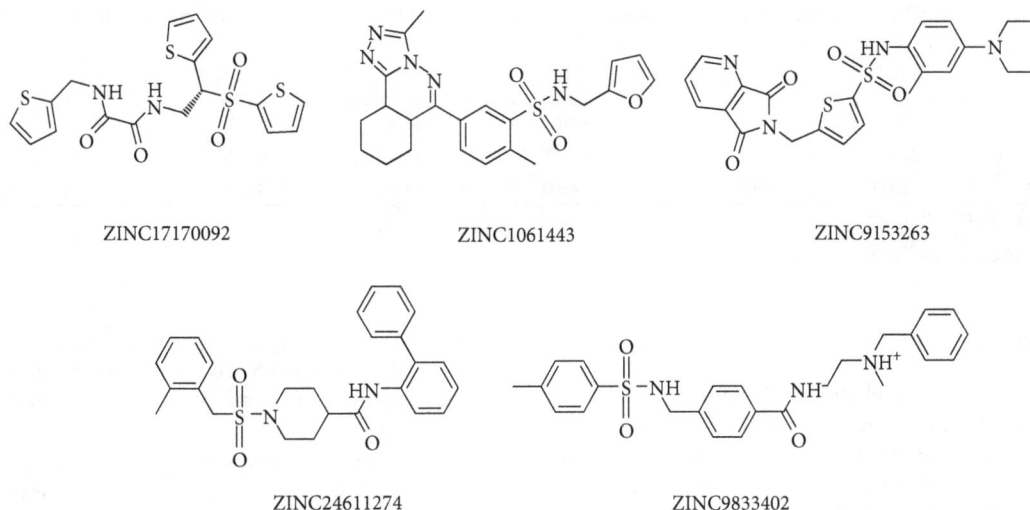

ZINC17170092

ZINC1061443

ZINC9153263

ZINC24611274

ZINC9833402

FIGURE 5: Chemical structures of top five virtual hits obtained through sequential virtual screening using Hypo1.

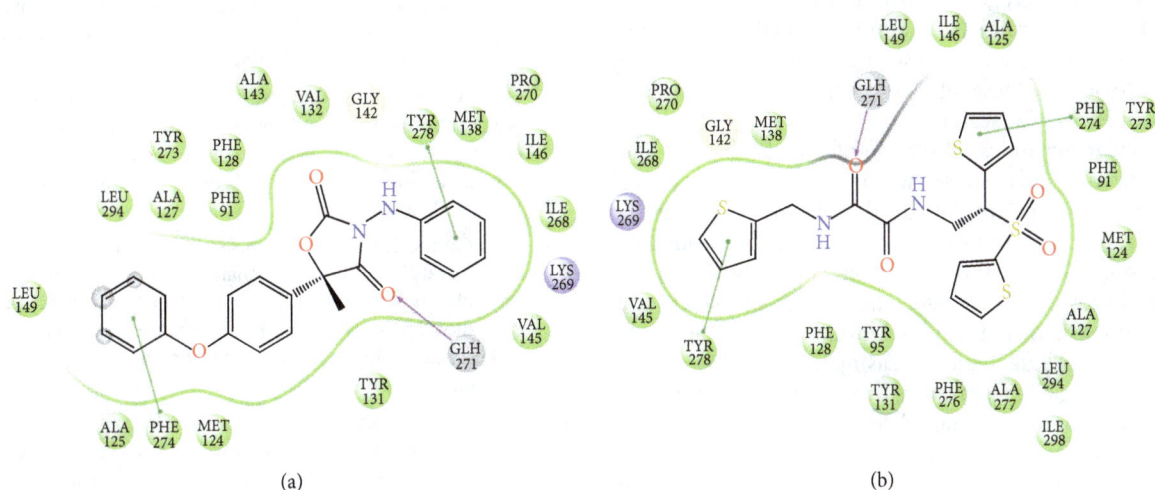

(a)

(b)

FIGURE 6: The 2D interactions plot of cocrystallized inhibitor (Famoxadone) and top virtual hit (ZINC17170092).

exhibited low backbone and ligand RMSD values, which indicate the high binding affinities of cytochrome *bc1* and inhibitors, further enhancing the credibility of the docking results.

Further, insights into the forces involved in the binding of inhibitors were obtained by analysis of the MM-GBSA-free energy contributions, as listed in Table 3. The calculated ΔG binding for the cytochrome *bc1* with top two virtual hit complexes was slightly higher than the value of the cytochrome *bc1*/and cocrystallized ligand complexes, demonstrating that the potential activity of top virtual hit is as high as the known potent inhibitors. Both, the intermolecular van der Waals and the electrostatic interaction energies have shown significant contributions in the binding, whereas polar solvation terms are calculated by GB counteract binding. Nonpolar solvation terms that correspond to the burial of the solvent-accessible surface area contribute slightly in binding. Comparing the van der Waals contributions with the

electrostatic contributions, we noticed that the association between cytochrome *bc1* and inhibitors is mainly driven by more favorable van der Waals interaction in the complex than in solution. The van der Waals/nonpolar contributions of the cytochrome *bc1*/inhibitors reveal that inhibitor fits more tightly within the active-site cavity. Taking all energy contributions into account, virtual hits present slightly higher potential activity than cocrystallized ligand. Hence, inspired by the molecular dynamics studies, we conclude a possible strategy to design a new series of cytochrome *bc1* inhibitors with high potential activity, which is to retain the important hydrogen bond and enhance the hydrophobic interactions with the hydrophobic residues in the pocket. In our study, top virtual hits exhibit the most favorable affinity with cytochrome *bc1*, because it obeys the previously mentioned strategy that it retains important hydrogen bonds with Glu271 and increases the hydrophobic interactions with receptor.

Table 3: Binding-free energy and individual energy components calculated using MM-GBSA method for cocrystallized ligands and top two virtual hits.

Compounds	ΔE_{int}^{ele}	ΔE_{int}^{vdw}	ΔE_{sol}^{nonpol}	ΔG_{sol}^{ele}	ΔG_{sol}^{a}	ΔG_{ele}^{b}	ΔG_b
FMX	−18.16	−53.39	−4.02	36.45	32.43	18.29	−39.10
ZINC17170092	−25.08	−69.67	−6.60	51.60	45.00	26.52	−43.15
ZINC09153263	−19.00	−61.64	−4.62	44.96	40.34	25.96	−40.30

[a]The polar/nonpolar ($\Delta E_{sol}^{nonpol} + \Delta G_{sol}^{ele}$) contributions.
[b]The electrostatic ($\Delta E_{int}^{ele} + \Delta G_{sol}^{ele}$) contributions.

4. Conclusions

In this study, we have developed a structure-based pharmacophore model, which was validated to evaluate its predicting power over the diverse test set compounds. The best structure-based pharmacophore hypothesis consists of one HBA, one HY, and two HYAr features. This predictive hypothesis was further used in virtual screening to identify novel cytochrome *bc1* inhibitors. Molecular docking analysis reveals that hydrogen bond interaction with Glu271 is essential for cytochrome *bc1* inhibition. Finally, compounds were selected as positive hits based on the molecular docking analysis. Novelty of these hits was confirmed with PubChem and SciFinder scholar search tool.

Molecular dynamics simulation of cytochrome bc1 with cocrystallized ligands and top two virtual hits was performed for getting deeper insights into the driving forces between the inhibitors and cytochrome bc1. Free energy calculations were done by MM-GBSA method. Based on the observation, a new strategy is proposed to design a new series of cytochrome bc1 inhibitors. It includes the retention of hydrogen bond interaction with Glu271 and increasing hydrophobic interaction. Combining all these results, five novel compounds were identified as possible lead candidates to be used as a novel and potent cytochrome *bc1* inhibitors. Further, *in vitro* testing of the virtual hits will confirm the success rate of this study to optimize the hits thereafter.

Acknowledgment

The authors acknowledge financial support from the Department of Science and Technology (DST), New Delhi, India.

References

[1] P.-L. Zhao, L. Wang, X.-L. Zhu et al., "Subnanomolar inhibitor of cytochrome *bc1* complex designed by optimizing interaction with conformationally flexible residues," *Journal of the American Chemical Society*, vol. 132, no. 1, pp. 185–194, 2010.

[2] S. Iwata, J. W. Lee, K. Okada et al., "Complete structure of the 11-subunit bovine mitochondrial cytochrome *bc1* complex," *Science*, vol. 281, no. 5373, pp. 64–71, 1998.

[3] E. A. Berry, L.-S. Huang, Z. Zhang, and S.-H. Kim, "Structure of the avian mitochondrial cytochrome *bc1* complex," *Journal of Bioenergetics and Biomembranes*, vol. 31, no. 3, pp. 177–190, 1999.

[4] F. Muller, A. R. Crofts, and D. M. Kramer, "Multiple Q-cycle bypass reactions at the Qo site of the cytochrome *bc1* complex," *Biochemistry*, vol. 41, no. 25, pp. 7866–7874, 2002.

[5] G. A. Biagini, N. Fisher, N. Berry et al., "Acridinediones: selective and potent inhibitors of the malaria parasite mitochondrial *bc1* complex," *Molecular Pharmacology*, vol. 73, no. 5, pp. 1347–1355, 2008.

[6] I. K. Srivastava, J. M. Morrlsey, E. Darrouzet, F. Daldal, and A. B. Vaidya, "Resistance mutations reveal the atovaquone-binding domain of cytochrome b in malaria parasites," *Molecular Microbiology*, vol. 33, no. 4, pp. 704–711, 1999.

[7] P. Kazanjian, W. Armstrong, P. A. Hossler et al., "Pneumocystis carinii cytochrome b mutations are associated with atovaquone exposure in patients with AIDS," *Journal of Infectious Diseases*, vol. 183, no. 5, pp. 819–822, 2001.

[8] D. C. McFadden, S. Tomavo, E. A. Berry, and J. C. Boothroyd, "Characterization of cytochrome *b* from *Toxoplasma gondii* and Q$_o$ domain mutations as a mechanism of atovaquone-resistance," *Molecular and Biochemical Parasitology*, vol. 108, no. 1, pp. 1–12, 2000.

[9] A. R. Crofts, B. Barquera, R. B. Gennis, R. Kuras, M. Guergova-Kuras, and E. A. Berry, "Mechanistic aspects of the Qo-site of the bc1-complex as revealed by mutagenesis studies, and the crystallographic structure," in *The Phototrophic Prokaryotes*, G. A. Peschek, W. Loeffelhardt, and G. Schmetterer, Eds., pp. 229–239, Springer, 1999.

[10] L. Esser, B. Quinn, Y.-F. Li et al., "Crystallographic studies of quinol oxidation site inhibitors: a modified classification of inhibitors for the cytochrome *bc1* complex," *Journal of Molecular Biology*, vol. 341, no. 1, pp. 281–302, 2004.

[11] F. Wang, H. Li, L. Wang, W.-C. Yang, J.-W. Wu, and G.-F. Yang, "Design, syntheses, and kinetic evaluation of 3-(phenylamino)oxazolidine-2, 4-diones as potent cytochrome *bc1* complex inhibitors," *Bioorganic & Medicinal Chemistry*, vol. 19, no. 15, pp. 4608–4615, 2011.

[12] R. P. Gangwal, A. Bhadauriya, M. V. Damre, G. V. Dhoke, and A. T. Sangamwar, "p38 mitogen-activated protein kinase inhibitors: a review on pharmacophore mapping and QSAR Studies," *Current Topics in Medicinal Chemistry*, vol. 13, no. 9, pp. 1015–1035, 2013.

[13] *LigandScout, Version 3. 0*, Inte:Ligand GmbH, Clemesn-Maria-Hofbaurer-G, Maria Enzersdorf, Austria, 2010.

[14] *Discovery Studio Version 2. 5 (DS 2. 5) User Manual*, Accelrys, San Diego, Calif, USA, 2009.

[15] G. V. Dhoke, R. P. Gangwal, and A. T. Sangamwar, "A combined ligand and structure based approach to design potent PPAR-alpha agonists," *Journal of Molecular Structure*, vol. 1028, no. 28, pp. 22–30, 2012.

[16] T. Rodrigues, R. Moreira, J. Gut et al., "Identification of new antimalarial leads by use of virtual screening against cytochrome *bc1*," *Bioorganic & Medicinal Chemistry*, vol. 19, no. 21, pp. 6302–6308, 2011.

[17] C. Pidathala, R. Amewu, B. Pacorel et al., "Identification, design and biological evaluation of bisaryl quinolones targeting *Plasmodium falciparum* type II NADH: quinone oxidoreductase (PfNDH2)," *Journal of Medicinal Chemistry*, vol. 55, no. 5, pp. 1831–1843, 2012.

[18] V. Barton, N. Fisher, G. A. Biagini, S. A. Ward, and P. M. O'Neill, "Inhibiting Plasmodium cytochrome *bc1*: a complex issue," *Current Opinion in Chemical Biology*, vol. 14, no. 4, pp. 440–446, 2010.

[19] J. M. Bueno, P. Manzano, M. C. García et al., "Potent antimalarial 4-pyridones with improved physico-chemical properties," *Bioorganic & Medicinal Chemistry Letters*, vol. 21, no. 18, pp. 5214–5218, 2011.

[20] A. Cereto-Massagué, L. Guasch, C. Valls, M. Mulero, G. Pujadas, and S. Garcia-Vallvé, "DecoyFinder: an easy-to-use python GUI application for building target-specific decoy sets," *Bioinformatics*, vol. 28, no. 12, pp. 1661–1662, 2012.

[21] U. Singh, R. P. Gangwal, G. V. Dhoke, R. Prajapati, and A. T. Sangamwar, "3D QSAR pharmacophore-based virtual screening and molecular docking studies to identify novel matrix metalloproteinase 12 inhibitors," *Molecular Simulation*, vol. 39, no. 5, pp. 385–396, 2012.

[22] R. Brenk, A. Schipani, D. James et al., "Lessons learnt from assembling screening libraries for drug discovery for neglected diseases," *ChemMedChem*, vol. 3, no. 3, pp. 435–444, 2008.

[23] G. R. Bickerton, G. V. Paolini, J. Besnard, S. Muresan, and A. L. Hopkins, "Quantifying the chemical beauty of drugs," *Nature Chemistry*, vol. 4, no. 2, pp. 90–98, 2012.

[24] *Glide, Version 5. 5*, Schrödinger, New York, NY, USA, 2009.

[25] P. S. Ambure, R. P. Gangwal, and A. T. Sangamwar, "3D-QSAR and molecular docking analysis of biphenyl amide derivatives as p38 α mitogen-activated protein kinase inhibitors," *Molecular Diversity*, vol. 16, no. 2, pp. 377–388, 2012.

[26] U. Singh, R. P. Gangwal, G. V. Dhoke, R. Prajapati, M. Damre, and A. T. Sangamwar, "3D-QSAR and molecular docking analysis of (4-Piperidinyl)-piperazines as acetyl-CoA carboxylases inhibitors," *Arabian Journal of Chemistry*, 2012.

[27] *AMBER11*, University of California, San Francisco, Calif, USA, 2011.

[28] B. Kuhn and P. A. Kollman, "Binding of a diverse set of ligands to avidin and streptavidin: an accurate quantitative prediction of their relative affinities by a combination of molecular mechanics and continuum solvent models," *Journal of Medicinal Chemistry*, vol. 43, no. 20, pp. 3786–3791, 2000.

[29] A. Bhadauriya, G. Dhoke, R. Gangwal, M. Damre, and A. Sangamwar, "Identification of dual Acetyl-CoA carboxylases 1 and 2 inhibitors by pharmacophore based virtual screening and molecular docking approach," *Molecular Diversity*, vol. 17, no. 1, pp. 139–149, 2013.

[30] Y. Wang, E. Bolton, S. Dracheva et al., "An overview of the PubChem BioAssay resource," *Nucleic Acids Research*, vol. 38, no. 1, pp. D255–D266, 2009.

[31] A. B. Wagner, "SciFinder Scholar 2006: an empirical analysis of research topic query processing," *Journal of Chemical Information and Modeling*, vol. 46, no. 2, pp. 767–774, 2006.

11

Validation of Shape Context Based Image Registration Method Using Digital Image Correlation Measurement on a Rat Stomach

Donghua Liao,[1,2] Peng Wang,[3] Jingbo Zhao,[1,2] and Hans Gregersen[4,5]

[1] GIOME Academia, Institute of Clinical Medicine, Aarhus University Hospital, 8200 Aarhus, Denmark
[2] Mech-Sense, Department of Gastroenterology and Surgery, Aalborg University Hospital, 9000 Aalborg, Denmark
[3] Department of Mechanical and Manufacturing Engineering, Aalborg University, 9220 Aalborg, Denmark
[4] College of Bioengineering, Chongqing University, Chongqing 400050, China
[5] The GIOME Institute, Dubai, UAE

Correspondence should be addressed to Donghua Liao; liao.donghua@ki.au.dk

Academic Editor: Jackie Wu

Recently we developed analysis for 3D visceral organ deformation by combining the shape context (SC) method with a full-field strain (strain distribution on a whole 3D surface) analysis for calculating distension-induced rat stomach deformation. The surface deformation detected by the SC method needs to be further verified by using a feature tracking measurement. Hence, the aim of this study was to verify the SC method-based calculation by using digital image correlation (DIC) measurement on a rat stomach. The rat stomach exposed to distension pressures 0.0, 0.2, 0.4, and 0.6 kPa were studied using both 3D DIC system and SC-based image registration calculation. Three different surface sample counts between the reference and the target surfaces were used to gauge the effect of the surface sample counts on the calculation. Each pair of the surface points between the DIC measured target surface and the SC calculated correspondence surface was compared. Compared with DIC measurement, the SC calculated surface had errors from 5% to 23% at pressures from 0.2 to 0.6 kPa with different surface sample counts between the reference surface and the target surface. This indicates good qualitative and quantitative agreement on the surfaces with small dissimilarity and small sample count difference between the reference surface and the target surface. In conclusion, this is the first study to validate the 3D SC-based image registration method by using unique tracking features measurement. The developed method can be used in the future for analysing scientific and clinical data of visceral organ geometry and biomechanical properties in health and disease.

1. Introduction

Identifying corresponding points between two configurations is a common problem in medical image processing. Point matching-based surface registration using 3D shape context (SC) has recently emerged as an alternative to intensity-based nonlinear registration. The major contribution of SC lies in the global shape characterization at a local level for each single point. The point matching is based on 3D shape descriptors that characterize the shape of each point based on histograms of the distribution of points around them. Corresponding points on similar shapes will have similar shape contexts. In comparison to other point matching techniques, SC do not require an equal number of points for the shapes to be compared or segments with specific geometrical configurations [1, 2].

Studies on lung and cortical surfaces demonstrated that the SC matching approach-based nonlinear registration method is a well-suited method for a variety of soft tissue organ surfaces [1, 3–8]. Recently we developed a 3D SC-based nonlinear image registration by combining the image registration method with a full-field strain (strain distribution on a whole 3D surface) analysis for calculation of distension-induced rat stomach deformation [9]. Our study showed the dependency of the surface deformation estimation on the surface matching quality. Consequently, for exploring the developed method on estimations of *in vivo* visceral organs surface deformation, validation of the SC-based surface point matching is needed. Existing validation tests of 3D SC method were limited in (1) the matching experiments that were on synthetically transformed data (the target surface for the registration was mathematically transformed from a reference surface [5, 7, 8]), (2) the equal number of surface points that was selected between the reference surface and the target surface [7], and (3) only few surface points were selected manually for comparisons between the target surface and SC method calculated correspondence surface [2]. The configuration of the visceral organ changes with large deformation due to nonlinear tissue mechanical properties. Moreover, *in vivo* deformation of the visceral organ is location and orientation dependent due to the diseases caused tissue remodelling or heterogeneous tissue properties. Hence, *in vivo* movement or deformation in the visceral organs undergoes a complex and irregular configuration change, and it is difficult to map the deformed surface through a transformation from a reference surface.

From 3D surface reconstruction aspects of view, it is difficult to maintain the equal number of surface points on surfaces that are reconstructed from images at various geometric or mechanical states. Therefore, it is necessary to validate the 3D SC method by comparing if the calculated correspondence surface is identical to the measured target surface at each surface point. Only a feature tracking measurement, for example, 3D digital image correlation (DIC) photogrammetry, is able to follow each surface point between the reference surface and the target surfaces. DIC measurement obtains the deformation of a surface by comparison of digital images of the undeformed and deformed configuration shapes. The assumption is that there is direct correspondence between the motions of points in the image and motions of points on the object. With the use of two CCD cameras, the DIC measurement is becoming a popular and widely used tool for 3D deformation analysis [10]. Therefore, DIC measurement is an excellent tool for verifying the SC-based 3D model registrations *in vitro* [11].

In this study, a rat stomach exposed to distension pressures 0.0, 0.2, 0.4, and 0.6 kPa was investigated by the DIC measurement for capturing the correspondence surface points during the distensions. In the meantime, the correspondence surface points between pressure 0.0 and pressures 0.2, 0.4, and 0.6 kPa were estimated by SC method, in which the DIC measured surface at pressure 0.0 was used as a reference surface, and surfaces at pressures 0.2, 0.4, and 0.6 kPa were used as the target surfaces. The target surfaces were registering to the reference surface and the point-by-point correspondence between the reference surface and the target surface was established. The purpose of this study was to verify the surface point matching calculated by SC method from the DIC measurement on a distended rat stomach.

2. Materials and Methods

In this study, a rat stomach with marked black dots on the outer surface was used as an example to verify the accuracy of the 3D shape context- (SC-) based nonrigid image registration. The rat stomach was selected because, in our recent study, the 3D SC method combined with a full-field strain

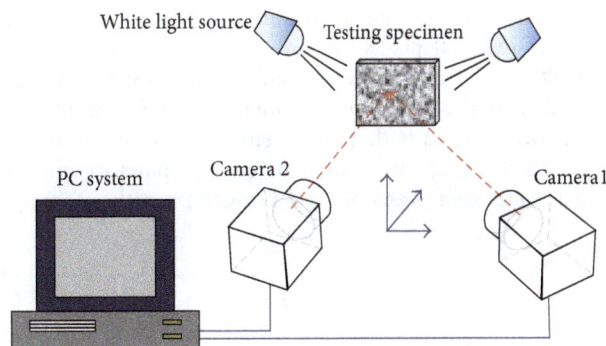

FIGURE 1: A schematic plot of DIC testing setup.

analysis method was introduced, and full-field strain analysis on a rat gastric model with distension pressures from 0.1 kPa to 0.8 kPa was obtained. We are hereby using DIC measurement to validate the 3D SC method described in our previous study [9].

2.1. Stomach Sample. The stomach of a Wistar rat weighing 300 g was used in this study. The rat was anaesthetised with Hypnorm 0.5 mg and Dormicum 0.25 mg per 100 g body weight. Following laparotomy, the whole stomach with the distal part of the oesophagus and the proximal part of the duodenum was excised. The stomach was rinsed with saline solution introduced into the lumen through the distal oesophagus. The rat was killed by a CO_2 inhalation overdose after the stomach was taken out of the abdominal cavity in accordance with guidelines and approval from the Danish Committee for Animal Experimentation. The experiment was conducted at room temperature.

2.2. Experimental Setup and Procedure. The stomach surface was gently dried and cleaned by tissue papers and was sprayed with white paint for making a white background. After a few seconds, the outer surface was sprayed with black dye to mark the stomach surface in a random dot pattern. The stomach was suspended (greater curvature down) in an organ bath by fixing the oesophageal end and the duodenal end vertically to a bar above the organ bath for avoiding rigid movement and rotation of the stomach during the distensions. The bar was then lowered to completely submerge the stomach into the organ bath. The organ bath was filled with saline solution. The duodenal end was closed after the pressure equilibration and the oesophageal end was connected via a tube to a fluid container containing saline solution. The container was used for applying static gastric luminal pressures of 0.0, 0.2, 0.4, and 0.6 kPa. Five minutes were allowed for equilibration at each pressure level.

The stomach was photographed at each pressure level using a 3D DIC system (ARAMIS 4 M, GOM GmbH, Germany) (Figure 1). A basic idea of this technique is to determine 3D coordinates of the points from a pair of pictures with two different cameras in same magnifications. The configuration of these two cameras was obtained by a calibration process with the aid of a calibration object. 3D DIC system measures the complete 3D surface displacement fields on curved or planar specimens, with accuracy on the order of ±0.01 pixels for the in-plane components and $Z/50000$ in the out-of-plane component, where Z is the distance from the object to the camera [9, 12]. In the present study, two cameras with 50 mm lenses and a resolution of 2048×2048 pixel2 were used to capture pairs of images at each distension pressure. The distance from the stomach to the camera was about 50 cm. The stomach surface with pressure of 0.0 kPa was used as the reference configuration. Each image was divided into many small computational units called facets or subsets. The detected stomach surface was reconstructed from the 3D coordinates of the centre of each facet. The distension which caused surface outwards displacement at each surface point was denoted as

$$D_i = \sqrt{\left(x_{i\_DIC} - X_{i\_DIC}\right)^2 + \left(y_{i\_Dic} - Y_{i-Dic}\right)^2 + \left(z_{i\_Dic} - Z_{i\_Dic}\right)^2}, \tag{1}$$

where x, y, z and X, Y, Z are surface point coordinates in $x, y,$ and z directions at the deformed state and the reference state, i_DIC is the surface points on the DIC measured surface, and $i = 1, 2, 3 \ldots n$ is number of the surface points.

2.3. SC Method-Based Calculations. The shape context (SC) is a shape descriptor that for a single surface captures the distribution of points over relative positions of the global shape points. In our recent study, we have extended the 2D SC to 3D and have developed the 3D SC by a combination to a 3D full-field surface strain calculation [9]. Details about SC method are described in Appendices A and B.

Based on the DIC measured surface at pressure 0.0 kPa, three references surfaces for SC method were reconstructed as reference surface 1 (RS 1), the same surface as that detected by DIC measurement; reference surface 2 (RS 2), the same surface as reference surface 1, but resampling with 90% surface sample counts of the RS 1 (selecting 9 surface points

in every 10 surface points); and reference surface 3 (RS 3), the same surface as reference surface 1, but resampling with 80% surface sample counts of the RS 1 (selecting four surface points in every five surface points). The DIC measured surfaces at pressures 0.2, 0.4, and 0.6 kPa were used as three target surfaces. For each reference surface, all three target surfaces were registering to align with the reference surface, and the point-by-point correspondence between the reference surface and the target surface was established by using the SC method-based nonlinear image registration analysis.

2.4. Accuracy of the SC Method-Based Calculations. The accuracy of the SC method was described as, with the same reference surface, the deviation of each pair of surface point between the DIC measurement (target surface) and the SC calculated correspondence surface as

$$\varepsilon_i\% = 100 * \frac{\sqrt{\left(x_{i\_DIC} - x_{i\_SC}\right)^2 + \left(y_{i\_Dic} - y_{i\_SC}\right)^2 + \left(z_{i\_Dic} - z_{i\_SC}\right)^2}}{D_i}, \tag{2}$$

where x, and y, z are surface point coordinates in $x, y,$ and z directions at the deformed state; i_DIC and i_SC are the surface points on the DIC measured surface and the SC calculated surface; D_i is the DIC measured displacement on the surface point as that presented in (1); $i = 1, 2, 3 \ldots n$ is number of the surface points; and n is equal to the surface sample counts at the selected reference surface.

2.5. Statistical Analysis. Data are expressed as means ± SD. Two-way ANOVA was used to distinguish difference in distension pressure 0.2, 0.4, and 0.6 kPa and with three reference surfaces. Differences were considered statistically significant if $P < 0.05$. All analyses were done by using the software package Sigma Stat 2.0 (SPSS Inc.).

3. Results

3.1. Experimental Results. Captured images at distension pressures of 0.0, 0.2, and 0.4 kPa are shown in Figure 2(a). As the larger section of the sample tended to collapse beyond

the viewing field of the cameras, only the patch marked with colour (Figures 2(b) and 2(c)) was analyzed. The colour graphics in Figures 2(b) and 2(c) represent the measured full-field strain distribution from DIC measurement. The stomach surface was distended with outwards displacement in ranges 0.51, 1.67 with mean value 0.95 ± 0.14, 1.12, 2.46 with mean value 1.72 ± 0.25 and 2.17, 4.67 with mean value 3.39 ± 0.51 mm in pressures 0.2, 0.4, and 0.6 kPa. Representative surface displacement, calculated from each correspondence surface point pairs, at distension pressure of 0.4 kPa showed a nonhomogeneous surface displacement on the detected stomach surface patches. The surface at the bottom displaced more than the rest of stomach patch (Figure 2(d)).

3.2. Accuracy of the SC Method-Based Calculations. The colour marked surface in Figure 2 was estimated using the SC method by matching the surface at the reference state (reference surface) to the distended state (target surface). For RS 1, that is, the same surface sample counts between the reference

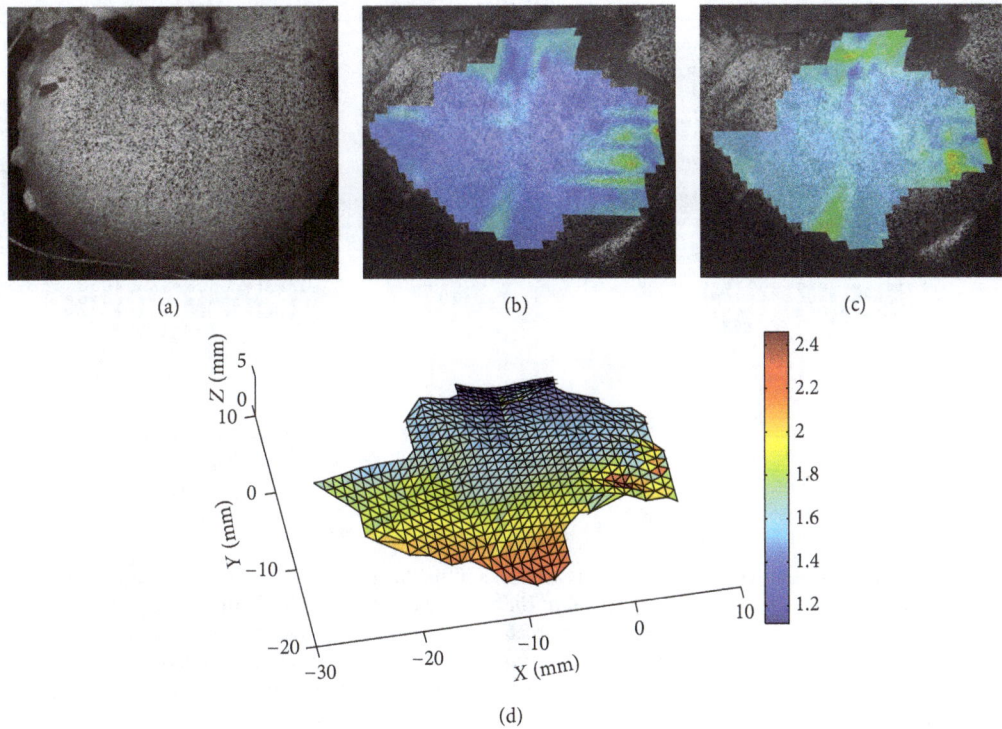

(a)   (b)   (c)

(d)

FIGURE 2: The stomach surface at distension pressure of 0.0 kPa (a), 0.2 kPa (b), 0.4 kPa (c), and the calculated 3D displacement distribution at pressure 0.4 kpa (d). The colour areas in figures (b) and (c) are DIC measured full-field strain distributions where images were obtained from the DIC system. The displacement distribution in (d) was calculated from (1), by using the DIC system recorded 3D coordinates of each correspondence surface point pairs between the reference surface (pressure = 0.0 kPa) and the target surface (pressure = 0.4 kPa). Colours from blue to red represent increasing values.

TABLE 1: Errors between the SD method calculation and DIC measurement.

Pressure/ε	RS 1 (Nr = Nt)	RS 2 (Nr = 90% × Nt)	RS 3 (Nr = 80% × Nt)
0.2 kPa	5% ± 8%	7% ± 15%	7% ± 12%
0.4 kPa	7% ± 11%	11% ± 16%	14% ± 18%
0.6 kPa	8% ± 11%	22% ± 19%	23% ± 20%

Notes: data are means ± SD; RS 1, RS 2, and RS 3: the reference surfaces 1, 2, and 3; Nr: the surface sample counts on the reference surface (surface at pressure = 0.0 kPa); and Nt: the surface sampling point on the DIC measured target surface (surface at pressures 0.2, 0.4, or 0.6 kPa).

surface and the target surface, the SC method calculated correspondence surface agreed well with the DIC measurement at all three pressure levels (Figure 3(a), Table 1). For RSs 2 and 3, increased pressure and surface sample counts differences resulted in bigger errors between the target surface and the correspondence surface (for factor 1 = pressure, $F = 197.1$, $P < 0.001$ and for factor 2 = different surface sample counts, $F = 127.04$, $P < 0.001$, Figure 3(b), Table 1). However, for pressure 0.2 kPa, the increased surface sample count difference likely did not affect the accuracy of the calculation.

4. Discussion

To the best of our knowledge, this is the first study to validate the 3D SC-based image registration method using a unique tracking features measurement. The accuracy of the SC method-based image registration was described by comparing the calculated 3D correspondence surface to the DIC measurement. Compared with previous validation studies on the SC method, we moved a step further by comparing the shape similarity between the target surface and correspondence surface for each single surface point. Hence we described quantitatively the accuracy of the SC calculations.

Exploration of disease-induced tissue remodelling in visceral organs will be improved dramatically by the introduction of medical imaging modalities such as Magnetic Resonance Imaging (MRI) and ultrasonography. The use of medical image derived, 3D-reconstructed numerical models needs further development in the photogrammetry-based tissue remodelling analysis. Previous studies have demonstrated associations between morphometric and kinematical abnormalities and diseases in visceral organs such as heart, lungs, and stomach [6, 13–19]. Our recent study demonstrated the feasibility to describe the kinematic activity of visceral organs by using combined SC-based nonrigid registration and full-field strain analysis. However, a limitation of SC method-based point matching was, because of global and local dissimilarity and existence of outliers, the significant amount of point mismatching occurring between the correspondence surface and the target surface. Visceral organs, such as stomach and bladder, undergo nonlinear and large deformation under physiological condition. For example, the volume of the stomach can be changed manifolds from empty

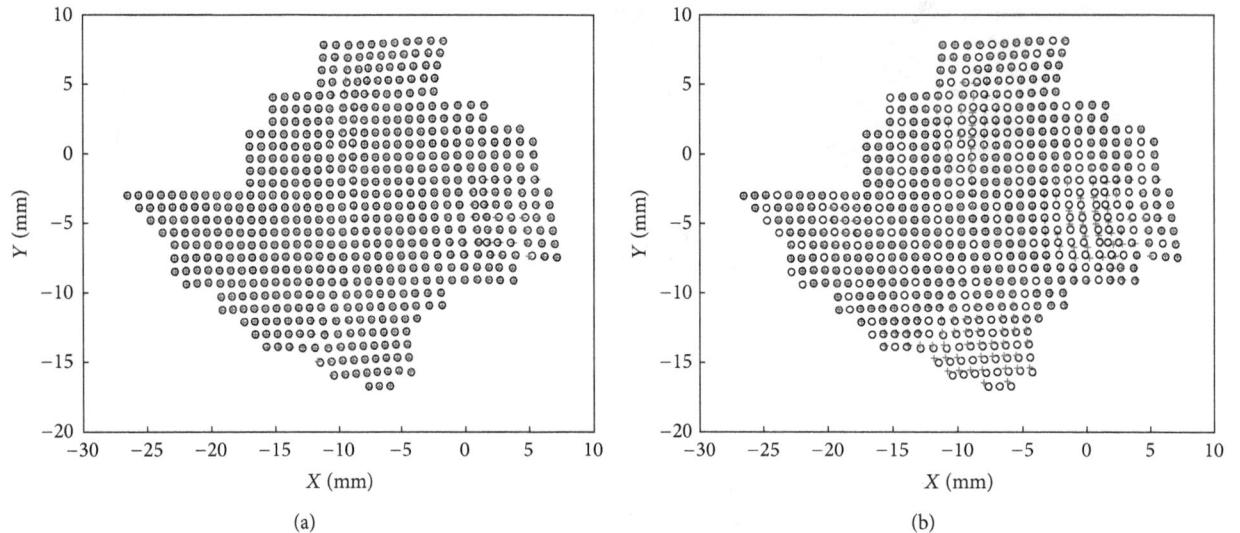

FIGURE 3: A representative DIC measured target surface (empty circles) and the SC method calculated correspondence surface (crosses) at pressure 0.4 kPa with the RS 1 (a) and RS 3 (b) for the SC calculation. The calculated corresponding surface with RS 1 showed a good agreement with the target surface. However, there are some surface points mismatching when the RS 3 was selected. RS 1, the reference surface that was detected by DIC measurement at pressure 0 kPa, and the RS 3, the same surface as the reference surface 1, but resampling with 80% surface sample counts of the RS 1 (selecting four surface points in every five surface points). Target surface, the surface measured by DIC at pressure 0.4 kPa.

to full. Moreover, heterogeneous distribution of the organ wall material will enhance deformation that caused local shape variation. Hence, using nonlinear image registration methods on living organs to define associations between the kinematical properties, tissue remodelling and diseases, it is important to determine the degree of how the method is an accurate representation of the real world from the perspective of the intended uses of the method [20].

Analysis in this study showed that the reference surface and the target surface with larger shape similarity had a better accuracy for surface point matching. Furthermore, a lower resolution of the reference surface (i.e., the reference surface has less surface sample count compared with that in the target surface) enlarges the error for the surface matching. Hence, matching between two large deformed surfaces should be achieved by a number of monotonic deformation paths, that is, by using the incremental deformation analysis. The errors caused due to the lower resolution of the reference surface can be improved in our near future studies by using soft assignments [5] or the soft shape context method [21]. This will allow multi-samples in the target surface to be assigned to one sample in the reference surface and hence will be more robust to distortions and the surfaces with different sample counts.

Some surface points with noncontinuous displacement were found in the DIC measurement (Figure 2(d)). Noncontinuous displacement could occur when some markers moved out of the gastric surface during the distension. However, the DIC system is limited in the fixed camera setting and thus resulting in loss of information and potentially increased measurement error on the surface points with those moved markers [12]. In this study, only a part of the stomach surface patch was captured by the DIC system. However, the surface patch covered the stomach body including the lesser and the great curvatures, where the major features of the distension that caused stomach deformation were represented [22]. Further studies with larger view scale on 3D measurement are needed for testing the whole 3D surface. Rotation invariance is not considered in this work as data sets are already in a similar position and orientation.

In conclusion, this is the first study to validate the 3D SC-based image registration method by using unique tracking features measurement. The influence of the shape similarity and the resolutions of the reference surface to the accuracy of point-by-point correspondence between two surfaces were investigated. Combination of the presented method and the recently developed combined SC and full-field strain analysis method will pave a way in the future to define the association between tissue remodelling and disease in more detail and will help to build a patient-based quantitative model for accessing disease induced remodelling *in vivo*.

Appendices

A. Point Matching

The shape context of a point is a measure of the distribution of relative positions with other points. The distribution is defined as a joint histogram where each histogram axis represents a parameter in a polar coordinate system. For a P on the shape, the histogram of the relative coordinates of the remaining N-1 points is defined to be the shape context of P. In a 3D shape context, a point histogram is built based on a 3D spherical coordinate system. For any two points (P_m and q_n) in different configurations, P_m belonging to point set

1 (reference state) and q_n belonging to point set 2 (deformed state), a measure of similarity between these two points can be computed as

$$C\left(p_m, q_n\right) = C_{mn} = \frac{1}{2}\sum_{l=1}^{L} \frac{\left(h_m\left(l\right) - h_n\left(l\right)\right)^2}{h_m\left(l\right) + h_n\left(l\right)}, \qquad \text{(A.1)}$$

where $h_m(l)$ and $h_n(l), l = 1, 2, \ldots L$ denote the L-bin normalized histogram (shape context) of P_m and q_n, $C(P_m, q_n) = C_{mn}$ is the cost of matching these two points. Therefore, a low cost value for two shape contexts means a high similarity between the two points.

On the basis of the previous description of (A.1), a cost matrix between all pairs of points P_m on the first shape and q_n on the second shape can be defined. Hence, the points in the first shape that best resembles the associate set of points in the second shape can be obtained by minimizing the total corresponding cost as

$$H = \min \sum_{\forall m, n} C_{mn}. \qquad \text{(A.2)}$$

The Hungarian method was used to minimize the cost function and enforce a one-to-one point matching. After completing the one-to-one matching search, the points which are set with high similarity are chosen as final correspondences.

B. Nonrigid Registration

On the basis of the points matching procedure described above, high similarity point pairs between the reference shape and the deformed shape were identified. For finding the entire matched points in these two shapes, the identified point pairs were used as a resource for the registration by mapping the entire points from the first configuration to the second configuration with a thin-plate spline method (TPS) [23]. The TPS model, describing a transformed 3D point (x', y', z') independently as a function of a source point (x, y, z), can be expressed as

$$\left(x', y', z'\right) = \left(f_x\left(x, y, z\right), f_y\left(x, y, z\right), f_z\left(x, y, z\right)\right),$$

$$f\left(x, y, z\right) = a_1 + a_2 x + a_3 y + a_4 z \qquad \text{(B.1)}$$

$$+ \sum w_i U\left(\left|P_i - \left(x, y, z\right)\right|\right),$$

where $U(r) = r^2 \log r$ is the kernel function and r is Euclidean-distance between 2 points. $P_i \; (i = 1, 2, \ldots, N)$ are points in the first shape; N is the total points number in the first shape. $a = \{a_1, a_2, a_3, a_4\}$ is the global affine coefficients of the transformation and $w = \{w_1, \ldots, w_n\}$ is the coefficients of the additional nonlinear deformation. The identified corresponding points are used to compute the coefficients of the TPS function by minimizing its bending energy as

$$E\left[f\right] = \iiint f \left|D^2 f\right|^2 dX, \qquad \text{(B.2)}$$

where $D^2 f$ is the matrix of second-order partial derivatives of f and $\left|D^2 f\right|^2$ is the sum of squares of the matrix entries. $dX = dx, dy, dz$.

With the obtained TPS function, a nonrigid wrap can thus be applied to the entire point of the referenced shape, and the registered deformed shape can be obtained with a smooth deformation field. For reducing the point mismatching in shape context analysis, the developed topological structure correction method (TSCM) [8] was used in this study.

Conflict of Interests

The authors declare that there is no conflict of interests regarding the publication of this paper.

Acknowledgment

The study was supported by grants from Karen Elise Jensens Foundation.

References

[1] O. Acosta, J. Fripp, V. Doré et al., "Cortical surface mapping using topology correction, partial flattening and 3D shape context-based non-rigid registration for use in quantifying atrophy in Alzheimer's disease," *Journal of Neuroscience Methods*, vol. 205, no. 1, pp. 96–109, 2012.

[2] J. Carballido-Gamio, J. S. Bauer, R. Stahl et al., "Inter-subject comparison of MRI knee cartilage thickness," *Medical Image Analysis*, vol. 12, no. 2, pp. 120–135, 2008.

[3] O. Acosta, J. Fripp, A. Rueda et al., "3D shape context surface registration for cortical mapping," in *Proceedings of the 7th IEEE International Symposium on Biomedical Imaging: From Nano to Macro (ISBI '10)*, pp. 1021–1024, April 2010.

[4] S. Belongie, J. Malik, and J. Puzicha, "Shape matching and object recognition using shape contexts," *IEEE Transactions on Pattern Analysis and Machine Intelligence*, vol. 24, no. 4, pp. 509–522, 2002.

[5] M. Kortgen, G. Park, M. Novotni et al., "3D shape matching with 3D shape contexts," in *Proceedings of the 7th Central European Seminar on Computer Graphics*, Budmerice, Slovakia, 2003.

[6] M. Urschler and H. Bischof, *Matching 3D Lung Surfaces with the Shape Context Approach*, 2004.

[7] M. Urschler and H. Bischof, "Assessing breathing motion by shape matching of lung and diaphragm surfaces," in *Medical Imaging 2005: Physiology, Function, and Structure from Medical Images*, Proceedings of SPIE, pp. 440–452, February 2005.

[8] D. Xiao, D. Zahra, P. Bourgeat et al., "An improved 3D shape context based non-rigid registration method and its application to small animal skeletons registration," *Computerized Medical Imaging and Graphics*, vol. 34, no. 4, pp. 321–332, 2010.

[9] D. Liao, J. Zhao, and H. Gregersen, "A novel 3D shape context method based strain analysis on a rat stomach model," *Journal of Biomechanics*, vol. 45, pp. 1566–1573, 2012.

[10] M. A. Sutton and J. Orteu, "Digital image correlation (DIC)," in *Image Correlation for Shape, Motion and Deformation Measurements*, H. Schreier and J. Jomas, Eds., Springer, New York, NY, USA, 2009.

[11] J. Tyson, T. Schmidt, and K. Galanulis, "Biomechanics deformation and strain measurements with 3D image correlation

photogrammetry," *Experimental Techniques*, vol. 26, no. 5, pp. 39–42, 2002.

[12] M. A. Sutton, "Digital image correlation for shape and deformation measurements," in *Springer Handbook of Experimental Solid Mechanics*, pp. 565–600, Springer, New York, NY, USA, 2008.

[13] E. Distrutti, F. Azpiroz, A. Soldevilla, and J.-R. Malagelada, "Gastric wall tension determines perception of gastric distention," *Gastroenterology*, vol. 116, no. 5, pp. 1035–1042, 1999.

[14] D. Liao, J. B. Frøkjær, J. Yang et al., "Three-dimensional surface model analysis in the gastrointestinal tract," *World Journal of Gastroenterology*, vol. 12, no. 19, pp. 2870–2875, 2006.

[15] H. Liu, H. Hu, C. L. Ken Wong, and P. Shi, "Cardiac motion analysis using nonlinear biomechanical constraints," in *Proceedings of the 27th Annual International Conference of the Engineering in Medicine and Biology Society*, vol. 2, pp. 1578–1581, 2005.

[16] G. Moragas, F. Azpiroz, J. Pavia, and J.-R. Malagelada, "Relations among intragastric pressure, postcibal perception, and gastric emptying," *American Journal of Physiology—Gastrointestinal and Liver Physiology*, vol. 264, no. 6, pp. G1112–G1117, 1993.

[17] X. Papademetris, A. J. Sinusas, D. P. Dione, and J. S. Duncan, "Estimation of 3D left ventricular deformation from echocardiography," *Medical Image Analysis*, vol. 5, no. 1, pp. 17–28, 2001.

[18] K. Schulze-Delrieu and S. S. Shirazi, "Pressure and length adaptations in isolated cat stomach," *American Journal of Physiology—Gastrointestinal and Liver Physiology*, vol. 252, no. 1, part 1, pp. G92–G99, 1987.

[19] P. Shi, A. J. Sinusas, R. T. Constable, and J. S. Duncan, "Volumetric deformation analysis using mechanics-based data fusion: applications in cardiac motion recovery," *International Journal of Computer Vision*, vol. 35, no. 1, pp. 87–107, 1999.

[20] H. B. Henninger, S. P. Reese, A. E. Anderson, and J. A. Weiss, "Validation of computational models in biomechanics," *Journal of Engineering in Medicine*, vol. 224, no. 7, pp. 801–812, 2010.

[21] D. Liu and T. Chen, "Soft shape context for iterative closest point registration," in *Proceedings of the International Conference on Image Processing (ICIP '04)*, pp. 1081–1084, October 2004.

[22] D. Liao, J. Zhao, and H. Gregersen, "Regional surface geometry of the rat stomach based on three-dimensional curvature analysis," *Physics in Medicine and Biology*, vol. 50, no. 2, pp. 231–246, 2005.

[23] F. L. Bookstein, "Principal warps: thin-plate splines and the decomposition of deformations," *IEEE Transactions on Pattern Analysis and Machine Intelligence*, vol. v, pp. 567–585, 1992.

12

An Object-Oriented Framework for Versatile Finite Element Based Simulations of Neurostimulation

Edward T. Dougherty[1] **and James C. Turner**[2]

[1]*Mathematics Department, Rowan University, Glassboro, NJ 08028, USA*
[2]*Mathematics Department, Virginia Polytechnic Institute and State University, Blacksburg, VA 24061, USA*

Correspondence should be addressed to Edward T. Dougherty; doughertye@rowan.edu

Academic Editor: Camillo Porcaro

Computational simulations of transcranial electrical stimulation (TES) are commonly utilized by the neurostimulation community, and while vastly different TES application areas can be investigated, the mathematical equations and physiological characteristics that govern this research are identical. The goal of this work was to develop a robust software framework for TES that efficiently supports the spectrum of computational simulations routinely utilized by the TES community and in addition easily extends to support alternative neurostimulation research objectives. Using well-established object-oriented software engineering techniques, we have designed a software framework based upon the physical and computational aspects of TES. The framework's versatility is demonstrated with a set of diverse neurostimulation simulations that (i) reinforce the importance of using anisotropic tissue conductivities, (ii) demonstrate the enhanced precision of high-definition stimulation electrodes, and (iii) highlight the benefits of utilizing multigrid solution algorithms. Our approaches result in a framework that facilitates rapid prototyping of real-world, customized TES administrations and supports virtually any clinical, biomedical, or computational aspect of this treatment. Software reuse and maintainability are optimized, and in addition, the same code can be effortlessly augmented to provide support for alternative neurostimulation research endeavors.

1. Introduction

Transcranial electrical stimulation (TES) is a collection of noninvasive neurostimulation techniques that strategically modulate activity in regions of the brain with low magnitude electric current delivered through electrodes positioned on the scalp surface. Forms of TES include the commonly used transcranial direct current stimulation (tDCS), as well as transcranial alternating current stimulation (tACS) [1]. Recently, the use of numerous smaller sized electrodes, termed high-definition tDCS (HD-tDCS), has emerged as a form of TES that enhances electrical current focality [2, 3]. Clinical and biomedical research continue to demonstrate the capabilities of TES as a medical treatment. For example, Alzheimer and Parkinson's disease patients have demonstrated increased memory abilities [4–6]. In addition, TES has shown to alleviate symptoms of psychiatric disorders including depression [7, 8] and schizophrenia [9–11].

The efficacy and comprehension of TES have been enhanced with mathematical modeling and computational simulation. In particular, simulations can compute the current density distribution for a given patient and TES apparatus configuration [1, 12–15] and have demonstrated the importance of modulating treatment stimulation dosage [16]. Other simulations have illustrated the importance of incorporating anisotropic tissue conductivity data [17, 18], and numerical studies aid in identifying the computational solution methods most efficient in simulating TES mathematical models [19].

Object-oriented design is a software design approach that defines objects, which are simply software entities that encapsulate data and functionality and the relationships among objects. Features of object-oriented design can be utilized to maximize code reusability, simplify software maintenance, and promote application versatility [20]. The prevalence of object-oriented design in scientific and biomedical applications began in the 1990s, and its use has dramatically increased due to its advantages over procedural software implementations [21–26]. In particular, mathematical and physical attributes of a model can be naturally represented with objects [27, 28].

A common approach for simulating partial differential equation (PDE) based mathematical models is to use prebuilt simulation software programs. These "black-boxes" can simplify model implementation; however, there are limitations with this approach. A researcher is often confined to the numerical algorithms and programming controls offered by the simulation program; it can be very difficult, or perhaps not possible, to incorporate numerics and solution techniques not supported by the software. In addition, integrating a prebuilt software application with external data sources and applications can be very challenging, which obstructs the use of its simulations within larger software solutions.

An alternative strategy is to create custom software that utilizes numerical application programming interfaces (APIs). While this approach generally takes longer to implement, it allows the use of problem-specific algorithms and programming logic that facilitate accurate and expedient simulation results [28]. Coupling this philosophy with object-oriented software engineering techniques can produce a final product that is versatile, expandable, and computationally efficient. Interactions with external systems can be seamlessly integrated, and the ability to compile the software to executable machine code simplifies its deployment to alternative hardware platforms, for example, medical imaging machines.

In this paper, we present an object-oriented software framework for finite element based TES simulations. Multiple features of object-oriented design and programming are utilized to create a modular software architecture that encapsulates medical, mathematical, and computational attributes of TES. The result is a program that maximizes code reuse and TES simulation versatility. We demonstrate this versatility with several simulations, each with a distinct TES research focus. These simulations utilize MRI-derived three-dimensional head models, with physiologically based tissue conductivities and real-world electrode configurations. Finally, we show how the same software can be easily extended to address alternative neurostimulation research areas, such as deep brain stimulation (DBS). In addition, all components of the framework are available to the community as a supplement to this paper.

2. Materials and Methods

2.1. Governing Equations. The electric current density within the head and brain from neurostimulation can be modeled by the Poisson equation; namely, $-\nabla \cdot \mathbf{M}\nabla\Phi = f(\vec{x})$, where Φ is the electric potential, $\mathbf{M}$ is the tissue conductivity tensor, and $f(\vec{x})$ is a given electrical source term. For isotropic mediums, $\mathbf{M}$ can be represented as a scalar, which varies for different tissue types.

Electric current delivered by TES anode electrode(s) is given by the nonhomogeneous Neumann boundary condition $\vec{n} \cdot \mathbf{M}\nabla\Phi = I(\vec{x})$, where $I(\vec{x})$ represents the stimulation current density and $\vec{n}$ is the outward boundary normal vector.

Cathode electrode(s) are represented by the homogeneous Dirichlet condition $\Phi(\vec{x}) = 0$. All other points on the skin surface are insulated by the surrounding air; thus $\vec{n} \cdot \mathbf{M}\nabla\Phi = 0$.

Our governing equations are as follows:

$$-\nabla \cdot \mathbf{M}\nabla\Phi = f(\vec{x}), \quad \vec{x} \in \Omega, \tag{1a}$$

$$\Phi = 0, \quad \vec{x} \in \partial\Omega_C, \tag{1b}$$

$$\vec{n} \cdot \mathbf{M}\nabla\Phi = I(\vec{x}), \quad \vec{x} \in \partial\Omega_A, \tag{1c}$$

$$\vec{n} \cdot \mathbf{M}\nabla\Phi = 0, \quad \vec{x} \in \partial\Omega_S, \tag{1d}$$

where Ω is the head volume, $\partial\Omega_A$ and $\partial\Omega_C$ represent the areas on the scalp covered by anode and cathode electrodes, respectively, and $\partial\Omega_S$ is the remaining portion of the head surface. Note that, for TES simulations, there is no source term within the volume, and so $f(\vec{x}) = 0$ (1a). Alternatively, DBS is realized with an appropriate definition of $f(\vec{x})$ and the homogeneous Neumann boundary condition (1d) applied to the entire boundary; namely, $\partial\Omega_s = \partial\Omega$ [29].

The associated weak formulation (see Appendix) is to find $\Phi(\vec{x}) \in H_0^1(\Omega)$ given $f(\vec{x}) \in L_2(\Omega)$ such that

$$\int_\Omega \nabla v \cdot \mathbf{M}\nabla\Phi \, dx = \int_{\partial\Omega_A} vI \, ds + \int_\Omega fv \, dx, \tag{2}$$
$$\forall v(\vec{x}) \in H_0^1(\Omega),$$

where

$$H_0^1(\Omega) = \left\{ u \mid u \in H^1(\Omega), u = 0 \; \forall \vec{x} \in \partial\Omega_C \right\},$$

$$H^1(\Omega) = \left\{ u \mid u \in L_2(\Omega), \frac{\partial u}{\partial x_i} \in L_2(\Omega) \right\}, \tag{3}$$

$$L_2(\Omega) = \left\{ p \mid \int_\Omega |p|^2 \, dx < \infty \right\}.$$

2.2. Framework Design. The fundamental task in the design of the framework was to create objects based on attributes of TES and TES simulations. We refer to [30] for a detailed explanation of object-oriented design and provide just a brief overview of the key aspects utilized within our framework.

Objects encapsulate data and functions that operate on the data. A *class* provides the description of an object type by defining variable and function names, and an object is more formally viewed as a specific instance of a class. *Inheritance* is a class relationship and provides the ability to extend the functionality of a class with a so-called *subclass*. A subclass can contain data and functionality from a parent class and can define its own as well. Inheritance is a major object-oriented design concept that exploits code reuse, since all subclasses can reuse data constructs and functions from a parent class. *Polymorphism* enables a subclass to give specific functionality to an abstract function defined by a parent class. This powerful technique allows parent classes to encapsulate generic and broad ideas by delegating specific function implementations to subclasses [30].

We required that electrode configuration, stimulation parameters, tissue conductivity information, computational

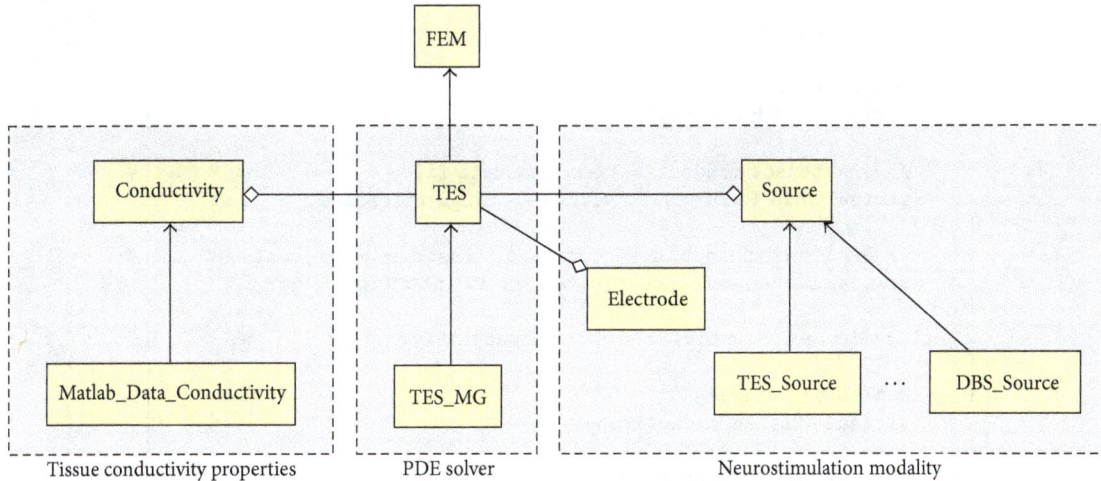

FIGURE 1: Software architecture and main classes in the object-oriented TES simulation framework. Classes are represented with boxes, and arrow and diamond tipped lines represent inheritance and aggregation, respectively.

domain, and numerical solution methods be specified via an input file. This permits customized TES simulations without the need to rewrite and recompile code. In addition, by mathematically retaining the source term, $f(\vec{x})$, in the weak formulation (2) and allowing this function to be defined by a user, different neurostimulation modalities, for example, DBS, can be simulated.

We choose to base our framework design on Diffpack [31], which is a numerical API library for solving PDEs. It is based on the C++ programming language [32] and possesses a vast collection of PDE solution algorithms [27, 28]. The C++ language incorporates well-established software engineering practices [33] and is compiled to machine code, resulting in fast execution speeds and portability to alternative hardware platforms. Despite our use of a specific numerical library and programming language, the object-oriented design and implementation strategies presented in this paper apply to any programming language and API package that supports an object-oriented approach.

Figure 1 displays the main software components in the TES simulation framework. Each box represents a class, and each arrow and diamond tipped line represents inheritance and aggregation, respectively. FEM is a class in the Diffpack library that offers fundamental finite element method data structures and algorithms. Class TES, which is the corner-stone of the framework, inherits FEM functionality to solve simulations given by system (1a)–(1d). Class TES_MG extends TES functionality so that multigrid (MG) algorithms can also be utilized in solving this system.

For TES simulations to be fully realized, tissue conductivity and electrode information are needed. These ideas have been encapsulated with respective classes, and TES possesses instances of each. Since conductivity data can come from a variety of sources with differing storage formats, the Conductivity class merely defines abstract function names that are viewed as common to all conductivity data sources. Then, specific functionality for specific conductivity data sources is implemented in subclasses, for example,

Matlab_Data_Conductivity, via polymorphism. This approach allows different conductivity data sources to be incorporated into the framework without needing to modify code in the TES and Conductivity classes. The boundary conditions are also managed by TES, using information from class Electrode, which maintains TES electrode location and size information. In addition, by retaining the source term $f(\vec{x})$ in the weak formulation (2) and encapsulating it as a class, namely, Source, assignments to $f(\vec{x})$ enable the simulation of alternative types of neurostimulation, such as DBS.

2.3. Framework Implementation. In this section, key software implementation aspects of the framework and related Diffpack concepts are described. For a complete guide to Diffpack, see [27].

2.3.1. Tissue Conductivity. Class Conductivity defines general function names but delegates the implementation of these functions to its subclasses (Code 1). MatlabConductivity inherits Conductivity and provides specific implementations of the loadConductivities and getConductivity functions based on a Matlab [34] binary data file format produced by the SimNIBS software package [35].

Two additional data members are defined by MatlabConductivity, namely, a MatlabHelper object, mh, which manages a runtime interface with the MatlabEngine [34], and a Matlab matrix, ct. These two members are needed by the MatlabConductivity subclass, not the parent Conductivity class, and are therefore included in only the subclass. The MatlabConductivity implementation of the loadConductivities function simply creates a Matlab command to load the anisotropic conductivity data source, executes this command within the MatlabEngine via the mh object, and then stores the anisotropic conductivity tensor data into the ct matrix which are then accessible throughout a TES simulation via the getConductivity function (Code 1).

```
class Conductivity
{
  Conductivity();
  virtual ~Conductivity();

  // Load tensor conductivities from data files
  virtual void loadConductivities (String& fileName);

  // Get ith component of conductivity tensor at pt (x,y,z)
  virtual double getConductivity (int i, int x, int y, int z);

class MatlabConductivity: public Conductivity
{
  MatlabConductivity();
  virtual ~MatlabConductivity();

  // Inherited from Conductivity
  virtual void loadConductivities(String& fileName);
  virtual double getConductivity(int i, int x, int y, int z);

  MatlabHelper* mh; // Mangage interface with the MatlabEngine
  mxArray* ct;      // Matrix with conductivity tensor data

void MatlabConductivity::loadConductivities(String& fileName){
  String name = "load('" + fileName + "');";
  engEvalString(mh->ep, name.c_str());
  ct = engGetVariable(mh->ep, "ct");
}
```

CODE 1: Class definitions for tissue conductivity data. Class Conductivity provides general function names, that is, loadConductivities and getConductivity. The MatlabConductivity subclass implements these functions for a particular data source. For example, its loadConductivities function loads a Matlab anisotropic conductivity data source into the ct matrix for use in a simulation.

The Conductivity-MatlabConductivity relationship demonstrates the advantages of object-oriented inheritance and polymorphism. Conductivity is used to define function names common to all conductivity data sources and serves as the bridge between these repositories and the framework. Polymorphism permits the MatlabConductivity subclass to implement specific loadConductivities and getConductivity functionality for its particular data format. Code within the Conductivity class and all other framework classes does not dependent on these subclass implementations. Thus, alternative conductivity data sources can be easily incorporated into the framework as a subclass of Conductivity, in an identical fashion, requiring no modification to any other framework component.

2.3.2. Source Term. Class Source is a software abstraction of the $f(\vec{x})$ source term (1a) and like Conductivity defines basic functionality to be implemented in subclasses (Code 2). Source inherits the Diffpack class FieldFunc which allows a scalar function to be defined over the domain. Different subclass implementations of the valuePt function can be used to model different neurostimulation modalities. For TES, valuePt in class TES_Source simply returns zero since $f(\vec{x}) = 0$ in this case (Code 2).

Main TES Class. Class TES is the main class in the framework. Code 3 presents the key elements of this class, which contains numerous objects, functions, and Diffpack concepts. Class TES inherits the Diffpack FEM class, giving it access to finite element data structures and functionality. Handle objects, which are pointers in Diffpack that include memory management features, are defined for the computational grid, grid, and electric potential and current density solution results, u and currDensity, respectively.

Several other class members are needed to implement TES simulations. Variables to store boundary condition values are included, as well as the anodes and cathodes vectors to store electrode information. The vector isoSigma and matrix sigma store isotropic and anisotropic conductivity data, and the choice of conductivity representation is determined by a user via the isotropic boolean variable. The mc data member is a reference to the Conductivity class, providing an interface to conductivity data. Note that mc is type Conductivity and not MatlabConductivity. The mc object can therefore use the loadConductivities and getConductivity functions of any Conductivity subclass, including MatlabConductivity. This design approach allows new Conductivity subclasses to be defined and utilized without the need to modify code in class TES.

```
class Source: public FieldFunc
{
  TES* data;                // Provides access to TES class members

  Source (){}
  virtual dpreal valuePt    // Source term value at pt. x; Abstract function
              (const Ptv(dpreal)& x, dpreal t = DUMMY) = 0;
};

dpreal TES_Source:: valuePt(const Ptv(dpreal)& x, dpreal t) {
  dpreal val = 0.0;
  return val;
}
```

CODE 2: Source term class definitions. The TES_Source subclass of Source enables TES simulations by defining its valuePt function to return a value of zero at all points.

```
class TES: public FEM
{
  // DATA TYPES:
  Handle(GridFE)      grid;         // Underlying finite element grid
  Handle(FieldFE)     u;            // Electric potential over grid
  Handle(FieldsFE)    currDensity;  // Electric Current density over grid

  dpreal              dirichlet_val1;  // Constant phi value at a boundary
  dpreal              dirichlet_val2;  // Constant phi value at boundary
  dpreal              robin_U0;        // Constants for Neumann boundary condition

  vector<Electrode>   anodes;       // Anode electrodes
  vector<Electrode>   cathodes;     // Cathode electrodes

  bool                isotropic;    // Isotrpoic or anisotropic bool control
  Vec(dpreal)         isoSigma;     // Isotropic brain tissue conductance values
  MatSimple(dpreal)   sigma;        // Anisotropic conductivity tensor matrix
  Conductivity*       mc;           // Interface class for anisotropic conductivities

  Handle(FieldFunc)   source;        // Source term for initializing f(x)
  Handle(FieldFunc)   alternatingStim;  // Object to model non-direct TES, i.e. tACS

  // FUNCTIONS:
  // Standard finite element functions inherited from class FEM
  virtual void fillEssBC ();              // Set dirichlet boundary conditions
  virtual void calcElmMatVec              // Compute FE coefficient matrix and load vector
              (int e, ElmMatVec& elmat, FiniteElement& fe);
  virtual void integrands                 // Implement weak formulation integrand
              (ElmMatVec& elmat, const FiniteElement& fe);
  virtual void integrands4side            // Neumann boundary integral
              (int side, int boind, ElmMatVec& elmat, const FiniteElement& fe);
}
```

CODE 3: Main elements within the TES class. Handles are Diffpack pointers that include memory management features. The class definition contains a Handle for the computational grid (grid) and electric potential (u) and current density (currDensity) solution results. Next, variables store boundary condition values and anode (anodes) and cathode (cathodes) electrode information. Support for both isotropic and anisotropic conductivity data is provided, as well as functions for source and nonconstant anode stimulation. Functions inherited from FEM are required to perform finite element calculations.

```
void TES:: integrands (ElmMatVec& elmat, const FiniteElement& fe)
{
  int i,j,q;                         // Loop control variables
  const int nbf = fe.getNoBasisFunc(); // no of nodes/basis functions
  dpreal detJxW = fe.detJxW();         // Numerical integration weight
  const int nsd = fe.getNoSpaceDim();  // Number of spatial dimensions

  // Get conductivity tensor for the current element.
  updateConductivityTensors(fe);

  // Get a point in the global domain represented by elemnt fe.
  Ptv(NUMT) x(nsd);
  fe.getGlobalEvalPt(x);

  // Get the source term, f(x), for this element.
  dpreal f_val;
  if (source.ok())
    f_val = source->valuePt(x);
  else f_val = 0;

  // Compute weak formulation
  dpreal gradNi_gradNj;
  for (i = 1; i <= nbf; i++) {
    for (j = 1; j <= nbf; j++) {
      gradNi_gradNj = 0;
      for (q = 1; q <= nsd; q++){
        // Compute inner product of grad(N_i) and grad(N_j).
        gradNi_gradNj += sigma(q,q) * fe.dN(i,q) * fe.dN(j,q);
      }

      // Update linear system coefficient matrix.
      elmat.A(i,j) += gradNi_gradNj*detJxW;
    }
    // Update linear system RHS (load vector).
    elmat.b(i) += fe.N(i)*f_val*detJxW;
  }
}
```

CODE 4: TES class integrands function for computing weak formulation volume integrals. Conductivity and source term values for finite element `fe` are retrieved with calls to the `updateConductivityTensors` and source `valuePt` functions. Finite element basis functions are then iterated to compute the volume integrals.

There is also a reference to a Source object, for example, TES_Source, as well as a field function for nonconstant stimulation currents, for example, tACS. Finally, TES inherits functions from FEM to perform finite element computations, including `fillEssBC` to set Dirichlet boundary conditions, `calcElmMatVec` to assemble the finite element linear system coefficient matrix and load vector, and the `integrands` and `integrands4side` functions to evaluate the weak formulation volume and boundary integrals, respectively.

2.3.3. Weak Formulation Integration. The weak formulation volume integrals (2) are computed in the TESintegrands function (Code 4). The Diffpack linear system assembler automatically calls this function as it iterates over the finite elements in the computational grid. Conductivity values for the current element are attained with a call to

the `updateConductivityTensors` function, which determines if isotropic or anisotropic conductivities are desired and then populates the `sigma` matrix accordingly.

The source term $f(\vec{x})$ over the current element is retrieved via a call to the `valuePt` function in a Source class. Then, the finite element basis functions for this element are iterated over, and the weak formulation is computed. Note that, in this implementation, `sigma` is assumed to be diagonal; however, this can be generalized with the incorporation of an additional loop. Finally, the coefficient matrix, A, and load vector, b, are updated. The boundary integral in the weak formulation is computed similarly in the `integrands4side` function, and its contribution is incorporated into b.

2.3.4. Multigrid. Multigrid is a linear system solution algorithm that utilizes multiple computational grid resolutions to

```
class TES_MG: public TES
{
    int                 no_of_grids;
    Handle(MGtools)     mgtools;

    // Set boundary condtion on grid level specified by space
    virtual void mgFillEssBC (SpaceId space);
```

CODE 5: New members of TES_MG class definition. The mgtools object references the Diffpack multigrid toolbox. The no_of_grids integer stores the number of MG grid levels, and the mgFillEssBC function sets the essential boundary condition on all grid levels.

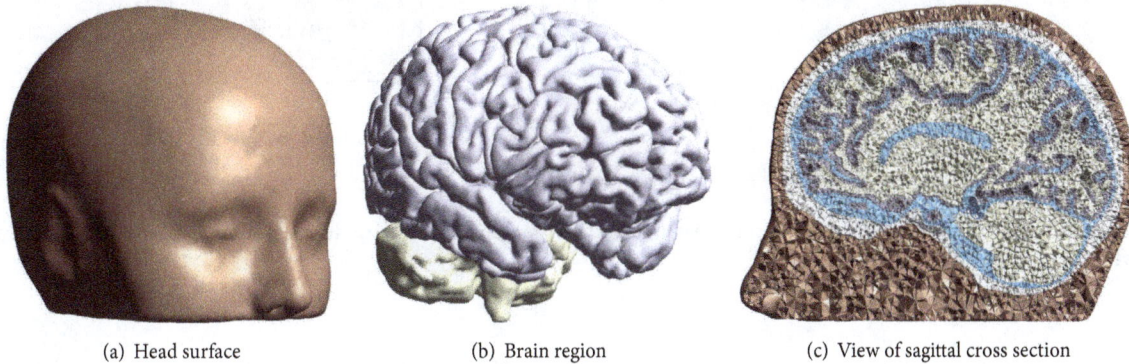

(a) Head surface   (b) Brain region   (c) View of sagittal cross section

FIGURE 2: Computational domain used in numerical simulations.

achieve fast solution convergence [36]. By performing just a few iterations on each grid and then changing between finer and coarser grids, large portions of the error are efficiently removed [37]. In addition, as a preconditioner to the commonly used conjugate gradient (CG) method, MG is highly effective at solving linear systems that result from finite element based TES simulations [38]. Two commonly used MG cycles are the V-cycle and the W-cycle, and identifying the optimal cycle type for a given PDE system, in addition to other MG parameters including the number of grid levels, can be challenging [38].

As a subclass of TES, very few new data members and functions are needed in TES_MG (Code 5), since the entirety of TES is efficiently reused. The new members in TES_MG are a reference to the Diffpack multigrid toolbox, mgtools, and an integer representing the number of MG grid levels, no_of_grids. Finally, just one new function, mgFillEssBC, is needed to set the essential boundary condition (1b) on all grid levels.

2.4. Computational Tools. Numerical simulations were performed on a three-dimensional mesh (Figure 2) generated from human MRI images by the SimNIBS software package [35]. The mesh contains the skin, skull, cerebral spinal fluid (CSF), gray matter (GM), and white matter (WM) tissues of the head. Gmsh [39] enabled mesh visualization, identification of electrode coordinates, and grid conversion to a form supported by Diffpack. Electric potential and current density results were exported from Diffpack and visualized with ParaView [40] and gnuplot [41]. Anisotropic conductivity data for the GM and WM regions are provided by SimNIBS in

a Matlab binary data file; these data are accessed by the MatlabEngine [34] via the MatlabHelper object of the MatlabConductivity class (Code 1).

2.5. Computational Simulations. Multiple simulations were performed with the TES framework. Simulations were selected to demonstrate the framework's versatility and ability to target medical, biophysical, and computational research objectives. Finally, to illustrate how alternative forms of neurostimulation can be simulated with the same software, we show a trivial extension to the framework that enables support for DBS applications.

Simulation 1 (comparison of isotropic and anisotropic conductivity data). Previous research suggests that incorporating anisotropic, rather than isotropic, brain tissue conductivity data is important for most accurately modeling TES electrical current distribution [17, 42]. To evaluate the impact that these two conductivity representations have on simulation results, TES simulations were performed with isotropic and anisotropic data. The three-dimensional domain shown in Figure 2 was used with approximately 2.8 million linear tetrahedra finite elements.

Anode and cathode electrodes were positioned at C3 and C4 [43], respectively, each with a surface area of approximately $16\,cm^2$, and the anode electric current magnitude was set to 1.0 mA. This montage has been used to stimulate the motor cortex ipsilateral to the C3 anode electrode [44, 45]. First, isotropic electrical conductivities were assigned to different tissues: skin = 0.465, skull = 0.010, CSF = 1.654, GM = 0.276, and WM = 0.126, each with units (S/m) [46].

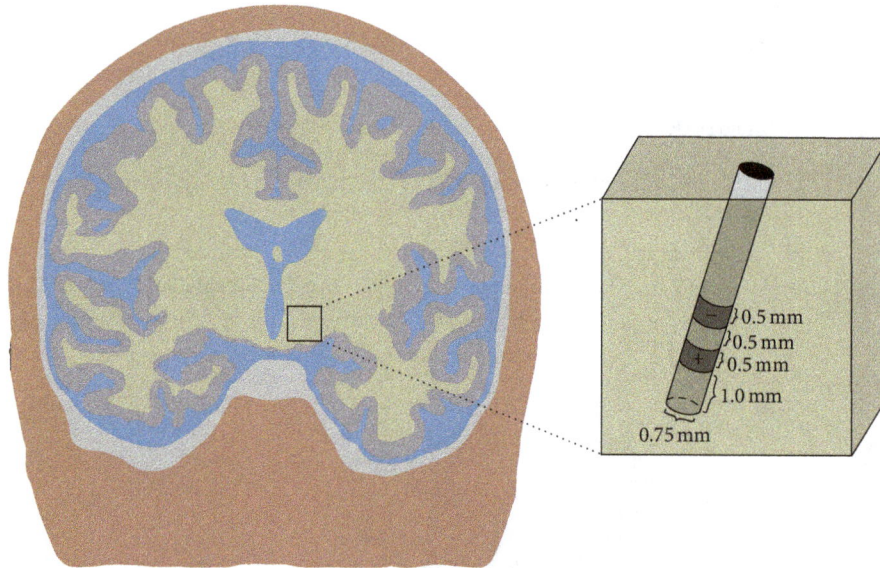

FIGURE 3: Simulation 4, DBS electrode positioning (subthalamic nucleus) and dimensions. Anode and cathode contacts are denoted with "+" and "−" symbols, respectively.

Then, anisotropic conductivity data were used via the `MatlabConductivity` class as previously described (see Code 1).

Simulation 2 (comparison of tDCS and HD-tDCS electrode montages). High-definition TES electrodes have demonstrated a greater ability to focus its electrical current on a targeted brain region than traditional tDCS, which uses two larger electrodes [2, 3]. Using the same computational grid as Simulation 1, the current densities produced by tDCS and HD-tDCS were compared.

For tDCS, the anode was positioned over C3 and the cathode over the contralateral supraorbital, each with a surface area of approximately 16 cm^2. In comparison, high-definition electrodes, each circular with a 12 mm diameter, were positioned according to a 4 × 1 configuration; a single anode was positioned over C3, and four cathodes were placed approximately 5 cm radially from the anode, forming a square. Both of these montages are known to target the motor cortex region ipsilateral to the anode electrode [15, 47–50]. Anode stimulation strength for each simulation was once again 1.0 mA, and both utilized anisotropic conductivities.

Simulation 3 (comparison of finite element linear system solvers). Finite element based simulations of TES require the solution of large systems of linear equations, which can become a computational bottleneck for simulations performed on very fine meshes. Therefore, the effectiveness of a TES simulation is directly related to the efficiency of the chosen linear solver. The CG method is ideal for solving these linear systems and appropriate preconditioning can rapidly accelerate numerical results [36, 38].

The numerical efficiency of the preconditioned CG method was evaluated with TES simulations on the three-dimensional volume mesh (Figure 2), with approximately

29 million linear tetrahedra finite elements and roughly 5.1 million unknowns. The anode was positioned at CZ, with a stimulation strength of 1.0 mA, and the cathode at OZ [12, 51]. Simulations were performed with the CG method preconditioned with symmetric successive overrelaxation (SSOR), relaxed incomplete LU decomposition (RILU), and multigrid. The RILU relaxation parameter was set to 0.5 [27]. The MG preconditioner was simulated with a V-cycle with both two and three grid levels, and a W-cycle with three grid levels. The relative residual convergence tolerance was set to 10^{-8} for all numerical experiments.

Simulation 4 (impact of conductivity representation on DBS simulation results). The importance of incorporating anisotropic conductivities in TES simulations suggests that accurately simulating other neurostimulation modalities may depend on this conductivity representation as well. In this numerical experiment, we compared DBS simulation results using both isotropic and anisotropic conductivities. A single electrode was positioned in the subthalamic nucleus (STN), the most commonly targeted location for DBS [52]. The electrode is a simplified version of the Medtronic (Model 3387) electrode used in humans [53]. The lower 5.0 mm of the electrode was modeled. The anode is positioned 1.0 mm from the electrode tip and the cathode is separated by 0.5 mm from the anode. Both the anode and cathode are 0.5 mm in height, and the overall electrode diameter was set to 0.75 mm (Figure 3). The anode and cathode metal contacts were modeled as conductors by setting the electrical conductivities of these regions to 10^6 (S/m), and the remaining electrode shaft was modeled as an insulator with conductivity equal to 10^{-6} (S/m) [54]. Because DBS electric current is proximal to the electrode [29, 55], a 10.0 mm × 4.0 mm × 4.0 mm subset of tissue around the electrode was considered as the computational domain.

```
class DBS_Source: public Source
{
  DBS_Source(TES* data);
  virtual dpreal valuePt(const Ptv(dpreal)& x, dpreal t = DUMMY);
};

dpreal DBS_Source:: valuePt(const Ptv(dpreal)& x, dpreal t) {
  dpreal val = 0.0;

  if (4.625 <= x(1) && x(1) <= 5.375 &&
      4.625 <= x(2) && x(2) <= 5.375 &&
      3.500 <= x(3) && x(3) <= 4.000 ) {
    val = 0.001;
  }
```

CODE 6: DBS_Source class definition and sample code from its valuePt function.

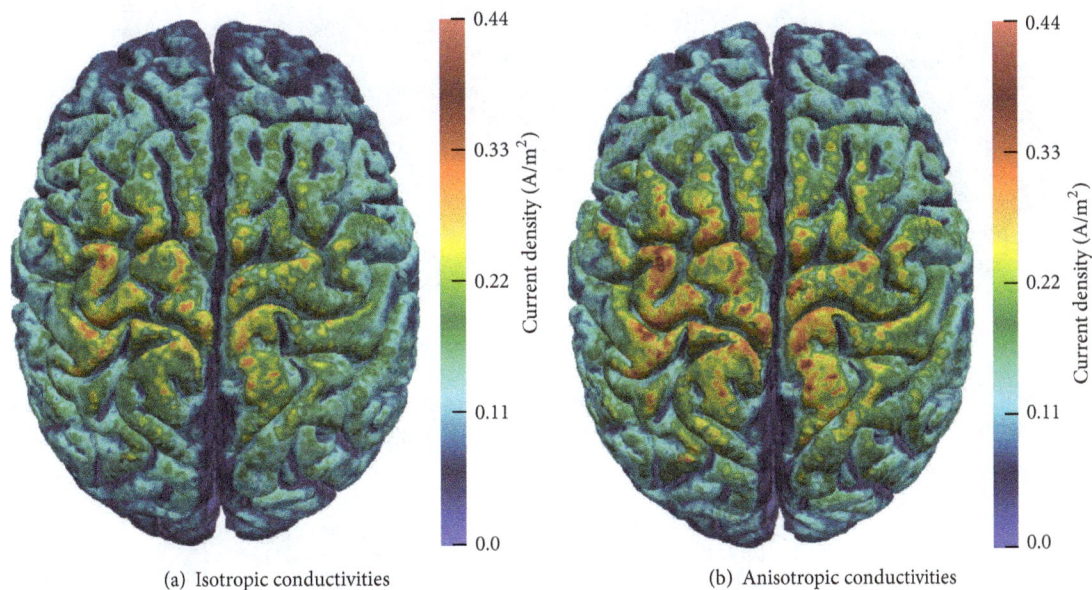

(a) Isotropic conductivities

(b) Anisotropic conductivities

FIGURE 4: Simulation 1, current density results viewed from above with the nasion facing up. Anode was placed at C3 and cathode at C4.

To simulate DBS with the existing TES software framework, no existing code required modification. Rather, the only addition was a new subclass of class Source that defines $f(\vec{x})$ (1a) for DBS; in total, less than ten lines of code were added. Code 6 displays this new subclass definition, Source_DBS, and highlights of its valuePt function implementation, which in this simplified scenario simply injects 1.0 mA of current from the anode contact into the surrounding tissue. In practice, DBS stimulations are time-varying pulses, and differing stimulation frequencies impact GM and WM tissue conductivities [56]. However, when examining electric field dispersion around a DBS electrode as in this simulation, a constant-valued source term in (1a) can be utilized [57].

3. Results and Discussion

3.1. Simulation 1. Electric current density results on the surface of the brain tissue are displayed in Figure 4. Viewing perspective is from above the head with the nasion facing up. As expected, the largest electric current density values are attained near the anode and cathode locations. Despite an overall similar pattern of electric current distribution, the simulated current densities, particularly in the motor cortex ipsilateral to the anode electrode, are significantly different between the isotropic and anisotropic simulations. For example, the maximal anisotropic current density value (0.434 (A/m^2)) is approximately 18.2% higher than in the isotropic case (0.367 (A/m^2)). Similar discrepancies are observed throughout the top surface of the brain, including a substantial impact on the paracentral lobule contralateral to the anode. In addition, these discrepancies extend to the GM and WM interiors. These results reinforce the importance of using anisotropic conductivities to most accurately model TES administrations and in addition showcase the capabilities of the object-oriented framework to support both isotropic and anisotropic TES simulations.

(a) tDCS electric potential

(b) HD-tDCS electric potential

(c) tDCS electric current density

(d) HD-tDCS electric current density

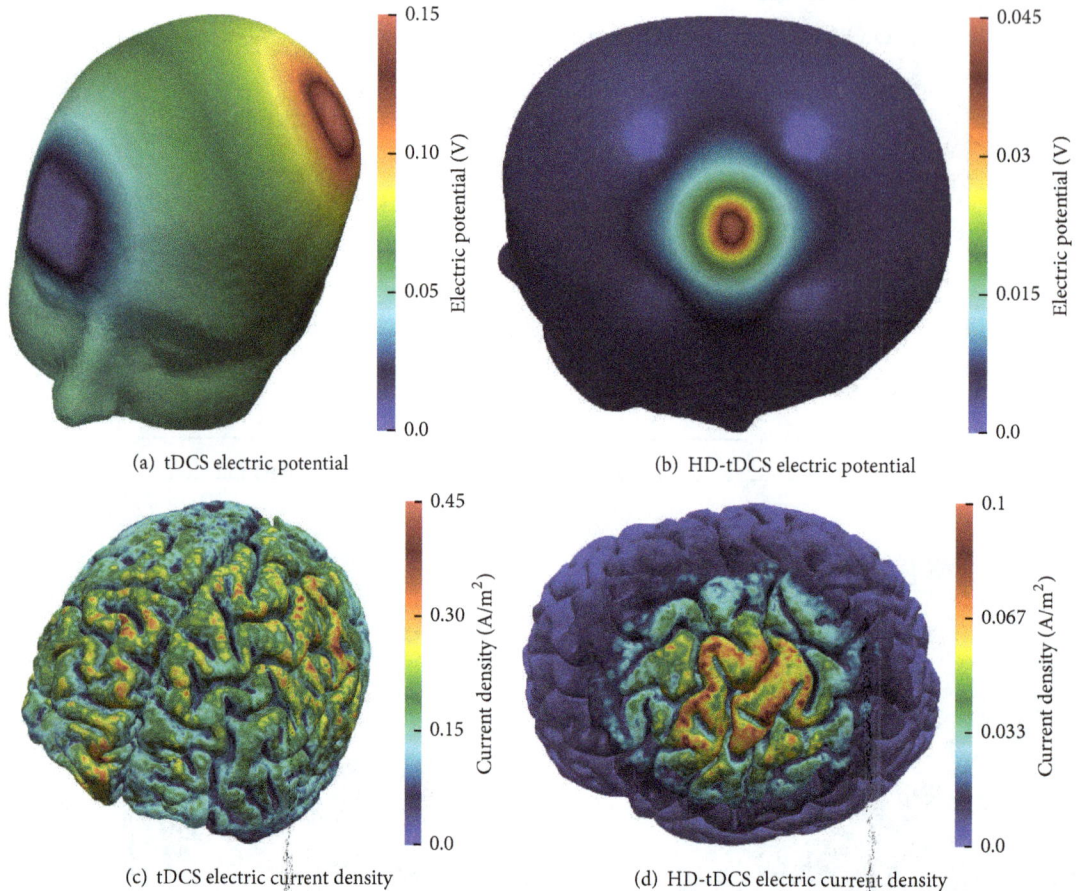

FIGURE 5: Simulation 2, electric potential and current density results. The tDCS montage positioned the anode at C3 and the cathode over the contralateral supraorbital. A 4×1 configuration was used for HD-tDCS with a single anode positioned over C3.

3.2. Simulation 2. Electric potential and electric current density results are displayed in Figure 5. The tDCS montage results in a noticeably larger range of electric potential values (Figures 5(a) and 5(b)). However, the focus of the tDCS current density on the targeted region, in this case the motor cortex under C3, is much less than the HD-tDCS electrode montage (Figures 5(c) and 5(d)). Specifically, the brain tissue outside of the square formed by the HD-tDCS cathodes is virtually unstimulated, whereas tDCS results in a much greater electric current dispersion.

One limitation of this HD-tDCS electrode arrangement is the lower concentration of electric current that reaches the brain tissue. Specifically, the maximal electric current density in the brain from HD-tDCS is just approximately 23% of that achieved with traditional tDCS. The culprit for this effect is the shunting of the electric current around the poorly conducting skull; the HD-tDCS montage used in this simulation yields a minuscule amount of current that penetrates the skull to reach the CSF and brain tissues (Figure 6). Potential remedies for this behavior are a greater anode stimulation or positioning the cathodes at greater distances from the anode [3].

This simulation demonstrates the framework's ability to support varying TES electrode montages, including high-definition electrode configurations. Results of this simulation

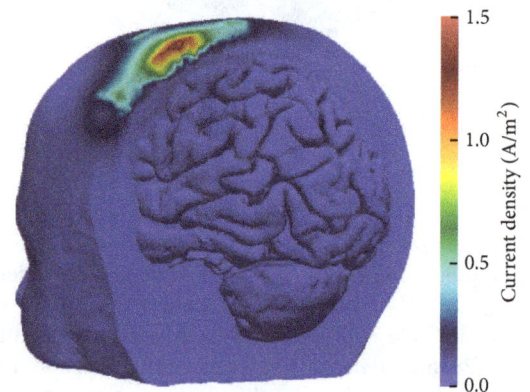

FIGURE 6: Simulation 2, HD-tDCS electric current density. Cross section is through two diagonally positioned cathodes.

corroborate that HD-tDCS offers greater electric current focality; however, its net stimulation of brain tissue is potentially much lower than tDCS.

3.3. Simulation 3. Electric potential and current density results on the head surface are displayed in Figure 7. Viewing

(a) Electric potential

(b) Current density

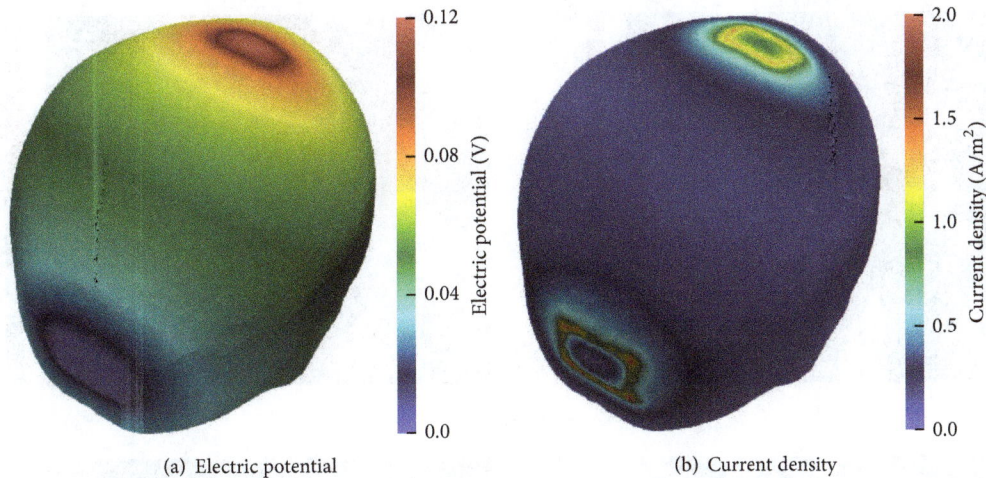

FIGURE 7: Simulation 3, electric potential and current density results viewed from the back of the head. The anode was positioned at CZ and the cathode at OZ.

perspective is from behind the head, and as anticipated, maximal and minimal electric potential and current density values occur at the anode and cathode, respectively. The shunting of the electric current around the skull, due to its low electrical conductivity, results in the segregated current density pattern around the anode and cathode centers (Figure 7(b)). This phenomenon has been previously observed [1]; however, it is highlighted by the very fine mesh resolution used in this simulation.

Figure 8 displays convergence history curves and performance metrics for each CG preconditioning strategy. With no preconditioning, the CG method will eventually convergence but will accomplish this extremely slowly, requiring more than 6 hours to solve the linear system. The SSOR and RILU preconditioners demonstrate comparable performances, both in solution time and number of iterations. Multigrid preconditioning with two grid levels has far fewer iterations with 166 than both SSOR and RILU and yet has a greater run time. This observation can be explained by the fact that a single iteration of MG has embedded iterations on the different mesh refinements [37]. However, three-grid-level MG noticeably accelerates convergence rates, with both the V- and W-cycles outperforming the other preconditioners. Three-grid-level MG with a W-cycle pattern has slightly fewer iterations than its corresponding V-cycle, yet this V-cycle preconditioner is approximately 11.3% faster.

The ability of the framework to support numerically oriented TES research is presented in this simulation example. The results indicate that the CG method combined with an appropriately configured MG preconditioner is highly efficient in solving the linear systems produced in TES computational simulations.

3.4. Simulation 4. Figure 9 displays the electric current densities produced by the DBS electrode using isotropic (Figure 9(a)) and anisotropic (Figure 9(b)) conductivities. In both cases, the majority of the current density is proximal to the electrode, indicating that accurate placement of electrodes in DBS procedures is paramount [56]. While

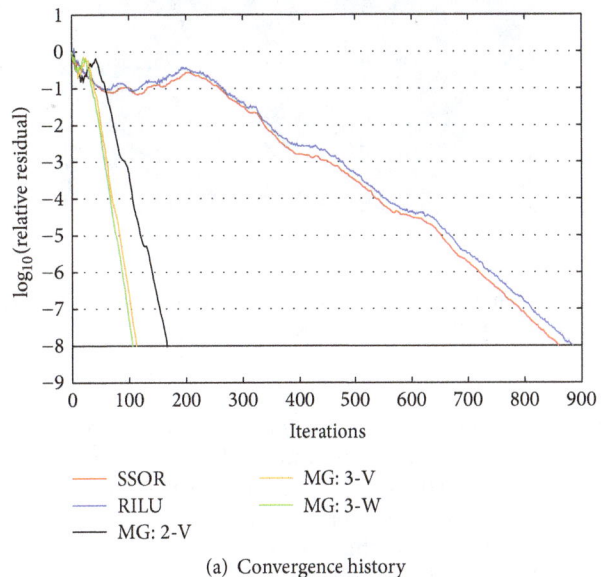

SSOR
RILU
MG: 2-V
MG: 3-V
MG: 3-W

(a) Convergence history

Preconditioner	Iterations	Time (min)
None	>5000	>360
SSOR	860	113.4
RILU	885	117.5
MG 2-grid V-cycle	166	126.4
MG 3-grid V-cycle	113	**57.4**
MG 3-grid W-cycle	**106**	64.7

(b) Numerical iterations and linear system solve time. Boldface values indicate best convergence results

FIGURE 8: Convergence performances of the preconditioned conjugate gradient methods.

the maximal current densities of the isotropic and anisotropic scenarios are similar, other differences between them are observable. First, the current density around the electrode is nonsymmetric in the anisotropic case, as is expected with directionally dependent conductivity data. In addition,

(a) Isotropic

(b) Anisotropic

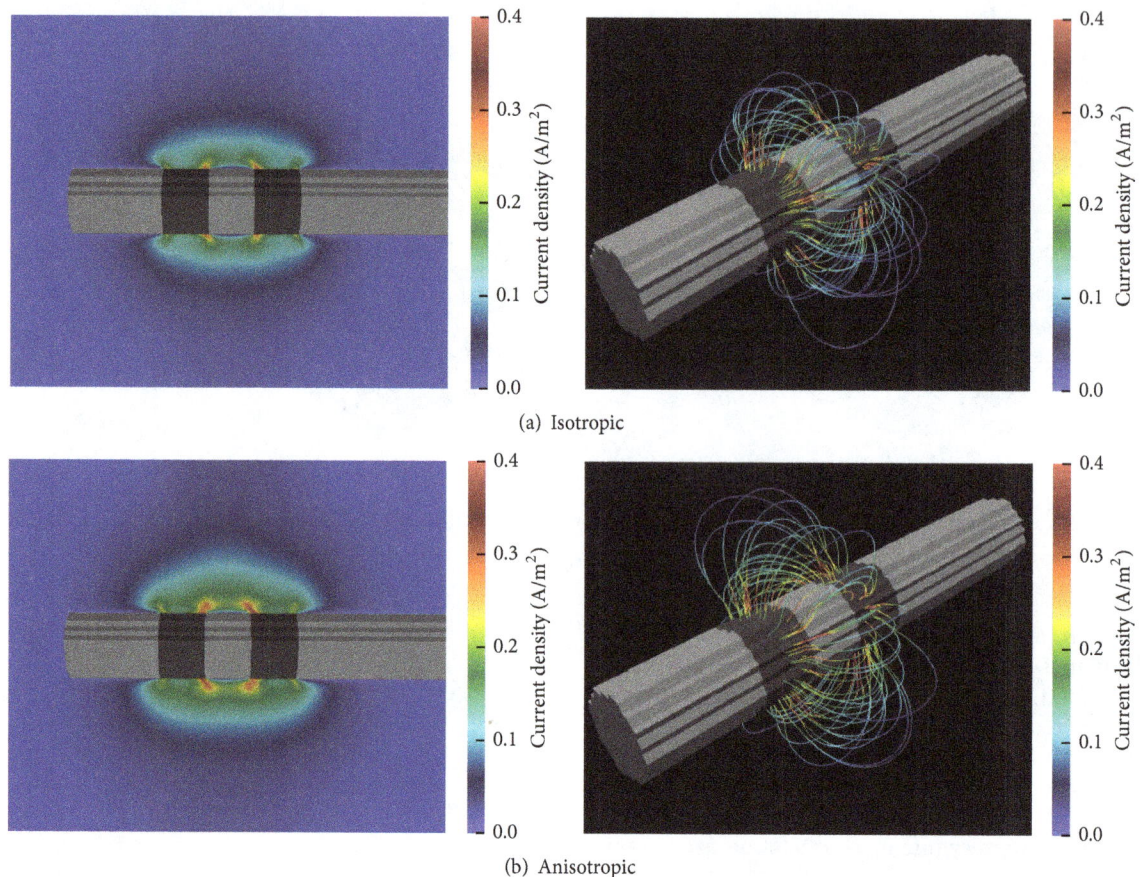

FIGURE 9: Simulation 4, electric current density magnitudes and field lines. Current densities in the figures on the left are from a coronal cross section through the electrode center.

anisotropic conductivities result in a greater electrical current intensity adjacent to the electrode and more dispersion into the neighbouring tissue. This is also observed in the electrical field lines, where anisotropic conductivities produce a more intense and further-reaching current.

With a straightforward extension, DBS was simulated with the object-oriented TES framework. The entirety of the framework is reused in the DBS simulation, which demonstrates how object-oriented design can produce efficient and scalable software implementations. This particular example further reinforces the importance that anisotropic conductivities play in accurately modeling neurostimulation.

While this DBS scenario utilizes a constant source term to assess electrode electric field dispersion [57], alternative applications may demand the use of time-dependent pulses, such as those that examine temporal neuronal responses to nonconstant electric current administrations. In these cases, different stimulation frequencies have an impact on the electrical impedance; specifically, WM and GM conductivities are frequency dependent where an increase in stimulation frequency yields an increase in electrical conductivity.

Applications such as these are supported by the software framework. First, since isotropic tissue conductivity values are specified within the configuration input file, and not hard-coded in the software, alternative DBS pulses can

be accurately simulated by modifying these values. For anisotropic data, modifications to support frequency-dependent conductivities can be made within the Conductivity classes. For example, the SimNIBS software package volume normalizes the WM and GM anisotropic conductivities such that the mean conductivity value of each tensor is maintained to the associated tissue's isotropic value [35]. Therefore, for different DBS frequencies, tensors could be updated to be normalized to different isotropic values within the framework's Conductivity components. To implement the time-varying source itself, the existing definition of the valuePt function in class Source contains an argument for time, namely, dpreal t. Thus, implementations of valuePt in the Source_DBS class can be based on time, and system (1a)–(1d) can then be iteratively solved for with time-based source values.

4. Conclusions

Computational simulations of neurostimulation are a valuable tool that enable researchers to investigate this form of brain therapy *in silico*, and as simulations become more refined, their utility to medical and biomedical research grows. While prebuilt simulation software programs can simplify and expedite TES model implementation, they possess application and portability limitations. In addition, recreating custom software as applications and research objectives change is inefficient, error-prone, and tedious to maintain.

Since the mathematics and physiology that govern all forms of neurostimulation are the same, a single, well-designed software code can support a versatile range of neurostimulation simulations. In this paper, we have presented one such software framework, described its design and implementation, and demonstrated its abilities to support diverse neurostimulation research objectives. The cornerstone of the design stage was to encapsulate general neurostimulation concepts into modular software objects. In doing so, a multitude of TES simulation areas are supported, and in addition, alternative forms of neurostimulation, for example, DBS, can be simulated with the same software.

Simulation results show the importance of using anisotropic conductivities in both TES and DBS. This is especially important for simulations utilized in selecting patient-specific neurostimulation parameters. In addition, results demonstrate the ability of HD-tDCS to focus the electrical current on a specific brain region; however, this capability must be balanced with a potentially low concentration of electric current actually reaching the target. The object-oriented TES framework is an ideal tool for this scenario, enabling different permutations of HD-tDCS electrode montages and stimulation strengths to be conveniently investigated to identify an optimal configuration for a particular patient's data and therapeutic objectives.

Results also illustrate that appropriately configured multigrid preconditioning can achieve superior convergence rates. It is conceivable that hundreds of simulations could be run to identify an optimal electrode montage and neurostimulation parameters for a particular patient. Hence, efficiently solving the linear system of equations resulting from TES finite element simulations is crucial, and MG can be used in this capacity to greatly decrease simulation run times. Finally, we demonstrated how a minor addition to the object-oriented TES framework enables simulations of DBS. The DBS simulation example that was performed utilizes a constant stimulation source term; however, the software framework description and simulation ensemble presented in this paper motivate how the framework could be used to address DBS research related to electrode placement and parameter values.

In future work, we plan to extend the framework to support anisotropic transcranial magnetic stimulation (TMS), in a similar fashion as was demonstrated for DBS. In addition, we plan to utilize the framework to more thoroughly investigate correlations between HD-tDCS interelectrode distances and electric current distributions.

Appendix

Weak Formulation

We multiply (1a) by a test function $v = v(\vec{x})$ and integrate over Ω to obtain

$$-\int_\Omega v\left(\nabla \cdot (\mathbf{M}\nabla\Phi)\right) dx = \int_\Omega vf\, dx, \qquad \text{(A.1)}$$

and using Green's theorem we have

$$\int_\Omega \nabla v \cdot \mathbf{M}\nabla\Phi\, dx = \int_{\partial\Omega} v\left(\mathbf{M}\nabla\Phi \cdot \vec{n}\right) ds + \int_\Omega vf\, dx. \quad \text{(A.2)}$$

Expanding the surface integral gives

$$\begin{aligned}
\int_\Omega \nabla v \cdot \mathbf{M}\nabla\Phi\, dx &= \int_{\partial\Omega_C} v\left(\mathbf{M}\nabla\Phi \cdot \vec{n}\right) ds \\
&+ \int_{\partial\Omega_A} v\left(\mathbf{M}\nabla\Phi \cdot \vec{n}\right) ds \\
&+ \int_{\partial\Omega_S} v\left(\mathbf{M}\nabla\Phi \cdot \vec{n}\right) ds \\
&+ \int_\Omega vf\, dx,
\end{aligned} \qquad \text{(A.3)}$$

and substituting the boundary conditions (1c) and (1d) yields

$$\begin{aligned}
\int_\Omega \nabla v \cdot \mathbf{M}\nabla\Phi\, dx &= \int_{\partial\Omega_C} v\left(\mathbf{M}\nabla\Phi \cdot \vec{n}\right) ds \\
&+ \int_{\partial\Omega_A} vI\, ds + \int_\Omega vf\, dx.
\end{aligned} \qquad \text{(A.4)}$$

For these integrals to exist, we require $v, \Phi \in H^1(\Omega)$ and $f \in L_2(\Omega)$, where

$$\begin{aligned}
H^1(\Omega) &= \left\{ u \mid u \in L_2(\Omega), \frac{\partial u}{\partial x_i} \in L_2(\Omega) \right\}, \\
L_2(\Omega) &= \left\{ p \mid \int_\Omega |p|^2\, dx < \infty \right\},
\end{aligned} \qquad \text{(A.5)}$$

and we enforce the Dirichlet boundary condition (1b) on our solution space by further stipulating that $v, \Phi \in H_0^1 = \{u \mid u \in H^1(\Omega), u = 0 \text{ for } \vec{x} \in \partial\Omega_C\}$.

Consequently, we have the following weak formulation.

Given $f(\vec{x}) \in L_2(\Omega)$, find $\Phi(\vec{x}) \in H_0^1(\Omega)$ such that

$$\begin{aligned}
\int_\Omega \nabla v \cdot \mathbf{M}\nabla\Phi\, dx &= \int_{\partial\Omega_A} vI\, ds + \int_\Omega fv\, dx, \\
&\forall v(\vec{x}) \in H_0^1(\Omega).
\end{aligned} \qquad \text{(A.6)}$$

Conflict of Interests

The authors declare that there is no conflict of interests regarding the publication of this paper.

Acknowledgments

The authors would like to acknowledge Frank Vogel and the entire inuTech team for their assistance with Diffpack. The authors would also like to acknowledge the financial support received from Virginia Tech's Open Access Subvention Fund.

References

[1] A. Datta, X. Zhou, Y. Su, L. C. Parra, and M. Bikson, "Validation of finite element model of transcranial electrical stimulation using scalp potentials: implications for clinical dose," *Journal of Neural Engineering*, vol. 10, no. 3, Article ID 036018, 2013.

[2] A. Datta, V. Bansal, J. Diaz, J. Patel, D. Reato, and M. Bikson, "Gyri-precise head model of transcranial direct current stimulation: improved spatial focality using a ring electrode versus conventional rectangular pad," *Brain Stimulation*, vol. 2, no. 4, pp. 201–207, 2009.

[3] P. Faria, M. Hallett, and P. C. Miranda, "A finite element analysis of the effect of electrode area and inter-electrode distance on the spatial distribution of the current density in tDCS," *Journal of Neural Engineering*, vol. 8, no. 6, Article ID 066017, 2011.

[4] P. S. Boggio, R. Ferrucci, S. P. Rigonatti et al., "Effects of transcranial direct current stimulation on working memory in patients with Parkinson's disease," *Journal of the Neurological Sciences*, vol. 249, no. 1, pp. 31–38, 2006.

[5] P. S. Boggio, L. P. Khoury, D. C. S. Martins, O. E. M. S. Martins, E. C. de Macedo, and F. Fregni, "Temporal cortex direct current stimulation enhances performance on a visual recognition memory task in Alzheimer disease," *Journal of Neurology, Neurosurgery and Psychiatry*, vol. 80, no. 4, pp. 444–447, 2009.

[6] P. S. Boggio, C. A. Valasek, C. Campanhã et al., "Non-invasive brain stimulation to assess and modulate neuroplasticity in Alzheimer's disease," *Neuropsychological Rehabilitation*, vol. 21, no. 5, pp. 703–716, 2011.

[7] R. Ferrucci, M. Bortolomasi, M. Vergari et al., "Transcranial direct current stimulation in severe, drug-resistant major depression," *Journal of Affective Disorders*, vol. 118, no. 1–3, pp. 215–219, 2009.

[8] P. S. Boggio, S. P. Rigonatti, R. B. Ribeiro et al., "A randomized, double-blind clinical trial on the efficacy of cortical direct current stimulation for the treatment of major depression," *International Journal of Neuropsychopharmacology*, vol. 11, no. 2, pp. 249–254, 2008.

[9] P. Homan, J. Kindler, A. Federspiel et al., "Muting the voice: a case of arterial spin labeling-monitored transcranial direct current stimulation treatment of auditory verbal hallucinations," *The American Journal of Psychiatry*, vol. 168, no. 8, pp. 853–854, 2011.

[10] J. Brunelin, M. Mondino, F. Haesebaert, M. Saoud, M. F. Suaud-Chagny, and E. Poulet, "Efficacy and safety of bifocal tDCS as an interventional treatment for refractory schizophrenia," *Brain Stimulation*, vol. 5, no. 3, pp. 431–432, 2012.

[11] A. Antal and W. Paulus, "Transcranial alternating current stimulation (tACS)," *Frontiers in Human Neuroscience*, vol. 7, article 317, 2013.

[12] T. Neuling, S. Wagner, C. H. Wolters, T. Zaehle, and C. S. Herrmann, "Finite-element model predicts current density distribution for clinical applications of tDCS and tACS," *Frontiers in Psychiatry*, vol. 3, article 83, 2012.

[13] F. Gasca, L. Marshall, S. Binder, A. Schlaefer, U. G. Hofmann, and A. Schweikard, "Finite element simulation of transcranial current stimulation in realistic rat head model," in *Proceedings of the 5th International IEEE/EMBS Conference on Neural Engineering (NER 2011)*, pp. 36–39, IEEE, Cancun, Mexico, May 2011.

[14] P. C. Miranda, M. Lomarev, and M. Hallett, "Modeling the current distribution during transcranial direct current stimulation," *Clinical Neurophysiology*, vol. 117, no. 7, pp. 1623–1629, 2006.

[15] E. M. Caparelli-Daquer, T. J. Zimmermann, E. Mooshagian et al., "A pilot study on effects of 4 × 1 high-definition tDCS on motor cortex excitability," in *Proceedings of the IEEE Annual International Conference of the Engineering in Medicine and Biology Society (EMBC '12)*, vol. 735, pp. 735–738, San Diego, Calif, USA, September 2012.

[16] S. K. Kessler, P. Minhas, A. J. Woods, A. Rosen, C. Gorman, and M. Bikson, "Dosage considerations for transcranial direct current stimulation in children: a computational modeling study," *PLoS ONE*, vol. 8, no. 9, Article ID e76112, 2013.

[17] H. S. Suh, W. H. Lee, and T.-S. Kim, "Influence of anisotropic conductivity in the skull and white matter on transcranial direct current stimulation via an anatomically realistic finite element head model," *Physics in Medicine and Biology*, vol. 57, no. 21, pp. 6961–6980, 2012.

[18] S. Wagner, S. M. Rampersad, Ü. Aydin et al., "Investigation of tDCS volume conduction effects in a highly realistic head model," *Journal of Neural Engineering*, vol. 11, no. 1, Article ID 016002, 2014.

[19] S. Lew, C. H. Wolters, T. Dierkes, C. Röer, and R. S. MacLeod, "Accuracy and run-time comparison for different potential approaches and iterative solvers in finite element method based EEG source analysis," *Applied Numerical Mathematics*, vol. 59, no. 8, pp. 1970–1988, 2009.

[20] W. Aquino, "An object-oriented framework for reduced-order models using proper orthogonal decomposition (POD)," *Computer Methods in Applied Mechanics and Engineering*, vol. 196, no. 41–44, pp. 4375–4390, 2007.

[21] R. I. Mackie, "An object-oriented approach to fully interactive finite element software," *Advances in Engineering Software*, vol. 29, no. 2, pp. 139–149, 1998.

[22] R. Sampath and N. Zabaras, "An object-oriented framework for the implementation of adjoint techniques in the design and control of complex continuum systems," *International Journal for Numerical Methods in Engineering*, vol. 48, no. 2, pp. 239–266, 2000.

[23] M. Hakman and T. Groth, "Object-oriented biomedical system modeling—the rationale," *Computer Methods and Programs in Biomedicine*, vol. 59, no. 1, pp. 1–17, 1999.

[24] S. C. Lee, K. Bhalerao, and M. Ferrari, "Object-oriented design tools for supramolecular devices and biomedical nanotechnology," *Annals of the New York Academy of Sciences*, vol. 1013, pp. 110–123, 2004.

[25] S. Tuchschmid, M. Grassi, D. Bachofen et al., "A flexible framework for highly-modular surgical simulation systems," in *Biomedical Simulation*, vol. 4072 of *Lecture Notes in Computer Science*, pp. 84–92, Springer, Berlin, Germany, 2006.

[26] A. Doronin and I. Meglinski, "Online object oriented Monte Carlo computational tool for the needs of biomedical optics," *Biomedical Optics Express*, vol. 2, no. 9, pp. 2461–2469, 2011.

[27] H. P. Langtangen, *Computational Partial Differential Equations: Numerical Methods and Diffpack Programming*, Texts in Computational Science and Engineering, Springer, Berlin, Germany, 2003.

[28] H. P. Langtangen and A. Tveito, *Advanced Topics in Computational Partial Differential Equations: Numerical Methods and Diffpack Programming*, Lecture Notes in Computational Science and Engineering, Springer, Berlin, Germany, 2003.

[29] M. Åström, L. U. Zrinzo, S. Tisch, E. Tripoliti, M. I. Hariz, and K. Wårdell, "Method for patient-specific finite element modeling and simulation of deep brain stimulation," *Medical and Biological Engineering and Computing*, vol. 47, no. 1, pp. 21–28, 2009.

[30] T. Budd, *An Introduction to Object-Oriented Programming*, Addison-Wesley, Boston, Mass, USA, 2002.

[31] A. M. Bruaset and H. P. Langtangen, "Diffpack: a software environment for rapid prototyping of PDE solvers," in *Proceedings of the 15th IMACS World Congress on Scientific Computation, Modeling and Applied Mathematics*, pp. 553–558, Berlin, Germany, August 1997.

[32] B. Stroustrup, *The C++ Programming Language*, Addison-Wesley, Upper Saddle River, NJ, USA, 2013.

[33] S. Prata, *C++ Primer Plus*, Addison-Wesley, Upper Saddle River, NJ, USA, 2012.

[34] *MATLAB Version 8.2.0.701 (R2013b)*, MathWorks, Natick, Mass, USA, 2013.

[35] M. Windhoff, A. Opitz, and A. Thielscher, "Electric field calculations in brain stimulation based on finite elements: an optimized processing pipeline for the generation and usage of accurate individual head models," *Human Brain Mapping*, vol. 34, no. 4, pp. 923–935, 2013.

[36] H. A. van der Vorst, *Iterative Krylov Methods for Large Linear Systems*, Cambridge Monographs on Applied and Computational Mathematics, Cambridge University Press, 2003.

[37] W. L. Briggs, *A Multigrid Tutorial*, SIAM, Philadelphia, Pa, USA, 2000.

[38] K. A. Mardal, G. W. Zumbusch, and H. P. Langtangen, "Software tools for multigrid methods," in *Advanced Topics in Computational Partial Differential Equations: Numerical Methods and Diffpack Programming*, H. P. Langtangen and A. Tveito, Eds., Lecture Notes in Computational Science and Engineering, pp. 97–152, Springer, Berlin, Germany, 2003.

[39] C. Geuzaine and J.-F. Remacle, "Gmsh: a 3-D finite element mesh generator with built-in pre- and post-processing facilities," *International Journal for Numerical Methods in Engineering*, vol. 79, no. 11, pp. 1309–1331, 2009.

[40] A. Henderson, J. Ahrens, and C. Law, *The Paraview Guide*, Kitware Inc, Clifton Park, NY, USA, 2004.

[41] T. Williams, C. Kelley et al., "Gnuplot 4.4: an interactive plotting program," March 2011.

[42] A. Opitz, M. Windhoff, R. M. Heidemann, R. Turner, and A. Thielscher, "How the brain tissue shapes the electric field induced by transcranial magnetic stimulation," *NeuroImage*, vol. 58, no. 3, pp. 849–859, 2011.

[43] M. A. Nitsche, L. G. Cohen, E. M. Wassermann et al., "Transcranial direct current stimulation: state of the art 2008," *Brain Stimulation*, vol. 1, no. 3, pp. 206–223, 2008.

[44] M. Okamoto, H. Dan, K. Sakamoto et al., "Three-dimensional probabilistic anatomical cranio-cerebral correlation via the international 10-20 system oriented for transcranial functional brain mapping," *NeuroImage*, vol. 21, no. 1, pp. 99–111, 2004.

[45] E. K. Kang and N.-J. Paik, "Effect of a tDCS electrode montage on implicit motor sequence learning in healthy subjects," *Experimental and Translational Stroke Medicine*, vol. 3, no. 1, article 4, 2011.

[46] A. Datta, J. M. Baker, M. Bikson, and J. Fridriksson, "Individualized model predicts brain current flow during transcranial direct-current stimulation treatment in responsive stroke patient," *Brain Stimulation*, vol. 4, no. 3, pp. 169–174, 2011.

[47] G. Schlaug, V. Renga, and D. Nair, "Transcranial direct current stimulation in stroke recovery," *Archives of Neurology*, vol. 65, no. 12, pp. 1571–1576, 2008.

[48] A. F. DaSilva, M. S. Volz, M. Bikson, and F. Fregni, "Electrode positioning and montage in transcranial direct current stimulation," *Journal of Visualized Experiments*, no. 51, 2011.

[49] A. Antal, D. Terney, C. Poreisz, and W. Paulus, "Towards unravelling task-related modulations of neuroplastic changes induced in the human motor cortex," *European Journal of Neuroscience*, vol. 26, no. 9, pp. 2687–2691, 2007.

[50] D. Q. Truong, G. Magerowski, G. L. Blackburn, M. Bikson, and M. Alonso-Alonso, "Computational modeling of transcranial direct current stimulation (tDCS) in obesity: impact of head fat and dose guidelines," *NeuroImage: Clinical*, vol. 2, no. 1, pp. 759–766, 2013.

[51] A. Antal, K. Boros, C. Poreisz, L. Chaieb, D. Terney, and W. Paulus, "Comparatively weak after-effects of transcranial alternating current stimulation (tACS) on cortical excitability in humans," *Brain Stimulation*, vol. 1, no. 2, pp. 97–105, 2008.

[52] S. Miocinovic, S. Somayajula, S. Chitnis, and J. L. Vitek, "History, applications, and mechanisms of deep brain stimulation," *JAMA Neurology*, vol. 70, no. 2, pp. 163–171, 2013.

[53] L. M. Zitella, K. Mohsenian, M. Pahwa, C. Gloeckner, and M. D. Johnson, "Computational modeling of pedunculopontine nucleus deep brain stimulation," *Journal of Neural Engineering*, vol. 10, no. 4, Article ID 045005, 2013.

[54] S. Miocinovic, M. Parent, C. R. Butson et al., "Computational analysis of subthalamic nucleus and lenticular fasciculus activation during therapeutic deep brain stimulation," *Journal of Neurophysiology*, vol. 96, no. 3, pp. 1569–1580, 2006.

[55] C. C. Mcintyre and T. J. Foutz, "Computational modeling of deep brain stimulation," *Handbook of Clinical Neurology*, vol. 116, pp. 55–61, 2013.

[56] D. Tarsy, *Deep Brain Stimulation In Neurological And Psychiatric Disorders*, Humana Press, Totowa, NJ, USA, 2008.

[57] M. Astrom, *Modelling, simulation, and visualization of deep brain stimulation [Ph.D. thesis]*, Linköping University, Linköping, Sweden, 2011.

13

A Hertzian Integrated Contact Model of the Total Knee Replacement Implant for the Estimation of Joint Contact Forces

Tien Tuan Dao and Philippe Pouletaut

Sorbonne Universités, Université de Technologie de Compiègne, CNRS, UMR 7338 Biomécanique et Bioingénierie, Centre de Recherche Royallieu, CS 60 319, 60 203 Compiègne, France

Correspondence should be addressed to Tien Tuan Dao; tien-tuan.dao@utc.fr

Academic Editor: Darryl D. D'Lima

The prediction of lower limb muscle and contact forces may provide useful knowledge to assist the clinicians in the diagnosis as well as in the development of appropriate treatment for musculoskeletal disorders. Research studies have commonly estimated joint contact forces using model-based muscle force estimation due to the lack of a reliable contact model and material properties. The objective of this present study was to develop a Hertzian integrated contact model. Then, *in vivo* elastic properties of the Total Knee Replacement (TKR) implant were identified using *in vivo* contact forces leading to providing reliable material properties for modeling purposes. First, a patient specific rigid musculoskeletal model was built. Second, a STL-based implant model was designed to compute the contact area evolutions during gait motions. Finally, a Hertzian integrated contact model was defined for the *in vivo* identification of elastic properties (Young's modulus and Poisson coefficient) of the instrumented TKR implant. Our study showed a potential use of a new approach to predict the contact forces without knowledge of muscle forces. Thus, the outcomes may lead to accurate and reliable prediction of human joint contact forces for new case study.

1. Introduction

Total Knee Replacement (TKR) implant has been commonly prescribed for patients with severe knee joint damage (e.g., osteoarthritis) associated with progressive pain and impaired function [1, 2]. The implant with distal femoral and proximal tibial compartments is usually created with biocompatible materials [3, 4]. Besides, TKR implant may include patella-femoral interaction which helps the knee joint to be functionally stabilized. It is important to emphasize that the knee contact force behaviors are activity-specific and the optimal design of the TKR may lead to maximizing the clinical outcomes. However, the implant design may be optimized when its effect on the musculoskeletal tissues and structures could be elucidated [5]. Joint contact forces play an important role in the understanding of the effect of the implant on the joint behavior and musculoskeletal load [6]. Finite element modeling may provide reliable information on the joint contact force behavior. However, the lack of accurate muscle modeling and reliable definition of boundary and loading conditions may affect the contact force computation [7, 8]. Research studies demonstrated a deeper knowledge of hip implant effect thanks to computational rigid-body models and available *in vivo* experimental data measured directly within the instrumented hip implant [9–11]. Recently, *in vivo* knee contact forces can be measured from a new knee device [12, 13]. Thus, for the first time, computational rigid musculoskeletal models, used to facilitate the surgical and functional rehabilitation treatments of the musculoskeletal disorders, may be evaluated for their predictive capacities related to muscle force estimation and knee contact load by using these available experimental data [14, 15]. Thus, these models may be potentially accepted in a clinical routine procedure in the future [9, 16]. Moreover, an open and free access database (http://www.orthoload.com/) of the orthopedic implant loads was also provided leading to promoting extensive research activities in this field of study.

The prediction of *in vivo* muscle and contact forces, especially within a Total Knee Replacement, is a challenging task for biomechanical engineers/researchers. Model-based estimation of these forces has been commonly performed [17–19]. Thus, the redundant phenomena of the human neural control (i.e., the number of muscles is greater than the number of degrees of freedom) may be computationally solved using optimization techniques even if the best optimization strategy remains unknown. However, the prediction accuracy of such forces depends on the accurate modeling of musculoskeletal tissues (e.g., muscles, bone, tendons, ligaments, and cartilage) and structures (e.g., joint) as well as appropriate formulation of physical behaviors (e.g., joint contact or multi-body dynamics) [19, 20]. Model validation has been a challenging issue. Qualitative pattern of the muscle force was commonly validated against the EMG-based muscle activities.

In vivo knee contact forces may be computationally estimated with or without contact model. On the one hand, model-based efforts related to the use of inverse dynamics approach coupled with an elastic contact model. Within the scope of this vision, Kim et al. [21] developed two-stage simulation to compute the muscle forces and then combine them with ground reaction forces and fluoroscopic data within a Hertzian contact model to predict the knee contact forces. Moreover, Hast and Piazza [22] used a coupling between inverse dynamics, forward dynamics, and computed muscle control (CMC) algorithm within a spring-based contact model to compute the nodes-to-surface knee contact forces. On the other hand, knee contact forces have been predicted without contact model. Based on the muscle forces estimated from pseudoinverse method and constrained static optimization with Lagrange multipliers formulation and parameter reduction strategy [23], contact forces were computed. Moreover, Electromyography-(EMG-) driven muscle force estimation approach coupled with moment balancing algorithm has been used to predict the medial contact force [24, 25]. Furthermore, a parametric numerical model including 9 equilibrium equations reflecting muscle activation levels, passive structure activation, joint moments, external joint forces, maximum physiological muscle moments, and forces has been also developed to predict the knee contact forces [26]. In fact, without contact model, the problem formulation and computational cost may be more advantageous than the use of a contact model. A recent comparison of predicted contact forces in the framework of the Knee Grand Challenge showed that the use of a contact model does not guarantee their accuracy [15]. However, a deformable contact model may provide useful knowledge about the interactions between the implant components and also those at bone-to-implant surface. It is important to note that the Knee Grand Challenge has been created to open a new dimension on the prediction of *in vivo* muscle and contact forces [14, 15]. Almost all available measurements ranging from medical imaging data to gait analysis and experimental contact forces were provided to enhance the research activities related to the prediction of these forces.

Previous studies used only simplified representation (e.g., one point contact or nodes-to-surface contact) of contact surface between implant components. Moreover, material properties of the implants were commonly provided by manufacturer. However, assumptions were commonly performed for musculoskeletal modeling. Thus, these properties need to be calibrated and fitted to the modeling assumption for predicting accurately the knee contact forces. In fact, predictive trends of numerical models are limited for clinical applications. Thus, the objectives of this present study are twofold: (1) the development of a Hertzian integrated contact model based on a global surface-to-surface interaction and (2) the use of *in vivo* contact forces and the developed contact model to identify the reliable and fitted elastic properties of the implant for modeling purpose.

2. Materials and Methods

2.1. Computational Workflow. A computational workflow was developed to identify the elastic properties of the instrumented TKR implant (Figure 1). The workflow consists of the following components: (1) a patient specific rigid musculoskeletal model to compute the knee kinematics from skin-mounted markers' trajectories; (2) a STL-based implant model to compute the contact area evolution during knee motion; and (3) a Hertzian integrated contact model for the *in vivo* identification of elastic properties (Young's modulus and Poisson coefficient) of the instrumented TKR implant using contact area information and *in vivo* measured joint contact forces.

2.2. Patient Data. The patient data from the fourth edition of the Knee Grand Challenge [14] was used in this present study. Imaging and gait data were acquired on a patient (male, 88 years old, 168 cm body height, 66.7 kg body mass, and 23.6 kg/m^2 Body Mass Index (BMI)) with knee implant instrumented in his right knee side (Figure 2(a)). The patient had Rockport flat bottom sneakers shoes during the gait data acquisition process. The patient performed an overground normal gait pattern, which was used as reference pattern. Then, 4 overground gait trials reflecting 4 gait modification strategies (bouncy, medial thrust, mild crouch, and mtp) were acquired using an 8-camera Vicon system (Table 1). All skin-mounted markers were posed using a modified Cleveland Clinic marker protocol [14]. *In vivo* knee contact forces were also obtained during the gait data acquisition. Four uniaxial load cell measurements (posterior-medial (PM), anterior-medial (AM), anterior-lateral (AL), and posterior-lateral (PL)) from the instrumented tibial prosthesis were performed (Figure 2(b)). The first generation of tray design (eKnee) was used. The main implant components were fabricated in CoCr, polyethylene, and titanium. Sampling frequency is 120 Hz. Furthermore, pre- and postsurgery CT data were also acquired on the patient using a Siemens CT machine; the slice thickness was set up as 0.6 mm. The matrix is 512 × 512 and the pixel resolution is 0.9 × 0.9 mm^2. The number of slices is 1900 for the whole scanned lower limb.

2.3. Patient Specific Rigid Musculoskeletal Model

2.3.1. Model Development. To compute the knee kinematics, a patient specific musculoskeletal model, which is provided

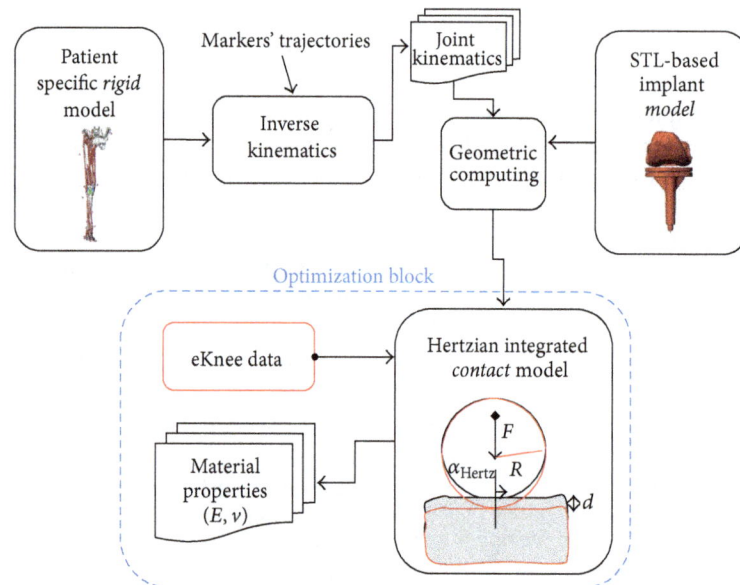

FIGURE 1: Workflow of the computational process to *in vivo* characterize the elastic properties of the instrumented TKR implant.

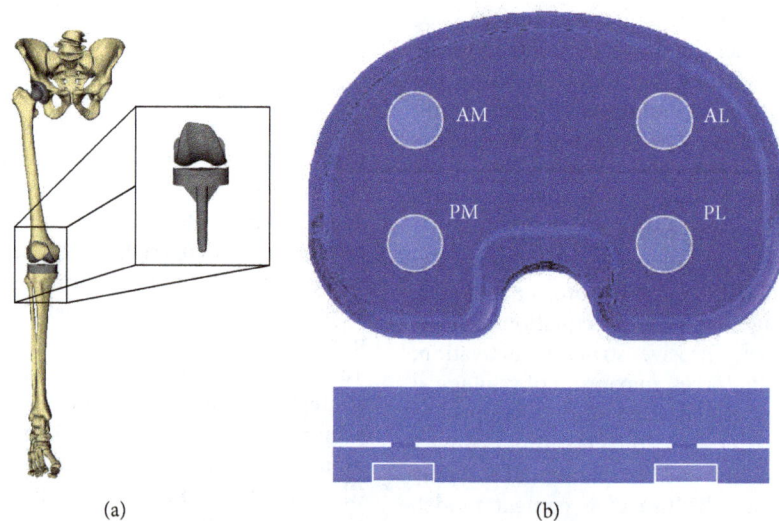

<table>
<tr><td>(a)</td><td>(b)</td></tr>
</table>

FIGURE 2: Geometrical components of the TKR implant within the skeletal model (a) and locations of 4 load cells (posterior-medial (PM), anterior-medial (AM), anterior-lateral (AL), and posterior-lateral (PL)) used to measure the contact forces (b).

TABLE 1: Description of normal gait and gait modification strategies.

Gait modifications	Description	Trial name: gait cycle times (start > end) (time in sec)
Ngait	Normal gait	Ngait_og1: 1.699 > 2.811 (1.112)
Bouncy	Increased superior-inferior translation of the pelvis	Bouncy1: 2.066 > 3.214 (1.148)
Medial thrust	Internally rotated hip of the stance leg	Medthrust2: 2.415 > 3.571 (1.156)
Midcrouch	Crouched position with a mild increase in knee flexion angle	Mildcrouch1: 10.822 > 11.901 (1.079)
Mtp	Gait with forefoot strike	Mtpgait2: 2.276 > 3.421 (1.145)

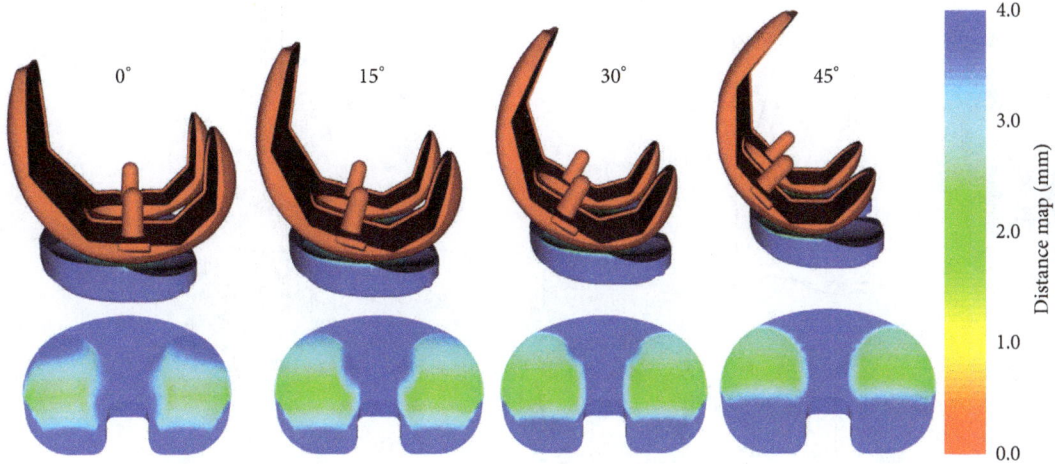

FIGURE 3: Illustration of knee contact area evolution map.

from the fourth edition of the Knee Grand Challenge [14], was used. This model has 8 segments (pelvis, right femur, femoral implant component, patella, tibial implant component, right tibia, right fibula, and right foot). Image segmentation using SliceOmatic (Montreal, Canada) was performed on the post- and presurgery CT data and laser-scan-based implant component to extract bony segments and implant components. STL-based surface geometries were created and imported into OpenSIM engine [27] to develop corresponding bony segments. The model has 24 degrees of freedom (DOF) (6-DOF ground-to-pelvis joint, 3-DOF hip joint, 6-DOF tibiofemoral joint, 6-DOF patellofemoral joint, 2-DOF ankle joint, and 1-DOF toes joint). The interaction between implant components and its respective bone was modeled using an OpenSIM weld joint. The interaction between implant components (femoral component, tibial tray, and patella/femoral component) was modeled using an OpenSIM reverse joint. All segment coordinate systems were based on the ISB recommendations [28]. The model has 22 skin-mounted virtual markers' cluster according to the real market cloud used in the motion capture acquisition. This model has 44 lower limb muscles. Each muscle was modeled as a Schutte muscle model [29]. Muscle attachment points and wrapping surface were created using an available lower limb model [30]. A transformation process using information from bone-to-bone alignment was performed to morph the patient specific musculature. Some attachments points and unrealistic intersection of muscle lines of action were manually adjusted.

2.3.2. Joint Angle Computing.
Based on skin-mounted marker's trajectories, inverse kinematics was performed to compute the knee joint angles of each gait pattern (normal, bouncy, medial thrust, mild crouch, and mtp). At each time step (i.e., frame of motion), generalized coordinate values were computed to put the model in a best-fitting pose in minimizing the deviation between the experimental markers'

and estimated coordinate values. The deviation is expressed as a weighted least squares problem as follows:

$$\min_{q} \left[\sum_{i \in \text{markers}} w_i \left\| x_i^{\text{exp}} - x_i(q) \right\|^2 \right], \tag{1}$$

where q is the vector of generalized coordinates; w_i is the marker weight; x_i^{exp} is the experimental position of the marker i; $x_i(q)$ is the position of the corresponding marker on the model.

2.4. STL-Based Implant Model and Contact Area Computing.
Based on the reconstructed implant components, a geometrical computing process was applied to compute the surface-to-surface contact area evolution according to each series of knee kinematics (e.g., flexion/extension). Threshold-based minimal distance principle was used to compute the implant-to-implant contact area: minimal distance map was computed and area under the threshold of 4 mm was calculated [31]. The threshold was calibrated using experimental data of the knee contact area [32]. An illustration of contact area map during knee flexion/extension from 0 to 90 degrees is shown in Figure 3.

2.5. Hertzian Integrated Contact Model

2.5.1. Contact Model.
To describe the physical relationships between the applied force and the contact behavior, a Hertzian linearly elastic contact model was formulated. This model describes conservative interaction forces [33]. Constitutive equation of this model is expressed as follows:

$$F_{\text{Hertz}} = \frac{2}{3R} \frac{E}{(1 - v^2)} \left(a_{\text{Hertz}} \right)^3, \tag{2}$$

where F_{Hertz} and a_{Hertz} are applied force and its respective contact radius. R is the radius of the contact cylinder

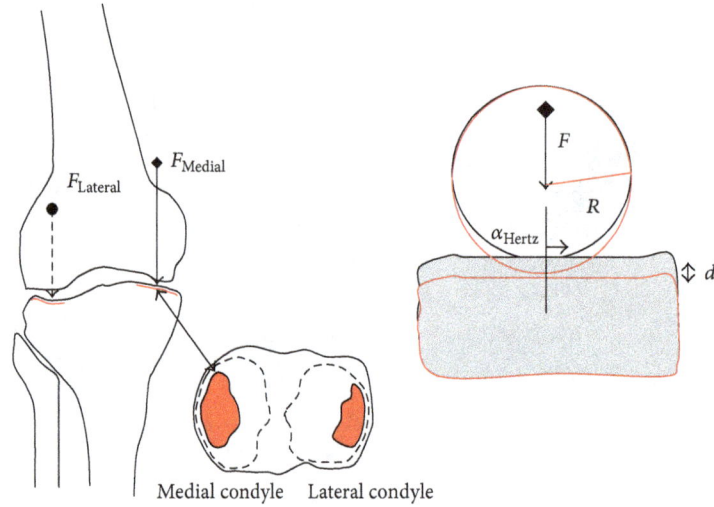

FIGURE 4: Schematic representation of a Hertzian elastic contact model.

(e.g., femoral condyle) (Figure 4). E and ν are Young's modulus and Poisson coefficient, respectively. It is assumed that R is constant for different knee flexion/extension angles.

2.5.2. Elastic Property Identification. To identify the appropriate values of the implant elastic material properties (E and ν), an optimization problem was formulated as follows:

$$\min_{u} \left\| F^{\text{Hertz}} - F^{\text{eKnee}} \right\|^2$$

$$\text{Subject to: } E > 0, \ 0 < \nu < 0.5 \tag{3}$$

$$a_{\text{Hertz}} = \sqrt{\frac{S}{\pi}},$$

where F^{eKnee} is the *in vivo* measured contact force. u is a set of knee angles. S is the total contact area computed by the method described in Section 2.4. To compute the value of R, a cylinder-fitting process was applied. The values of *in vivo* measured contact forces were calculated from the load cell measurements ($F_{\text{AM}}, F_{\text{PM}}, F_{\text{AL}}, F_{\text{PL}}$) (Figure 2(b)) by using the following validated regression equations [34]:

$$F^{\text{eKnee}} = F^{\text{Medial}} + F^{\text{Lateral}},$$

$$F^{\text{Medial}} = 0.9871 F_{\text{AM}} + 0.9683 F_{\text{PM}} + 0.0387 F_{\text{AL}}$$
$$+ 0.0211 F_{\text{PL}}, \tag{4}$$

$$F^{\text{Lateral}} = 0.0129 F_{\text{AM}} + 0.0317 F_{\text{PM}} + 0.9613 F_{\text{AL}}$$
$$+ 0.9789 F_{\text{PL}}.$$

The constrained optimization process was performed using a quasi-Newton approach implemented in the Optimization Toolbox in Matlab R2010b (Mathworks, USA).

3. Results

3.1. Determination of Contact Cylinder Radius R. The fitted cylinder used to compute the value of the radius R is shown

in Figure 5. It is important to note that two physiological condyles were assumed to be symmetric. Thus, the knee joint behavior functions like a hinge joint. A value of 37 mm was found with a mean error of 16.52 mm from 1024 points between the fitted cylinder and the external femoral surface of the implant component. Note this error is relatively high due to the assumption of constant R for different knee flexion/extension angles.

3.2. Knee Kinematics during Gait Motions. Figure 6 shows the evolution of knee flexion/extension angles during the normal gait with instrumented TKR implant. The total squared error between real markers' coordinates and virtual makers' coordinates computed by inverse kinematics process ranges from 0.00072 to 0.00215 mm for 326 frames. The same pattern was obtained for other gait patterns with a first peak-to-peak absolute deviation ranging from 5.6 to 18.5 degrees as well as a second peak-to-peak absolute deviation ranging from 1.8 to 8.52 degrees. It is important to note that these deviations are due to temporal shifts when modifying the gait patterns.

3.3. Implant-to-Implant Contact Area Evolution. The evolution of implant-to-implant contact area during the stance phase (60%) of the normal and modified gaits is illustrated in Figure 7. The peak contact area values range from 1016 to 1117 mm^2 for all gait patterns. According to the normal gait, the patterns of the contact area are different for all modified strategies, except for the Medthrust. These differences are directly related to the differences in the kinematics patterns of these modified strategies.

3.4. In Vivo Contact Forces and Implant's Elastic Properties. The *in vivo* medial contact forces during the normal and 4 modified gaits are shown in Figure 8. Root mean square errors (RMSE) between the normal gait and bouncy, medial thrust, mild crouch, mtp gaits are 222.5, 192.8, 132.3, and 1777.7 N, respectively, for the medial side. On the other hand,

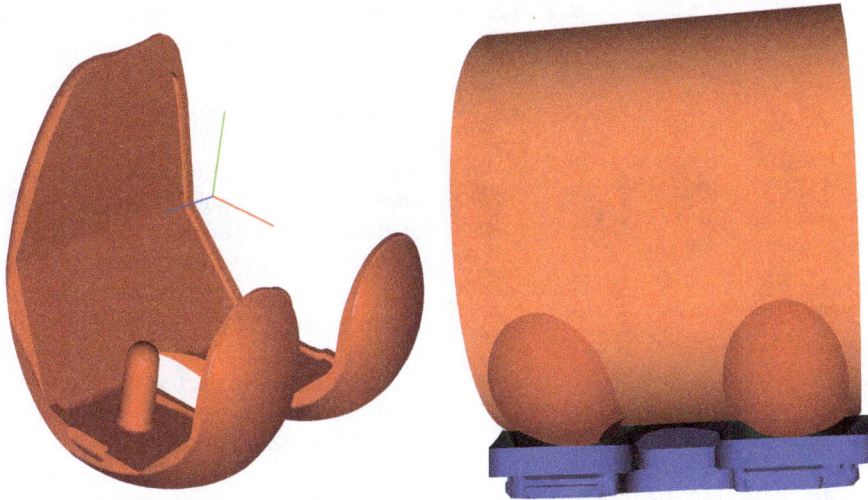

FIGURE 5: Fitted cylinder of the femoral implant component.

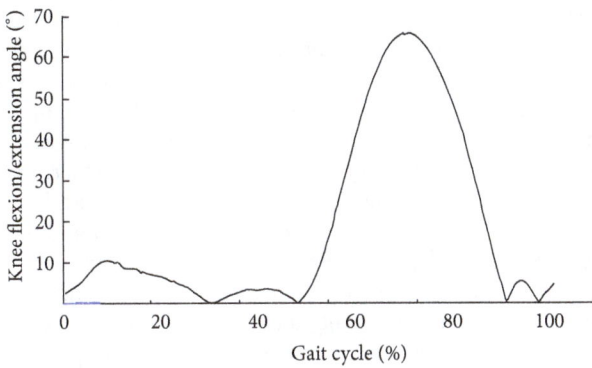

FIGURE 6: Evolution of knee flexion/extension angles during the normal gait with instrumented TKR implant.

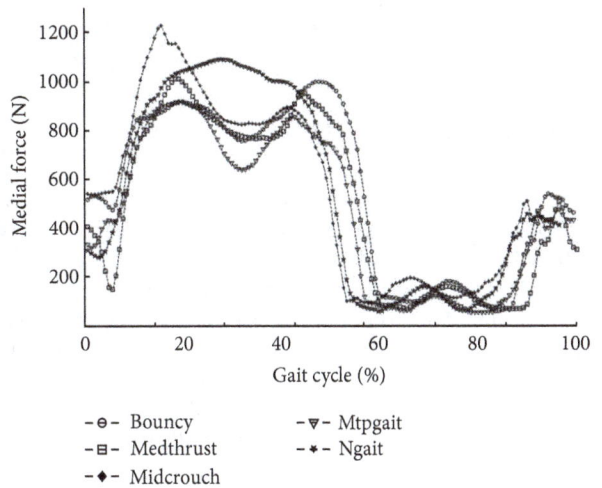

FIGURE 7: Implant-to-implant contact area evolutions during gait.

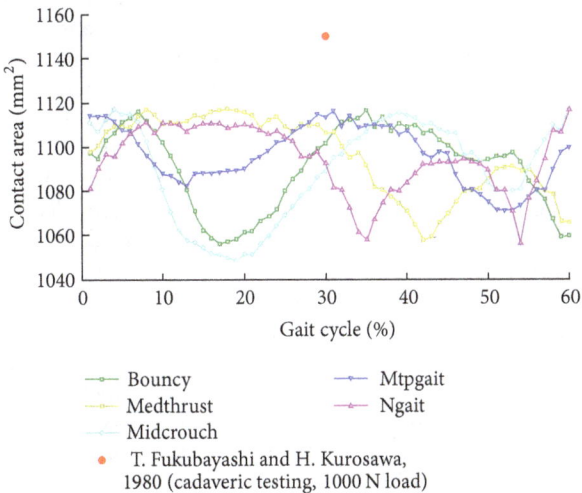

FIGURE 8: Evolutions of *in vivo* contact forces at the medial side of the TKR implant.

lateral side revealed a RMSE of 120.2, 122.6, 91.1, and 89.6 N for comparison between the normal and the bouncy, medial thrust, mild crouch, and mtp gaits, respectively. The maximal RMSE of the medial contact force is 222.5 N between the normal and the bouncy gaits. The maximal RMSE of the lateral contact force is 122.6 N between the normal and the medial thrust gaits. Using the total contact forces with the integrated contact model, the optimization process was converged after 6 iterations (3, 15, 30, 33, 36, 39, and 42 function calls, resp.) at the minimal objective function value of $1.16437e - 009$. Thus, optimal Young's modulus was 4.67 GPa and its respective Poisson coefficient was 0.25.

Figure 9 shows the evolutions of predicted contact forces using integrated contact model and experimental eKnee data for the normal gait. A good convergence (i.e., error between predicted results and experimental data leads nearly to 0) was

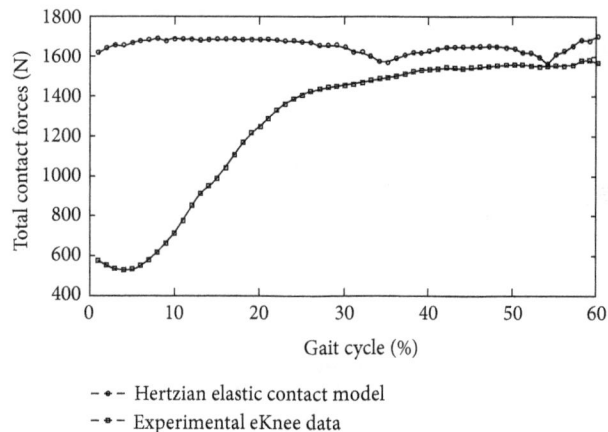

Figure 9: Comparisons between predicted contact forces using integrated contact model and experimental eKnee data for the normal gait.

noted over the 54% of the gait cycle. However, the amplitudes and trends of the predicted values were largely different in early phase of the gait cycle. This is due to the modeling assumption of the ideal symmetric contact model.

4. Discussion

The prediction of *in vivo* muscle and contact forces plays an important role in the objective and precise diagnosis and treatment of the musculoskeletal disorders in the future [9, 10, 14, 35, 36]. In fact, the use of computational models may allow the clinicians to perform a series of virtual treatment trials without any dangerous risk for the involved patients. Moreover, optimal treatment plan may be elucidated with objective data related to its effect on the musculoskeletal tissues and structures. However, the validation of model behavior/prediction against critical experimental data is extremely a challenging task, especially for *in vivo* estimated muscle and contact forces. Skeletal muscle with its multiscale architecture revealed a complex (e.g., anisotropic or heterogeneous) living material. Hill-based macroscopic rheological model has been commonly used to define the physiological force-length and force-velocity relationships [37]. Despite many efforts during the last several decades to estimate the *in vivo* muscle forces using inverse dynamics and optimization or EMG-driven approach [17, 19, 20, 24, 25, 29], the lack of *in vivo* experimental data for direct and quantitative validation purpose may be one of the obstacles to promote the use of computational musculoskeletal models in the clinical setting. Recently, technological progress allows measuring *in vivo* contact forces within instrumented implants (e.g., at the hip and knee levels) [9, 12, 13], which could be used to validate indirectly the muscle force estimation. However, these data are only available for patients with instrumented implant. Thus, the accurate and reliable prediction and its quantitative validation of these forces on the healthy subjects to prevent the musculoskeletal diseases remain a challenge for musculoskeletal modeling community.

Regarding the Knee Grand Challenge, a series of editions has been organized and many efforts have been investigated to predict the *in vivo* contact forces using different approaches [15, 21–26]. In fact, contact forces may be predicted with or without a contact model formulation. Even if the approach without a contact model revealed interesting results [26], this approach is based purely on the numerical power to find the statistical correlation pattern between the contact forces and other physically measurable or computable quantities such as EMG-based muscle activation levels or maximum physiological muscle moments. Besides, the use of a contact model may provide more descriptive and meaningful information inside the implant-to-implant interaction under musculoskeletal load. However, current approach based on Hertzian contact model has two disadvantages. The first one relates to the strong constraint of the use of muscle forces to predict the contact forces due to the lack of contact area information. The second one deals with the simplified representation of the contact interaction. Thus, nodes-to-surface approach is commonly used. However, the number and location of nodes may be sensitive factors influencing the prediction of the contact forces. This present study developed a Hertzian contact model integrating contact area information. Indeed, muscle forces are not necessary to predict the contact forces. Moreover, thanks to available *in vivo* contact forces, elastic properties (Young's modulus and Poisson coefficient) of the implant were numerically identified and then may be used for the further prediction of the new patient case. Furthermore, when the reliable contact forces are known, muscle forces may be further estimated in a reliable manner. In addition, the knowledge of the contact area may allow other contact properties such as contact pressure and surface energy to be computed, leading to better understanding of the effect of TKR implant on the musculoskeletal tissues and structures.

From methodological point of view, the fact that muscle forces are not required to predict the contact forces leads to avoiding the limitations of the muscle force estimation approaches. For example, inverse dynamics and static optimization showed high residual results due to dynamic inconsistencies between ground reaction forces (GFR) and captured kinematics [17, 19]. Kinematical errors coming from anatomical representation, marker registration, and soft tissue artifacts may alter the accuracy of the results [12]. Moreover, the inaccuracy may come from the noise in GRF or drift effect over time. Furthermore, the choice of the objective function may create nonuniqueness solutions. EMG-driven approach has computational complexity. In addition, the accuracy of estimated muscle forces depends on the accuracy of EMG signals related to electrode type and location. Furthermore, EMG signal processing approach may alter significantly the simulation results [38].

Regarding our identification process, the value of cylinder radius (R) fitted to the femoral implant component is very close to the value used in the literature (R = 40 mm) [21]. Moreover, a good agreement was also noted between our contact area and the literature value acquired from cadaveric testing with 1000 N of load (Figure 8) [32]. The contact evolution maps revealed a more descriptive surface-to-surface interaction between implant components.

The accuracy of our prediction depends strongly on the contact area estimation. Thus, the input data such as joint angle needs to be accurately computed. The use of a patient specific musculoskeletal model without scaling step may guarantee the minimal errors between virtual marker coordinates and the real marker ones during inverse kinematics process [19]. However, the lack of knowledge about the muscles forces may lead to the neglect of the contact force balance ratio between medial and lateral sides [14]. Moreover, the present definition of the contact model is global and its behavior is symmetric. Furthermore, from computational point of view, this contact area process is dissociated from the inverse kinematics analysis. Indeed, further work will be investigated for the cosimulation of these physics with asymmetric definition of the contact model integrated side-dependent kinematic data such as joint abduction/adduction patterns. In this case, advanced computational paradigm needs to be developed [18, 23]. Thus, available fluoroscopic data will provide precise and local information on the translation and rotation of the implant leading to possibly achieving this challenging goal.

In addition, the use of a Hertzian contact model allows only the description of conservative interaction forces via a linearly elastic behavior. More advanced contact models need to be investigated. For example, Derjaguin-Muller-Toporov (DMT) model [39] may provide elastic behavior and van der Waals forces outside the contact region. Moreover, Johnson-Kendall-Robert (JKR) model [40] allows defining the adhesion (i.e., short-range forces in the contact area) phenomena and this model may be used to predict infinite stress at edge of contact circle and nonconservative interaction forces. Furthermore, the model needs to be refined for other types of implants with different designs.

In conclusion, reliable elastic properties of the TKR implants were identified using a Hertzian integrated contact model and *in vivo* contact forces. The availability of contact area information allows the *in vivo* prediction of contact forces without knowledge of the muscle forces. Thus, our present study demonstrated a potential use of such approach in the accurate and reliable prediction of human joint contact forces leading to better diagnosis and a more suitable treatment prescription for patients with instrumented implants to recover locomotion function and to improve the quality of daily activities of life.

Conflict of Interests

The authors declare no conflict of interests.

Acknowledgment

The authors would like to thank the organizers of the Knee Grand Challenge for providing available useful data for research purposes.

References

[1] T. K. Fehring, S. Odum, W. L. Griffin, J. B. Mason, and M. Nadaud, "Early failures in total knee arthroplasty," *Clinical Orthopaedics and Related Research*, no. 392, pp. 315–318, 2001.

[2] E. A. Lingard, J. N. Katz, E. A. Wright, and C. B. Sledge, "Predicting the outcome of total knee arthroplasty," *The Journal of Bone & Joint Surgery—American Volume*, vol. 86, no. 10, pp. 2179–2186, 2004.

[3] C. E. H. Scott, M. J. Eaton, R. W. Nutton, F. A. Wade, P. Pankaj, and S. L. Evans, "Proximal tibial strain in medial unicompartmental knee replacements: a biomechanical study of implant design," *Bone and Joint Journal*, vol. 95, no. 10, pp. 1339–1347, 2013.

[4] P. Pankaj, "Patient-specific modelling of bone and bone-implant systems: the challenges," *International Journal for Numerical Methods in Biomedical Engineering*, vol. 29, no. 2, pp. 233–249, 2013.

[5] A. A. Oshkour, N. A. A. Osman, M. M. Davoodi et al., "Finite element analysis on longitudinal and radial functionally graded femoral prosthesis," *International Journal for Numerical Methods in Biomedical Engineering*, vol. 29, no. 12, pp. 1412–1427, 2013.

[6] B. J. Fregly, "Design of optimal treatments for neuromusculoskeletal disorders using patient-specific multibody dynamic models," *International Journal of Computational Vision and Biomechanics*, vol. 2, no. 2, pp. 145–154, 2009.

[7] J. P. Halloran, A. J. Petrella, and P. J. Rullkoetter, "Explicit finite element modeling of total knee replacement mechanics," *Journal of Biomechanics*, vol. 38, no. 2, pp. 323–331, 2005.

[8] M. Taylor, R. Bryan, and F. Galloway, "Accounting for patient variability in finite element analysis of the intact and implanted hip and knee: a review," *International Journal for Numerical Methods in Biomedical Engineering*, vol. 29, no. 2, pp. 273–292, 2013.

[9] M. O. Heller, G. Bergmann, J.-P. Kassi, L. Claes, N. P. Haas, and G. N. Duda, "Determination of muscle loading at the hip joint for use in pre-clinical testing," *Journal of Biomechanics*, vol. 38, no. 5, pp. 1155–1163, 2005.

[10] G. Bergmann, F. Graichen, A. Rohlmann et al., "Realistic loads for testing hip implants," *Bio-Medical Materials and Engineering*, vol. 20, no. 2, pp. 65–75, 2010.

[11] V. Schwachmeyer, P. Damm, A. Bender, J. Dymke, F. Graichen, and G. Bergmann, "In vivo hip joint loading during postoperative physiotherapeutic exercises," *PLOS ONE*, vol. 8, no. 10, Article ID e77807, 2013.

[12] D. D. D'Lima, C. P. Townsend, S. W. Arms, B. A. Morris, and C. W. Colwell Jr., "An implantable telemetry device to measure intra-articular tibial forces," *Journal of Biomechanics*, vol. 38, no. 2, pp. 299–304, 2005.

[13] B. Kirking, J. Krevolin, C. Townsend, C. W. Colwell Jr., and D. D. D'Lima, "A multiaxial force-sensing implantable tibial prosthesis," *Journal of Biomechanics*, vol. 39, no. 9, pp. 1744–1751, 2006.

[14] B. J. Fregly, T. F. Besier, D. G. Lloyd et al., "Grand challenge competition to predict in vivo knee loads," *Journal of Orthopaedic Research*, vol. 30, no. 4, pp. 503–513, 2012.

[15] A. L. Kinney, T. F. Besier, D. D. D'Lima, and B. J. Fregly, "Update on grand challenge competition to predict *in vivo* knee loads," *Journal of Biomechanical Engineering*, vol. 135, no. 2, Article ID 021005, 2013.

[16] J. Li, A. C. Redmond, Z. Jin, J. Fisher, M. H. Stone, and T. D. Stewart, "Hip contact forces in asymptomatic total hip replacement patients differ from normal healthy individuals: implications for preclinical testing," *Clinical Biomechanics*, vol. 29, no. 7, pp. 747–751, 2014.

[17] A. Erdemir, S. McLean, W. Herzog, and A. J. van den Bogert, "Model-based estimation of muscle forces exerted during movements," *Clinical Biomechanics*, vol. 22, no. 2, pp. 131–154, 2007.

[18] Y.-C. Lin, J. P. Walter, S. A. Banks, M. G. Pandy, and B. J. Fregly, "Simultaneous prediction of muscle and contact forces in the knee during gait," *Journal of Biomechanics*, vol. 43, no. 5, pp. 945–952, 2010.

[19] T. T. Dao, F. Marin, P. Pouletaut, F. Charleux, P. Aufaure, and M. C. Ho Ba Tho, "Estimation of accuracy of patient-specific musculoskeletal modelling: case study on a post polio residual paralysis subject," *Computer Methods in Biomechanics and Biomedical Engineering*, vol. 15, no. 7, pp. 745–751, 2012.

[20] T. T. Dao, P. Pouletaut, F. Charleux et al., "Estimation of patient specific lumbar spine muscle forces using multi-physical musculoskeletal model and dynamic MRI," in *Knowledge and Systems Engineering*, vol. 245 of *Advances in Intelligent Systems and Computing*, pp. 411–422, Springer, 2014.

[21] H. J. Kim, J. W. Fernandez, M. Akbarshahi, J. P. Walter, B. J. Fregly, and M. G. Pandy, "Evaluation of predicted knee-joint muscle forces during gait using an instrumented knee implant," *Journal of Orthopaedic Research*, vol. 27, no. 10, pp. 1326–1331, 2009.

[22] M. W. Hast and S. J. Piazza, "Dual-joint modeling for estimation of total knee replacement contact forces during locomotion," *Journal of Biomechanical Engineering*, vol. 135, no. 2, Article ID 021013, 2013.

[23] F. Moissenet, L. Chèze, and R. Dumas, "A 3D lower limb musculoskeletal model for simultaneous estimation of musculo-tendon, joint contact, ligament and bone forces during gait," *Journal of Biomechanics*, vol. 47, no. 1, pp. 50–58, 2014.

[24] K. Manal and T. S. Buchanan, "An electromyogram-driven musculoskeletal model of the knee to predict *in vivo* joint contact forces during normal and novel gait patterns," *Journal of Biomechanical Engineering*, vol. 135, no. 2, Article ID 021014, 7 pages, 2013.

[25] P. Gerus, M. Sartori, T. F. Besier et al., "Subject-specific knee joint geometry improves predictions of medial tibiofemoral contact forces," *Journal of Biomechanics*, vol. 46, no. 16, pp. 2778–2786, 2013.

[26] H. J. Lundberg, C. Knowlton, and M. A. Wimmer, "Fine tuning total knee replacement contact force prediction algorithms using blinded model validation," *Journal of Biomechanical Engineering*, vol. 135, no. 2, Article ID 021008, 2013.

[27] S. L. Delp, F. C. Anderson, A. S. Arnold et al., "OpenSim: open-source software to create and analyze dynamic simulations of movement," *IEEE Transactions on Biomedical Engineering*, vol. 54, no. 11, pp. 1940–1950, 2007.

[28] G. Wu, S. Siegler, P. Allard et al., "ISB recommendation on definition of joint coordinate system of various joints for the reporting of human joint motion—part 1 ankle, hip, and spine," *Journal of Biomechanics*, vol. 35, no. 4, pp. 543–548, 2002.

[29] L. M. Schutte, M. Rodgers, F. E. Zajac, and R. M. Glaser, "Improving the efficacy of electrical stimulation-induced leg cycle ergometry: an analysis based on a dynamic musculoskeletal model," *IEEE Transactions on Rehabilitation Engineering*, vol. 1, no. 2, pp. 109–125, 1993.

[30] E. M. Arnold, S. R. Ward, R. L. Lieber, and S. L. Delp, "A model of the lower limb for analysis of human movement," *Annals of Biomedical Engineering*, vol. 38, no. 2, pp. 269–279, 2010.

[31] T. T. Dao, P. Pouletaut, J.-C. Goebel, A. Pinzano, P. Gillet, and M. C. Ho Ba Tho, "In vivo characterization of morphological properties and contact areas of the rat cartilage derived from high-resolution MRI," *IRBM*, vol. 32, no. 3, pp. 204–213, 2011.

[32] T. Fukubayashi and H. Kurosawa, "The contact area and pressure distribution pattern of the knee: a study of normal and osteoarthrotic knee joints," *Acta Orthopaedica Scandinavica*, vol. 51, no. 1–6, pp. 871–879, 1980.

[33] H. Hertz, "On the contact of rigid elastic solids," *Journal für die Reine und Angewandte Mathematik*, vol. 92, pp. 156–171, 1896.

[34] D. Zhao, S. A. Banks, D. D. D'Lima, C. W. Colwell Jr., and B. J. Fregly, "In vivo medial and lateral tibial loads during dynamic and high flexion activities," *Journal of Orthopaedic Research*, vol. 25, no. 5, pp. 593–602, 2007.

[35] S. S. Blemker, D. S. Asakawa, G. E. Gold, and S. L. Delp, "Image-based musculoskeletal modeling: applications, advances, and future opportunities," *Journal of Magnetic Resonance Imaging*, vol. 25, no. 2, pp. 441–451, 2007.

[36] S. F. Bensamoun, T. T. Dao, F. Charleux, and M.-C. Ho Ba Tho, "Estimation of muscle force derived from *in vivo* MR elastography tests: a preliminary study," *Journal of Musculoskeletal Research*, vol. 16, no. 3, Article ID 1350015, 10 pages, 2013.

[37] F. E. Zajac, "Muscle and tendon: properties, models, scaling, and application to biomechanics and motor control," *Critical Reviews in Biomedical Engineering*, vol. 17, no. 4, pp. 359–411, 1989.

[38] D. Staudenmann, K. Roeleveld, D. F. Stegeman, and J. H. van Dieën, "Methodological aspects of SEMG recordings for force estimation—a tutorial and review," *Journal of Electromyography and Kinesiology*, vol. 20, no. 3, pp. 375–387, 2010.

[39] B. V. Derjaguin, V. M. Muller, and Y. P. Toporov, "Effect of contact deformations on the adhesion of particles," *Journal of Colloid And Interface Science*, vol. 53, no. 2, pp. 314–326, 1975.

[40] K. L. Johnson, K. Kendall, and A. D. Roberts, "Surface energy and the contact of elastic solids," *Proceedings of the Royal Society of London Series A: Mathematical and Physical Sciences*, vol. 324, no. 1558, pp. 301–313, 1971.

14

Musculoskeletal Simulation for Assessment of Effect of Movement-Based Structure-Modifying Treatment Strategies

Tien Tuan Dao

Sorbonne Universités, Université de Technologie de Compiègne, CNRS, UMR 7338, Biomécanique et Bioingénierie, Centre de Recherche Royallieu, CS 60 319, 60 203 Compiègne, France

Correspondence should be addressed to Tien Tuan Dao; tien-tuan.dao@utc.fr

Academic Editor: Camillo Porcaro

The better understanding of the complex mechanism between neural motor control and its resulting joint kinematics and muscle forces allows a better elucidation of the mechanisms behind body growth, aging progression, and disease development. This study aimed at investigating the impact of movement-based structure-modifying treatment strategies on joint kinematics, muscle forces, and muscle synergies of the gait with instrumented implant. A patient-specific musculoskeletal model was used to quantitatively assess the deviations of joint and muscle behaviors between the normal gait and 4 gait modifications (bouncy, medial thrust, midcrouch, and mtp (i.e., gait with forefoot strike)). Moreover, muscle synergy analysis was performed using EMG-based nonnegative matrix factorization. Large variation of 19 degrees and 190 N was found for knee flexion/extension and lower limb muscle forces, respectively. EMG-based muscle synergy analysis revealed that the activation levels of the vastus lateralis and tibialis anterior are dominant for the midcrouch gait. In addition, an important contribution of semimembranosus to the medial thrust and midcrouch gaits was also observed. In fact, such useful information could allow a better understanding of the joint function and muscle synergy strategies leading to deeper knowledge of joint and muscle mechanisms related to neural voluntary motor commands.

1. Introduction

Accurate simulation of the human dynamics movement is one of the most challenging research topics in the last two decades in the biomechanics field. Most of the research projects focused on the *in vivo* estimation of joint kinematics and muscle forces during motion [1–6]. Such information could be of great clinical interest to objectively evaluate the mechanical functions of the musculoskeletal system in normal as well as in pathological conditions [7–9]. In the case of orthopedic device prescription especially, the joint kinematics and muscle force information could allow an optimal design to be performed leading to maximizing the benefit of the involved patient [10, 11]. In addition, structure-modifying treatment modalities such as voluntary gait modification strategies have been studied to alter the medial knee joint load leading to decreasing the external knee adduction moment (KAM) [12–14]. This conservative nonpharmacologic management allows symptoms or disease

progression to be alleviated for degenerative joint disorders such as osteoarthritis (OA).

A recent review study [15] showed kinetic and kinematic changes by using some gait modifications such as increases of step width or cadence or knee flexion or mediolateral trunk lean or weight transfer to the medial foot or hip internal rotation or toe-out or speed as well as reductions of vertical acceleration and initial contact or stride length or toe-off or speed or using gait aids (e.g., ipsilateral/contralateral cane) and applications of specific gait patterns (medial knee thrust or Tai Chi gait). These gait modifications have shown their efficiencies in the management of knee joint disease. In fact, the use of contralateral cane and the increase of trunk lean lead to reducing the early-stance KAM. Besides, the increase of toe-out modification leads to reducing the late-stance KAM. Particularly, the medial knee thrust gait altered dynamically knee alignment and thus KAM lever arm leading to the reduction of KAM during gait cycle. Despite their great potentials, further investigation is needed to elucidate

TABLE 1: Description of normal gait and gait modification strategies.

Gait modifications	Description	Marker's number	Trial name: gait cycle times (start > end) (time in sec)
Ngait	Normal gait	56	Ngait_og1: 1.699 > 2.811 (1.112)
Bouncy	Increased superior-inferior translation of the pelvis	52	Bouncy1: 2.066 > 3.214 (1.148)
Medial thrust	Internally rotated hip of the stance leg	52	Medthrust2: 2.415 > 3.571 (1.156)
Midcrouch	Crouched position with a mild increase in knee flexion angle	56	Mildcrouch1: 10.822 > 11.901 (1.079)
Mtp	Gait with forefoot strike	52	Mtpgait2: 2.276 > 3.421 (1.145)

the effect of voluntary gait modifications on the muscle force, which is still not fully understood.

There exist many cutting-edge computational approaches to estimate the joint kinematics and muscle force. The first one related to inverse dynamics and static optimization [4, 16]. This approach used skin-mounted marker's trajectories and ground reaction forces within a musculoskeletal model. The second approach deals with the EMG-driven forward dynamic. In this case, the surface electromyography is commonly used to define the muscle activation pattern [17] to reproduce the observed motion. The third approach is the dynamic optimization using muscle activation-driven pattern to generate the body motion [18, 19]. This approach is computationally complex, but the results are practically equivalent to the static optimization [20]. The choice of the appropriate approach depends on the specific objective as well as on the availability of input data. However, the interaction between neural motor command and musculoskeletal structures remains a challenging issue. One of the current most-used strategies related to the replacement of the neural motor command by the hypothesis of the performance strategies of the human body. In fact, the optimization of muscle metabolic function is one of the most used hypotheses when using inverse dynamics and static optimization approach. Thus, the understanding of this underlying interaction could allow a deeper knowledge of the mechanical function of the human body, especially in the cases of muscle weakness or spasticity and muscle synergies.

Motor cortex is involved in planning, control, and execution of voluntary motions. The motor cortex gradually performs the coordination of several muscles in the control of body forces and motions when the human being learns a new complex locomotion pattern. The understanding of this complex coordination mechanism may be elucidated by brain-based electrical stimulation [21, 22]. Moreover, Barroso et al. [23] studied the muscle coordination strategy by muscle synergy analysis during walking and running. In fact, muscle synergies relate to the coordinated and temporal recruitment of muscle groups to perform a specific task. However, muscle synergies have not yet been compared between the normal gait and voluntary gait modification patterns. The question of how the module function (i.e., muscle synergy) changes from the normal gait to other voluntary altered gaits is still misunderstood. The response to this question may provide

some elucidation for robotic application using neural control strategies or for testing and optimizing the implant effect on the human locomotor function. In fact, the objectives of this present study were to (1) quantitatively assess the effect of voluntary neural command through 4 altered gait modifications (bouncy, medial thrust, midcrouch, and mtp (i.e., gait with forefoot strike)) on the joint kinematics and muscle force estimation and (2) find muscle synergy patterns related to the normal gait as well as these altered gait modifications.

2. Materials and Methods

2.1. Patient Data. The patient data used in this present study were extracted from the fourth edition of the Knee Grand Challenge [24]. All used data are briefly summarised here. Data acquisition was performed on a patient (male, 88 years old, 168 cm body height, 66.7 kg body weight, and 23.6 kg/m^2 Body Mass Index (BMI)) with knee implant instrumented in his right knee side. The patient had Rockport flat bottom sneakers shoes during the gait data acquisition process. The patient performed an overground normal gait pattern, which was used as reference pattern. Then, 4 overground gait trials reflecting 4 gait modification strategies (bouncy, medial thrust, mild crouch, and mtp (i.e., gait with forefoot strike)) were acquired using an 8-camera Vicon system. All skin-mounted markers were posed using a modified Cleveland Clinic marker protocol [24]. Kinematical sampling frequency is 120 Hz. Ground reaction forces were acquired using 3 AMTI force plates. Sampling frequency of the ground reaction forces is 1000 Hz. Moreover, during each acquisition trial, surface electromyography (EMG) of 15 lower limbs muscles (semimembranosus, biceps femoris, vastus medialis, vastus lateralis, rectus femoris, medial gastrocnemius, lateral gastrocnemius, tensor fascia latae, tibialis anterior, peroneus longus, soleus, adductor magnus, gluteus maximus, gluteus medius, and sartorius) was also monitored using Delsys Bagnoli EMG System. The description of the normal gait and these gait modification strategies is depicted in Table 1. Furthermore, pre- and postsurgery CT data were also acquired on the patient using a Siemens CT machine; the slice thickness was set up as 0.6 mm. The matrix is 512 × 512 and the pixel resolution is 0.9 × 0.9 mm^2. The number of slices is 1900 for the whole scanned lower limb.

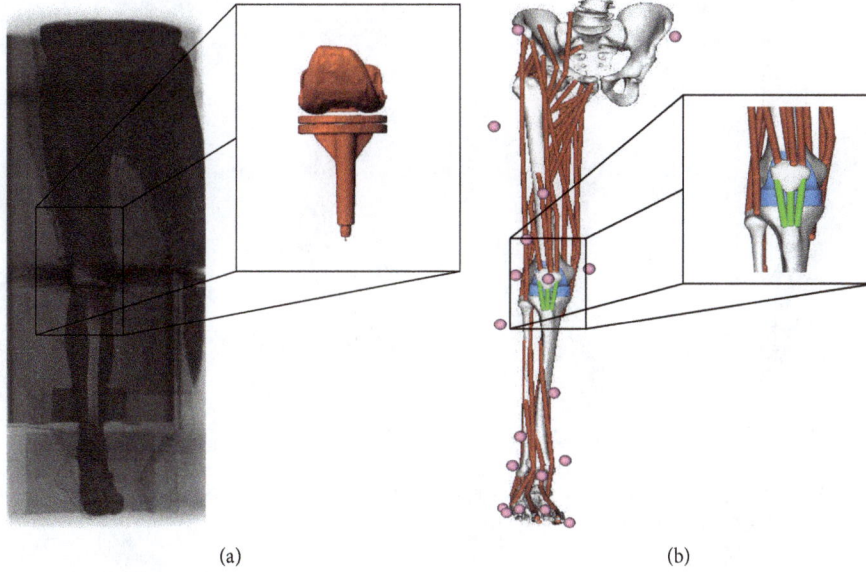

FIGURE 1: Patient-specific rigid musculoskeletal model: CT-based visualization of the lower limb with implant (a) and its respective OpenSIM model (b).

2.2. Patient-Specific Rigid Musculoskeletal Model. An available 7-segment patient-specific OpenSIM musculoskeletal model was utilized to compute gait kinematics and muscle forces for normal gait and gait modification patterns [25] (Figure 1). The model composed of the pelvis and right leg of the patient under investigation. Post- and presurgery CT data and laser-scan-based implant component were used to develop geometric model. The model development process is briefly described here. Image segmentation using SliceOmatic (Montreal, Canada) was performed to extract bony segments (pelvis, femur, patella, tibia, fibula, talus, calcaneus, and phalanges) and implant components (femoral component, tibial tray). Data from postsurgery (spanned from the proximal end of the pelvis to the distal tips of the toes) was aligned with those from presurgery data (approximately 15 cm above and below the joint line). STL-based surface geometries were created and imported into OpenSIM to develop corresponding bony segments. The model has 24 degrees of freedom (DOF) (6 DOF ground-to-pelvis joint, 3 DOF hip joint, 6 DOF tibiofemoral joint, 6 DOF patellofemoral joint, 2 DOF ankle joint, and 1 DOF toes joint). The interaction between implant components and its respective bone was modeled using a weld joint. The interaction between implant components (femoral component, tibial tray, and patella/femoral component) was modeled using a reverse joint. All segment coordinate systems were based on the ISB recommendations [26]. The model has 22-skin-mounted virtual marker's cluster according to the real market cloud used in the motion capture acquisition. Mass and inertial properties of segmental bodies were scaled using the data from Arnold et al. [27].

44 lower limb muscles were integrated into the bony model. Each muscle was modeled as a Schutte muscle model [28]. Muscle attachment points and wrapping surface were created using an available lower limb model [27].

A transformation process using information from bone-to-bone alignment was performed to morph the patient-specific musculature. Some attachments' points and unrealistic intersection of muscle lines of action were manually adjusted.

2.3. Estimation of Joint Kinematics and Muscle Forces. Based on skin-mounted marker's trajectories, inverse kinematics was performed to compute the joint kinematics. Then, inverse dynamics and static optimization [2, 4, 16] were applied to estimate the muscle forces according to the normal gait and each gait modification pattern. All these algorithms were performed using OpenSIM 3.1 version on a Dell computer (Precision T3500, 2.8 Ghz, 3 GB RAM). Inverse dynamic aims at estimating net joint moments from tracked segment kinematics. Static optimization allows the estimation of the muscle forces to be performed using the equilibrium principle between net joint moments, muscle lever arms, and muscle forces. In this present study, the optimization problem is expressed as follows:

$$\text{minimize} \quad F_{\text{obj}}$$

$$\text{subject to} \quad R(q) F^{TM} = T_{MT} \tag{1}$$

$$0 \leq F^{TM} \leq F_M^0,$$

where q is the joint angles set for n joints; $R(q)$ is the muscle moment arms $(n \times m)$ matrix; F^{TM} are the muscle force $(m \times 1)$ matrix; T_{MT} is the muscular joint moments $(n \times 1)$ matrix; F_M^0 is the peak isometric muscle force deriving from the cross-sectional area of the muscle; and F_{obj} is an activation-based objective function as follows:

$$F_{\text{obj}} = \left(\sum_{j=1}^{N} a_j(t_i) \right)^2, \tag{2}$$

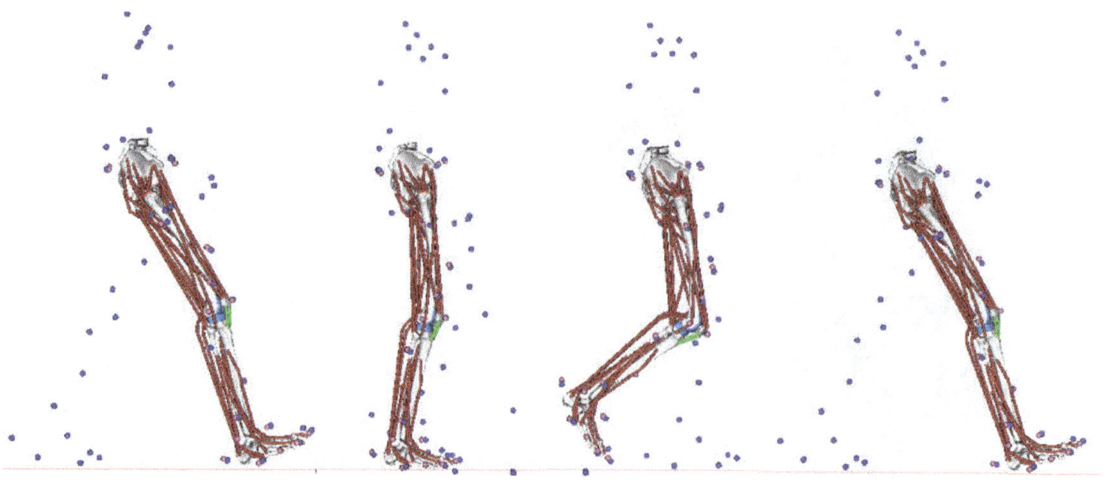

FIGURE 2: Visualization of the normal gait motion of the patient-specific model superposed with the experimental 56-skin-mounted (blue color) and virtual 22-skin-mounted (pink color) marker clusters.

where a_j is the activation level of the muscle j and N (= 44) is the number of muscles of interest.

To assess the kinematical deviation, a peak-to-peak absolute error was computed for each pair of comparison between the normal gait pattern and each gait modification pattern. The deviation of muscle forces was quantified using root mean square error (RMSE) and its relative error (RE) according to the maximal value. These quantities were calculated for each pair of comparison between the normal gait pattern and each gait modification pattern. Respective mathematical equations of these errors are expressed as follows:

$$\text{RMSE} = \sqrt{\frac{\sum_i (X_i - Y_i)^2}{N}},$$

$$\text{RE} = \frac{\text{RMSE}}{\max(\max(X_i), \max(Y_i))}, \tag{3}$$

where X_i and Y_i ($i \in \{1, \ldots, N\}$) are time series of two data sets used for the comparison. All postprocessing steps were performed using MATLAB R2010b (MathWorks, USA).

2.4. Muscle Synergy Analysis. The muscle synergies during the normal gait and respective gait modifications were computed using nonnegative matrix factorization method [29–31]. This multivariate analysis and linear algebra tool allows transforming the EMG signals into muscle synergy features in reducing their dimensionality [32]. The respective equation of this feature transformation is expressed as follows:

$$\text{EMG}_{nm} = W_{np} \times H_{pm} + R_m, \tag{4}$$

where EMG_{nm} is the matrix of EMG signals of m muscles; W_{np} is the synergy matrix in which vector columns correspond to relative muscle activation levels; p is the number of synergies; n is the number of time steps; H_{pm} is the synergy activation vector reflecting the EMG-to-force behavior; and R_m is the factorization residual vector. The nonnegative matrix factorization method was implemented using MATLAB R2010b (MathWorks, USA).

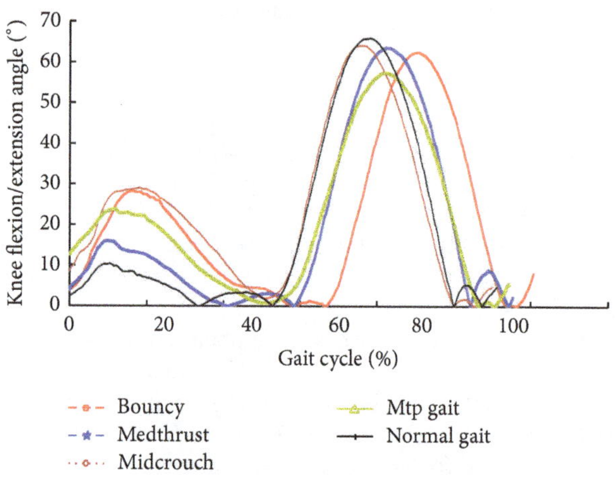

FIGURE 3: Evolution of the patient right knee flexion/extension within his instrumented implant during normal gait and altered gait modifications.

3. Results

3.1. Kinematical Deviation. A motion of the patient-specific model within the knee implant during his normal gait cycle is shown in Figure 2. The duration of his normal gait cycle is around 1.112 sec. The time durations of the bouncy, medial thrust, midcrouch, and mtp (i.e., gait with forefoot strike) gaits are around 1.148, 1.156, 1.079, and 1.145 sec, respectively. The evolutions of the knee flexion/extension within his instrumented implant during normal and modified gaits are illustrated in Figure 3. The 1st and 2nd peak-to-peak deviations of the knee flexion/extension motion of each modified gait according to the normal gait are depicted in Table 2. The 1st peak-to-peak deviation showed an increase of flexion/extension angle ranging from 5.6 (medial thrust) to 18.5 (midcrouch) degrees for all comparisons. The 2nd peak-to-peak deviation showed a decrease of flexion/extension angle ranging from 1.8 (midcrouch) to 8.52 (mtp) degrees for all comparisons. It is important to emphasize that, due to

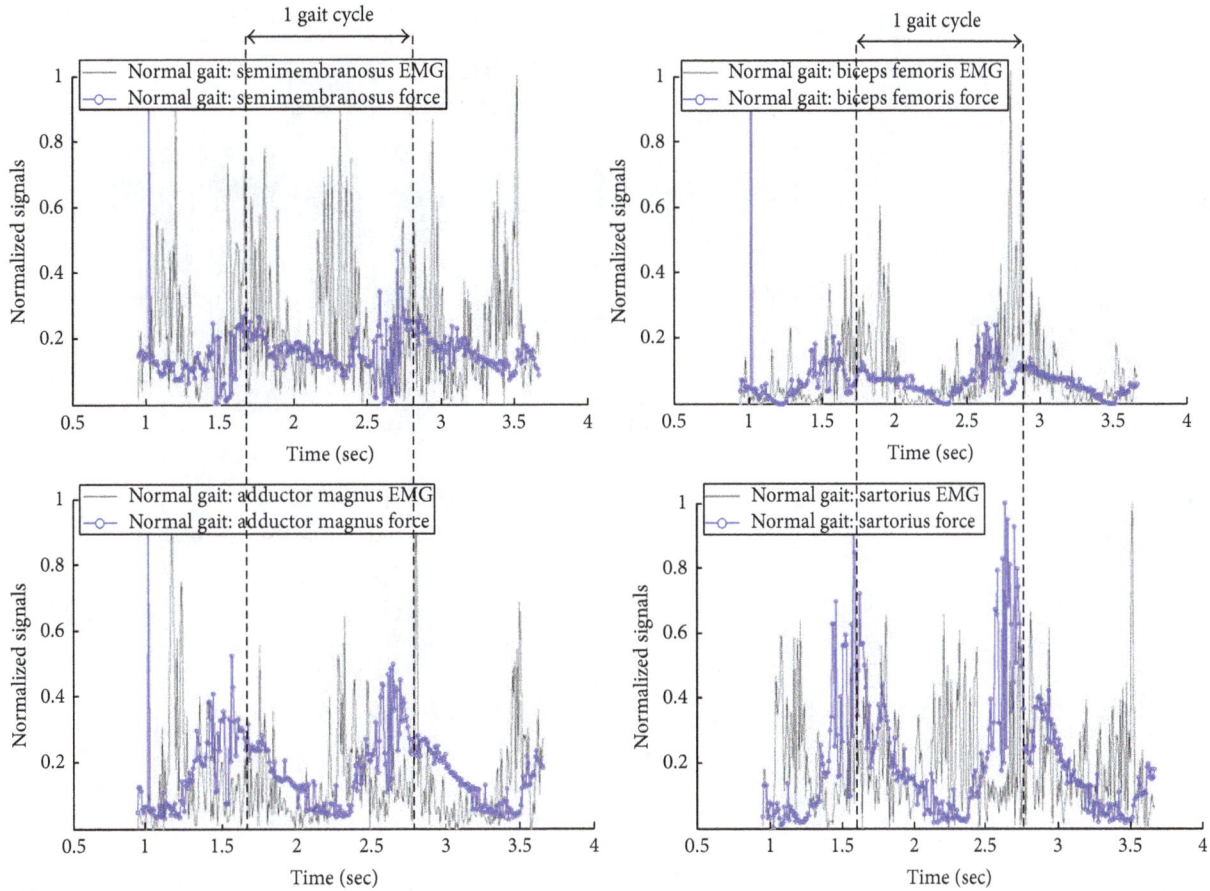

FIGURE 4: Lower limb muscle behaviors during the normal gait: normalized tensile forces versus EMG signals.

TABLE 2: Kinematical deviations between the normal gait and modification gait patterns.

	1st peak-to-peak deviation (°)	2nd peak-to-peak deviation (°)
Bouncy versus normal gait	17.7	−3.44
Medthrust versus normal gait	5.6	−2.42
Midcrouch versus normal gait	18.5	−1.8
Mtpgait versus normal gait	13.4	−8.52

the instrumented knee implant, these gait patterns fall out of normality with some cusps effects according to conventional gait patterns.

3.2. Muscle Force Deviation. Muscle force and EMG evolutions of the lower limb muscle during the normal gait and the medial thrust gaits are shown in Figures 4 and 5. Overall, the comparisons revealed a fair qualitative agreement between muscle force and EMG-based patterns of each muscle during the normal gait and also medial thrust gait. The same observations were found for the bouncy, midcrouch, and mtp gait modifications. However, at some periods over the gait cycle, the high EMG activity does not perfectly correspond to the muscle peak force.

When analyzing the difference between each gait modification according to the normal gait, we observed altered muscle force ranges (Figure 6 and Table 3). Root mean square errors range from 7.9 to 139 N, from 7.4 to 189.1 N, from 5.7 to 101.3 N, and from 7.4 to 126.2 N for the comparisons between the normal gait and the bouncy, medial thrust, midcrouch, and mtp gait modifications, respectively. Moreover, overall quantitative assessment revealed a root mean square error ranging from 5.5 to 189.1 N for all comparisons. The maximal deviation arises from the gluteus medius muscle during the medial thrust gait modification. The peroneus longus showed a minimal deviation during the midcrouch gait modification. Regarding the relative deviation, the overall range is from 10 to 34%. The medial gastrocnemius revealed a minimal deviation during midcrouch gait modification while the sartorius showed a maximal deviation during the mtp gait modification.

3.3. Muscle Synergies. Muscle synergies extracted from the EMG signals during the midcrouch gait modifications are illustrated in Figure 7. We noted that the activation levels of the vastus lateralis and tibialis anterior are dominant for the midcrouch gait. The comparison between the muscle synergies patterns of the normal gait and other gait modifications is shown in Figure 8. We observed a large faction

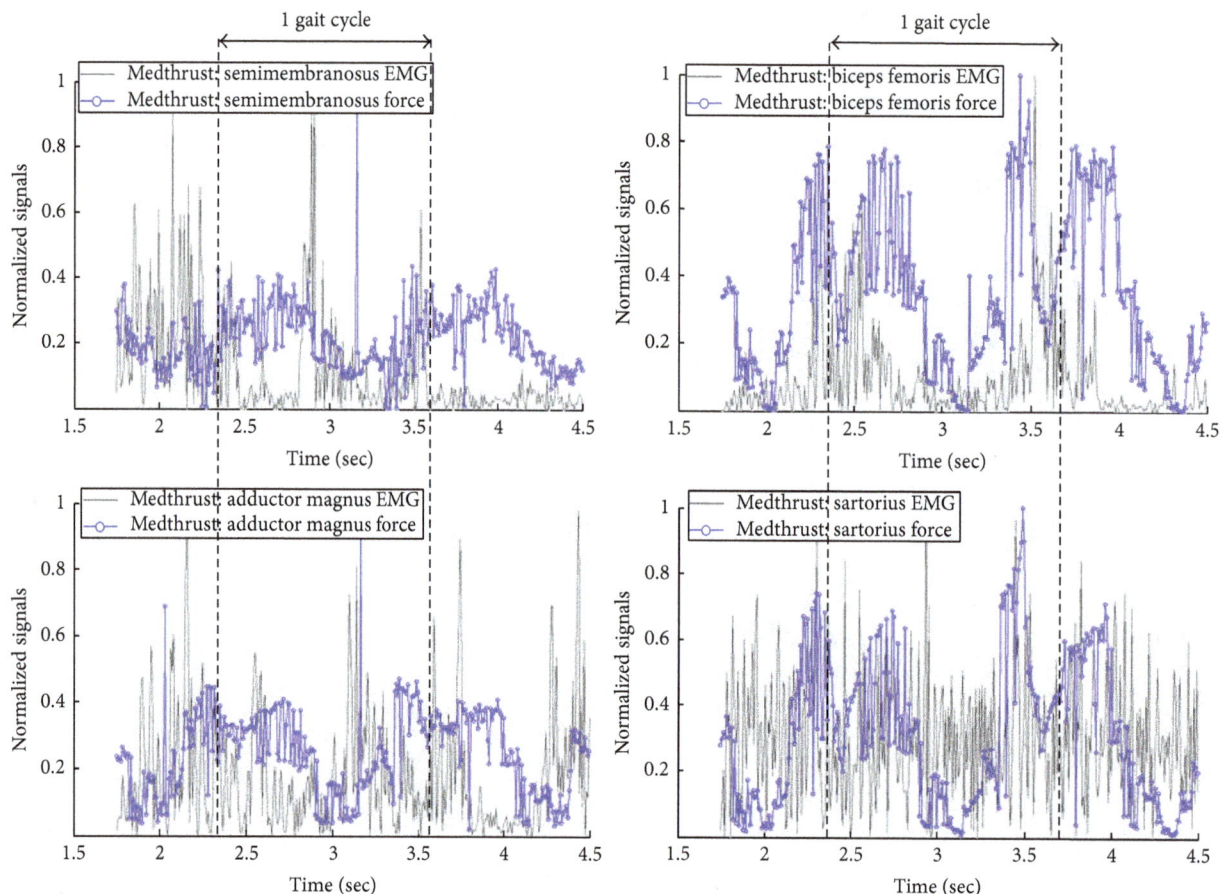

FIGURE 5: Lower limb muscle behaviors during the medial thrust gait: normalized tensile forces versus EMG signals.

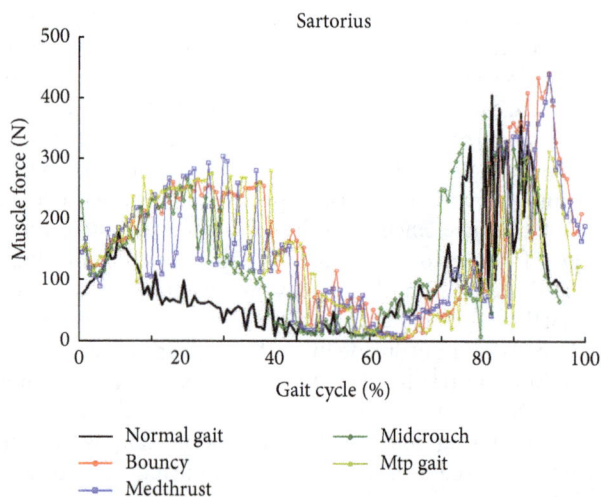

FIGURE 6: Evolution patterns of the thigh muscle (semimembranosus, biceps femoris, rectus femoris, and sartorius) forces: normal gait versus modification gait patterns.

of variation in the muscle patterns between the normal gait and all gait modifications. It is important to note that a small number of 4 synergies are sufficient to generate the functional output of muscle patterns. It is important to

emphasize that one of the main objectives is to reach this number as small as possible when analyzing an important number of signals. Moreover, the activation level of the semimembranosus is more important for medial thrust and midcrouch gait modifications than other gaits.

4. Discussion

Neural motor control and its resulting joint kinematics and muscle forces provide basic knowledge of locomotion function of the human body in the normal as well as in the pathophysiological conditions [16, 33, 34]. Moreover, the better understanding of this complex underlying mechanism allows a better elucidation of the mechanisms behind body growth, aging progression, and disease development [3, 23]. This may lead to a precise and accurate diagnosis of the musculoskeletal diseases. Furthermore, this provides also important knowledge in the fight (e.g., more efficient treatment prescription) against these musculoskeletal diseases. In this present study, the impact of the voluntary altered gait modifications on joint kinematics, muscle forces, and muscle synergies was assessed. Our findings contributed to the understanding of how the motor cortex changes voluntarily the motion patterns and its resulting effect on the joint and muscle mechanics. In fact, a large kinematic

TABLE 3: Muscle force deviations between the normal gait and modification gait patterns: root mean square error (N) and relative error (%).

	Semimem N (%)	Bflh N (%)	Rf N (%)	Gasmed N (%)	Gaslat N (%)	Perlong N (%)	Soleus N (%)	Addmag N (%)	Glmax N (%)	Glmed N (%)	Sart N (%)
Bouncy versus normal gait	94.9 (22.4)	88.1 (25.8)	62.1 (20.9)	47.2 (27.3)	23.2 (22.9)	7.9 (31.9)	72.4 (24)	72.2 (26)	17.3 (26.3)	122.9 (19.9)	136.4 (30.4)
Medthrust versus normal gait	119.5 (11.3)	82.7 (25.8)	43.8 (19.5)	46.1 (27.3)	33 (15.2)	7.4 (21.6)	67.8 (26.3)	79.9 (14)	19.4 (20.3)	**189.1** (19.1)	119.1 (31)
Midcrouch versus normal gait	74.9 (21.2)	68.8 (25.8)	56.5 (19.7)	50.2 (9.6)	18 (14)	**5.7** (31.9)	58.7 (21.2)	80.2 (11)	14.4 (26.3)	101.3 (14.7)	95.4 (33.8)
Mtpgait versus normal gait	97.6 (22.7)	82 (25.8)	65.1 (18.9)	42.5 (27.3)	24.6 (25.7)	7.4 (31.8)	70 (25.9)	73.3 (26)	15.1 (26)	117.7 (19.9)	126.2 (33.8)

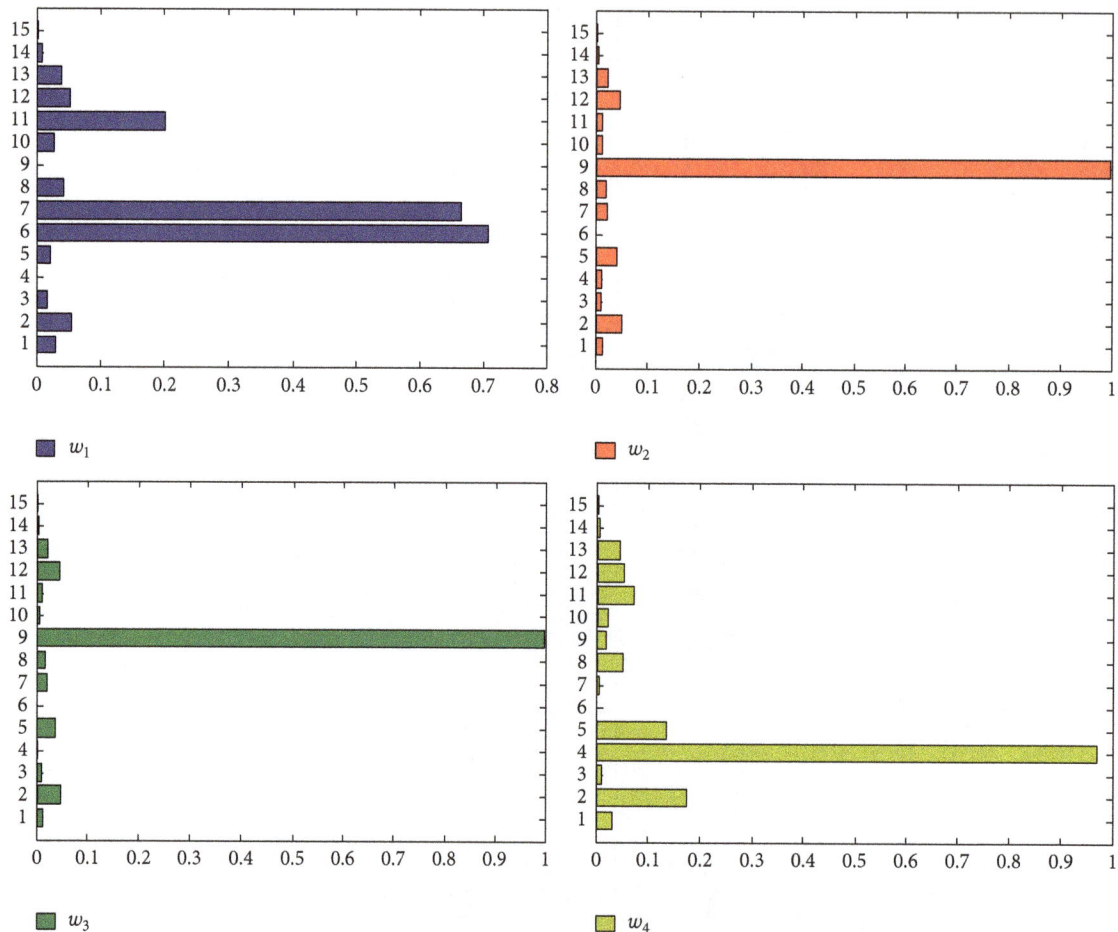

FIGURE 7: Muscle synergies matrix (w—activation level) identified from the nonnegative matrix factorization based on the EMG signals collected during the midcrouch gait: (1) semimembranosus, (2) biceps femoris, (3) vastus medialis, (4) vastus lateralis, (5) rectus femoris, (6) medial gastrocnemius, (7) lateral gastrocnemius, (8) tensor fascia latae, (9) tibialis anterior, (10) peroneus longus, (11) soleus, (12) adductor magnus, (13) gluteus maximus, (14) gluteus medius, and (15) sartorius. Each column of muscle synergies (w_1, w_2, w_3, and w_4) includes a vector of relative level of muscle activations of 15 analyzed muscles illustrated by horizontal bars.

deviation of around 19 degrees for knee flexion/extension was found between the normal gait and 4 other gait modifications (bouncy, medial thrust, midcrouch, and mtp). A significant change of 190 N for the lower limb muscle forces was also noted. In fact, our used musculoskeletal model was sensitive enough to detect the changes of the motor control strategies and their resulting effects on the joint and muscle behaviors. Motor commands may be generated through muscle synergy mechanism. Healthy human being is able to adapt a set of muscle synergies to effectively control body movements and stabilities. Nonetheless, abnormal gait (e.g., gait with instrumented implant in this present study) showed a large variation in the joint kinematics and muscle force patterns across a variety of gait modifications strategies. This could be explained by the fact that the implant may influence the decision-making process of the motor cortex leading to the joint and muscle adaptation behaviors, which are specific to each motion pattern.

In addition to the effect on the joint kinematics and muscle forces, EMG-based muscle synergy analysis revealed an important contribution of semimembranosus to the medial thrust and midcrouch gaits. Thus, this advanced multivariate analysis allows recognizing functional output of muscle activation patterns for each specific motion pattern [32]. In fact, we demonstrated that different altered motor behaviors may be constructed by a common set of muscle synergies (as results shown in Figures 7 and 8). Our findings support prior works related to the changes in the modular organization of different motion patterns of healthy and pathological subjects [35, 36].

At the moment, cutting-edge computational approaches such as inverse dynamics, static and dynamic optimization, and EMG-driven forward dynamics are commonly used to elucidate the neurophysiological relationships between the motor cortex, the muscle, and the joint mechanics [4]. Each approach has underlying advantages as well as disadvantages. Inverse dynamics and static optimization showed high residual results due to dynamic inconsistencies between ground reaction forces (GFR) and captured kinematics. Kinematical errors coming from anatomical representation, marker

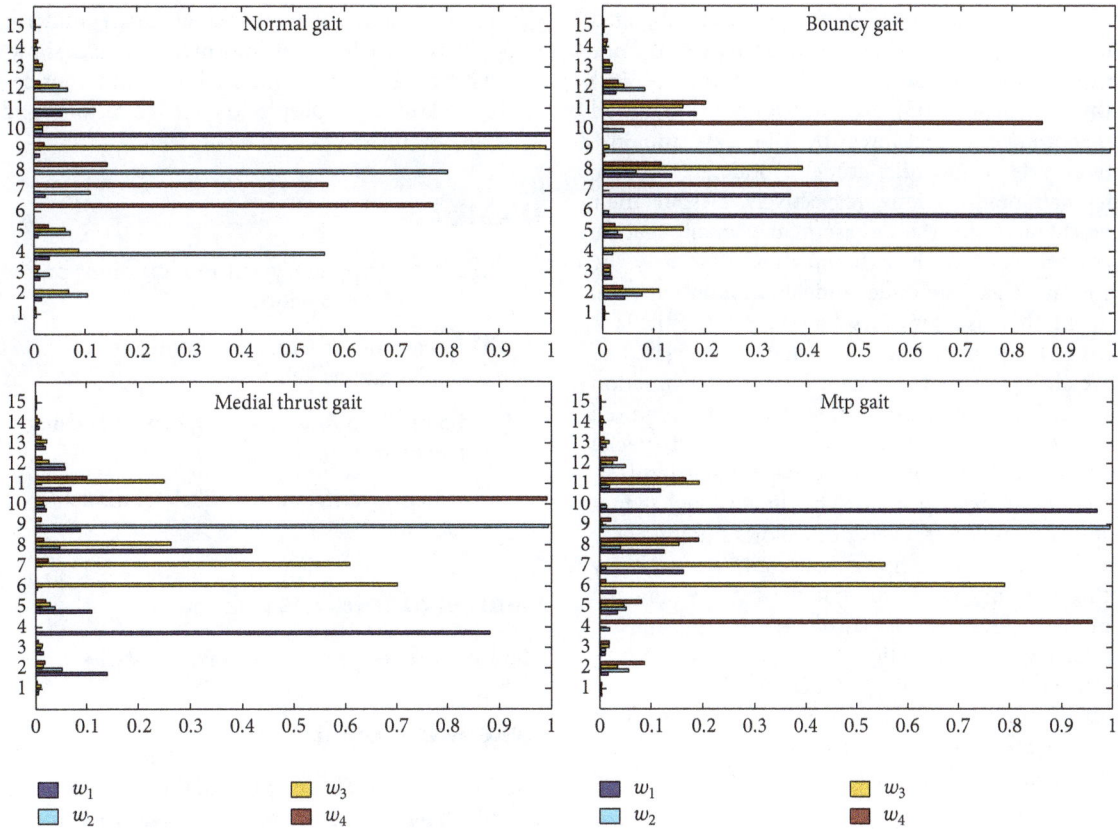

FIGURE 8: Comparison of all muscle synergies matrix (w—activation level) between the normal gait and other gait modifications: (1) semimembranosus, (2) biceps femoris, (3) vastus medialis, (4) vastus lateralis, (5) rectus femoris, (6) medial gastrocnemius, (7) lateral gastrocnemius, (8) tensor fascia latae, (9) tibialis anterior, (10) peroneus longus, (11) soleus, (12) adductor magnus, (13) gluteus maximus, (14) gluteus medius, and (15) sartorius. Each gait pattern corresponds to the visualization of all 15 muscles of interest and their associated synergies. Each column of muscle synergies (w_1, w_2, w_3, and w_4) includes a vector of relative level of muscle activations of 15 analyzed muscles illustrated by horizontal bars.

registration, and soft tissue artifacts may alter the accuracy of the results [16]. Moreover, the inaccuracy may come from the noise in GRF or drift effect over time. Furthermore, the choice of the objective function may create nonuniqueness solutions. However, this approach has a short computing time and this may be appropriately suitable for real-time simulation. Forward dynamics and dynamic optimization have computational complexity. The accuracy of EMG signals due to electrode location and signal processing approach may alter significantly the simulation results [37]. Another challenge is how to deal with the recruitment mechanism of related motor units in pathological muscles. Thus, the estimation of muscle forces using optimization deals with nonuniqueness cost function and this approach may be invalid for movement disorders. The EMG-driven approach is challenging, but there are many disadvantageous factors related to the cross talk effect and noise or uncertain muscle model parameters. Moreover, it is especially difficult to acquire accurately deep muscle excitations in noninvasive manner. In fact, the choice of the appropriate approaches depends on the specific objective of study. In this present study, inverse dynamics and static optimization were applied to estimate the lower limb muscle forces. The comparisons

between muscle force patterns and EMG-based activation patterns showed a good agreement (Figures 4 and 5) for the normal gait pattern. This finding confirmed the reasonable accuracy of the used approach in the estimation of *in vivo* patient-specific healthy muscle forces [6, 20]. However, it is important to emphasize that the use of EMG signals allows only a qualitative validation of the estimated muscle forces to be achieved. Consequently, the present study showed some disagreements between estimated muscle forces and EMG signals, especially for modified gait patterns. This phenomenon could be explained by the fact that the modeling of abnormal muscle behaviors, especially with instrumented implant devices, remains a challenging issue. Moreover, the use of an activation-based optimization function may be not well appropriate for these modified gaits. In perspective, further works related to the definition of new optimization functions for abnormal gaits need to be performed to improve the simulation outcomes. Furthermore, electrical activities of the semimembranosus and adductor magnus muscles do not match the EMG profiles of the healthy subjects [38]. The differences may be explained by the fact that the instrumented implant changed the muscle behaviors. In fact, more works are needed to elucidate this point.

The medial thrust gait allows the footpath to be changed during gait cycle. Recent study showed decreases of knee adduction torque (−34%) and hip abduction torque (−15%) by using this gait pattern [13]. Another study [39] showed the increases of knee contact forces by 23%, 29%, and 36% in the lateral side using mild crouch, moderate crouch, and bouncy gait modifications, respectively. Despite their inexpensive character for the disease management, specific gait patterns such as crouch or bouncy and especially the medial knee thrust gait are quite complex motion patterns. At the moment, there is no universal method due to the lack of long-term effectiveness study. The challenges related to these gait-retaining strategies remain in the determination of optimal strategy and magnitude of modifications required to maximize beneficial effects and an efficient and special training method with real-time biofeedback is needed [14]. Muscle synergies analysis based on the dimensional reduction principle (i.e., matrix factorization) allows studying how the nervous system reduces movement control complexity [40]. In this present study, the muscle synergy analysis provides muscle activation pattern of each specific muscle related to each gait modification (bouncy, medial thrust, mild crouch, and mtp) leading to determining its effect on the muscle biomechanics. Moreover, our findings are in agreement with the literature works showing that only 3–7 neural commands (i.e., number of muscle synergies) are required for walking activities [39].

The use of a single subject with instrumented implant is the main limitation of this study. Consequently, more subjects are needed to generalize our findings. However, this present study provided unique and important information about the effect of voluntary gait modification strategies on the muscle biomechanics (e.g., activations and forces). The validation of the musculoskeletal simulation results is also a current challenging issue. This modeling problem depends upon objective and context of the research question and how modeling hypotheses are performed. At the moment, new experimental technologies and protocols need to be developed to provide new exploitable data for validation and verification purpose. In the scope of this objective, a Knee Grand Challenge has been organized to validate the joint loading and muscle forces by using joint reaction forces measured from instrumented implants. This provides a large panel of experimental data for musculoskeletal modeling purposes. In this present study, muscle force patterns were provided for the normal gait and 4 gait modifications. Then, EMG-based activation patterns were compared to muscle force patterns to evaluate the accuracy of the developed model. These data will be used to validate the joint reaction forces by a new approach of validation based on musculoskeletal simulation results and machine learning technique.

5. Conclusions

This present study showed an important variation of kinematical and muscle force behaviors under the voluntary altered gait patterns. Our findings allowed also muscle synergies to be recognized for the normal gait as well as 4

gait modifications (bouncy, medial thrust, midcrouch, and mtp). In fact, such useful information could allow a better understanding of the joint function and muscle synergy strategies leading to deeper knowledge of joint and muscle mechanisms related to neural commands.

Highlights

(i) Effect of voluntary gait modifications on the human knee joint behaviors.

(ii) Impact of structure-modifying treatment strategies on the muscle behaviors.

(iii) Lower limb muscle synergy analysis using nonnegative matrix factorization.

(iv) Patient-specific musculoskeletal modeling and simulation.

Conflict of Interests

The author reports no conflict of interests.

Acknowledgment

The author would like to thank all the organizers of the Knee Grand Challenge for the available data used in this present study.

References

[1] S. J. Piazza and S. L. Delp, "The influence of muscles on knee flexion during the swing phase of gait," *Journal of Biomechanics*, vol. 29, no. 6, pp. 723–733, 1996.

[2] M. G. Pandy, "Computer modeling and simulation of human movement," *Annual Review of Biomedical Engineering*, vol. 3, pp. 245–273, 2001.

[3] T. S. Buchanan, D. G. Lloyd, K. Manal, and T. F. Besier, "Neuromusculoskeletal modeling: estimation of muscle forces and joint moments and movements from measurements of neural command," *Journal of Applied Biomechanics*, vol. 20, no. 4, pp. 367–395, 2004.

[4] A. Erdemir, S. McLean, W. Herzog, and A. J. van den Bogert, "Model-based estimation of muscle forces exerted during movements," *Clinical Biomechanics*, vol. 22, no. 2, pp. 131–154, 2007.

[5] E. M. Arnold, S. R. Hamner, A. Seth, M. Millard, and S. L. Delp, "How muscle fiber lengths and velocities affect muscle force generation as humans walk and run at different speeds," *Journal of Experimental Biology*, vol. 216, no. 11, pp. 2150–2160, 2013.

[6] T. T. Dao, P. Pouletaut, F. Charleux et al., "Estimation of patient specific lumbar spine muscle forces using multi-physical musculoskeletal model and dynamic MRI," *Advances in Intelligent and Soft Computing*, vol. 245, pp. 411–422, 2014.

[7] A. S. Arnold, M. Q. Liu, M. H. Schwartz, S. Õunpuu, L. S. Dias, and S. L. Delp, "Do the hamstrings operate at increased muscle-tendon lengths and velocities after surgical lengthening?" *Journal of Biomechanics*, vol. 39, no. 8, pp. 1498–1506, 2006.

[8] J. L. Hicks, S. L. Delp, and M. H. Schwartz, "Can biomechanical variables predict improvement in crouch gait?" *Gait and Posture*, vol. 34, no. 2, pp. 197–201, 2011.

[9] P. Gerus, M. Sartori, T. F. Besier et al., "Subject-specific knee joint geometry improves predictions of medial tibiofemoral contact forces," *Journal of Biomechanics*, vol. 46, no. 16, pp. 2778–2786, 2013.

[10] H. J. Kim, J. W. Fernandez, M. Akbarshahi, J. P. Walter, B. J. Fregly, and M. G. Pandy, "Evaluation of predicted knee-joint muscle forces during gait using an instrumented knee implant," *Journal of Orthopaedic Research*, vol. 27, no. 10, pp. 1326–1331, 2009.

[11] M. W. Hast and S. J. Piazza, "Dual-joint modeling for estimation of total knee replacement contact forces during locomotion," *Journal of Biomechanical Engineering*, vol. 135, no. 2, Article ID 021013, 9 pages, 2013.

[12] B. J. Fregly, J. A. Reinbolt, K. L. Rooney, K. H. Mitchell, and T. L. Chmielewski, "Design of patient-specific gait modifications for knee osteoarthritis rhabilitation," *IEEE Transactions on Biomedical Engineering*, vol. 54, no. 9, pp. 1687–1695, 2007.

[13] B. Fregly, "Computational assessment of combinations of gait modifications for knee osteoarthritis rehabilitation," *IEEE Transactions on Biomedical Engineering*, vol. 55, no. 8, pp. 2104–2106, 2008.

[14] B. J. Fregly, "Gait modification to treat knee osteoarthritis," *HSS Journal*, vol. 8, no. 1, pp. 45–48, 2012.

[15] M. Simic, R. S. Hinman, T. V. Wrigley, K. L. Bennell, and M. A. Hunt, "Gait modification strategies for altering medial knee joint load: a systematic review," *Arthritis Care and Research*, vol. 63, no. 3, pp. 405–426, 2011.

[16] T. T. Dao, F. Marin, P. Pouletaut, F. Charleux, P. Aufaure, and M. C. Ho Ba Tho, "Estimation of accuracy of patient-specific musculoskeletal modelling: case study on a post polio residual paralysis subject," *Computer Methods in Biomechanics and Biomedical Engineering*, vol. 15, no. 7, pp. 745–751, 2012.

[17] K. Manal and T. S. Buchanan, "An electromyogram-driven musculoskeletal model of the knee to predict in vivo joint contact forces during normal and novel gait patterns," *Journal of Biomechanical Engineering*, vol. 135, no. 2, Article ID 021007, 2013.

[18] D. T. Davy and M. L. Audu, "A dynamic optimization technique for predicting muscle forces in the swing phase of gait," *Journal of Biomechanics*, vol. 20, no. 2, pp. 187–201, 1987.

[19] F. C. Anderson and M. G. Pandy, "Dynamic optimization of human walking," *Journal of Biomechanical Engineering*, vol. 123, no. 5, pp. 381–390, 2001.

[20] F. C. Anderson and M. G. Pandy, "Static and dynamic optimization solutions for gait are practically equivalent," *Journal of Biomechanics*, vol. 34, no. 2, pp. 153–161, 2001.

[21] M. S. A. Graziano, C. S. R. Taylor, and T. Moore, "Complex movements evoked by microstimulation of precentral cortex," *Neuron*, vol. 34, no. 5, pp. 841–851, 2002.

[22] I. Stepniewska, P.-C. Fang, and J. H. Kaas, "Microstimulation reveals specialized subregions for different complex movements in posterior parietal cortex of prosimian galagos," *Proceedings of the National Academy of Sciences of the United States of America*, vol. 102, no. 13, pp. 4878–4883, 2005.

[23] F. O. Barroso, D. Torricelli, J. C. Moreno et al., "Shared muscle synergies in human walking and cycling," *Journal of Neurophysiology*, vol. 112, no. 8, pp. 1984–1998, 2014.

[24] B. J. Fregly, T. F. Besier, D. G. Lloyd et al., "Grand challenge competition to predict in vivo knee loads," *Journal of Orthopaedic Research*, vol. 30, no. 4, pp. 503–513, 2012.

[25] S. L. Delp, F. C. Anderson, A. S. Arnold et al., "OpenSim: opensource software to create and analyze dynamic simulations of movement," *IEEE Transactions on Biomedical Engineering*, vol. 54, no. 11, pp. 1940–1950, 2007.

[26] G. Wu, S. Siegler, P. Allard et al., "ISB recommendation on definitions of joint coordinate system of various joints for the reporting of human joint motion—part I: ankle, hip, and spine," *Journal of Biomechanics*, vol. 35, no. 4, pp. 543–548, 2002.

[27] E. M. Arnold, S. R. Ward, R. L. Lieber, and S. L. Delp, "A model of the lower limb for analysis of human movement," *Annals of Biomedical Engineering*, vol. 38, no. 2, pp. 269–279, 2010.

[28] L. M. Schutte, M. Rodgers, F. E. Zajac, and R. M. Glaser, "Improving the efficacy of electrical stimulation-induced leg cycle ergometry: an analysis based on a dynamic musculoskeletal model," *IEEE Transactions on Rehabilitation Engineering*, vol. 1, no. 2, pp. 109–125, 1993.

[29] P. Paatero and U. Tapper, "Positive matrix factorization: a non-negative factor model with optimal utilization of error estimates of data values," *Environmetrics*, vol. 5, no. 2, pp. 111–126, 1994.

[30] D. D. Lee and H. S. Seung, "Learning the parts of objects by non-negative matrix factorization," *Nature*, vol. 401, no. 6755, pp. 788–791, 1999.

[31] J. Kim and H. Park, "Fast nonnegative matrix factorization: an active-set-like method and comparisons," *SIAM Journal on Scientific Computing*, vol. 33, no. 6, pp. 3261–3281, 2011.

[32] D. J. Berger and A. d'Avella, "Effective force control by muscle synergies," *Frontiers in Computational Neuroscience*, vol. 8, no. 1, article 46, 2014.

[33] A. S. Arnold, M. Q. Liu, M. H. Schwartz, S. Õunpuu, L. S. Dias, and S. L. Delp, "Do the hamstrings operate at increased muscle-tendon lengths and velocities after surgical lengthening?" *Journal of Biomechanics*, vol. 39, no. 8, pp. 1498–1506, 2006.

[34] H. J. Lundberg, C. Knowlton, and M. A. Wimmer, "Fine tuning total knee replacement contact force prediction algorithms using blinded model validation," *Journal of Biomechanical Engineering*, vol. 135, no. 2, Article ID 021008, 2013.

[35] L. Gizzi, J. F. Nielsen, F. Felici, Y. P. Ivanenko, and D. Farina, "Impulses of activation but not motor modules are preserved in the locomotion of subacute stroke patients," *Journal of Neurophysiology*, vol. 106, no. 1, pp. 202–210, 2011.

[36] K. L. Rodriguez, R. T. Roemmich, B. Cam, B. J. Fregly, and C. J. Hass, "Persons with Parkinson's disease exhibit decreased neuromuscular complexity during gait," *Clinical Neurophysiology*, vol. 124, no. 7, pp. 1390–1397, 2013.

[37] D. Staudenmann, K. Roeleveld, D. F. Stegeman, and J. H. van Dieen, "Methodological aspects of SEMG recordings for force estimation—a tutorial and review," *Journal of Electromyography and Kinesiology*, vol. 20, no. 3, pp. 375–387, 2010.

[38] J. Perry and J. M. Burnfield, *Gait Analysis: Normal and Pathological Function*, SLACK Incorporated, Thorofare, NJ, USA, 2010.

[39] A. L. Kinney, T. F. Besier, A. Silder, S. L. Delp, D. D. D'Lima, and B. J. Fregly, "Changes in in vivo knee contact forces through gait modification," *Journal of Orthopaedic Research*, vol. 31, no. 3, pp. 434–440, 2013.

[40] J. P. Walter, A. L. Kinney, S. A. Banks et al., "Muscle synergies may improve optimization prediction of knee contact forces during walking," *Journal of Biomechanical Engineering*, vol. 136, no. 2, Article ID 021031, 2014.

15

Automatic Segmentation of Medical Images Using Fuzzy c-Means and the Genetic Algorithm

Omid Jamshidi and Abdol Hamid Pilevar

Medical Intelligence Lab, Department of Computer Engineering, Bu Ali Sina University, Hamedan, Iran

Correspondence should be addressed to Omid Jamshidi; o.jamshidi@gmail.com

Academic Editor: Hiroshi Watabe

Magnetic resonance imaging (MRI) segmentation is a complex issue. This paper proposes a new method for estimating the right number of segments and automatic segmentation of human normal and abnormal MR brain images. The purpose of automatic diagnosis of the segments is to find the number of divided image areas of an image according to its entropy and with correctly diagnose of the segment of an image also increased the precision of segmentation. Regarding the fact that guessing the number of image segments and the center of segments automatically requires algorithm test many states in order to solve this problem and to have a high accuracy, we used a combination of the genetic algorithm and the fuzzy c-means (FCM) method. In this method, it has been tried to change the FCM method as a fitness function for combination of it in genetic algorithm to do the image segmentation more accurately. Our experiment shows that the proposed method has a significant improvement in the accuracy of image segmentation in comparison to similar methods.

1. Introduction

Image segmentation is one of the difficult issues in the field of image processing. Image segmentation is the process of assigning a label to every pixel in an image so that pixels with the same label share certain visual characteristics. Many applications such as object identification, feature extraction, and object position identifications and classification require accurate image segmentation. Several methods of medical image segmentation have been proposed, such as edge based, region based, or a combination of both. The purpose of medical image segmentation is to provide a more meaningful image which can be more easily understood and analyzed.

The edge-based methods use edge information in an image to determine the boundaries of objects and, hence, to form closed regions that determine different objects in an image. In some image segmentation methods, this method has been consistently used with the edge of the area for segmenting magnetic resonance imaging (MRI).

Chun and Yang performed image segmentation according to the edge information [1]. In addition to edge information, they made use of a similarity measure which was obtained as the median pixel variance parameters. The method used a fuzzy validity function as well as genetic algorithms and tried to find limit and suitable search space for image segmentation. Finding the main edges and removing redundant edges were the main issues in this method. Moreover, atlas-based segmentation methods were successfully employed for different applications. For instance, Heckemann segmented 67 brain images using 29 marked images [2].

On the other hand, k-means and the fuzzy c-means (FCM) are two successful region-based approaches. FCM can be obtained by a little modification in the k-means algorithm. FCM has been successfully used for MR image segmentation.

Neural network method needs a large number of training data and long time required for network training. For many experts, manual image segmentation is difficult and time consuming, and this leads to the use of automatic method.

Among the image segmentation methods, the FCM is more popular. Vast usage of it is due to its simplicity and accuracy. However, FCM has weaknesses in noise detection; many attempts are done for covering this weakness. In [3],

$j-1$	NW $x_{i-1,j-1}$	N $x_{i,j-1}$	NE $x_{i+1,j-1}$
j	W $x_{i-1,j}$	$x_{i,j}$	E $x_{i-1,j-1}$
$j+1$	SW $x_{i-1,j+1}$	S $x_{i,j+1}$	SE $x_{i+1,j+1}$
	$i-1$	i	$i+1$

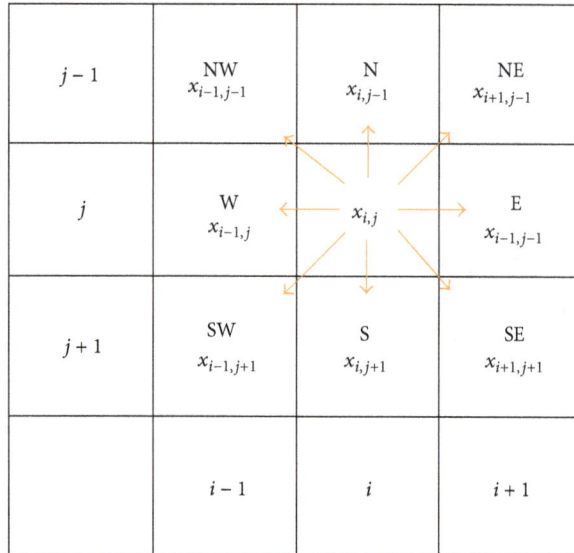

FIGURE 1: Definition of eight directions.

with using the objective function FCM and the use of neighbor pixels in addition to the pixel and also pixel division have been used. In [4–6], FCM method is used, and for improving the accuracy in image segmentation, membership function is changed. The defined object function in FCM is used, the local and nonlocal data segmentation are done, and the effect of each neighbor in the objective function is tested [7]. According to the total biases and gradient of sparse matrix, the FCM objective function has been changed [8]. The weight of local points in the objective function is calculated, and fuzzy clustering algorithm and continuity of local areas are used to make a better classification [9–11]. In [12], it is tried to change the FCM method to improve image segmentation. In order to reduce noise impact, local and nonlocal information have been used for image segmentation. In this paper, a new method is used to determine the dissimilarity with respect to local and nonlocal distances of each pixel. An algorithm based on histogram and using predefined window class centers was introduced. Then, the modified FCM method that in its neighboring areas are also used, and ultimately a new technique that is called a neighborhood-based membership ambiguity correction is used to eliminate small noises [13]. In [14], a hierarchical genetic method is used. In this method, chromosome is divided into two parts; that is, randomly placed one section of chromosomes with center point and the other with a random value of zero. The centers are determined by enabling or disabling. In [15], the genetic method and LVQ network for hierarchical classification of MR images are used. In this method, each chromosome is divided into two parts: one part is LVQ network weight and the other is determined by enabling or disabling the neurons of the LVQ network. In [16], a combination of statistical expectation maximization (EM) and pulse coupled neural network (PCNN) for segmentation of MR images has been used.

In most of the articles in the area of FCM segmentation, they believe that it is an effective method.

2. The Presented Method

Noise is inevitable in medical images. Therefore, this is essential to reduce the effect of noise prior to image segmentation. Since the method presented in this paper is based on FCM, we can perform noise reduction after noise detection and then perform image segmentation. Alternatively, we can estimate the probability of presence of noise in each pixel and change the effect of that pixel in FCM method accordingly. In this paper, we apply noise reduction to improve the image and, hence, to obtain a more reliable image segmentation.

2.1. Method to Reduce Noise on the Image. In this paper, we distinguish noise with respect to local neighborhood of each pixel. In addition, we consider the neighboring pixels while detection of noise. Considering the fact that we aim at a fast image segmentation method, we need to make use of a fast noise reduction method.

2.1.1. Detection of the Noisy Pixels. To detect a noisy pixel with the help of neighboring pixels, we followed the method proposed by [17] and defined the neighborhood of a pixel as shown in Figure 1.

Distance of central pixel with one of 8 first-order neighbors is calculated using

$$\text{Distance with NW} = \left| x_{i-1,j-1} - x_{i,j} \right|. \tag{1}$$

The distance of the corresponding pixel from all its neighbors was obtained. These distances were sorted in an ascending order, and 5 neighbors with the longest distances are selected. If the average of these 5 values was greater than a certain threshold, it means that at least five of the neighboring pixels have been very different so that the pixel is not considered as an edge position, and it is probably a noisy pixel. As we will discuss later, even if a pixel was wrongly detected as noisy, it would not affect much the algorithm as the noise correction method we use can usually handle it.

2.1.2. Correction of the Noisy Pixels. When a pixel was identified as noisy, we use its neighboring pixels to correct it. The reason we use neighboring pixels lies in the fact that a pixel is expected to be similar to its surrounding pixel. To do this, we select the pixel where total distance of its neighbor pixels with neighboring pixels of noisy pixel is less; this means that Euclidean distance between each neighboring pixel selected from the neighboring pixel in the same position of noisy pixel is calculated. Pixels to produce the lowest value means that their neighbors are more like together. Two pixels with similar neighbor values are expected to be close to each other, and, hence, the pixel can be replaced by the noisy pixel.

2.2. Image Segmentation. Given the fact that FCM method is simple and accurate and also due to the fuzzy nature of the image segmentation, many works on segmentation have used this method. Different works have tried to tackle some of the weaknesses associated with FCM. An important problem in image segmentation is to guess the number of parts of an image. Some of the methods in the literature have ignored this factor and performed image segmentation with a predefined number of segments. However, in some specific cases such as MR images, the number of segments of an image can be guessed. But even in medical images, sometimes when image quality is low or variant or there exist tumors in the image, it is not possible to estimate the number of segments. Having an accurate estimate of the number of segments in an image is crucial as parameters that determine accuracy as boundary overlaps highly depend on that.

In this work, we try segment to increase the accuracy in image segmentation in an automatic manner and without expert aid. In [18], objective function is based on the distance of each point from determined centers, and the extent of membership of each point to these centers is used to determine the centers in the next steps.

By considering the predefined parameters and number of segments and by using the principle of maximum entropy and genetic algorithm, we try to improve the existing parameters. In this method, the value of the membership of each pixel is clearly observable. Differences in the number of segments of an image directly affect the membership of each pixel. The method proposed in this paper utilizes the genetic algorithm and the FCM objective function and automatically estimates the number of segments for each given image.

2.2.1. Chromosome Representation.
The values corresponding to segment centers are placed in each chromosome. Hence, the length of a chromosome shows the number of different groups of data or, in other words, the number of segments in an image. We can control the maximum number of segments by measuring the length of each chromosome. Each cell of chromosomes can be initialized according to pixel values in the range of 0 to 255. For the first initialization, these numbers will be randomly generated. Table 1 is an example of a chromosome whose values are randomly generated.

If the chromosomes are initialized in the range 0 to 255, it means that the number of segments is equal to the length of the chromosome. But we want to set the number of image segments automatically. Some cells of chromosomes should have values that can show that they are not valid centers. To represent this, we can use negative values. The negative values of a cell correspond to the fact that this cell should not be considered as a data center. Hence, the number of nonnegative values in a chromosome determines the number of data centers. Some examples of chromosomes with length 6 are given in Table 2.

The first chromosome in Table 2 shows three centers with the values of 150.7, 121.1, and 94.3. The second chromosome shows six valid centers, whereas the third one contains four valid centers.

2.2.2. Initial Population.
We construct the initial population using the method described earlier. To do this, we create arbitrary number of randomly initialized chromosomes. Also, we want to assign negative value to some allele of chromosomes. As mentioned, the negative values are not considered as centers of data. The number of valid data can

be different in each chromosome. According to a fixed and predetermined probability, the values of chromosome alleles will change to negative. The number of valid data in each chromosome can be at least 2 and at most equal to its total length.

2.2.3. Fitness Computation.
With respect to the accuracy of FCM method, we leverage this method to calculate the compatibility. For each chromosome, using the estimated data centers and the pixel values of the image, we construct a matrix u that consists of membership values for each pixel. The elements of this matrix are calculated according to

$$u_{ij} = \frac{1}{\sum_{k=1}^{c} \left(\left\| x_i - c_j \right\| / \left\| x_i - c_k \right\| \right)^{2/(m-1)}}. \qquad (2)$$

The objective function of Formula (2) is defined as

$$J_m = \sum_{i=1}^{N} \sum_{j=1}^{C} u_{ij}^m \left\| x_i - c_j \right\|^2, \quad 1 \le m < \infty, \qquad (3)$$

where m is any real number greater than 1, u_{ij} is the degree of membership of x_i in the data center j, x_i is the ith dimension of the d-dimensional measured data, c_j is the d-dimension center of the data center, and $\| * \|$ is any norm expressing the similarity between any measured data and the center, while c_j are set of centers that are stored in chromosomes.

With respect to J_m value that is considered as fitness, the best value of the J_m occurs when each data center is placed in the center of data sets, and this causes J_m be small, therefore as much J_m be smaller, then the approach is better, and we are try to get the smallest amount for J_m.

If all of the data for the chromosome are a valid set of data centers or that the entire chromosome is equal to the number of valid data, J_m is calculated according to the aforementioned method that is acceptable, but with respect to the fact that in each chromosome, the number of valid data as class centers is different, the value of J_m obtained for comparing chromosomes fitness value is not proper and proportional to the number of the centers, and the fitness should be corrected such that the comparison between chromosomes becomes possible.

It should be noted that with increasing the number of centers, the distance of each x_i from the nearest center decreases, and it is expected that by increasing centers and decreasing the distance of each x_i with nearest center, the J_m value is reduced, and because the J_m is generally less in chromosome with more valid numbers, usually chromosomes with high number of centers are selected, but our favorite state is when data centers are being guessed in the centers of data sets and automatically determine the minimum required number of data centers with respect to data entropy. Based on the importance of the J_m value, we need to add another parameter to correct fitness value according to the changes in the number of the centers. For improvement of the presented method, we assign a penalty factor for recognizing the increment of the number of data centers. We add y to show the factor of penalty. Parameter y is obtained from the total

TABLE 1: A sample chromosome with length of 6.

Value in each chromosome, are the data centers. Thus, the length of each chromosome shows the number of different categories or in other words shows the number of segment of image. We can control the maximum number of the data sets with controlling the length of chromosomes. Each cell of chromosomes initialized can be in the range of 0 to 255. In the first place, the numbers will be randomly generated. An example of randomly generated chromosome is shown in here.	20.7	42	92.8	120	198

TABLE 2: Three chromosomes of the initial population generated randomly.

−170	150.7	−170	121.1	−170	94.3
83.1	73.5	159.7	196.7	63.3	224.9
111.7	−170	−170	38.1	187.1	65.2

TABLE 3: Different modes of pixels.

	True class	
	Abnormal	Normal
Detected class		
Abnormal	N_{tp}	N_{fp}
Normal	N_{fn}	N_{tn}

length of the valid data of each chromosome to total length of chromosome according to

$$y = \frac{\text{length of valid data of chromosome}}{\text{total length of chromosome}}. \quad (4)$$

Then, with multiplying, J_m in y fitness is calculated for each chromosome according to

$$J_m = \sum_{i=1}^{N} \sum_{j=1}^{C} u_{ij}^m \|x_i - c_j\|^2 \times y, \quad 1 \leq m < \infty. \quad (5)$$

2.2.4. Selection. We use the roulette wheel technique to produce the mating pool of chromosomes. The main idea of the roulette wheel technique is to associate more chance to better chromosomes.

2.2.5. Crossover. Crossover is the next step after the selection of parent chromosomes. In this step, a new offspring is generated as a result of combining two parents.

2.2.6. Mutation. Each allele of the chromosome changes according to the probability P_m. Mutation is used to perform a search over the entire range of answers. Figure 2 shows an overview of our approach to segmentation.

3. Results

To evaluate the proposed method, we use an MR image of brain of size 217×181 pixels, each of whose pixels range from zero to 255 (256 gray level). The number of initial population is set to 20 and the maximum number of generations to 100. The number of individuals to be replaced in each generation

TABLE 4: Parameters for genetic operations.

Representation	Bit representation
Crossover type	One point crossover
Crossover rate	0.7
Mutation type	Bit mutation
Mutation rate	0.1

is set to 40% of the total population. As mentioned earlier, we utilize roulette wheel selection technique. Images obtained by the proposed method determine the appropriate number of segments and the estimated center for each.

In the resulting segments, in order to verify the correctness of segments which are in the same group, we use different colors which are random.

Figure 3 shows the output of the proposed method for automatic segmentation of the original MR image.

In order to verify the performance of our algorithm, we use sensitivity, specificity, Jaccard, and k index parameters measures. If A and B are the automatic and manual segmentations of an image, respectively, then $T_p = B \cap A$ will be the true positive, and $F_p = A - B$, $F_n = B - A$ will be the false positive and false negative, respectively.

According to Table 3, sensitivity is defined as [19]

$$\text{Sensitivity} = \frac{N_{tp}}{N_{tp} + N_{fn}}. \quad (6)$$

Specificity as

$$\text{Specificity} = \frac{N_{tn}}{N_{fp} + N_{tn}}. \quad (7)$$

Similarity is defined as [20]

$$k(A, B) = \frac{2|A \cap B|}{|A + B|} \times 100\% = \frac{2T_p}{|B| + |A|} \times 100\%. \quad (8)$$

Jaccard index is defined as

$$J(A, B) = \frac{|A \cap B|}{A \cup B} \times 100\% = \frac{|T_p|}{|T_p| + |F_n| + |F_p|} \times 100\%. \quad (9)$$

The parameters settings for the genetic operations in this experiment are determined as shown in Table 4. Table 5 shows the performance of the proposed method when the initial number of chromosomes is set to 20 and 100 generations.

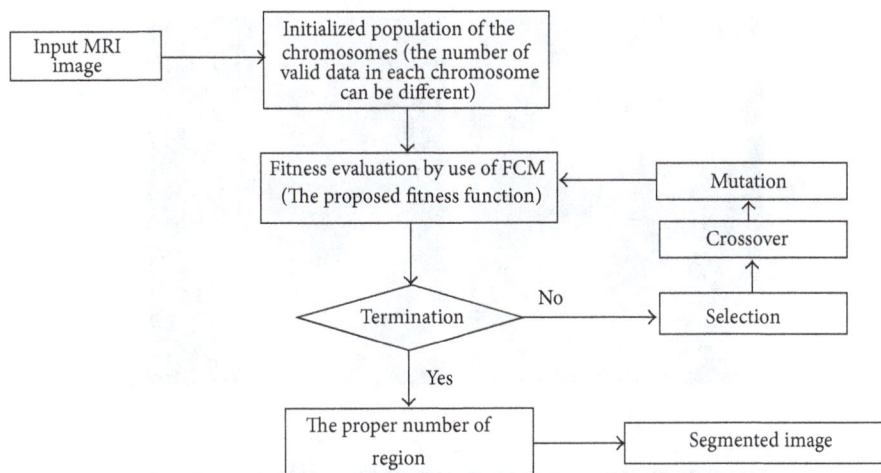

FIGURE 2: The schematic flow chart of segmentation.

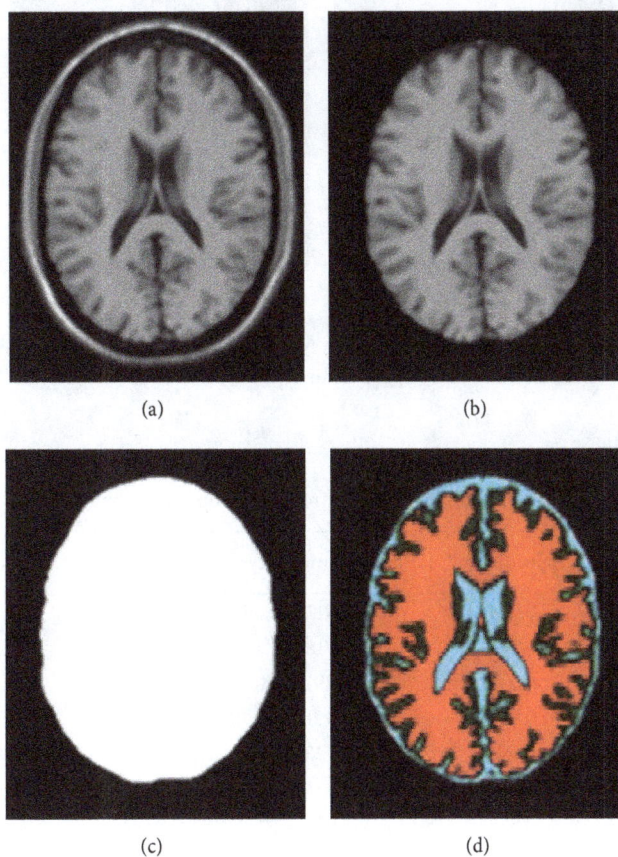

FIGURE 3: Automatic segmentation results of our algorithm. (a) is the original image, (b) is the brain for segmentation, (c) is the background of the image removed from brain, and (d) is MR brain image which is divided into 3 segments (shown with 3 different colors).

As shown in Table 5, every time we increase the length of the chromosomes, the output results become more accurate. The answers are different in each run of the algorithm because the chromosomes are initialized randomly in each run of algorithm. Also, maximum number of iteration of the genetic algorithm is 100.

In addition, in Figure 4, we show the performance of our algorithm on a noisy image.

The overall results of our method on a noisy image are given in Table 6.

4. Suggestions

Given that the proposed method is based on the inner class distance, it has been attempted to act according to

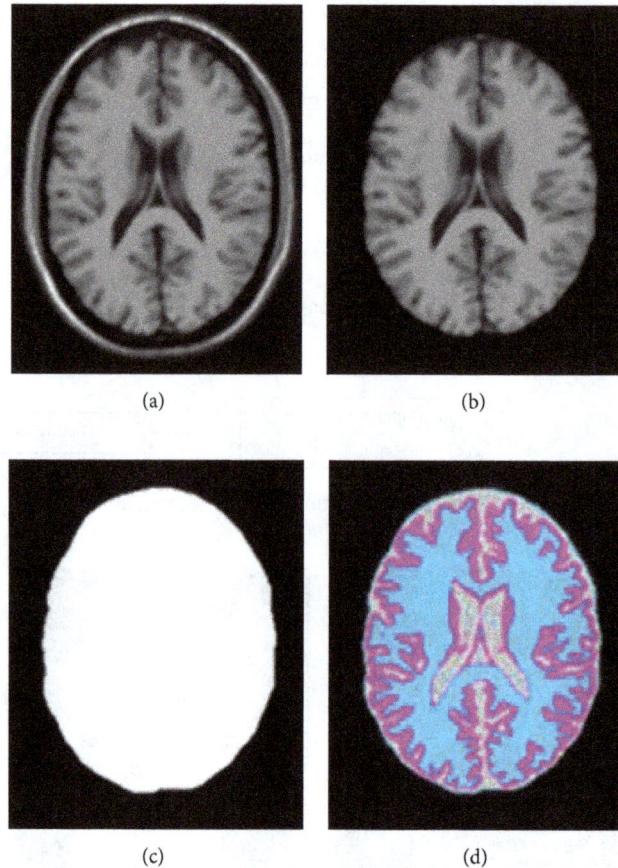

(a)   (b)

(c)   (d)

FIGURE 4: Performance of our algorithm on an image with 3% noise. Image (a) is the original image, (b) is the brain for segmentation, (c) is the background of the image removed from brain, and (d) is MR brain image which is divided into 3 segments (shown with 3 different colors).

TABLE 5: Results obtained from the proposed method.

Initial number of chromosome length	Sensitivity	Specificity	Jaccard similarity	k index	CPU time (s)	Number of final center
5	0.967	0.974	0.913	0.919	12.5	3
5	0.961	0.964	0.912	0.921	12.9	3
5	0.971	0.978	0.891	0.895	12.7	3
5	0.966	0.959	0.921	0.931	10.5	3
6	0.963	0.941	0.928	0.933	11.8	3
6	0.968	0.959	0.933	0.945	12.9	3
6	0.973	0.976	0.935	0.937	14.4	3
6	0.970	0.967	0.938	0.827	14.7	3
7	0.979	0.977	0.944	0.958	15.8	3

the distance with the nearest center and correction center. However, one can think of using outer class distance to obtain increased classification accuracy. In this case, in addition to each pixel belonging to the nearest center, the parameter of being distant from the other points is also taken into account. With respect to these two parameters, the precision of medical image segmentation methods can be expected to be increased.

5. Conclusion

FCM is a popular clustering method and has been widely applied for medical image segmentation. However, traditional FCM always suffers from noise in the images. Although many researchers have developed various extended algorithms based on FCM, none of them are flawless. A method based on genetic algorithm with use of FCM is proposed in

TABLE 6: Results obtained from the proposed method.

Initial number of chromosome length	Sensitivity	Specificity	Jaccard similarity	k index	CPU time (s)	Number of final centers
5	0.960	0.964	0.911	0.913	12.4	3
5	0.954	0.962	0.912	0.919	12.8	3
5	0.959	0.965	0.892	0.897	12.9	3
5	0.961	0.955	0.918	0.927	11.4	3
6	0.958	0.943	0.925	0.931	11.8	3
6	0.962	0.954	0.931	0.940	13.1	3
6	0.965	0.967	0.932	0.935	14.2	3
6	0.961	0.965	0.929	0.932	14.9	3
7	0.968	0.972	0.938	0.949	16.3	3

this paper. In our algorithm, local neighbor pixels are used. We tested our algorithm on simulated MR images. In this method, we obtained the right number of the segments fully automatically. We reduced the number of iterations of genetic algorithm and increased the convergence speed by applying proposed technique.

References

[1] D. N. Chun and H. S. Yang, "Robust image segmentation using genetic algorithm with a fuzzy measure," *Pattern Recognition*, vol. 29, no. 7, pp. 1195–1211, 1996.

[2] R. A. Heckemann, J. V. Hajnal, P. Aljabar, D. Rueckert, and A. Hammers, "Automatic anatomical brain MRI segmentation combining label propagation and decision fusion," *NeuroImage*, vol. 33, no. 1, pp. 115–126, 2006.

[3] Z. M. Wang, Y. C. Soh, Q. Song, and K. Sim, "Adaptive spatial information-theoretic clustering for image segmentation," *Pattern Recognition*, vol. 42, no. 9, pp. 2029–2044, 2009.

[4] S. R. Kannan, S. Ramathilagam, R. Devi, and E. Hines, "Strong fuzzy c-means in medical image data analysis," *Journal of Systems and Software*, vol. 85, no. 11, pp. 2425–2438, 2012.

[5] S. R. Kannan, S. Ramathilagam, R. Devi, and A. Sathya, "Robust kernel FCM in segmentation of breast medical images," *Expert Systems with Applications*, vol. 38, no. 4, pp. 4382–4389, 2011.

[6] S. R. Kannan, A. Sathya, S. Ramathilagam, and R. Devi, "Novel segmentation algorithm in segmenting medical images," *Journal of Systems and Software*, vol. 83, no. 12, pp. 2487–2495, 2010.

[7] B. Caldairou, N. Passat, P. A. Habas, C. Studholme, and F. Rousseau, "A non-local fuzzy segmentation method: application to brain MRI," *Pattern Recognition*, vol. 44, no. 9, pp. 1916–1927, 2011.

[8] Y. He, M. Y. Hussaini, J. Ma, B. Shafei, and G. Steidl, "A new fuzzy c-means method with total variation regularization for segmentation of images with noisy and incomplete data," *Pattern Recognition*, vol. 45, no. 9, pp. 3463–3471, 2012.

[9] Z.-X. Ji, Q.-S. Sun, and D. S. Xia, "A framework with modified fast FCM for brain MR images segmentation," *Pattern Recognition*, vol. 44, no. 5, pp. 999–1013, 2011.

[10] Z.-X. Ji, Q.-S. Sun, and D. S. Xia, "A modified possibilistic fuzzy c-means clustering algorithm for bias field estimation and segmentation of brain MR image," *Computerized Medical Imaging and Graphics*, vol. 35, no. 5, pp. 383–397, 2011.

[11] Z. Ji, Q. Sun, Y. Xia, Q. Chen, D. Xia, and D. Feng, "Generalized rough fuzzy c-means algorithm for brain MR image segmentation," *Computer Methods and Programs in Biomedicine*, vol. 108, no. 2, pp. 644–655, 2011.

[12] J. Wang, J. Kong, Y. Lu, M. Qi, and B. Zhang, "A modified FCM algorithm for MRI brain image segmentation using both local and non-local spatial constraints," *Computerized Medical Imaging and Graphics*, vol. 32, no. 8, pp. 685–698, 2008.

[13] K. Sikka, N. Sinha, P. K. Singh, and A. K. Mishra, "A fully automated algorithm under modified FCM framework for improved brain MR image segmentation," *Magnetic Resonance Imaging*, vol. 27, no. 7, pp. 994–1004, 2009.

[14] C.-C. Lai and C.-Y. Chang, "A hierarchical evolutionary algorithm for automatic medical image segmentation," *Expert Systems with Applications*, vol. 36, no. 1, pp. 248–259, 2009.

[15] J. Y. Yeh and J. C. Fu, "A hierarchical genetic algorithm for segmentation of multi-spectral human-brain MRI," *Expert Systems with Applications*, vol. 34, no. 2, pp. 1285–1295, 2008.

[16] J. C. Fu, C. C. Chen, J. W. Chai, S. T. C. Wong, and I. C. Li, "Image segmentation by EM-based adaptive pulse coupled neural networks in brain magnetic resonance imaging," *Computerized Medical Imaging and Graphics*, vol. 34, no. 4, pp. 308–320, 2010.

[17] H.-C. Chen and W.-J. Wang, "Efficient impulse noise reduction via local directional gradients and fuzzy logic," *Fuzzy Sets and Systems*, vol. 160, no. 13, pp. 1841–1857, 2009.

[18] W.-B. Tao, J.-W. Tian, and J. Liu, "Image segmentation by three-level thresholding based on maximum fuzzy entropy and genetic algorithm," *Pattern Recognition Letters*, vol. 24, no. 16, pp. 3069–3078, 2003.

[19] A. R. Van Erkel and P. M. T. Pattynama, "Receiver operating characteristic (ROC) analysis: basic principles and applications in radiology," *European Journal of Radiology*, vol. 27, no. 2, pp. 88–94, 1998.

[20] J. K. Udupa, V. R. LeBlanc, Y. Zhuge et al., "A framework for evaluating image segmentation algorithms," *Computerized Medical Imaging and Graphics*, vol. 30, no. 2, pp. 75–87, 2006.

16

Molecular Docking Study on the Interaction of Riboflavin (Vitamin B$_2$) and Cyanocobalamin (Vitamin B$_{12}$) Coenzymes

Ambreen Hafeez,[1] Zafar Saied Saify,[2] Afshan Naz,[1] Farzana Yasmin,[3] and Naheed Akhtar[1]

[1] *Biophysics Research Unit, Department of Biochemistry, University of Karachi, Karachi 75270, Pakistan*
[2] *International Center for Biological and Chemical Sciences, HEJ Research Institute of Chemistry, University of Karachi, Karachi 75270, Pakistan*
[3] *Biomedical Engineering Department, NED University of Engineering and Technology, Karachi 75270, Pakistan*

Correspondence should be addressed to Ambreen Hafeez; ambreenfv@hotmail.com

Academic Editor: Rocky Goldsmith

Cobalamins are the largest and structurally complex cofactors found in biological systems and have attracted considerable attention due to their participation in the metabolic reactions taking place in humans, animals, and microorganisms. Riboflavin (vitamin B$_2$) is a micronutrient and is the precursor of coenzymes, FMN and FAD, required for a wide variety of cellular processes with a key role in energy-based metabolic reactions. As coenzymes of both vitamins are the part of enzyme systems, the possibility of their mutual interaction in the body cannot be overruled. A molecular docking study was conducted on riboflavin molecule with B$_{12}$ coenzymes present in the enzymes glutamate mutase, diol dehydratase, and methionine synthase by using ArgusLab 4.0.1 software to understand the possible mode of interaction between these vitamins. The results from ArgusLab showed the best binding affinity of riboflavin with the enzyme glutamate mutase for which the calculated least binding energy has been found to be −7.13 kcal/mol. The results indicate a significant inhibitory effect of riboflavin on the catalysis of B$_{12}$-dependent enzymes. This information can be utilized to design potent therapeutic drugs having structural similarity to that of riboflavin.

1. Introduction

B$_{12}$ cofactors play important roles in the metabolism of microorganisms, animals, and humans. They are involved in the metabolism of almost every cell of the body specifically the DNA synthesis and regulation. The structure and reactivity of B$_{12}$ derivatives and structural aspects of their interactions with proteins and nucleotides are crucial for the efficient catalysis by the important B$_{12}$-dependent enzymes [1]. Biologically active cobalamins, adenosylcobalamin (AdoCbl), and methylcobalamin (MeCbl) are cofactors for many enzyme systems, containing a metal carbon bond involved in enzyme catalyzed reactions [2]. They catalyze enzymatic reactions which involve the making and breaking of the C–Co bond of these cofactors. The X-ray structures of B$_{12}$-enzyme complexes revealed that the B$_{12}$-cofactor undergoes a major conformational change on binding to the apoenzyme in AdoCbl and MeCbl containing enzymes such

as isomerases, eliminases, and methyltransferases [3]. A key step in the catalytic mechanism of coenzyme-B$_{12}$ containing enzymes is the homolysis of Co–C organometallic bond that leads to the intricate pathways of B$_{12}$ metabolic functions and the catalysis of related chemical reactions [4]. The Co–C bond undergoes homolytic cleavage in B$_{12}$-dependent enzymes more quickly as compared to that of the isolated cofactor in aqueous solution [5] which is a clue to the catalytic role of vitamin B$_{12}$.

Coenzyme B$_{12}$-dependent enzymes may bind to their cofactors in two possible modes, "base-on" or "base-off" modes. In base-on mode, the original 5,6-dimethylbenzimidazole base coordinates cobalt as the α-ligand at the lower side in the enzyme-coenzyme complex, while in base-off binding mode, the 5,6-dimethylbenzimidazole moiety is displaced and substituted by an exogenous ligand, such as histidine residue of the protein which coordinates the Co-atom as α-ligand, that is, base-off/His-on mode [6].

Cobalamins in the +3 oxidation state exist usually in the base-on form with the axial ligand X (Ado, CH_3, or CN) coordinated on the β side (upper side) of the octahedral cobalt compound, while in the +2 oxidation state, it has no β ligand and is called cob(II)alamin or B12r and in the +1 oxidation state it has been assigned a name co(I)alamin or B12s, in the base-off form along with the absence of β ligand [7].

The objective of the current study was to evaluate the binding affinity of riboflavin with B_{12} coenzymes by *molecular docking* technique to find out its effect on the inhibition or acceleration of enzyme activity. This depends on the interaction of the functional groups of riboflavin with those amino acid residues of B_{12} enzymes that are present in the active site cavity or take part in enzyme catalysis indirectly.

Molecular docking techniques are used to predict how a protein interacts with small vitamin-like molecules. This ability governs a significant part of the protein's dynamics which may enhance/inhibit its biological function [8]. Two factors are of paramount importance in molecular docking studies: optimizing the candidate ligand for the correct native conformation in the presence of which it can achieve a best fit orientation to bind with a protein of interest, and the conformational flexibility of ligand and protein [9]. Thus, the accurate prediction of the binding modes between the ligand and protein is of fundamental importance in modern structure-based drug design. Computer-based molecular modeling aims to speed up drug discoveries by predicting potential effectiveness of ligand-protein interactions prior to laborious experiments and costly preclinical trials.

Numerous software packages have been developed with the implementation of various molecular docking algorithms based on different search methods [10]. The present work of molecular docking has been done using commercially available software, ArgusLab 4.0.1. It is a molecular modeling, graphics, and drug designing program based on genetic algorithm. It is implemented with exhaustive search methods, the Argus Dock docking engine and AScore scoring function [11]. It is also capable of performing molecular geometry calculations and molecular structure visualization.

2. Materials and Methods

2.1. Computational Methodology

2.1.1. Data Set. Three-dimensional (3D) experimentally known protein-ligand complexes were obtained from Brookhaven Protein Data Bank (PDB) [12] (http://www.rcsb.org/). These were the structures of enzymes from three major enzyme families with bound coenzyme B_{12}: glutamate mutase from isomerases [13], diol dehydratase from lyases [14], and methionine synthase from transferases [15] having PDB codes 1CCW, 1EGM, and 3IV9, respectively.

2.1.2. Input File Preparations for Energy Minimization of Protein. For each of the protein-ligand complexes chosen for the study, a "clean input file" was generated by removing water molecules, ions, ligands, and subunits not involved in ligand binding from the original structure file. Water molecules were removed because ArgusLab sometimes failed to dock the compounds having water molecules at their binding sites [16]. All hydrogen atoms in the protein were allowed to optimize. The hydrogen locations are not specified by the X-ray structure but these are necessary to improve the hydrogen bond geometries, at the same time maintaining the protein conformation very close to that observed in the crystallographic model. The resulting receptor model was saved to a PDB file. Minimization was performed by geometry convergence function of ArgusLab software performed according to Hartree-Fock calculation method.

2.1.3. Ligand Input File Preparation and Optimization. Ligand input structure was drawn using Marvin Sketch software. The structure was cleaned in 3D format and energy was minimized using Marvin sketch software. The resulting structure was then saved in "mdl mol" and "sdf" file formats for molecular docking studies

2.2. Docking Methodology. After the preparation of the protein and ligand, molecular docking studies were performed by ArgusLab 4.0.1 to evaluate the interactions.

2.2.1. ArgusLab 4.0.1. ArgusLab is implemented with shape-based search algorithm. Docking has been done using "Argus Dock" exhaustive search docking function of ArgusLab with grid resolution of 0.40 Å. Docking precision was set to "Regular precision" and "Flexible" ligand docking mode was employed for each docking run. The stability of each docked pose was evaluated using ArgusLab energy calculations and the number of hydrogen bonds formed [17].

2.2.2. Molecular Docking Study. To perform docking one first needs to define atoms that make up the ligand and the binding sites of the protein where the ligand should bind. The prepared 3D structures of 1ccw, 1egm, and 3iv9 proteins were downloaded into the ArgusLab program and binding sites were made by choosing "Make binding site for this protein" option. The ligand (cleaned riboflavin molecule) was then introduced and docking calculation was allowed to run using shape-based search algorithm and AScore scoring function. The scoring function is responsible for evaluating the energy between the ligand and the protein target. Flexible docking was allowed by constructing grids over the binding sites of the protein and energy-based rotation is set for that ligand's group of atoms that do not have rotatable bonds. For each rotation, torsions are created and poses (conformations) are generated during the docking process [11]. For each complex, 10 independent runs were conducted and one pose was returned for each run. The best docking model was selected according to the lowest AScore calculated by ArgusLab, and the most suitable binding conformation was selected on the basis of hydrogen bond interactions between the ligand and protein near the substrate binding site. The lowest energy poses indicate the highest binding affinity as high energy produces the unstable conformations.

TABLE 1: Binding energies of riboflavin coenzyme B_{12} containing enzyme complex by AScore scoring function of ArgusLab.

S. no.	Enzyme name (pdb code)	AScore (kcal/mol)
1	Glutamate mutase (1ccw)	−7.13
2	Diol dehydratase (1egm)	−6.98
3	Methionine synthase (3iv9)	−6.07

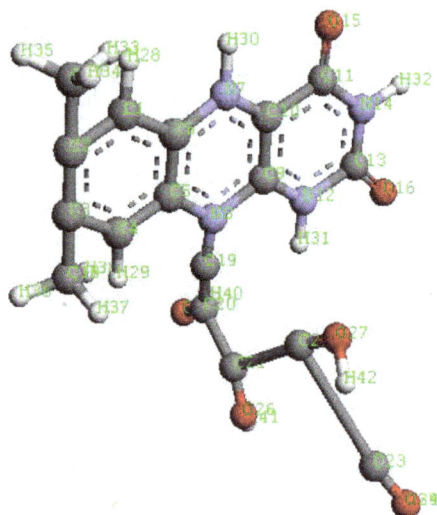

FIGURE 1: Minimized structure of riboflavin. Atoms in red are oxygen, blue are nitrogen, grey are carbon, and white are hydrogen. The number of hydrogen atoms is indicated in light green color.

3. Results and Discussion

Minimized structure of riboflavin is given in Figure 1. Docking studies of the compound riboflavin with each of the three enzymes having PDB codes *1ccw, 1egm,* and *3iv9* were carried out by ArgusLab 4.0.1. The least binding energy exhibits the highest activity which has been observed by the ranking of poses generated by AScore scoring function of ArgusLab and is given in Table 1.

List of hydrogen bonds between riboflavin and coenzyme B_{12}-dependent enzymes is given in Table 2. The best fitted poses adopted by riboflavin docked into enzymes 1ccw, 1egm, and 3iv9 are shown in Figures 2, 3, and 4, respectively.

In the present study, cyanocobalamin coenzyme was taken as an active ligand instead of cocrystallized inhibitor D-tartaric acid, to bind with the compound riboflavin in order to examine a possible mode of interaction between these two vitamins in an enzyme system. The docked binding mode of riboflavin was manually inspected in order to verify that it effectively binds to the catalytic site. The docking results of riboflavin with each of the individual enzymes are as follows.

3.1. Glutamate Mutase. The compound riboflavin interacted with enzyme glutamate mutase (in complex with coenzyme B_{12} and the inhibitor, D-tartaric acid) by least binding energy of −7.13 kcal/mol. In Figure 2 riboflavin seemed to bind at the lower axial end of the coenzyme B_{12} with the base 5,6-dimethylbenzimidazole (DMB) by replacing water

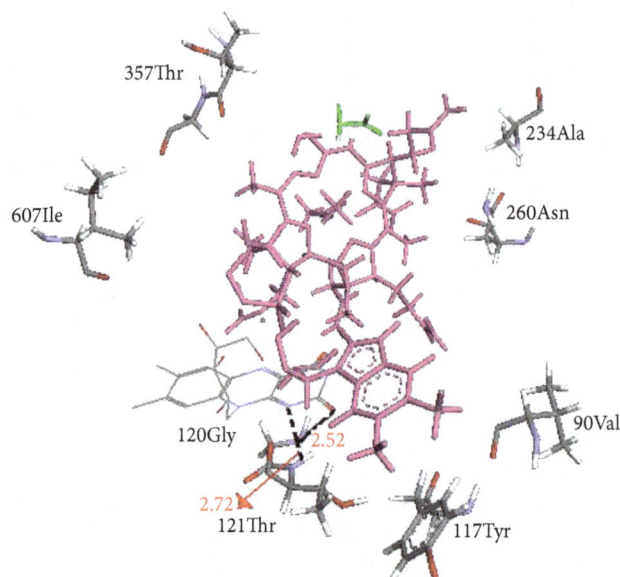

FIGURE 2: Docking of riboflavin into enzyme glutamate mutase [13]. Riboflavin and protein binding sites are shown in element colors in wireframe and thick stick models, respectively, whereas cyanocobalamin is represented in pink stick model. Inhibitor TAR is seen in green color in thick stick.

molecules. The oxygen (O2) of carbonyl group of riboflavin binds with nitrogen atom (NH) of amino acid residue Gly120. The hydrogen bond distance between these groups is 2.52 Å. Another hydrogen bond was formed between the nitrogen atom (N1) of riboflavin and NH of amino acid Thr121 at a distance of 2.72 Å. No interaction was observed between the riboflavin and cocrystallized inhibitor, D-tartaric acid. In glutamate mutase, the elongation of Co–N bond probably contributes to the weakening of Co–C bond in the coenzyme [13]. Therefore, the docked position and conformation of riboflavin revealed that the compound may inhibit the usual catalytic process of the enzyme by altering the conformational change in the nucleotide base, which plays an important role in initiating the Co–C bond cleavage and thus hinders the continuous progress of radical reactions. The relative conformation and arrangement of cofactor and substrate also play a part in this aspect. The calculated AScore shows a significant affinity of riboflavin towards the enzyme glutamate mutase.

3.2. Diol Dehydratase. In Figure 3, deep analysis of the docked structure of riboflavin revealed that the molecule seemed to bind in between the enzyme's active site, that is, the E-subunit and B_{12}-cofactor binding domain as indicated by the presence of amino acid residues Thr222, Val300, Phe374, and Gln336. These amino acid residues have been found to form the hydrophobic contacts with the inhibitor 1, 2-propanediol and play an important role in holding the substrate in the active site [14]. Three hydrogen bonds were formed with this enzyme; the nitrogen atom (N5) of riboflavin interacted with the sulphur (SH) of amino acid residue Cys302. The hydrogen bond distance between these groups was found to be 2.50 Å. Another two hydrogen bonds

TABLE 2: List of hydrogen bonds between riboflavin and coenzyme B_{12} containing enzymes.

S. no	Enzyme name	No. of H-bonds	Amino acid residue atom	Ligand atom	H-bond distance (Å)
1	Glutamate mutase (1ccw)	2	Gly120 (NH)	(O2)	2.52
			Thr121 (NH)	(N1)	2.72
2	Diol dehydratase (1egm)	3	Cys302 (SH)	(N5)	2.50
			Ser301 (O)	(N1)	2.96
			Arg699 (N)	(O2)	2.82
3	Methionine synthase (3iv9)	2	His759 (NH)	(O4)	2.68
			His1145 (NH)	(O2)	2.72

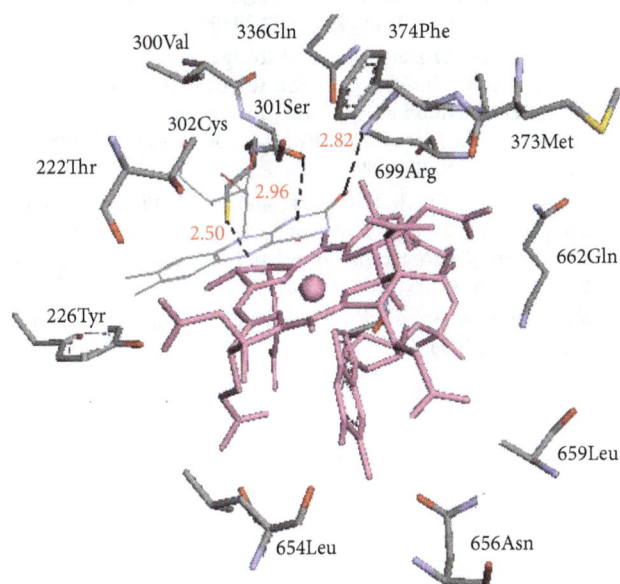

FIGURE 3: Docking of riboflavin into enzyme diol dehydratase [14]. Riboflavin and protein binding sites are shown in element colors in wireframe and thick stick models, respectively, whereas cyanocobalamin is represented in pink color in thick stick.

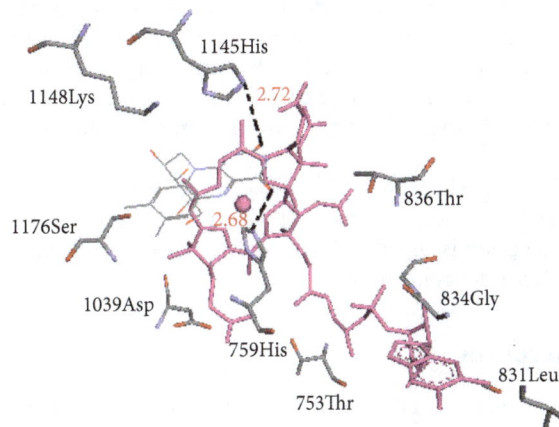

FIGURE 4: Docking of riboflavin into enzyme methionine synthase [15]. Riboflavin and protein binding sites are shown in element colors in wireframe and thick stick models, respectively, whereas cyanocobalamin is represented in pink color in thick stick.

were formed between the nitrogen (N1) of riboflavin and oxygen atom of Ser301 at a distance of 2.96 Å and between nitrogen of Arg699 and oxygen atom (O2) of riboflavin at a distance of 2.82 Å. The E-subunit comprises of active site of the enzyme which has been found to pack against the upper face of B_{12} cofactor and may facilitate the transfer of 5′-adenosyl radical from cofactor to substrate. Therefore, it may be assumed that the riboflavin may interfere with the catalytic process of the enzyme by binding at the interface of cofactor B_{12} and the enzyme's active site and thus inhibit the radical shuttling mechanism. The AScore value obtained for this complex was −6.98 kcal/mol which indicates that riboflavin significantly binds with the enzyme diol dehydratase.

3.3. Methionine Synthase. Figure 3 shows the binding of riboflavin near the cofactor making contact with amino acid residue His 759. The oxygen atom (O4) of the carbonyl group of riboflavin was hydrogen bonded to N-atom of the His 759 at a distance of 2.68 Å. Another hydrogen bonding

was seen between the N-atom of His1145 and the carbonyl oxygen (O2) of riboflavin at a distance of 2.72 Å. The docking AScore of the ligand-protein complex was −6.07 kcal/mol. The crystal structure of methionine synthase revealed that the enzyme is present in "base-off" or "His-on" form with His759 as the lower axial ligand. His759 has been found to act as transient intermediate in the reductive reactivation and conformational transition of cobalt following methylation in methionine synthase-dependent enzyme catalysis [15]. Therefore, we may assume that riboflavin may inhibit the important catalytic step of the enzyme, that is, reactivation and methylation probably by making contact with the same amino acid residue (His759) that is involved in the reaction. The binding energy also shows a significant ligand-receptor complex with this enzyme.

4. Conclusion

By analyzing the docking results we hypothesized that riboflavin might have inhibitory activity against cobalamin coenzymes. The enzyme glutamate mutase has been found to be the most susceptible protein target for the studied ligand and the riboflavin showed the best binding affinity with this enzyme having least binding energy of −7.13 kcal/mol.

Glutamate mutase and diol dehydratase can be considered as important targets for the development of antibiotics. Other useful therapeutic drugs can also be synthesized to enhance the function of enzyme methionine synthase as it converts homocystein into methionine and requires methylcobalamin coenzyme for its function. Inactivation of this coenzyme leads to the elevated levels of homocystein in blood and urine and may result in clotting and in long-term damage to the arteries (stroke and heart attack). Therefore, the interaction of vitamin B_2 and B_{12} and their role in important metabolic reactions in the body should be considered before preparing multivitamin complexes.

The fact that riboflavin participates in energy-based metabolic reactions may play an important role in enzyme catalysis which depends on a delicate energy balance for different reaction pathways. The local amino acids and substrates in the active sites of the enzymes may function in this respect.

Further experimental approaches can be adopted to probe the effect of structural alterations of flavin group of compounds in the catalytic properties of coenzyme B_{12}-dependent enzymes.

References

[1] K. Gruber, B. Puffer, and B. Krautler, "Vitamin B_{12}-derivatives-enzyme cofactors and ligands of proteins and nucleic acids," *Chemical Society Reviews*, vol. 40, no. 8, pp. 4346–4363, 2011.

[2] L. Randaccio, S. Geremia, N. Demitri, and J. Wuerges, "Vitamin B_{12}: unique metalorganic compounds and the most complex vitamins," *Molecules*, vol. 15, no. 5, pp. 3228–3259, 2010.

[3] R. Banerjee and S. W. Ragsdale, "The many faces of vitamin B_{12}: catalysis by cobalamin-dependent enzymes," *Annual Review of Biochemistry*, vol. 72, pp. 209–247, 2003.

[4] R. G. Matthews, "Cobalamin and corrinoid dependent enzymes," in *Metal Ions in Life Sciences*, A. Sigel, H. Sigel, and R. K. O. Sigel, Eds., vol. 6, pp. 53–114, Royal Society of Chemistry, Cambridge, UK, 2009.

[5] P. J. Kasper and U. Ryde, "How the Co-C bond is cleaved in coenzyme B_{12} enzymes: a theoretical study," *Journal of the American Chemical Society*, vol. 127, no. 25, pp. 9117–9128, 2005.

[6] L. Randaccio, S. Geremia, and J. Wuerges, "Crystallography of vitamin B_{12} proteins," *Journal of Organometallic Chemistry*, vol. 692, no. 6, pp. 1198–1215, 2007.

[7] B. Kräutler, "Organometallic chemistry of B_{12} coenzymes," in *Metal Ions in Life Sciences*, A. Sigel, H. Sigel and R. K. O. Sigel, Eds., vol. 6, pp. 1–51, Royal Society of Chemistry, Cambridge, UK, 2009.

[8] A. Kahraman, R. J. Morris, R. A. Laskowski, and J. M. Thornton, "Shape variation in protein binding pockets and their ligands," *Journal of Molecular Biology*, vol. 368, no. 1, pp. 283–301, 2007.

[9] S. F. Sousa, P. A. Fernandes, and M. J. Ramos, "Protein-ligand docking: current status and future challenges," *Proteins: Structure, Function and Genetics*, vol. 65, no. 1, pp. 15–26, 2006.

[10] R. D. Taylor, P. J. Jewsbury, and J. W. Essex, "A review of protein-small molecule docking methods," *Journal of Computer-Aided Molecular Design*, vol. 16, no. 3, pp. 151–166, 2002.

[11] M. A. Thompson, "Molecular docking using ArgusLab, an efficient shape-based search algorithm and AScore scoring function," in *Proceedings of the ACS Meeting*, Philadelphia, Pa, USA, March-April 2004, 172, CINF 42.

[12] R. Wang, X. Fang, Y. Lu, and S. Wang, "The PDBbind database: collection of binding affinities for protein-ligand complexes with known three-dimensional structures," *Journal of Medicinal Chemistry*, vol. 47, no. 12, pp. 2977–2980, 2004.

[13] R. Reitzer, K. Gruber, G. Jogl et al., "Glutamate mutase from Clostridium cochlearium: the structure of a coenzyme B_{12}-dependent enzyme provides new mechanistic insights," *Structure*, vol. 7, no. 8, pp. 891–902, 1999.

[14] N. Shibata, J. Masuda, T. Tobimatsu et al., "A new mode of B_{12} binding and the direct participation of a potassium ion in enzyme catalysis: X-ray structure of diol dehydratase," *Structure*, vol. 7, no. 8, pp. 997–1008, 1999.

[15] M. Koutmos, S. Datta, K. A. Pattridge, J. L. Smith, and R. G. Matthews, "Insights into the reactivation of cobalamin-dependent methionine synthase," *Proceedings of the National Academy of Sciences of the United States of America*, vol. 106, no. 44, pp. 18527–18532, 2009.

[16] S. Joy, P. S. Nair, R. Hariharan, and M. R. Pillai, "Detailed comparison of the protein-ligand docking efficiencies of GOLD, a commercial package and arguslab, a licensable freeware," *In Silico Biology*, vol. 6, no. 6, pp. 601–605, 2006.

[17] M. Thompson, *ArgusLab 4.0.1.*, Planaria software LLC, Seattle, Wash, USA, 2004.

Molecular Docking Assessment of Efficacy of Different Clinically Used Arsenic Chelator Drugs

Durjoy Majumder and Sayan Mukherjee

Department of Physiology, West Bengal State University, Berunanpukuria, P.O. Malikapur, Barasat, North 24 Parganas, Kolkata 700126, India

Correspondence should be addressed to Durjoy Majumder; durjoy@rocketmail.com

Academic Editor: Jeon-Hor Chen

Arsenic contamination of ground water has become a global problem affecting specially, south-east Asian countries like Bangladesh and eastern parts of India. It also affects South America and some parts of the US. Different organs of the physiological system are affected due to contamination of inorganic arsenic in water. Animal studies with different chelators are not very conclusive as far as the multi/differential organ effect(s) of arsenic is concerned. Our docking study establishes the molecular rationale of blood test for early detection of arsenic toxicity; as arsenic has a high affinity to albumin, a plasma protein and actin, a structural protein of all cells including Red Blood Cells. This study also shows that there is a little possibility of male reproductive organs toxicity by different forms of inorganic arsenic; however, female reproductive system is very much susceptible to sodium-arsenite. Through comparative analysis regarding the chelating effectiveness among the available arsenic chelator drugs, meso-2,3 dimercaptosuccinic acid (DMSA) and in some cases lipoic acid is the most preferred choice of drug for removing of arsenic deposits. This computational method actually reinforces the clinical finding regarding DMSA as the most preferred drug in removal of arsenic deposits from majority of the human tissues.

1. Introduction

The source of arsenic poisoning comes through drinking water and has now become a major concern throughout the globe. It affects a large population of Bangladesh [1] and eastern part of India. Arsenic occurs in nature in both organic and inorganic forms; the latter being more toxic. Inorganic form combines mainly with oxygen and sulfur. In drinking water, it is mainly present as arsenious acid in trivalent [As(III)] state [2]. Arsenic trioxide (ATO) (As_2O_3) dissolves in water under conditions dependent on pH, presence of redox chemicals, reducing bacteria, and so on to produce this arsenious acid [3]. Arsenic rarely occurs in the zero valent metalloid state and mostly occurs in the trivalent state and occasionally in the pentavalent state. Pentavalent arsenic compounds tend to decompose into trivalent state when ingested. Within physiological system, pentavalent arsenic uses ADP and uncouple oxidative phosphorylation to change to trivalent arsenic [4]. So, the main toxicity of inorganic arsenic comes from trivalent arsenic. The toxicity of trivalent arsenic [As(III)] arises from the fact that it binds to free thiol (–SH) groups in proteins, especially vicinal thiol groups [5].

Clinical reports suggest that arsenic toxicity affects a variety of organs, having highest concentrations in tissue where proteins have *sulfhudryl* (thiol) groups like skin, nails, and hair. When larger doses of arsenic are ingested, the tissue distribution appears to change. The LD_{50} for oral administration to mice are as follows: 3 mg/kg for arsine; 14 mg/kg for arsenite [As(III)]; 20 mg/kg for arsenate [As(V)]; 700–1800 mg/kg for monomethylarsonic acid (MMA), 700–2600 mg/kg for dimethylarsinic acid (DMA); and >10000 mg/kg for arsenobetaine and arsenocholine showing that inorganic arsenic is much more toxic [6] and the ingested dose determines the duration of chelation therapy combined or alone like with BAL (British Anti Lewsite) or dimercaprol (DMC) [7]. Many studies have been performed on humans after fatal arsenic poisoning. Results of these studies showed widespread distribution of arsenic in all organs; the highest concentrations is in the liver and kidneys, which had, respectively, 10- and 3-fold higher concentrations than in the other organs like brain, cerebellum, lung, heart, pancreas, spleen, muscle, and skin [8].

To understand arsenic removal from the physiological system and detoxification processes, experimental animal models are treated with acute intoxicating doses of inorganic arsenic and followed for hepatic and renal tissue distribution. These studies indicate the role of these organs in the detoxification and elimination of arsenic. These studies reveal that the liver is the site of inorganic arsenic methylation that helps in detoxification and elimination of arsenic [9]. Initial study showed that methyltransferases present in liver, transfers methyl group from S-adenosylmethionine to arsenite, thus forming monomethylarsonic acid (MMA) [10]. Further studies revealed that the high concentrations of arsenic are deposited in muscle and heart—the third and fourth highest arsenic concentrations after the liver and kidneys tissue. Therefore, the fatal rhabdomyolysis observed in animals treated with arsenic poisoning is followed by heart failure [8, 11–14]. Table 1 summarizes a list of affected organs by arsenic poisoning and the abundant protein(s) that are present in that organ. In case of ingestion of pentavalent arsenic [As(V)], toxicity occurs primarily by reduction to trivalent arsenic [As(III)].

Chelation is the process by which the metal is leached out of the body, for a long time the mainstay was BAL; then 2,3 Dimercapto propane-1-sulfonic acid (DMPS) and Dimercapto succinic acid (DMSA). The former drug was administered by intramuscular injection while the latter drugs can be easily administered through oral route. DMSA is also known as succimer; its various analogs like MonoisoamylDMSA (MiADMSA), MonomethylDMSA (MmDMSA), and Mono-cyclohexylDMSA (MchDMSA) were developed. A good chelating agent should be expected to have the following qualities:

(i) greater affinity for the metal,

(ii) same distribution as the metal,

(iii) low toxicity,

(iv) ability to compete with natural chelators,

(v) ability to penetrate cell membranes,

(vi) rapid elimination of the toxic metal,

(vii) high water solubility,

(viii) capacity to form nontoxic complexes [11].

In experimental models, tested chelators are DMSA, DMPS as its sodium salt, BAL, and Lipoic acid. The relative effectiveness of these dimercapto compounds in protecting mice from the lethal effects of an LD_{99} of sodium arsenite (SAN) $(NaAsO_2)$ is DMSA > DMPS > BAL [15]. No direct comparison with alpha lipoic acid (α-LA) has been made. BAL, however, increases the arsenic content of the brain of rabbits injected with sodium arsenite. These results raise an issue regarding the appropriateness of BAL as the treatment for systemic arsenic poisoning. DMPS and DMSA have effectiveness as prophylactics for the prevention of the vesicant

TABLE 1: Organs affected by arsenic and the most abundant protein(s) in that organ.

Affected organ by arsenic	Abundant protein of the organ
Skin [18]	Collagen
Heart muscle [19]	Lactate dehydrogenase (LDH)
Reproduction, carcinogenicity [20]	Estrogen receptor alpha (ER-α)
Liver [21]	Thioredoxin reductase (TDR)
Liver [22]	Glutathione reductase (GTH)
Energy metabolism in all cells [23]	Pyruvate dehydrogenase (PDH)
Cytoskeletal structure [24]	Tubulin
Cytoskeletal structure [25]	Actin
Blood (serum) [16, 26]	Albumin
Liver, kidney and brain [17, 21, 26]	Spermine and spermidine

effect of Lewisite. The sodium arsenite inhibition of the pyruvate dehydrogenase (PDH) complex can be prevented and reversed *in vitro* or *in vivo* by these chelators and for this action, DMPS is most potent. Otherwise, DMSA is the most potent chelator of arsenic in clinical practice. Lipoic acid, also an arsenic chelator, is used for its excellent blood brain barrier permeability to leach out brain deposits of arsenic [16, 17]. Different chelator drugs that are in use in arsenic toxicity are evaluated through empirically based observations of animal experimentations. Here, we explore the computational/quantitative rationale of those clinically used chelator drugs at molecular level.

2. Methods

Present study is aimed to make a computational assessment of the efficacy of different chelator drugs in different tissues involved with open source software on a Linux platform. Molecular docking of small molecule was done using Autodock3 which is free for academic user. For performing molecular docking procedures, we have chosen several proteins from the organs that are reported to be affected by arsenic toxicity (Table 1). The name and the collected source of structural detailing of the proteins in the PDB format are mentioned in Table 2. The chosen drug molecules and collected structures are mentioned in Table 3. The detailing steps of the molecular docking processes [27] are as follows.

(1) The PDB files of receptor (macromolecule) and ligand were obtained from the Protein Data Bank and the Drug bank or from any other source as mentioned in Tables 2 and 3.

(2) Preparing the receptor PDB files, as the PDB files often contained added waters, the files were read in the GUI of ADT, water selected as HOH* from a string and deleted after the warning.

(3) Preparation of the macromolecular files—Polar hydrogens were then added with no bond order. ADT was then used to add charges, and Kollman

charges added (by default; ADT adds Kollman charges for a peptide (determined by checking whether all of its component residue names appear in the standard set of 20 commonly occurring amino acids) and Gasteiger charges if not so). Finally, solvation parameters were added and the files were saved as molecule.pdbqs (where "q" and "s" represent charge and solvation, resp.).

(4) Preparation of the ligand file. Generally all hydrogens are added and nonpolar hydrogens are merged. Gasteiger were charges added unless the ligand is also a peptide, in which case the above procedure would be followed. ADT automatically takes care of solvation and checks for aromatic carbon atoms and hence lone pairs and nonpolar hydrogens merged. ADT then determined the best root (the best root is the atom in the ligand with the smallest or largest subtree; in case of a tie, if either atom is in a cycle, it is picked as the root, and if neither or both is in a cycle, the first to be found is picked). Next we defined rotatable bonds in the ligand, making all amide bonds nonrotatable, and set the number of active torsions to fewest atoms. The ligand file was then saved with a ligand.out.pdbq extension ("q" representing charge).

(5) Preparation of the grid and the grid parameter file. For the calculation of docking interaction energy, it is necessary to create 3D box (grid) in which the protein molecule is enclosed. The grid volume should be large enough to allow the ligand to rotate freely, even when the ligand is in its most fully extended conformation. The parameters required to create such a grid are stored in the grid parameter file, molecule.gpf.

(6) Now, autogrid3 was run to create a map for every atom type in the ligand and create the corresponding macromolecular file with the extension molecule.glg either from Run of the GUI or the command line autogrid3 -p molecule.gpf -l molecule.glg and when finished, it writes Successful Completion.

(7) Preparation of Docking Parameter File. The macromolecular pdbqs and ligand.out.pdbq files are read. The search methods of AutoDock include the Monte Carlo simulated annealing method, the genetic algorithm, local search, and the hybrid genetic algorithm with local search. The latter is also referred to as the Lamarckian genetic algorithm because offsprings are allowed to inherit the local search adaptations of their parents, and this was the chosen algorithm for the analysis. The docking job can similarly be run from Run of the GUI or from command line autodock3 -p molecule.dpf -l molecule.dlg, and

(8) When finished and Successful Completion is written, the PDB file and Analyze open docking log are done and choosing different color for receptor and ligand, the conformations can be played by energy. The dlg files can be opened in a terminal and each run's (the number of runs can be fixed by the user) final docked energy, Gibbs free energy, Inhibition

TABLE 2: Sources of PDB files of proteins in our study.

Protein	PDB ID/otherwise ID	Reference
Thioredoxin reductase	2CFY (edited)	[29]
Glutathione reductase	1GRT (edited, A34E + R37W mutant)	[29]
Collagen	1BKV (edited)	[29]
Actin	1J6Z (edited)	[29]
Estrogen receptor alpha (ER-Alpha)	1X7E (edited)	[29]
Pyruvate dehydrogenase	2BUB (edited)	[29]
Albumin	2BXI (edited)	[29]
Tubulin	2HXH (edited)	[29]
Keap1 (Keich-like ECH-associated protein-1)	3ADE (edited)	[29]
Kallikerin/KLK-7	3BSQ (edited)	[29]
Lactate dehydrogenase	3H3F (edited)	[29]
Spermine	HMDB, Acc no. HMDB01256	[30]
Spermidine	HMDB, Acc no. HMDB01257	[30]

TABLE 3: Sources of PDB files of ligands in our study.

Ligand	Accession no.	Reference
Arsenic trioxide (ATO)	DB01169	[31]
Sodium arsenite (SAN)	CID443495	[32]
Lipoic acid (α-LA) (ALA)	DB00166	[31]
Dimercaprol (BAL)	DB06782	[31]
DMSA (Dimercapto succinic acid) or succimer	DB00566	[31]
DMPS (2,3 Dimercapto propane-1-sulfonic acid)	12405pdb	[33]

Constant is written. Also, given in the file are the RMSD values. A conformation can be chosen and it's coordinates written to run the next set of docking and this should be done till Gibb's free energy is no longer significantly reduced.

(9) Diagrams are drawn with the protein and the ligand attached to it in its lowest energy conformer. Protein and ligand can be made of different width and color and the background white. The image can be saved in various formats of which we chose the tif format [28].

3. Results

3.1. Gibb's Free Energy and Binding Energy. The output results of AutoDock as mentioned in previous section are denoted by ΔG. AutoDock gives us the most important parameter in studying a closed system and it's minimum value of Gibbs Free energy or ΔG for every conformer of the ligand docked to the protein, also, calculating the equilibrium binding constant K in each case as these are related by the simple relation $\Delta G = -RT \ln K$.

TABLE 4: Minimum Gibbs' free energy (ΔG) in Kcal/mol.

Receptor/protein	Drug					
	ATO	SAN	ALA	DMC	DMPS	DMSA
TDR	−1.42	−1.81	−3.97	−2.99	−4.23	−4.93
Collagen	−0.91	−1.37	−4.09	−2.21	−3.14	−4.27
GTR	−1.48	−2.11	−4.61	−3.29	−4.87	−5.88
Actin	−1.66	−2.19 (Figure 2)	−5.33	−2.67	−4.94	−5.12
ER-Alpha	−1.61	−2.23 (Figure 2)	−6.01	−3.00	−4.28	−6.42
PDH	−1.35	−2.17	−4.92 (Figure 3)	−3.53	−4.85	−5.88
Albumin	−1.94 (Figure 1)	−1.99	−5.68 (Figure 3)	−3.02	−4.95	−5.85
Tubulin	−1.73	−2.08	−5.55	−3.06	−5.82 (Figure 4)	−5.90 (Figure 4)
Keap1	−1.84	−2.22	−7.03	−3.15	−5.12	−8.55
KLK−7	−1.91 (Figure 1)	−1.88	−6.37	−3.48	−6.17	−7.25
LDH	−1.48	−1.9	−6.67	−3.23	−4.32	−8.30
Spermine	−0.26	−0.36	−6.68	−0.89	−0.27	−8.95
Spermidine	−0.26	−0.34	−6.74	−0.98	−0.26	−9.92

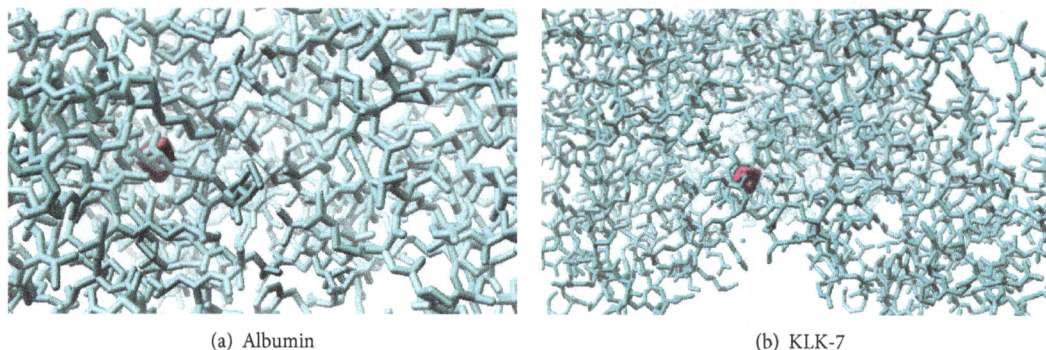

(a) Albumin   (b) KLK-7

FIGURE 1: ATO binding with albumin (a) and KLK-7 (b).

The most thermodynamically stable conformer in a bunch of conformers (say 20 or 50 runs) as that will have the minimum value of Gibb's free energy as per the two laws of thermodynamics. Thus, docking a ligand onto a protein we can predict it's most stable conformer and if there are a variety of ligands which ligand binds the best as in this case. Ligand docking (natural and drug) method was used to establish the rationale of long term toxicity of different adjuvant drugs of breast cancer [34].

Table 4 shows the minimum docked energy of different ligands (drugs) to the different protein molecules. Table 4 shows that arsenic trioxide (ATO) most strongly binds with the albumin protein and after that KLK-7, a tissue protein that is expressed on bacterial infection (Figure 1). It is to be noted here that experimental finding of arsenic toxicity and efficacies of different arsenic chelators are also revealed with sodium arsenite [15]. Hence, we make a comparative assessment between binding affinity of sodium arsenite (SAN) and ATO with the same proteins. Table 4 reveals that binding affinity of SAN is a little bit higher than ATO for most of the studied proteins (except KLK-7) due to more ionization potential. Among the studied proteins, SAN binds most strongly with ER-alpha and moderately with actin, a structural protein that is present in cells (Figure 2).

Docking study reveals further that DMSA and ALA (alpha-lipoic acid) binding to albumin are more than arsenic (Figure 3) (Table 4). Hence, they may be capable of removing arsenic from blood. In this connection, ALA could also become potent chelator of removing arsenic from tissue, as it binds strongly with actin, a structural protein of the cell. Of the available chelators, DMSA is the most potent and for chelation of arsenic from tubulin, a combination of DMPS and DMSA, would be effective (Figure 4). Arsenic chelation potentiality of DMSA is also helpful in protecting PDH, an important enzyme system of mitochondrial TCA cycle and the next most effective chelator for this enzyme system is the ALA (Figure 3) (Table 4).

ER-alpha is mostly affected by SAN as binding energy to this receptor protein is much more compared to other proteins studied. Our docking study also collaborate the experimental finding regarding the efficacy of different chelators in the order of DMSA > DMPS > DMC in protecting against SAN as these chelators have more affinity to ER-alpha [15].

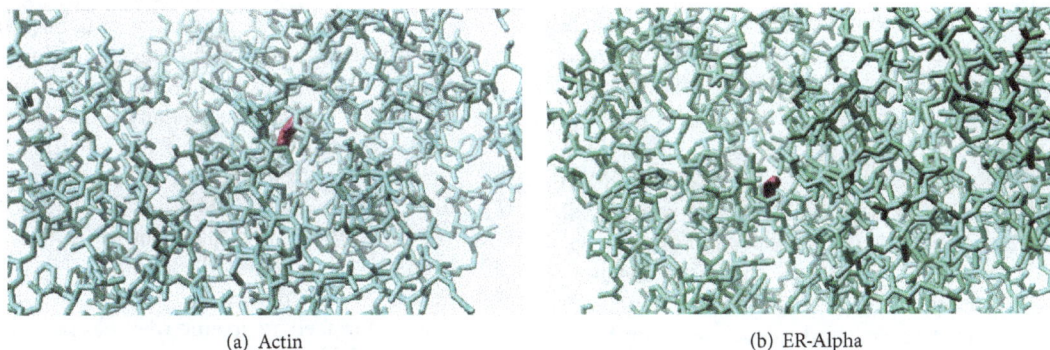

(a) Actin

(b) ER-Alpha

FIGURE 2: SAN binding with actin (a) and ER-alpha (b).

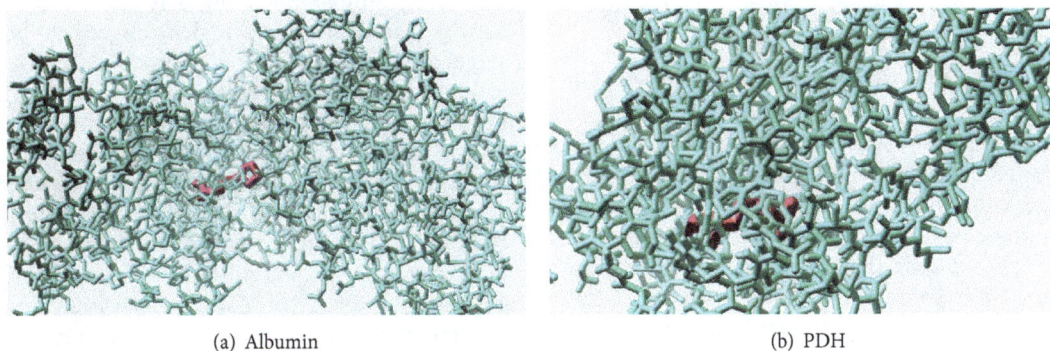

(a) Albumin

(b) PDH

FIGURE 3: α-LA binding with albumin (a) and PDH (b).

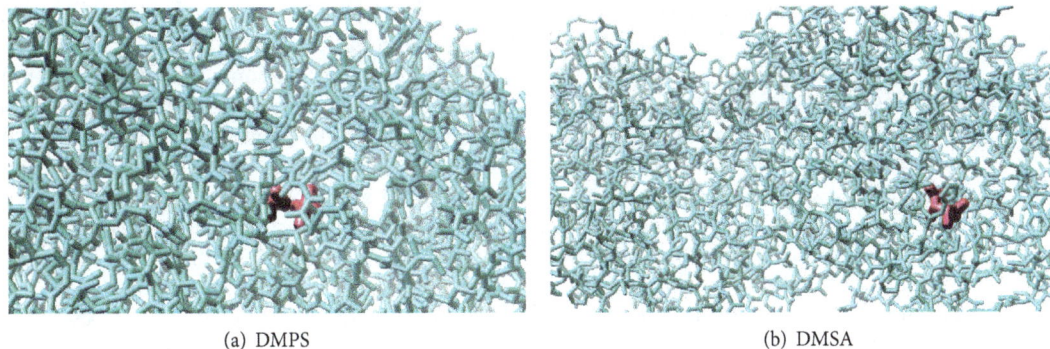

(a) DMPS

(b) DMSA

FIGURE 4: DMPS (a) and DMSA (b) binding with the tubulin.

4. Discussion

The concern of this paper is to find out suitable arsenic chelator for arsenic toxicity due to repeated drinking of contaminated ground water. Inorganic form of arsenic is the major cause of arsenic poisoning through drinking of ground water. In drinking water arsenious acid in trivalent [As(III)] state is the major source for arsenic toxicity. Arsenious acid is produced from arsenic trioxide under conditions dependent on pH, presence of redox chemicals, and reducing bacteria [3]. Hence, arsenic toxicity may occur primarily due to arsenic trioxide (ATO) and inorganic arsenic produces more toxicity compared to organic form of arsenic [6]. However, understanding of toxic effect of arsenic and determination of the efficacies of different arsenic chelators in different experimental animal model are carried out with sodium arsenite (SAN), a component of pesticide [15, 32]. Hence, binding affinity of both ATO and SAN is carried out for different proteins.

Arsenic trioxide has poor affinity towards spermine and spermidine and highest towards albumin. Arsenic toxicity by repeated drinking of contaminated ground water is often detected by a low serum albumin/globulin ratio [35]. Arsenic tends to lower serum album and cause albuminuria. Hence, any chelating agent with higher affinity for the protein can wash out arsenic from that protein. Our study indicates that DMSA followed by ALA would be the most potent drug for removing arsenic bound to the albumin as the binding energy of these drugs are more than the binding energy of arsenic.

Arsenic binds with thioredoxin reductase, a thiol enzyme present in liver cytosol and binding of arsenic to this protein can be removed away most effectively by DMPS, or succimer (DMSA). However, for collagen, succimer is the best. Bound arsenic to the liver enzyme glutathione reductase, a detoxifying enzyme can be washed by dimercaprol, DMPS or DMSA. It is noteworthy that ALA can also work in all the above-mentioned cases. Actin is involved in cytoskeletal structure of all cells and for this protein, the potent chelators would be DMPS, succimer, and ALA (Lipoic acid) added to remove brain deposits. An exact similar case arises for tubulin and pyruvate dehydrogenase. In all these cases, dimercaprol works as a less potent chelator. Arsenic chelating efficiency from these proteins is in the order of DMSA (succimer) > DMPS ≫ dimercaprol (DMC) (BAL). Moreover, the efficacy of these chelators also collaborate the experimental finding with SAN as these chelators has also more affinity to ER-alpha [15].

For estrogen receptors, most potent chelator would be DMSA (succimer) and for deposits in the brain, DMSA in combination with lipoic acid are used for the treatment especially for the cases of chronic arsenic poisoning. For the bacterial infected cells that secrete a serine protease Kallikerin/KLK-7, DMSA is a very potent chelator. DMSA is also effective for the removal of arsenic bound to Keap1 protein, a signalling protein. For lactate dehydrogenase which occurs in muscle, heart, and brain, DMSA is a very potent chelator compared to other chelators and Lipoic acid (ALA) is also the next best chelator so that it can be added to remove brain deposits of arsenic as it can cross the BBB (blood brain barrier) [36]. Reports suggest that other chelators when mixed with lipoic acid can pass the blood brain barrier easily and chelate brain deposits of arsenic due to the excellent lipophilic nature of lipoic acid [11].

Combination therapy was also suggested where two structurally different chelating agents are incorporated one is lipophilic and another is lipophobic simultaneously to chelate out both intracellular and extracellular metal deposits. Different antioxidants N-Acetyl cysteine, taurine, vitamin C, vitamin E, Zn, and Se enhance the effectiveness of different heavy metals chelation including arsenic by reducing the drug dose, preventing pro-oxidative damage, carcinogenic signalling is cut off and thus prevents tissue damage [11].

Arsenic binds to ER-α, the binding affinity of SAN is more than ATO. It might also get incorporated into spermine and spermidine, two peptides produced from the genital organs with high mitotic index and rapid turnover [37]. However, our study shows these peptides are less susceptible to arsenic toxicity (Table 4). Hence, male reproductive organ is less susceptible by both SAN and ATO; however, the female reproductive organ is more susceptible to SAN. Spermine and spermidine are interconvertible and occur in various organs like liver, kidneys, and cerebral regions of the brain. Dimercaprol and DMPS are both very poor chelators. Though trivalent arsenic has little affinity for spermine and spermidine; however, theoretically, DMSA is an extremely potent chelator as lipoic acid, and a combination of these would leach out arsenic very well from these two peptides. EDTA would

be a poor chelator for arsenic, the logic can be found looking at the periodic table as it best chelates d and f block elements.

Arsenic, in the form of sodium arsenite is one of the most extensively studied metals that induce ROS generation and results in oxidative stress. Experimental results show that superoxide radical ion and H_2O_2 are produced after exposure to arsenite in various cellular systems [38]. Arsenic is known not only to produce ROS but also, nitric oxide ($NO^\bullet$) [39], dimethylarsinic peroxyl radicals ($(CH_3)_2AsOO^\bullet$), and also the dimethylarsinic radical ($(CH_3)_2As^\bullet$) [40]. Oxidative DNA lesions induced by arsenic were observed both *in vivo* and *in vitro* [41]. The molecular cause may be due to reduced activation of glutathione reductase (GTR). Our docking study indicates that SAN is more potent in binding with GTR than ATO. Similar observation is also made with lactate dehydrogenase and pyruvate dehydrogenase—both enzyme system are involved with energy production.

Our computational prediction of chelators of a heavy metal poisoning, especially useful when practical or experimental data is scanty or it is not known that which proteins would be affected by a specific toxin. Comparative analysis of interaction between a toxin with its known protein and to its off-targets (unknown protein) may indicate a weak interaction of toxin to its off-targets. Though the interactions are weak, however, the docking algorithm and computer simulation may provide the molecular rationale of long-term toxicity [34]. Our study further indicates that different forms of inorganic arsenic strongly bind with albumin (plasma protein) and/or actin (structural component of all cells including red blood cells). Hence, blood analysis could be the first hand indicator of arsenic toxicity and reinforces the earlier clinical investigation of blood for detection of arsenic toxicity [16, 26]. So, we suggest that albumin and actin (blood test) testing should be done for the detection of early arsenic poisoning. Present study also reinforces the clinical finding regarding the effectiveness of DMSA or succimer as the most potent arsenic chelator. And if any sort of arsenic toxicity is found, DMSA alone or in combination of lipoic acid is the first hand choice of treatment.

Clinical medicine can come to way after a considerable number of experimentations with animal model; however, with the objections raised by different animal ethical committee across the globe restrict the use of animal for biological experimentation [42–44]. It is to be noted here that our previous study [34] and the present study indicate a close alignment with the clinical findings. Therefore, it can be proposed that docking could be an alternative method of animal uses in the assessment of toxicity of an agent and/or pharmacological evaluation of a drug.

References

[1] A. H. Smith, E. O. Lingas, and M. Rahman, "Contamination of drinking-water by arsenic in Bangladesh: a public health emergency," *Bulletin of the World Health Organization*, vol. 78, no. 9, pp. 1093–1103, 2000.

[2] S. Barlow, "Scientific facts on arsenic-details on arsenic level 2," *GreenFacts*, 2004, http://www.greenfacts.org/en/arsenic/l-2/index.htm#0.

[3] D. MacRae, "How does arsenic get into the groundwater?" http://www.civil.umaine.edu/macrae/arsenic_gw.htm.

[4] S. M. Gorby, "Clinical conference on arsenic poisoning," *Western Journal of Medicine*, vol. 149, pp. 308–315, 1998.

[5] N. A. Rey, O. W. Howarth, and E. C. Pereira-Maia, "Equilibrium characterization of As(III)-cysteine and As(III)-glutathione systems in aqueous solution," *Journal of Inorganic Biochemistry*, vol. 98, no. 6, pp. 1151–1159, 2004.

[6] R. L. Tatken and R. J. Lewis, Eds., *Registry of Toxic Effects Chemical Substances*, US Department of Health and Human Services, Cincinnati, Ohio, USA, 1983.

[7] A. M. Hays, R. C. Lantz, L. S. Rodgers et al., "Arsenic-induced decreases in the vascular matrix," *Toxicologic Pathology*, vol. 36, no. 6, pp. 805–817, 2008.

[8] J. T. Hindmarsh and R. F. McCurdy, "Clinical and environmental aspects of arsenic toxicity," *Critical Reviews in Clinical Laboratory Sciences*, vol. 23, no. 4, pp. 315–347, 1986.

[9] J. P. Buchet and R. Lauwerys, "Role of thiols in the *in-vitro* methylation of inorganic arsenic by rat liver cytosol," *Biochemical Pharmacology*, vol. 37, no. 16, pp. 3149–3153, 1988.

[10] H. V. Aposhian, "Enzymatic methylation of arsenic species and other new approaches to arsenic toxicity," *Annual Review of Pharmacology and Toxicology*, vol. 37, pp. 397–419, 1997.

[11] S. J. S. Flora and V. Pachauri, "Chelation in metal intoxication," *International Journal of Environmental Research and Public Health*, vol. 7, no. 7, pp. 2745–2788, 2010.

[12] L. Benramdane, M. Accominotti, L. Fanton, D. Malicier, and J. J. Vallon, "Arsenic speciation in human organs following fatal arsenic trioxide poisoning—a case report," *Clinical Chemistry*, vol. 45, no. 2, pp. 301–306, 1999.

[13] E. Marafante, J. Rade, E. Sabbioni, F. Bertolero, and V. Foa, "Intracellular interaction and metabolic fate of arsenite in the rabbit," *Clinical Toxicology*, vol. 18, no. 11, pp. 1335–1341, 1981.

[14] G. M. Bogdan, A. Sampayo-Reyesb, and H. Vasken-Aposhian, "Arsenic binding proteins of mammalian systems: I. isolation of three arsenite-binding proteins of rabbit liver," *Toxicology*, vol. 93, no. 2-3, pp. 175–193, 1994.

[15] H. V. Aposhian, D. E. Carter, T. D. Hoover, C. A. Hsu, R. M. Maiorino, and E. Stine, "DMSA, DMPS, and DMPA—as arsenic antidotes," *Fundamental and Applied Toxicology*, vol. 4, no. 2, pp. S58–S70, 1984.

[16] H. Jiang, J. Ding, P. Chang, Z. Chen, and G. Sun, "Determination of the interaction of arsenic and human serum albumin by online microdialysis coupled to LC with hydride generation atomic fluorescence spectroscopy," *Chromatographia*, vol. 71, no. 11-12, pp. 1075–1079, 2010.

[17] S. Shila, M. Subathra, M. A. Devi, and C. Panneerselvam, "Arsenic intoxication-induced reduction of glutathione level and of the activity of related enzymes in rat brain regions: reversal by DL-alpha-lipoic acid," *Archives of Toxicology*, vol. 79, no. 3, pp. 140–146, 2005.

[18] W. T. Klimecki, A. H. Borchers, R. E. Egbert, R. B. Nagle, D. E. Carter, and G. T. Bowden, "Effects of acute and chronic arsenic exposure of human-derived keratinocytes in an *in vitro* human skin equivalent system: a novel model of human arsenicism," *Toxicology in Vitro*, vol. 11, no. 1-2, pp. 89–98, 1997.

[19] M. R. Karim, K. A. Salam, E. Hossain et al., "Interaction between chronic arsenic exposure via drinking water and plasma lactate dehydrogenase activity," *Science of the Total Environment*, vol. 409, no. 2, pp. 278–283, 2010.

[20] J. C. Davey, J. E. Bodwell, J. A. Gosse, and J. W. Hamilton, "Arsenic as an endocrine disruptor: effects of arsenic on estrogen receptor-mediated gene expression *in vivo* and in cell culture," *Toxicological Sciences*, vol. 98, no. 1, pp. 75–86, 2007.

[21] S. Lin, L. M. Del Razo, M. Styblo, C. Wang, W. R. Cullen, and D. J. Thomas, "Arsenicals inhibit thioredoxin reductase in cultured rat hepatocytes," *Chemical Research in Toxicology*, vol. 14, no. 3, pp. 305–311, 2001.

[22] S. Maiti and A. K. Chatterjee, "Effects on levels of glutathione and some related enzymes in tissues after an acute arsenic exposure in rats and their relationship to dietary protein deficiency," *Archives of Toxicology*, vol. 75, no. 9, pp. 531–537, 2001.

[23] T. Samikkannu, C. H. Chen, L. H. Yih et al., "Reactive oxygen species are involved in arsenic trioxide inhibition of pyruvate dehydrogenase activity," *Chemical Research in Toxicology*, vol. 16, no. 3, pp. 409–414, 2003.

[24] Y. H. Ling, J. D. Jiang, J. F. Holland, and R. Perez-Soler, "Arsenic trioxide produces polymerization of microtubules and mitotic arrest before apoptosis in human tumor cell lines," *Molecular Pharmacology*, vol. 62, no. 3, pp. 529–538, 2002.

[25] M. Izdebska, A. Grzanka, M. Ostrowski, A. Zuryń, and D. Grzanka, "Effect of arsenic trioxide (Trisenox) on actin organization in K-562 erythroleukemia cells," *Folia Histochemica et Cytobiologica*, vol. 47, no. 3, pp. 453–459, 2009.

[26] E. K. Silbergeld, "Toxicology," in *ILO Encyclopedia of Occupational Health & Safety*, chapter 33, part 4, International Labour Office, Washington, DC, USA, 4th edition, 1998.

[27] R. Huey and G. Morris, "Using autodock 3 with autodock-tools 3.05 a tutorial by the Scripps Research Institute," 2006, http://autodock.scripps.edu/faqs-help/tutorial/using-autodock-with-autodocktools/UsingAutoDockWithADT_v2e.pdf.

[28] R. Huey and G. Morris, "Using autodock 3 with autodock-tools 3.05 a tutorial by the Scripps Research Institute," 2008, http://autodock.scripps.edu/faqs-help/tutorial/using-autodock-tools/UsingAutoDock4WithADT_1.4.5d.pdf.

[29] H. M. Berman, J. Westbrook, Z. Feng et al., "The protein data bank," *Nucleic Acids Research*, vol. 28, no. 1, pp. 235–242, 2000.

[30] HMDB: The Human Metabolome Database, http://www.hmdb.ca/.

[31] D. S. Wishart, C. Knox, A. C. Guo et al., "Drugbank: a comprehensive resource for in silico drug discovery and exploration," *Nucleic Acids Research*, vol. 1, pp. 34–36, 2006.

[32] "PubChem," http://pubchem.ncbi.nlm.nih.gov/.

[33] "Gnu-darwin," http://molecules.gnu-darwin.org/mod/e-e-more.html.

[34] S. Mukherjee and D. Majumder, "Computational molecular docking assessment of hormone receptor adjuvant drugs: breast cancer as an example," *Pathophysiology*, vol. 16, no. 1, pp. 19–29, 2009.

[35] M. M. Khan, M. K. Hossain, K. Kobayashi et al., "Levels of blood and urine chemicals associated with longer duration of having arsenicosis in Bangladesh," *International Journal of Environmental Health Research*, vol. 15, no. 4, pp. 289–301, 2005.

[36] Y. Gilgun-Sherki, E. Melamed, and D. Offen, "Oxidative stress induced-neurodegenerative diseases: the need for antioxidants that penetrate the blood brain barrier," *Neuropharmacology*, vol. 40, no. 8, pp. 959–975, 2001.

[37] H. Antrup and N. Seiler, "On the turnover of polyamines spermidine and spermine in mouse brain and other organs," *Neurochemical Research*, vol. 5, no. 2, pp. 123–143, 1980.

[38] S. J. Flora, S. Bhadauria, S. C. Pant, and R. K. Dhaked, "Arsenic induced blood and brain oxidative stress and its response to some thiol chelators in rats," *Life Sciences*, vol. 77, no. 18, pp. 2324–2337, 2005.

[39] J. Pi, S. Horiguchi, Y. Sun et al., "A potential mechanism for the impairment of nitric oxide formation caused by prolonged oral exposure to arsenate in rabbits," *Free Radical Biology and Medicine*, vol. 35, no. 1, pp. 102–113, 2003.

[40] H. Shi, X. Shi, and K. J. Liu, "Oxidative mechanism of arsenic toxicity and carcinogenesis," *Molecular and Cellular Biochemistry*, vol. 255, no. 1-2, pp. 67–78, 2004.

[41] A. S. Andrew, J. L. Burgess, M. M. Meza et al., "Arsenic exposure is associated with decreased DNA repair *in vitro* and in individuals exposed to drinking water arsenic," *Environmental Health Perspectives*, vol. 114, no. 8, pp. 1193–1198, 2006.

[42] "Times of India," http://articles.timesofindia.indiatimes.com/ 2012-04-17.

[43] "Humane society International," http://www.hsi.org/issues/ biomedical_research/facts/news_eu_law.html.

[44] "Report from the Commission to the European Parliament & the Council," Tech. Rep., Brussels, Belgium, 2011.

18

Reducing the Inconsistency between Doppler and Invasive Measurements of the Severity of Aortic Stenosis Using Aortic Valve Coefficient: A Retrospective Study on Humans

Anup K. Paul,[1] Rupak K. Banerjee,[1] Arumugam Narayanan,[2] Mohamed A. Effat,[2] and Jason J. Paquin[2]

[1] School of Dynamic Systems, Mechanical Engineering Program, University of Cincinnati, Cincinnati, OH 45221, USA
[2] Division of Cardiovascular Diseases, University of Cincinnati, Cincinnati, OH 45221, USA

Correspondence should be addressed to Jason J. Paquin; paquinjj@mail.uc.edu

Academic Editor: Marek Belohlavek

Background. It is not uncommon to observe inconsistencies in the diagnostic parameters derived from Doppler and catheterization measurements for assessing the severity of aortic stenosis (AS) which can result in suboptimal clinical decisions. In this pilot study, we investigate the possibility of improving the concordance between Doppler and catheter assessment of AS severity using the functional diagnostic parameter called aortic valve coefficient (AVC), defined as the ratio of the transvalvular pressure drop to the proximal dynamic pressure. *Method and Results.* AVC was calculated using diagnostic parameters obtained from retrospective chart reviews. AVC values were calculated independently from cardiac catheterization ($AVC_{catheter}$) and Doppler measurements ($AVC_{doppler}$). An improved significant correlation was observed between Doppler and catheter derived AVC ($r = 0.92$, $P < 0.05$) when compared to the correlation between Doppler and catheter measurements of mean pressure gradient ($r = 0.72$, $P < 0.05$) and aortic valve area ($r = 0.64$, $P < 0.05$). The correlation between Doppler and catheter derived AVC exhibited a marginal improvement over the correlation between Doppler and catheter derived aortic valve resistance ($r = 0.89$, $P < 0.05$). *Conclusion.* AVC is a refined clinical parameter that can improve the concordance between the noninvasive and invasive measures of the severity of aortic stenosis.

1. Introduction

Aortic stenosis (AS) is a type of valvular heart disease that results from abnormal narrowing of the aortic valve opening. A stenotic aortic valve creates an increased pressure gradient between the left ventricle and the aorta. The resulting increased ventricular workload and associated increased ventricular wall stress may contribute to left ventricular dysfunction and heart failure over time. AS is typically caused by progressive degeneration and calcification of the aortic valve; hence, the prevalence of calcific aortic valve disease increases with age [1, 2]. Calcific aortic valve disease ranges from mild valve thickening with minimal flow obstruction termed aortic sclerosis to severe calcification and flow obstruction termed AS. Generally, aortic valve replacement is indicated for symptomatic severe AS, since the outcome without valve replacement is poor with survival rates as low as 50% at two years [3–5]. Accurate assessment of the severity of stenosis is critical for clinical decision making in patients with AS. Severity of AS is currently assessed by one or more diagnostic indices obtained by Doppler echocardiography and/or cardiac catheterization [6, 7].

Severity of AS is currently assessed by Doppler echocardiography using a combination of transvalvular pressure gradients, aortic jet velocity, stenotic aortic valve area, and aortic valve resistance [6, 7]. The hydrodynamic principle of flow through stenotic orifices indicates progressive acceleration and convergence of flow field through the stenosis. The point of maximum convergence is termed *vena contracta* and usually lies just distal to the orifice area. Doppler measures the jet velocity at the *vena contracta* of the valve and velocity in the left ventricular outflow tract ($\widetilde{V}_{LVOT}$). The cross-sectional

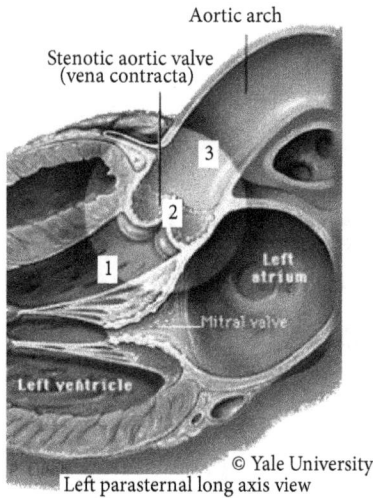

1 → Left ventricle outflow tract (LVOT)
2 → Stenotic aortic valve (AoV)
3 → Ascending aorta (AA),
      after pressure recovery

$$V_{\text{LVOT}} = V_1$$
$$\Delta p_{\text{catheter}} = P_1 - P_3$$
$$\Delta p_{\text{doppler}} = 4V_{\text{jet}}^2 = 4V_2^2$$

FIGURE 1: Anatomical location of diagnostic parameters for assessment of the severity of aortic stenosis [9].

area at the left ventricular outflow tract is also approximately calculated using 2D echo. The obtained velocities and the left ventricular outflow tract area are then used to calculate the mean transvalvular pressure gradient ($\Delta \widetilde{p}_{\text{doppler}}$), aortic valve area ($\widetilde{\text{AVA}}_{\text{doppler}}$), and aortic valve resistance (AVR) [7, 8]. The corresponding anatomical locations of the *vena contracta* and the left ventricular outflow tract are shown in Figure 1.

Invasive cardiac catheterization is the other common method used for determining the diagnostic end-points to assess AS severity. The mean transvalvular pressure gradient ($\Delta \widetilde{p}_{\text{catheter}}$) is directly measured during catheterization. The $\Delta \widetilde{p}_{\text{catheter}}$ is the pressure difference between the left ventricle and the ascending aorta after pressure-recovery [3] as shown in Figure 1. The cardiac output (CO) is measured using Fick's principle and/or the thermodilution method. The aortic valve area ($\widetilde{\text{AVA}}_{\text{catheter}}$) is then determined from the measured pressure gradient and CO using the Gorlin equation [10].

One of the most common causes for misclassification is due to the pressure-recovery phenomenon in the ascending aorta [3, 11–14]. The extent of pressure-recovery depends on the ratio of the *vena contracta* area to the cross-sectional area of the ascending aorta (Figure 1). A relatively larger pressure-recovery in relation to the overall pressure gradient is seen in subjects with mild to moderate stenosis and in subjects with small aorta [13, 15, 16]. Doppler measurements are taken at the *vena contracta* just distal to the aortic valve orifice and do not account for the pressure-recovery in the aorta, whereas catheterization measures the pressure difference between the left ventricle and a point in the aorta well beyond the aortic

valve where the pressure is, in general, completely recovered. Thus, there are significant differences between the pressure gradient obtained by Doppler and catheterization. While $\Delta \widetilde{p}_{\text{doppler}}$ will often overestimate the AS severity, $\Delta \widetilde{p}_{\text{catheter}}$ is typically recorded after pressure-recovery and therefore it usually represents the net pressure drop due to AS. The $\widetilde{\text{AVA}}_{\text{catheter}}$ does not represent the anatomical valve area but is one that reflects the hemodynamic consequence of the stenosis [13]. Moreover, $\Delta \widetilde{p}_{\text{doppler}}$ and $\widetilde{\text{AVA}}_{\text{doppler}}$ are quantities derived from velocity and measured area using simplified forms of the Bernoulli's equation which ignore the pressure loss due to frictional (viscous) effects and momentum change due to area reduction. Previous studies have shown that the Doppler and catheter measurements of the aortic valve area can vary up to 50% depending on the size of the aorta and the severity of AS [3, 15, 17].

We hypothesize that the proposed hemodynamic diagnostic parameter, based on fundamental fluid dynamics principles, will improve the concordance between Doppler and catheter assessment of AS severity. The proposed functional diagnostic index, aortic valve coefficient (AVC), is defined as the ratio of the mean net transvalvular pressure gradient to the mean proximal dynamic pressure (0.5 × blood density × $\widetilde{V}_{\text{LVOT}}^2$). The mean net transvalvular pressure gradient is the $\Delta \widetilde{p}_{\text{doppler}}$ corrected for pressure-recovery or the $\Delta \widetilde{p}_{\text{catheter}}$ and is represented by $P_1 - P_3$ in Figure 1. AVC, in general, is a nondimensional parameter that accounts for the resistance to the flow due to the area reduction caused by the stenosed valve and also the frictional loss. In this study, the correlation between Doppler and catheter derived mean transvalvular pressure gradient, aortic valve area, AVR, and AVC is examined to determine the potential of the proposed diagnostic index to reduce the variability in the assessment of the severity of AS between the two diagnostic methods.

2. Methods

2.1. Study Patients. The study population consisted of 36 patients that were selected by a retrospective review of patient records. The study protocol was approved by the Institutional Review Board at University of Cincinnati. The selected patients were aged 42–92 years with suspected AS who underwent precatheterization 2D transthoracic Doppler echocardiograms and left heart catheterizations from 2010 to 2012. Data from thirteen patients with inconsistent pressure-flow measurements (e.g., 1 patient with procedural error as catheterization transducer was not properly zeroed, 1 patient with $\Delta \widetilde{p}_{\text{catheter}} = 4 \times \Delta \widetilde{p}_{\text{doppler}}$, and 1 patient with Doppler measurement taken after cardiac arrest) and incomplete data (e.g., 10 patients with poor quality or incomplete Doppler measurements) were excluded. Three patients with bioprosthetic aortic valves were also excluded.

2.2. Data Analysis. The values of jet velocity ($\widetilde{V}_{\text{jet}}$), $\widetilde{V}_{\text{LVOT}}$, aortic root area ($\text{CSA}_{\text{aorta}}$), $\widetilde{\text{AVA}}_{\text{doppler}}$, and $\Delta \widetilde{p}_{\text{doppler}}$ (superscript "~" indicates mean values) were obtained from the standard Doppler echocardiography reports. Similarly, $\Delta \widetilde{p}_{\text{catheter}}$

and $\widehat{AVA}_{catheter}$ were obtained from standard catheterization reports. AVR, defined as the ratio of the mean pressure gradient to the mean flow rate expressed in units of $N \cdot s \cdot m^{-5}$ [7, 8], was calculated independently from Doppler ($AVR_{doppler}$) and catheterization measurements ($AVR_{catheter}$). The proposed hemodynamic diagnostic parameter, AVC, was calculated independently from Doppler ($AVC_{doppler}$) and catheterization ($AVC_{catheter}$) measurements, where $\Delta \widetilde{p}_{doppler\text{-}r}$ is the pressure-recovery corrected Doppler transvalvular pressure gradient and ρ is the density of blood (1050 kg/m^3). $\Delta \widetilde{p}_{doppler\text{-}r}$ was calculated from the Doppler measured $\Delta \widetilde{p}_{doppler}$ based on fluid mechanics theory [7, 11, 12, 14]. Consider

$$AVC_{doppler} = \frac{\Delta \widetilde{p}_{doppler\text{-}r}}{0.5 \times \rho \times \widetilde{V}_{LVOT}^2}$$

$$\Delta \widetilde{p}_{doppler\text{-}r}$$

$$= \Delta \widetilde{p}_{doppler} \left(1 - \left(2 \frac{\widehat{AVA}_{doppler}}{CSA_{aorta}} \left(1 - \frac{\widehat{AVA}_{doppler}}{CSA_{aorta}} \right) \right) \right)$$

$$AVC_{catheter} = \frac{\Delta \widetilde{p}_{catheter}}{0.5 \times \rho \times \widetilde{V}_{LVOT}^2}.$$

$$(1)$$

The velocity is not measured during standard of care catheterization and hence Doppler measured $\widetilde{V}_{LVOT}$ was used to calculate $AVR_{catheter}$ and $AVC_{catheter}$ in this retrospective study.

2.3. Statistical Analysis. A linear regression analysis was performed on data from the 20 patients to assess significant linear correlations between the Doppler and catheterization derived parameters. Data from 1 patient was found to be a significant outlier and excluded from the data analysis. Thus, 19 patients (7 females) were included in this retrospective study. A probability value of $P < 0.05$ was considered statistically significant. Statistical data analysis was performed using SAS version 9.3 (SAS Institute, NC). All diagnostic parameters are represented as mean $\pm$ SE unless otherwise specified.

3. Results and Discussion

Table 1 summarizes the Doppler and catheter data obtained by retrospective review of the records of 19 patients included in this study. For the patient group analyzed, there was no significant difference between the mean $\Delta \widetilde{p}_{doppler}$ (4506 $\pm$ 373 Pa) and the mean $\Delta \widetilde{p}_{catheter}$ (4680$\pm$307 Pa), with $P = 0.72$. Following AHA guidelines [6] for classifying AS severity by $\Delta \widetilde{p}_{doppler}$, 4 patients had mild AS (less than 3333 Pa), 9 patients had moderate AS (3333 to 5333 Pa), and 6 patients had severe (greater than 5333 Pa) AS. Categorizing the patient group based on $\Delta \widetilde{p}_{catheter}$, 5 patients had mild AS, 10 patients had moderate AS, and 4 patients had severe AS.

The results of the linear regression analysis between Doppler and catheter derived diagnostic parameters are presented in Figures 2, 3, 4, and 5(a). The $\Delta \widetilde{p}_{doppler}$ correlated

TABLE 1: Mean values and range of blood pressure and Doppler and catheterization measured diagnostic parameters obtained retrospectively ($n = 19$).

	Mean	Range
Systolic blood pressure [Pa]	17625 ± 667	11732–23065
$\widetilde{V}_{jet}$ [m/s]	2.76 ± 0.09	2.0–3.55
$\widetilde{V}_{LVOT}$ [m/s]	0.61 ± 0.036	0.42–0.93
$\Delta \widetilde{p}_{doppler}$ [Pa]	4506 ± 373	2666–7599
$\Delta \widetilde{p}_{catheter}$ [Pa]	4680 ± 307	1560–7866

$\widetilde{V}_{jet}$: Doppler measured mean jet velocity at the vena contracta of the aortic valve; $\widetilde{V}_{LVOT}$: Doppler measured mean left ventricular outflow tract velocity; $\Delta \widetilde{p}_{doppler}$: Doppler measured mean pressure gradient; $\Delta \widetilde{p}_{catheter}$: catheterization measured mean pressure gradient.

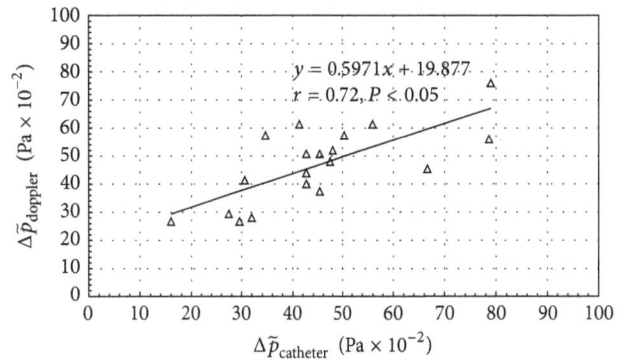

FIGURE 2: Relationship between Doppler measured mean pressure gradient ($\Delta \widetilde{p}_{doppler}$) and catheterization measured mean pressure gradient ($\Delta \widetilde{p}_{catheter}$).

moderately with the $\Delta \widetilde{p}_{catheter}$ ($r = 0.72$, $P < 0.05$; Figure 2). Similarly, $\widehat{AVA}_{doppler}$ also correlated moderately with $\widehat{AVA}_{catheter}$ ($r = 0.64$, $P < 0.05$; Figure 3). However, $AVR_{doppler}$ exhibits a superior correlation with $AVR_{catheter}$ ($r = 0.89$, $P < 0.05$; Figure 4). Similarly, $AVC_{doppler}$ also exhibits a statistically improved significant correlation with $AVC_{catheter}$ ($r = 0.92$, $P < 0.05$; Figure 5(a)). Thus, the correlation between Doppler and catheter derived AVC shows significant improvement when compared to Doppler and catheter derived $\Delta \widetilde{p}$ and $\widehat{AVA}$ and a marginal improvement when compared to Doppler and catheter derived AVR. Additionally, the agreement between the Doppler and catheter derived AVC was assessed using the Bland-Altman test (Figure 5(b)). The mean of the differences between the $AVC_{doppler}$ and $AVC_{catheter}$ is -2.7 ± 6.6 (mean $\pm$ SD) and the limits of agreement are -15.7 to 10.3. The Bland-Altman analysis reveals neither bias nor trend between the differences and magnitude of the measurements of AVC.

It is well known that, in flow through constrictions like arterial lesions and valvular stenosis, the mean pressure gradient ($\Delta \widetilde{p}$) is related to the mean velocity ($\widetilde{V}$) as $\Delta \widetilde{p} = A \times \widetilde{V} + B \times \widetilde{V}^2$, where A is the linear coefficient of viscous (frictional) loss and B is the nonlinear coefficient of pressure loss due to momentum change caused by area reduction [18]. At the higher Reynolds numbers ($\sim$5000)

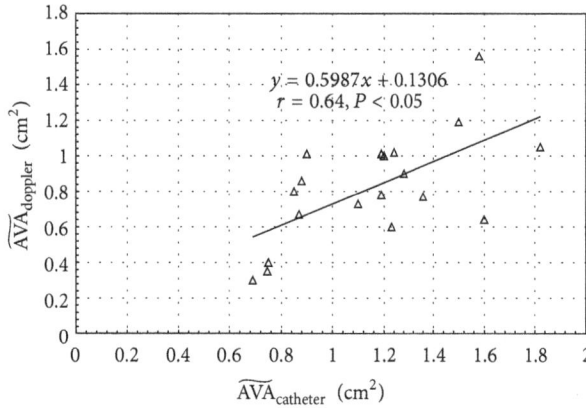

FIGURE 3: Relationship between Doppler derived mean aortic valve area ($\widetilde{\text{AVA}}_{\text{doppler}}$) and catheterization derived mean aortic valve area ($\widetilde{\text{AVA}}_{\text{catheter}}$).

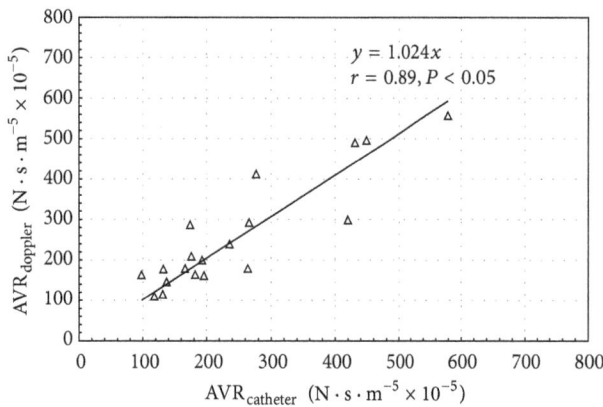

FIGURE 4: Correlation of Doppler derived aortic valve resistance ($\text{AVR}_{\text{doppler}}$) with catheterization derived aortic valve resistance ($\text{AVR}_{\text{catheter}}$).

that are typically observed in the human ascending aorta [19], the flow is transitional to turbulent and the nonlinear pressure loss due to the momentum change caused by aortic stenosis is generally more than the linear pressure loss due to viscous effects. Therefore, it should be noted that AVC (1) is a nondimensional diagnostic parameter that better accounts for the predominantly nonlinear pressure loss in stenosed aortic valves. In contrast, AVR is a dimensional flow dependent diagnostic parameter with limited prognostic value [7, 8] and it primarily represents the linear pressure loss due to frictional effects that is commonly observed in diffused arterial lesions.

The results of this retrospective study show a significant improvement in the correlation between Doppler and catheter derived AVR when compared to that between $\Delta\tilde{p}$ and $\widetilde{\text{AVA}}$ (Figures 2, 3, and 4). In addition, with the application of pressure-recovery correction, further improvement in the correlation between Doppler and catheter derived AVC is observed (Figure 5(a)), although there is only a marginal difference in Doppler-catheter correlations of AVC and AVR

(Figures 4 and 5(a)). The mean difference of −2.7 between Doppler and catheter derived AVC observed in the Bland-Altman analysis (Figure 5(b)) can be attributed to the small sample size of this study. Moreover, $\text{AVC}_{\text{catheter}}$ was calculated using $\tilde{V}_{\text{LVOT}}$ obtained retrospectively from Doppler echocardiography. Nevertheless, the results of this retrospective study support our hypothesis that AVC would further reduce the inconsistency between Doppler and catheter measurements. Further prospective studies are needed to confirm these results.

A diagnostic parameter pressure loss coefficient (ratio of the peak transvalvular pressure gradient to the peak outflow tract dynamic pressure), which is similar to AVC, has been previously evaluated for in vivo assessment of the degree of stenosis in both pulmonary and aortic valves [20]. Pressure loss coefficient was found to be independent of the blood velocity and its value of 15 was proposed as the cut-off value for decision on surgical procedure. Similarly, the hemodynamic parameter pressure drop coefficient (CDP), which is also similar to AVC, has been previously evaluated for assessing the severity of epicardial coronary artery stenosis by our group and shown to be independent of the hemodynamic influence of heart rate fluctuations [21–23]. Hence, AVC is expected to be largely independent of the variations in cardiac output, preload, and afterload and can better delineate the different grades of AS severity.

Recent studies have evaluated the parameter energy loss coefficient (ELCo) to reconcile Doppler and catheterization measurements [24]. The theoretical energy loss (EL) between the left ventricular outflow tract (LVOT) and the ascending aorta is defined as $(P_1 - P_3) + 0.5\rho(V_1^2 - V_3^2)$, where subscripts 1, 2, and 3 represent the LVOT, vena contracta, and ascending aorta after pressure recovery, respectively, as shown in Figure 1 [15]. Ignoring the net change in kinetic energy $[0.5\rho(V_1^2 - V_3^2)]$, which is typically negligible compared to $(P_1 - P_3)$ for patients with AS, theoretically, the EL, $\Delta\tilde{p}_{\text{doppler-}r}$ (r: indicating pressure after recovery), and $\Delta\tilde{p}_{\text{catheter}}$ represent the net pressure gradient, that is, $(P_1 - P_3)$. However, the ELCo, developed from the modified Bernoulli's equation, is a dimensional parameter with an atypical unit of cm^2 and is very similar to the valve area derived from catheterization data using the Gorlin equation [15, 24]. On the contrary, the AVC proposed in this study (1) is a nondimensional parameter where the normalization of the net pressure gradient is based on the differential mass and momentum equations [22]. Moreover, the EL is calculated from Doppler measurements [15] under the assumption of the limiting high Reynolds number condition where only loss due to momentum change caused by aortic stenosis is significant (Supplement A, [22]). This assumption may not be accurate for low flow or low Reynolds number conditions (for example, in patients with left ventricular dysfunction due to myocardial disease or hypertrophy). However, the $\Delta\tilde{p}$ in AVC includes both the frictional (viscous) loss and pressure loss due to momentum change irrespective of the flow status. Further, the normalization of the net pressure gradient with the native LVOT velocity in AVC is fundamentally more accurate from a fluid dynamic perspective and can provide

(a)

(b)

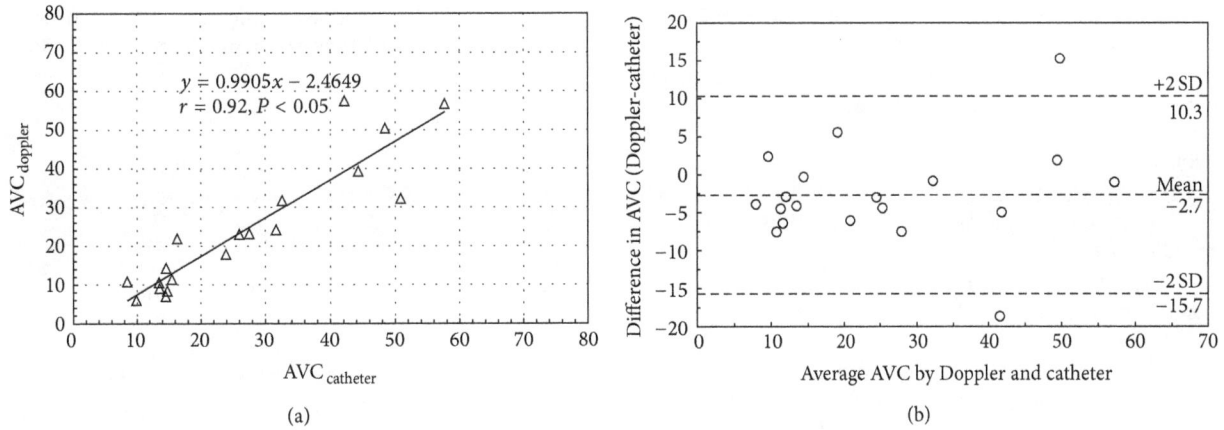

FIGURE 5: (a) Correlation of Doppler derived aortic valve coefficient ($AVC_{doppler}$) with catheterization derived aortic valve coefficient ($AVC_{catheter}$). (b) Bland-Altman plot of $AVC_{doppler}$ and $AVC_{catheter}$.

a wider range and enhanced delineation of aortic stenosis severity [23].

3.1. Study Limitations. The primary limitation of this retrospective study was the nonavailability of left ventricular outflow tract velocity from standard of care cardiac catheterization. Hence, $AVR_{catheter}$ and $AVC_{catheter}$ were calculated using the Doppler measured $\tilde{V}_{LVOT}$. True $AVR_{catheter}$ and $AVC_{catheter}$ should be evaluated in a prospective study where the pressure gradient and proximal velocity are measured simultaneously during catheterization.

4. Conclusion

This preliminary retrospective study has confirmed that AVC with the pressure-recovery correction has the potential to minimize the inconsistency between Doppler and catheter assessment of AS severity. As traditional surgical methods have improved and since the introduction of less invasive techniques for treatment like transcatheter aortic valve implantation (TAVI) technology, it is essential that more accurate diagnostic end-points be pursued. Presently, the inconsistencies in the diagnostic parameters derived from Doppler and catheterization measurements for assessing the severity of AS can result in suboptimal clinical decisions. Using a wide range of values, it is expected that AVC will be able to provide consistent and reproducible assessment of AS severity independent of the diagnostic method. In the future, it is of interest to conduct a prospective study to evaluate the specificity and sensitivity of AVC in delineating the severity of AS.

Conflict of Interests

The authors report no financial relationships or conflicts of interest regarding the content herein.

Authors' Contribution

Rupak K. Banerjee and Jason J. Paquin contributed equally to this work.

References

[1] J. Heikkilä, M. Kupari, R. Tilvis, and M. Lindroos, "Prevalence of aortic valve abnormalities in the elderly: an echocardiographic study of a random population sample," *Journal of the American College of Cardiology*, vol. 21, no. 5, pp. 1220–1225, 1993.

[2] R. V. Freeman and C. M. Otto, "Spectrum of calcific aortic valve disease: pathogenesis, disease progression, and treatment strategies," *Circulation*, vol. 111, no. 24, pp. 3316–3326, 2005.

[3] P. Pibarot and J. G. Dumesnil, "New concepts in valvular hemodynamics: implications for diagnosis and treatment of aortic stenosis," *Canadian Journal of Cardiology*, vol. 23, supplement B, pp. 40B–47B, 2007.

[4] F. Schwarz, P. Baumann, J. Manthey et al., "The effect of aortic valve replacement on survival," *Circulation*, vol. 66, no. 5, pp. 1105–1110, 1982.

[5] S. J. Lester, B. Heilbron, K. Gin, A. Dodek, and J. Jue, "The natural history and rate of progression of aortic stenosis," *Chest*, vol. 113, no. 4, pp. 1109–1114, 1998.

[6] R. O. Bonow, B. A. Carabello, K. Chatterjee et al., "ACC/AHA 2006 guidelines for the management of patients with valvular heart disease: a report of the American College of Cardiology/American Heart Association Task Force on Practice Guidelines (Writing Committee to Revise the 1998 Guidelines for the Management of Patients with Valvular Heart Disease)—developed in collaboration with the Society of Cardiovascular Anesthesiologists," *Circulation*, vol. 48, no. 3, pp. e1–e148, 2006.

[7] H. Baumgartner, J. Hung, J. Bermejo et al., "Echocardiographic assessment of valve stenosis: EAE/ASE recommendations for clinical practice," *Journal of the American Society of Echocardiography*, vol. 22, no. 1, pp. 1–23, 2009.

[8] F. Antonini-Canterin, P. Faggiano, D. Zanuttini, and F. Ribichini, "Is aortic valve resistance more clinically meaningful than valve area in aortic stenosis?" *Heart*, vol. 82, no. 1, pp. 9–10, 1999.

[9] C. C. Patrick, J. Lynch, and C. C. Jaffe, *Introduction to Cardiothoracic Imaging*, Yale University, 2006.

[10] R. Gorlin and S. G. Gorlin, "Hydraulic formula for calculation of the area of the stenotic mitral valve, other cardiac valves, and central circulatory shunts. I," *American Heart Journal*, vol. 41, no. 1, pp. 1–29, 1951.

[11] C. Clark, "The fluid mechanics of aortic stenosis. I. Theory and steady flow experiments," *Journal of Biomechanics*, vol. 9, no. 8, pp. 521–528, 1976.

[12] C. Clark, "The fluid mechanics of aortic stenosis. II. Unsteady flow experiments," *Journal of Biomechanics*, vol. 9, no. 9, pp. 567–573, 1976.

[13] A. E. Weyman and M. Scherrer-Crosbie, "Aortic stenosis: physics and physiology—what do the numbers really mean?" *Reviews in Cardiovascular Medicine*, vol. 6, no. 1, pp. 23–32, 2005.

[14] P. Gjertsson, K. Caidahl, G. Svensson, I. Wallentin, and O. Bech-Hanssen, "Important pressure recovery in patients with aortic stenosis and high Doppler gradients," *The American Journal Cardiology*, vol. 88, no. 2, pp. 139–144, 2001.

[15] D. Garcia, P. Pibarot, J. G. Dumesnil, F. Sakr, and L.-G. Durand, "Assessment of aortic valve stenosis severity: a new index based on the energy loss concept," *Circulation*, vol. 101, no. 7, pp. 765–771, 2000.

[16] W. A. Schöbel, W. Voelker, K. K. Haase, and K.-R. Karsch, "Extent, determinants and clinical importance of pressure recovery in patients with aortic valve stenosis," *European Heart Journal*, vol. 20, no. 18, pp. 1355–1363, 1999.

[17] D. Garcia and L. Kadem, "What do you mean by aortic valve area: geometric orifice area, effective orifice area, or Gorlin area?" *Journal of Heart Valve Disease*, vol. 15, no. 5, pp. 601–608, 2006.

[18] K. L. Gould, "Pressure-flow characteristics of coronary stenoses in unsedated dogs at rest and during coronary vasodilation," *Circulation Research*, vol. 43, no. 2, pp. 242–253, 1978.

[19] P. D. Stein and H. N. Sabbah, "Turbulent blood flow in the ascending aorta of humans with normal and diseased aortic valves," *Circulation Research*, vol. 39, no. 1, pp. 58–65, 1976.

[20] S. Hanya, M. Sugawara, H. Inage, and A. Ishihara, "A new method of evaluating the degree of stenosis using a multisensor catheter. Application of the pressure loss coefficient," *Heart and Vessels*, vol. 1, no. 1, pp. 36–42, 1985.

[21] R. K. Banerjee, K. D. Ashtekar, T. A. Helmy, M. A. Effat, L. H. Back, and S. F. Khoury, "Hemodynamic diagnostics of epicardial coronary stenoses: in-vitro experimental and computational study," *BioMedical Engineering Online*, vol. 7, article 24, 2008.

[22] R. K. Banerjee, A. Sinha Roy, L. H. Back, M. R. Back, S. F. Khoury, and R. W. Millard, "Characterizing momentum change and viscous loss of a hemodynamic endpoint in assessment of coronary lesions," *Journal of Biomechanics*, vol. 40, no. 3, pp. 652–662, 2007.

[23] K. K. Kolli, R. K. Banerjee, S. V. Peelukhana et al., "Influence of heart rate on fractional flow reserve, pressure drop coefficient, and lesion flow coefficient for epicardial coronary stenosis in a porcine model," *The American Journal Physiology—Heart and Circulatory Physiology*, vol. 300, no. 1, pp. H382–H387, 2011.

[24] D. Garcia, J. G. Dumesnil, L.-G. Durand, L. Kadem, and P. Pibarot, "Discrepancies between catheter and doppler estimates of valve effective orifice area can be predicted from the pressure recovery phenomenon: practical implications with regard to quantification of aortic stenosis severity," *Journal of the American College of Cardiology*, vol. 41, no. 3, pp. 435–442, 2003.

19

Mathematical Modeling of Melanoma Cell Migration with an Elastic Continuum Model for the Evaluation of the Influence of Tumor Necrosis Factor-Alpha on Migration

Julia Vianna Gallinaro,[1] **Claudia Mirian de Godoy Marques,**[2] **Fernando Mendes de Azevedo,**[1] **and Daniela Ota Hisayasu Suzuki**[1]

[1] *Instituto de Engenharia Biomédica, Departamento de Engenharia Elétrica, CTC,*
 Universidade Federal de Santa Catarina, 88040-900 Florianópolis, SC, Brazil
[2] *Centro de Ciências da Saúde e do Esporte, Universidade do Estado de Santa Catarina, 88080-350 Florianópolis, SC, Brazil*

Correspondence should be addressed to Julia Vianna Gallinaro; juliavg@gmail.com

Academic Editor: Hiroshi Watabe

An elastic continuum mathematical model was implemented to study collective C8161 melanoma cell migration during a "scratch wound" assay, in control and under the influence of the proinflammatory cytokine tumour necrosis factor-alpha (TNF-α). The model has four constants: force that results from lamellipod formation (F), adhesion constant between cells and extracellular matrix (ECM) (b), cell layer elasticity modulus (k), and growth rate (ρ). A nonlinear regression routine was used to obtain the parameters of the model with data from an experiment made with C8161 melanoma cells, with and without TNF-α. Coefficient of determination for both situations was $R^2 = 0.89$ and $R^2 = 0.92$, respectively. The parameters values obtained were similar to the ones found in the literature. However, the adhesion constant value decreased with the introduction of TNF-α, which is not in accordance with expected since the presence of TNF-α is associated with an increased expression of integrins that would promote an enhanced adhesion among cells. The model was used in a study relating to the adhesion constant and cell migration, and the results suggested that cell migration decreases with higher adhesion, which is also not in accordance with expected. These differences would not occur if it was considered that TNF-α increases the elasticity modulus of the cell layer.

1. Introduction

Skin cancer can be divided in two groups: melanoma and nonmelanoma. Melanoma initiates with an alteration in melanocytes, skin cells that produce melanin [1]. According to the World Health Organization data, there are worldwide currently 2 to 3 million nonmelanoma cases and 132 thousand melanoma cases. Although melanoma represents around 5% of total occurrences, it is responsible for most deaths of this type of cancer [2].

Melanoma has a radial growth phase that occurs in the epidermis. Radial growth phase cells can progress to vertical growth phase [3], in which cells grow beyond basal layer into the dermis, a vascularized region. Melanomas in radial growth phase can be surgically removed with high success rates, unlike vertical growth phase melanomas, which can become metastatic and have poor prognosis [4]. When melanoma is detected within initial stages, survival rate is of approximately 98%, decreasing to 16% in melanoma advanced stages [2].

Studies have shown a relationship between inflammatory processes and the appearance and development of different types of cancer, as well as lower incidence and mortality of several types of cancer through treatment with nonsteroidal anti-inflammatory agents [5–7]. During inflammatory processes, cytokines are produced such as TNF-α that promotes greater activation of adhesion molecule [8]. Cancer cell migration depends on the formation of focal complexes which promote adhesion between cell and ECM [9, 10]. Tumor cells can migrate in an individual or collective manner, and the way they do it is determined by their relation with the ECM. When compared to individual migration, collective migration, as in melanomas, presents higher dependence on cell-ECM adhesion [11]. In accordance with this statement, studies have shown that the presence of TNF-α increased melanoma cell migration [12–16].

When cutaneous melanoma is surgically removed, an inflammatory environment arises, which can favor local recurrences after surgery [15], and the exact area to be extracted during surgery is still a controversial theme. The area to be extracted is determined with classification, such as the Clark's levels, that establishes a relationship between tumor invasion level and patient's clinical prognosis, and the Breslow thickness, that refined Clark's levels by establishing a relationship between tumor thickness and patient survival prognosis [4]. According to the study developed by Kunishige et al. [17], the currently accepted extraction margin, based on a consensual opinion of 1992, is inadequate and might not be enough to completely extract cancer cells, increasing chances of recurrence, which should happen in up to 20% of cases.

Mathematical models can aid tumor growth and cell migration research since they allow simulations that are not easily obtained in *in vitro* or *in vivo* experiments. Mathematical models of tumor growth and cell migration have been developed in order to help treatment and diagnosis of several types of cancer [18–22]. Some of these models have a system of nondimensionalised equations [18, 19, 22], which complicates quantitative comparison with experimental work. Other models, such as the one developed by Eikenberry et al. [21], have dimensionalised equations; however, they do not quantitatively compare their results with experimental work. These facts lead to models that may indicate the way cell migration and tumor invasion occur but are not necessarily capable of describing experimentally obtained situation.

Most parts of current cancer cell migration models are based on a diffusion process [18, 19, 21, 22]. These studies present, generally, a principal variable: cancer cell concentration, which varies in time and space according to a diffusion equation based on Fick's law, with diffusion coefficient either constant or variable.

It is known that cell migration depends on the cell-to-ECM interaction through creation of adhesion complexes [9, 11]. Besides, it is also known that melanoma is a type of cancer that presents mostly collective migration [11], which implies in adherent junctions that promote cell-to-cell adhesion [23]. Diffusion processes by themselves do not account for these connections. Therefore, some models propose different manners of including parameters in the diffusion process that can represent cell-to-cell and cell-to-ECM connections, as in the model proposed by Chaplain [24].

Other models try to describe collective migration using agent-based models [25]. A study shown by Mi et al. [26] models a healing process using an elastic continuum model. This model was based on collective migration principles: during migration, cells do not separate from the edges, and no wholes are created on the cell layer. Mi et al. [26] proposed a mathematical model of enterocyte migration, during a healing process, in which cells undergo movement, deformation, and proliferation.

The aim of this work was to propose the use of a collective cell migration mathematical model that could be quantitatively compared to experimental data and allowed for an analysis on the influence of the pro-inflammatory cytokine TNF-α on melanoma cell migration.

2. Methods

2.1. Mathematical Model. The model proposed by Mi et al. [26] was a one-dimensional model that described migration of a cell layer after the opening of a wound on the layer, as in a "scratch wound" assay. The model followed some considerations: (1) it was based on a monolayer of cells, (2) there was connection between cells in the layer, (3) after the scratch (from the "scratch wound" assay), an external force was created as a result of lamellipod formation, (4) the cells in the interior of the layer did not form lamellipodia and hence were not directly actuating the motion, and (5) the cell layer came under deformation, movement, and material growth.

The variable s was used to describe the position of a cell on the original cell layer and the variable $x(t, s)$ the position at time instant t of the cell originally located at s. Variable $\hat{s}(t, s)$ represents the hypothetical position of cell located at s on the original layer at time instant t if all deformation from the layer was instantaneously removed. According to balance of momentum and neglecting its acceleration term, Mi et al. [26] showed that a segment of cells, which are the offsprings of cells between s and $s + ds$ of the original layer with ds assumed small, would have its motion described by the following equation:

$$
(x(t, s + ds) - x(t, s)) \\
* b * \frac{\partial x(t, s)}{\partial t} = f(t, s + ds) - f(t, s),
\tag{1}
$$

where b is the adhesion constant between cells and the surface and f the resultant force on a cross-section of the layer. In limit $ds \to 0$, (1) becomes

$$
b * \frac{\partial x}{\partial s} * \frac{\partial x}{\partial t} = \frac{\partial f}{\partial s}.
\tag{2}
$$

The strain (deformation gradient) in the cell layer can be described by the quantity

$$
\varepsilon = \frac{\partial x}{\partial \hat{s}} - 1,
\tag{3}
$$

with $\varepsilon > 0$ corresponding to stretch and $-1 < \varepsilon < 0$ corresponding to compression.

For the constitutive relation describing the dependence of f on ε, Mi et al. [26] used the equation

$$
f = k * \ln(\varepsilon + 1) = k \left[\ln\left(\frac{\partial x}{\partial s}\right) - \ln\left(\frac{\partial \hat{s}}{\partial s}\right) \right],
\tag{4}
$$

where k is the elasticity modulus of the cell layer.

Material growth from the layer was described using the growth gradient $g(t, s) = \partial \hat{s}/\partial s$ on the formula

$$
g(t, s) = \exp(\rho t),
\tag{5}
$$

where ρ is the growth rate.

From (2), (4), and (5), the following resulting equation was obtained:

$$\frac{\partial x}{\partial s} * \frac{\partial x}{\partial t} = \frac{k}{b} * \frac{\partial}{\partial s}\left(\ln\left(\frac{\partial x}{\partial s}\right) - \rho(s)\,t\right). \qquad (6)$$

Assuming that the location of the left boundary of the cell layer ($s = 0$) is fixed, the right boundary is free to move, and that the force applied at the right boundary is constant and equal to F, Mi et al. [26] proposed the use of the following initial and boundary conditions:

$$x(0, s) = 0, \quad \text{for } 0 \le s \le L, \qquad (7a)$$

$$x(t, 0) = 0, \quad \text{for } t \ge 0, \qquad (7b)$$

$$\frac{\partial x(t, 1)}{\partial s} = \exp\left[\left(\frac{F}{k}\right) + \rho t\right], \quad \text{for } t > 0. \qquad (7c)$$

Considering the growth rate ρ is spatially independent, (6) can be written as

$$\frac{\partial x}{\partial t} = \frac{k}{b} * \frac{\partial^2 x}{\partial s^2} * \left(\frac{\partial x}{\partial s}\right)^{-2}. \qquad (8)$$

From (3) and (5), the deformation gradient can be calculated with

$$\varepsilon = \frac{\partial x}{\partial s} * \exp(-\rho t) - 1. \qquad (9)$$

2.2. Calibration. A routine nonlinear minimization of the least square error was used to estimate the parameters. The constants k, b, and F appear on the problem only as the ratios $\kappa = k/b$ and $\varphi = F/k$. Therefore, regression was performed for the constants κ, φ, and ρ.

Experimental data used on calibration were based on the work by Redpath et al. [15]. Data were obtained from a study using C8161 human cutaneous melanoma, in control media culture and under the influence of pro-inflammatory cytokine TNF-α. The human C8161 melanoma line was established from an abdominal wall metastasis, which indicated that it was highly invasive.

Cells were seeded in culture plates in culture medium at a concentration of 4×10^4 cells/mL per well and were incubated for one day under standard culture conditions. On the second day, the culture medium was removed and replaced with an equal volume of fresh culture medium supplemented with TNF-α at a concentration of 800 U/mL. On the third day, a "scratch wound" for migration assay was made in each well using a plastic pipette tip, creating a cell-free zone in each well. The reduction of distance between the scratch edges at different time points (0, 2, 4, 6, and 8 hours) represented the migration of melanoma cells.

2.3. Simulation. A script was written in MATLAB to implement the model. Discretization both in time and space was obtained with the finite differences method [26]. Time and space steps were defined using the methodology proposed by Smith and Weaver [27], considering an error minor than 2% for the limits of this simulation. Time (dt) and space (ds) steps used were 1/120 h and 0.0125 μm, respectively.

TABLE 1: Parameter obtained from nonlinear regression. Values of the constants κ, φ, and ρ obtained during model calibration, based on experimental data from Redpath et al. [15].

Constants	Control	TNF-α
$\kappa = k/b$ (μm^2 h^{-1})	104.59	219.92
$\varphi = F/k$ (dimensionless)	0.096	0.13
ρ (h^{-1})	0.91	0.86

3. Results

The curves obtained with the mathematical model for the C8161 cell migration on control and under the influence of TNF-α after nonlinear regression showed determination coefficient of $R^2 = 0.89$ and $R^2 = 0.92$, respectively. The values of the constants obtained are shown in Table 1.

The values of the constants shown in Table 1 were used to study the influence of proliferation and deformation on control and TNF-α cell migration. The results are shown in Figure 2.

Figure 3 shows the influence of the adhesion constant on migration, considering a constant elasticity modulus.

A simulation was carried out to evaluate the influence of proliferation and deformation on cell migration, by studying the deformation gradient (Figure 4). Compression was considered to be related to proliferation due to the increase on the number of cells on the layer, and extension was considered to be related to deformation due to the tension applied by the cells on the border.

4. Discussion

A collective cell migration model was used to simulate melanoma cell migration during a "scratch wound" assay. The model was calibrated with experimental data that was obtained from a C8161 melanoma cell line, in control and under the influence of TNF-α.

Cell migration models based on diffusion have been used to model cancer cell migration [18, 19, 21, 22]. However, the coefficient values demonstrated by some of these models, such as by Eikenberry et al. [21] and Anderson et al. [18], are small (0.0009 mm^2 dia^{-1}~0.07 mm^2 dia^{-1}) when compared to diffusion coefficients experimentally obtained, for instance, by Lyng et al. [28] (50~80 mm^2 dia^{-1}). One possible explanation for this difference is that these models do not take the collective migration into account, as it is the case for melanoma cells. The elastic continuum model, proposed by Mi et al. [26], takes some collective migration aspects into consideration, and it is, therefore, a valid option for modeling "scratch wound" assays.

The values obtained during calibration are shown in Table 1. Since the parameters of interest k, b and F are presented on the model only as the ratios $\kappa = k/b$, and $\varphi = F/k$, nonlinear regression was performed for κ and φ. However, if a reference value is set for one of the three parameters of interest, it is possible to estimate the value of the other two. Mi et al. [26] modeled enterocyte migration during wound healing and showed a value of elasticity modulus k of approximately 44 nN. Considering melanoma cells migrating during the "scratch wound" assay demonstrate the same value of elasticity modulus, the cell layer would have, in control situation, force result from lamellipod formation F of approximately 4.22 nN and adhesion constant b of approximately 0.42 h nN/μm^2. Zhu et al. [12] showed that an increased integrin expression is observed in melanoma cells in the presence of TNF-α. When relating cell migration with integrin concentration, Mi et al. [26] discussed that the elasticity modulus of cell layer should be independent of integrin concentration. Therefore, considering that melanoma cells migrating in the assay under the influence of TNF-α show the same elasticity modulus k of the melanoma cells migrating in control situation, the cell layer would have force resulting from lamellipod formation F of approximately 5.72 nN and adhesion constant b of approximately 0.2 h nN/μm^2.

Based on the literature, values of protrusive force have measures that vary from 0.5 nN to 85 nN, depending on the method used for measuring and the place of the cell where the force was measured on [29–31]. Furthermore, the increased force observed from the control to the TNF-α situation is also in accordance with expected. It is known that the force with which the cell propels itself depends on the connections between the cell and the surface over which it moves and these connections are made by adhesion molecules, such as integrins [9, 29].

The values of the adhesion constant found in both situations are of the same magnitude of the ones demonstrated by Mi et al. [26] (approximately 0.11 h nN/μm^2). However, unlike what we expected, a decrease on the adhesion constant was observed with the introduction of TNF-α. The cytokine TNF-α is associated with an increased expression of integrins, which enhances cell adhesion [12]. Therefore, it would be expected that the value of the adhesion constant would increase with the addition of TNF-α, which did not happen. One hypothesis to explain this divergence would be that the elasticity modulus was not independent of the TNF-α concentration. It was considered that the elasticity modulus would remain the same with the introduction of TNF-α, based on the assumptions made by Mi et al. [26] in their work. However, in case the elasticity modulus increases with TNF-α introduction, the adhesion constant would increase as well.

A study was performed to analyze the influence of the adhesion constant on cell migration. For this study, cell migration was simulated for different values of the constant κ. The results can be seen in Figure 3. Considering the elasticity modulus on the layer is the same for all simulations, a decrease on the constant κ would mean an increase on the adhesion cell-to-ECM. The results show that an increase on the adhesion of the cells to ECM implies in a decrease in migration. However, Zhu et al. [12] have shown that an increase on adhesion would lead to increased migration, which is not in accordance with these results. Once again, one hypothesis to explain this divergence would be that the elasticity modulus was not independent of the TNF-α concentration. On the other hand, these results may be in accordance with another mathematical model proposed by DiMilla et al. [32], which showed a bell-shaped curve

to describe the relationship between migration speed and adhesion; that is, an increase on adhesion would lead to an increase on migration speed until a certain value, after which speed would stabilize and afterwards begin to decrease with an increase on adhesion. Thus, the values shown in Figure 3 could be located on the section of the graph in which the increase in adhesion implies decrease on migration speed.

Since the constants k, b, and F appear in the problem only as the ratios $\kappa = k/b$, and $\varphi = F/k$, the regression for parameter estimation was performed for the constants κ, φ, and ρ. Thus, the analysis of the constants k, b, and F requires that one of these values has to be fixed so the other two can be inferred. The previous discussion about the adhesion constant considers that the elasticity modulus is not altered when the integrin concentration increases, as suggested by Mi et al. [26], and this assumption can mathematically alter the results found about the adhesion constant. If the mathematical model allowed regression for the actual constants k, b, and F, this assumption would not need to be made and the role of TNF-α on adhesion and adhesion on migration according to the proposed model could be more precisely discussed.

Considering, for example, that the elasticity modulus would change with the introduction of TNF-α, there is the possibility that the adhesion constant would increase with the TNF-α, as expected. If the elasticity modulus increases with TNF-α, by a factor of at least 2.1, the adhesion constant would increase as well. In Figure 5, one can see the values of adhesion constant for different values of elasticity modulus, considering their ratio $\kappa = 219.92\ \mu$m^2 h^{-1} obtained with the nonlinear regression and shown in Table 1, for TNF-α. For values of elasticity modulus k greater than 92.37 nN, the adhesion constant b has values greater than the control situation, 0.42 h nN μm^{-2}. The adhesion constant is, on this model, related to the adhesion between the cells and the surface. It does not consider, however, the adhesion between cells observed on collective cell migration [23]. The elasticity modulus, on the other hand, could be related to the adhesion between cells on the layer, since it relates the force that is being applied and the deformation on the layer, as it is established on (4). If the TNF-α affects the adhesion between cells, as well as the adhesion between the cells and the surface, this could mean that the elasticity modulus would change with TNF-α, when compared to the control situation.

Table 1 shows there was a reduction in the growth rate when TNF-α was introduced. The role of TNF-α on cancer cell proliferation is still paradoxal [33]. In the present work, proliferation rate of melanoma cells decreased with the introduction of TNF-α. Kuninaka et al. [34] showed that TNF-α inhibited the growth of tumor cells and Marques [8] observed a reduction in C8161 cell viability in TNF-α-treated cells. In this proposed model, the proliferation rate accounts for both increase and decrease in the population cell number. Therefore, the results are in accordance with the results shown by Kuninaka et al. [34] and Marques [8], since both growth inhibition and cell viability reduction would lead to a decrease on the proliferation rate. Even though proliferation observed on the cells treated with TNF-α was smaller than the proliferation observed on the control

(a)

(b)

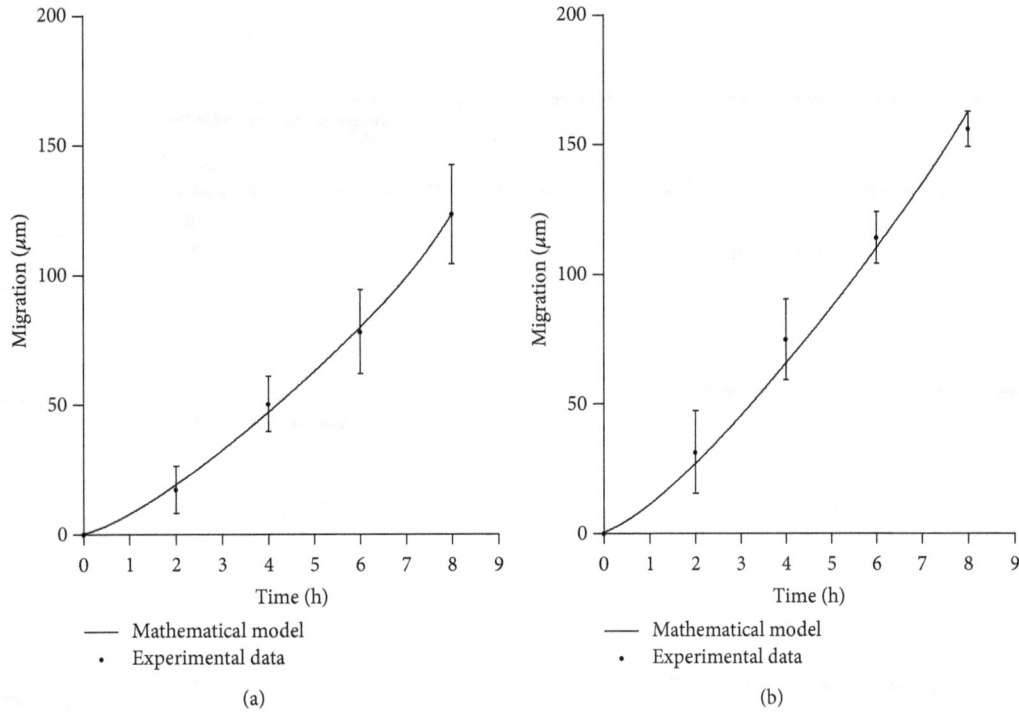

FIGURE 1: Mathematical model and experimental data after nonlinear regression. Curve obtained with the simulation of the mathematical model after nonlinear regression using experimental data from C8161 cell line on control situation (a), with $R^2 = 0.89$, and with TNF-α (b), with $R^2 = 0.92$. Experimental data are represented as mean ± standard deviation, $n = 7$.

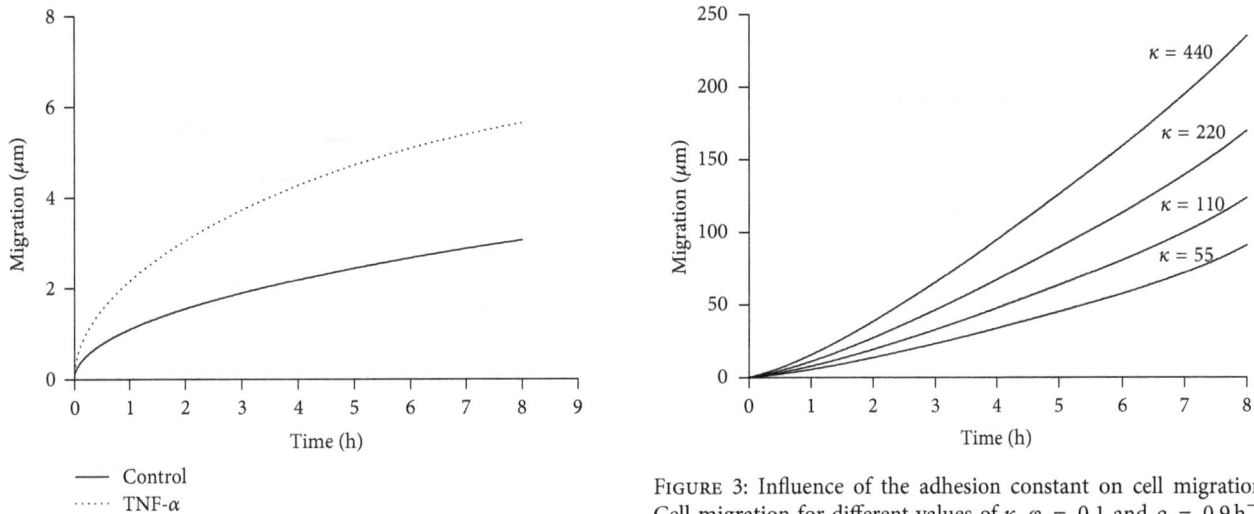

FIGURE 2: Migration due to deformation. Simulation of the model obtained for the hypothetical situation in which migration would occur exclusively due to deformation. The values of κ and φ used are the ones from Table 1. $\rho = 0\,\mathrm{h}^{-1}$ for both situations: control and TNF-α.

FIGURE 3: Influence of the adhesion constant on cell migration. Cell migration for different values of κ. $\varphi = 0.1$ and $\rho = 0.9\,\mathrm{h}^{-1}$. Considering a constant elasticity modulus, cell migration decreases with an increase on adhesion. All values of κ are expressed in $\mu\mathrm{m}^2\,\mathrm{h}^{-1}$.

situation, the final migration was greater for these cells due to the greater deformation observed in Figure 2.

As observed in Figure 4, migration is, at the beginning, more dependent on deformation, becoming more dependent

on proliferation after a while. At the same time, constant proliferation rate gives the migration an exponential characteristic. On "scratch wound" assays of cell migration, this is not always the case. In some of these assays, the migration curve has a saturation shape [8, 35, 36], which is not in accordance with the exponential shape observed in Figure 1. Studies suggest that the proliferation rate in "scratch wound"

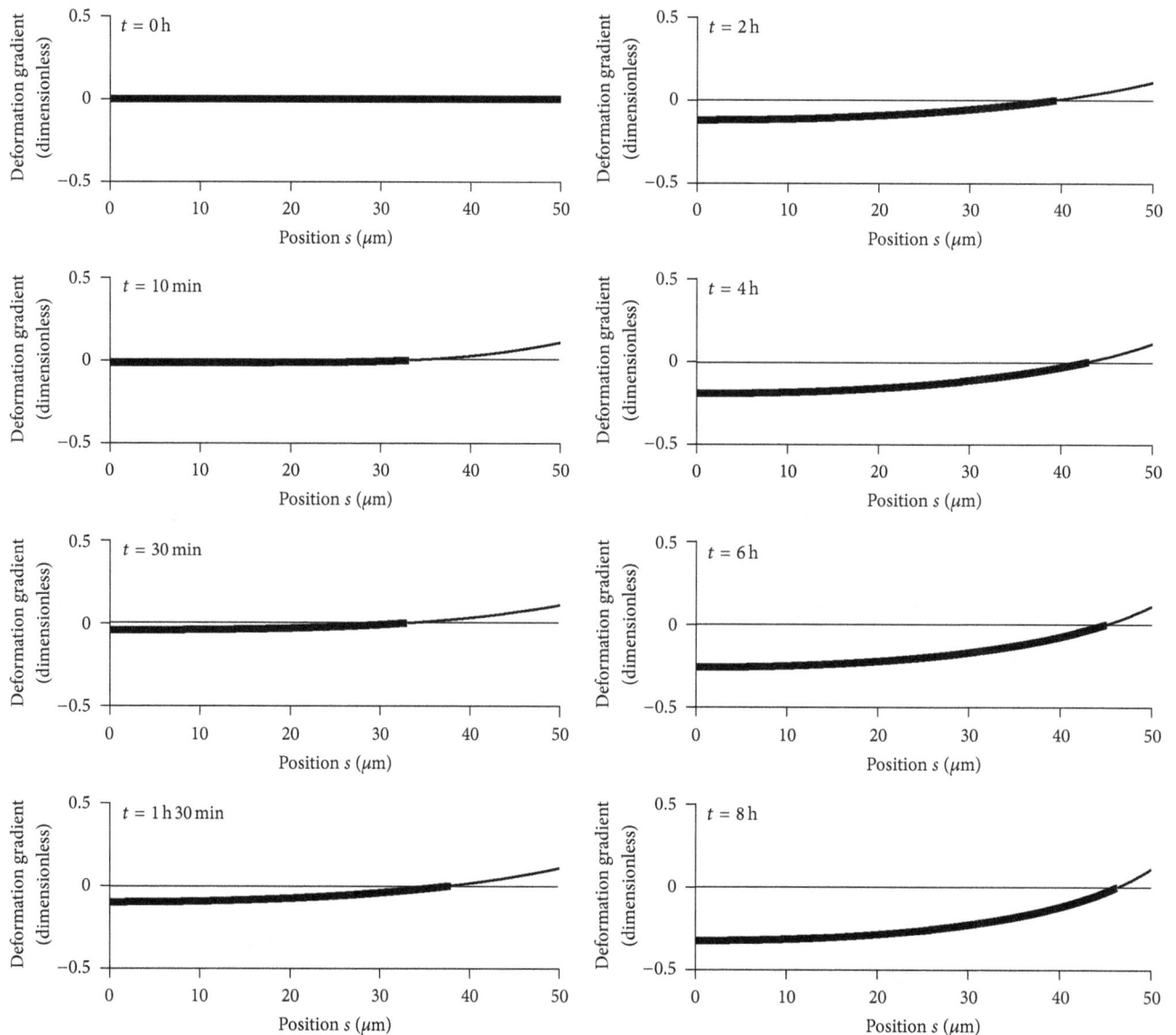

FIGURE 4: Deformation gradient of cell as a function of their position on the original layer in different time instants. Thick and thin lines indicate cells in compression and extension, respectively, except on $t = 0$ h, when the cells are in rest. On the beginning (left column), movement is dominated by deformation, causing extension on the cells near the border. After some time (right column), movement is dominated by proliferation, increasing compression on the layer as a whole. For this simulation, $\varphi = 0.1$, $\kappa = 440\,\mu m^2\,h^{-1}$, and $\rho = 0.1\,h^{-1}$.

assays can vary, depending on time and on the location on the cell layer [26]. More studies could be made to determine if the constant proliferation rate is indeed to be adequate for this kind of assay. A nonconstant proliferation rate could also alter the adhesion constant values, with and without TNF-α, found with regression. This could be another hypothesis for the differences between model and experimental results discussed previously.

Although the numerical method used to solve the model is the one proposed by Mi et al. [26] and the results are mostly in accordance with experimental values found in the literature, as discussed previously, it is important to analyze the influence of discretization on the obtained results. The analysis was performed according to the methodology proposed by Smith and Weaver [27], and, for the limits of this

simulation, the greater error found was of less than 2% on the migration curve.

5. Conclusion

A collective cell migration model was used to simulate melanoma cell migration in a "scratch wound" assay. The model takes into consideration aspects of collective cell migration, such as the adhesion between cells on the cell layer, which is not the case for the most part of current tumor growth models, based on simple diffusion process. With some exceptions, great part of tumor growth models is nondimensionalised, which does not allow quantitative analysis. In this work, a dimensionalised model was implemented and calibrated based on the experimental data, resulting in parameters that

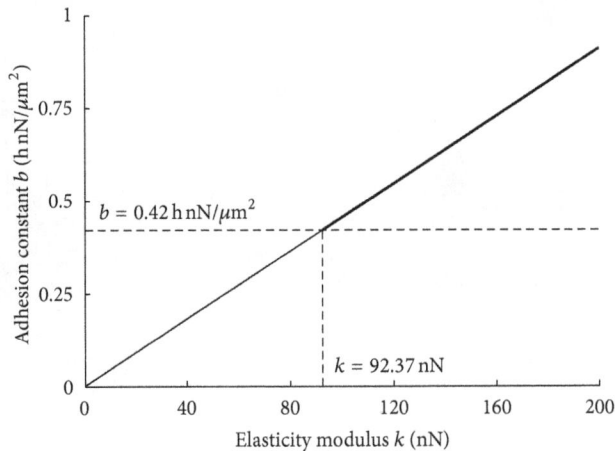

FIGURE 5: Adhesion constant for different values of elasticity modulus, considering their ratio $\kappa = 219.92\ \mu m^2\ h^{-1}$ obtained with the nonlinear regression and showed in Table 1, for TNF-α. The thick line shows values of adhesion constant that are greater than the value of the control adhesion constant ($0.42\ h\ nN\ \mu m^{-2}$). This happens for values of elasticity modulus greater than 92.37 nN.

have values comparable to experimental work, in most cases. The main differences found, involving the adhesion constant and migration with the introduction of TNF-α, could be related to the mathematical model itself or the proliferation rate used. These differences would not happen in case the TNF-α would affect and increase the elasticity modulus of the layer. Further analysis on the proliferation rate and a model that allowed for regression directly of the adhesion constant and the elasticity modulus could provide more insights on the differences found.

Acknowledgment

The authors thank CNPq (National Counsel of Technological and Scientific Development, Brazil) for the financial support.

References

[1] American Cancer Society, "Melanoma Skin Cancer Overview," 2011, http://www.cancer.org/Cancer/SkinCancer-Melanoma/index.

[2] American Cancer Society, "Cancer Facts & Figures," 2011, http://www.cancer.org/Research/CancerFactsFigures/Cancer-FactsFigures/cancer-facts-figures-2011.

[3] V. Gray-Schopfer, C. Wellbrock, and R. Marais, "Melanoma biology and new targeted therapy," *Nature*, vol. 445, no. 7130, pp. 851–857, 2007.

[4] A. Breslow, "Thickness, cross-sectional areas and depth of invasion in the prognosis of cutaneous melanoma," *Annals of Surgery*, vol. 172, no. 5, pp. 902–908, 1970.

[5] A. Mantovani, P. Allavena, A. Sica, and F. Balkwill, "Cancer-related inflammation," *Nature*, vol. 454, no. 7203, pp. 436–444, 2008.

[6] S. Ben-Eliyahu, "The promotion of tumor metastasis by surgery and stress: immunological basis and implications for psychoneuroimmunology," *Brain, Behavior, and Immunity*, vol. 17, supplement 1, pp. S27–S36, 2003.

[7] F. Balkwill and L. M. Coussens, "Cancer: an inflammatory link," *Nature*, vol. 431, no. 7007, pp. 405–406, 2004.

[8] C. M. G. Marques, *Tissue Engineered Human Skin Models to Study the Effect of Inflammation on Melanoma Invasion*, University of Sheffield, Sheffield, UK, 2010.

[9] D. A. Lauffenburger and A. F. Horwitz, "Cell migration: a physically integrated molecular process," *Cell*, vol. 84, no. 3, pp. 359–369, 1996.

[10] A. J. Ridley, M. A. Schwartz, K. Burridge et al., "Cell migration: integrating signals from front to back," *Science*, vol. 302, no. 5651, pp. 1704–1709, 2003.

[11] P. Friedl and K. Wolf, "Tumour-cell invasion and migration: diversity and escape mechanisms," *Nature Reviews Cancer*, vol. 3, no. 5, pp. 362–374, 2003.

[12] N. Zhu, P. C. Eves, E. Katerinaki et al., "Melanoma cell attachment, invasion, and integrin expression is upregulated by tumor necrosis factor α and suppressed by α melanocyte stimulating hormone," *Journal of Investigative Dermatology*, vol. 119, no. 5, pp. 1165–1171, 2002.

[13] N. Zhu, R. Lalla, P. Eves et al., "Melanoma cell migration is upregulated by tumour necrosis factor-α and suppressed by α-melanocyte-stimulating hormone," *British Journal of Cancer*, vol. 90, no. 7, pp. 1457–1463, 2004.

[14] E. Katerinaki, J. W. Haycock, R. Lalla et al., "Sodium salicylate inhibits TNF-α-induced NF-κB activation, cell migration, invasion and ICAM-1 expression in human melanoma cells," *Melanoma Research*, vol. 16, no. 1, pp. 11–22, 2006.

[15] M. Redpath, C. M. G. Marques, C. Dibden, A. Waddon, R. Lalla, and S. MacNeil, "Ibuprofen and hydrogel-released ibuprofen in the reduction of inflammation-induced migration in melanoma cells," *British Journal of Dermatology*, vol. 161, no. 1, pp. 25–33, 2009.

[16] I. Cantón, P. C. Eves, M. Szabo et al., "Tumor necrosis factor α increases and α-melanocyte-stimulating hormone reduces uveal melanoma invasion through fibronectin," *Journal of Investigative Dermatology*, vol. 121, no. 3, pp. 557–563, 2003.

[17] J. H. Kunishige, D. G. Brodland, and J. A. Zitelli, "Surgical margins for melanoma in situ," *Journal of the American Academy of Dermatology*, vol. 66, no. 3, pp. 438–444, 2012.

[18] A. Anderson, M. Chaplain, E. Newman, R. Steele, and A. Thompson, "Mathematical modelling of tumour invasion and metastasis," *Journal of Theoretical Medicine*, vol. 2, no. 2, pp. 129–151, 2000.

[19] A. R. A. Anderson, "A hybrid mathematical model of solid tumour invasion: the importance of cell adhesion," *Mathematical Medicine and Biology*, vol. 22, no. 2, pp. 163–186, 2005.

[20] P. Ciarletta, L. Foret, and M. B. Amar, "The radial growth phase of malignant melanoma: multi-phase modelling, numerical simulations and linear stability analysis," *Journal of the Royal Society Interface*, vol. 8, no. 56, pp. 345–368, 2011.

[21] S. Eikenberry, C. Thalhauser, and Y. Kuang, "Tumor-immune interaction, surgical treatment, and cancer recurrence in a mathematical model of melanoma," *PLoS Computational Biology*, vol. 5, no. 4, Article ID e1000362, 2009.

[22] S. Tohya, A. Mochizuki, S. Imayama, and Y. Iwasa, "On rugged shape of skin tumor (basal cell carcinoma)," *Journal of Theoretical Biology*, vol. 194, no. 1, pp. 65–78, 1998.

[23] P. Friedl and D. Gilmour, "Collective cell migration in morphogenesis, regeneration and cancer," *Nature Reviews Molecular Cell Biology*, vol. 10, no. 7, pp. 445–457, 2009.

[24] M. A. J. Chaplain, "Multiscale mathematical modelling in biology and medicine," *IMA Journal of Applied Mathematics*, vol. 76, no. 3, pp. 371–388, 2011.

[25] M. L. Wynn, P. M. Kulesa, and S. Schnell, "Computational modelling of cell chain migration reveals mechanisms that sustain follow-the-leader behaviour," *Journal of the Royal Society, Interface*, vol. 9, no. 72, pp. 1576–1588, 2012.

[26] Q. Mi, D. Swigon, B. Rivière, S. Cetin, Y. Vodovotz, and D. J. Hackamz, "One-dimensional elastic continuum model of enterocyte layer migration," *Biophysical Journal*, vol. 93, no. 11, pp. 3745–3752, 2007.

[27] K. C. Smith and J. C. Weaver, "Electrodiffusion of molecules in aqueous media: a robust, discretized description for electroporation and other transport phenomena," *IEEE Transactions on Bio-Medical Engineering*, vol. 59, no. 6, pp. 1514–1522, 2012.

[28] H. Lyng, O. Haraldseth, and E. K. Rofstad, "Measurement of cell density and necrotic fraction in human melanoma xenografts by diffusion weighted magnetic resonance imaging," *Magnetic Resonance in Medicine*, vol. 43, no. 6, pp. 828–836, 2000.

[29] R. Ananthakrishnan and A. Ehrlicher, "The forces behind cell movement," *International Journal of Biological Sciences*, vol. 3, no. 5, pp. 303–317, 2007.

[30] C. A. Brunner, A. Ehrlicher, B. Kohlstrunk, D. Knebel, J. A. Käs, and M. Goegler, "Cell migration through small gaps," *European Biophysics Journal*, vol. 35, no. 8, pp. 713–719, 2006.

[31] M. Prass, K. Jacobson, A. Mogilner, and M. Radmacher, "Direct measurement of the lamellipodial protrusive force in a migrating cell," *Journal of Cell Biology*, vol. 174, no. 6, pp. 767–772, 2006.

[32] P. A. DiMilla, K. Barbee, and D. A. Lauffenburger, "Mathematical model for the effects of adhesion and mechanics on cell migration speed," *Biophysical Journal*, vol. 60, no. 1, pp. 15–37, 1991.

[33] G. M. Anderson, M. T. Nakada, and M. DeWitte, "Tumor necrosis factor-α in the pathogenesis and treatment of cancer," *Current Opinion in Pharmacology*, vol. 4, no. 4, pp. 314–320, 2004.

[34] S. Kuninaka, T. Yano, H. Yokoyama et al., "Direct influences of pro-inflammatory cytokines (IL-1β, TNF-α, IL-6) on the proliferation and cell-surface antigen expression of cancer cells," *Cytokine*, vol. 12, no. 1, pp. 8–11, 2000.

[35] A. B. Beshir, G. Ren, A. N. Magpusao, L. M. Barone, K. C. Yeung, and G. Fenteany, "Raf kinase inhibitor protein suppresses nuclear factor-κB-dependent cancer cell invasion through negative regulation of matrix metalloproteinase expression," *Cancer Letters*, vol. 299, no. 2, pp. 137–149, 2010.

[36] O. Debeir, V. Mégalizzi, N. Warzée, R. Kiss, and C. Decaestecker, "Videomicroscopic extraction of specific information on cell proliferation and migration in vitro," *Experimental Cell Research*, vol. 314, no. 16, pp. 2985–2998, 2008.

20

SAR and Computer-Aided Drug Design Approaches in the Discovery of Peroxisome Proliferator-Activated Receptor γ Activators: A Perspective

Vaibhav A. Dixit and Prasad V. Bharatam

Department of Medicinal Chemistry, National Institute of Pharmaceutical Education and Research (NIPER), S. A. S. Nagar, Punjab 160062, India

Correspondence should be addressed to Prasad V. Bharatam; pvbharatam@niper.ac.in

Academic Editor: Michele Migliore

Activators of PPARγ, Troglitazone (TGZ), Rosiglitazone (RGZ), and Pioglitazone (PGZ) were introduced for treatment of Type 2 diabetes, but TGZ and RGZ have been withdrawn from the market along with other promising leads due cardiovascular side effects and hepatotoxicity. However, the continuously improving understanding of the structure/function of PPARγ and its interactions with potential ligands maintain the importance of PPARγ as an antidiabetic target. Extensive structure activity relationship (SAR) studies have thus been performed on a variety of structural scaffolds by various research groups. Computer-aided drug discovery (CADD) approaches have also played a vital role in the search and optimization of potential lead compounds. This paper focuses on these approaches adopted for the discovery of PPARγ ligands for the treatment of Type 2 diabetes. Key concepts employed during the discovery phase, classification based on agonistic character, applications of various QSAR, pharmacophore mapping, virtual screening, molecular docking, and molecular dynamics studies are highlighted. Molecular level analysis of the dynamic nature of ligand-receptor interaction is presented for the future design of ligands with better potency and safety profiles. Recently identified mechanism of inhibition of phosphorylation of PPARγ at SER273 by ligands is reviewed as a new strategy to identify novel drug candidates.

1. Introduction to Diabetes

Diabetes is a metabolic disorder caused mainly by insulin resistance and obesity. It is now recognized as a major health problem worldwide and affects adults of working age in developing countries. WHO estimates of global prevalence are expected to increase from 171 million in 2000 to 366 million in 2030, and 21.7% (i.e., ~8 crores) of these will be Indians [1]. The chronic nature of this disease leads to metabolic complications like kidney failure and cardiac problems. Early diagnosis and controlled diet combined with physical exercise of just thirty minutes have been shown to provide control in the progression of the disease.

Increasing technological advancements and decreasing proportion of physical activities in routine life are promoting sedentary lifestyle. Thus pharmacological intervention may remain the only choice in certain group of subjects. In addition lack of proper treatment and delayed diagnosis are the two major reasons for the increased economic burden and prevalence of diabetes in the developing countries.

Diabetes is generally classified into three classes: (1) Type 1—caused by complete lack of insulin production, (2) Type 2—due to insulin resistance and ineffective downstream signaling in the cell, and (3) gestational diabetes—affects 4% of all pregnant women and is rarely fatal. Almost 90% of all cases of diabetes are Type 2 class. All these facts and figures have forced most of the governments and scientists world over to look for effective therapies, resulting in a mammoth of efforts in the discovery and development of novel drug candidates.

These efforts have been based on a variety of drug targets and have led to introduction of a few drugs in the market. These drugs and their targets are briefly mentioned in

TABLE 1: Current treatment against Type 2 diabetes mellitus.[*]

Compounds	Examples	Mechanism	Adverse effects
Secretagogues (sulfonylureas, nonsulfonylureas)	Glibenclamide, meglitinide	Increase of insulin secretion	Hypoglycaemia, hyperinsulinaemia, weight gain, and vomiting
Biguanides	Metformin	Decrease of hepatic glucose output	Diarrhoea, vomiting, and lactic acidosis
α-Glucosidase inhibitors	Acarbose miglitol, voglibose	Inhibition of carbohydrate absorption	Flatulence, diarrhoea, and abdominal pain
GLP1, GIP, and DPP IV	Exenatide, LAF-237 Liraglutide, CJ-1131,	Incretin effect improvement of β-cell function	Vomiting, nausea
Thiazolidinediones	Pioglitazone, and Rosiglitazone	PPARγ activation	Weight gain, oedema

[*]Modified from [2].

Section 2. The focus of this paper is to highlight the major SAR and CADD studies performed on PPARγ. Readers interested in other targets are suggested to consult some of the excellent recent and older reviews published on these topics [3–5]. A brief literature search shows that a large amount of work has been done for the identification and testing of novel scaffolds for antidiabetic drug discovery in the PPAR arena. A review on PPARγ ligands was published with focus on dual, pan, and SPPARMs based strategy in 2008 [6]. As discussed in the Section 3.2 a large number of crystal structure have been published for PPARγ-ligand complexes, but a thorough understanding about the links between receptor-ligand interactions and antidiabetic benefits is far from complete. Thus an expert perspective and overall assessment of these efforts are urgently required to give proper direction to these attempts.

This paper begins with a brief introduction to current therapies for Type 2 diabetes followed by PPARγ localization, structure, and its ligands (natural and synthetic). This is followed by a brief classification of the ligands based on their agonistic character. Next, in an attempt to fill the gaps in the understanding of structure and function of PPARγ and its ligands, this review is divided into sections on (i) SAR studies performed in the past twelve years. An attempt has been made to present these studies in the chronological order, but some exceptions are allowed to maintain connectivity between selected studies. Majority of these studies involved classical medicinal chemistry approach to build SAR that is to modify the substituents on a structural scaffold using mostly biochemical intuition till the desired activity/affinity is observed. (ii) Rational drug design approaches using computational methods are then discussed. In this section also a chronological order has been followed, with some exceptions, and QSAR (2D, 3D, and higher-dimensional methods), pharmacophore mapping, molecular docking, and structure-based, ligand based, and *de novo* drug design approaches employed are discussed.

Despite the large number of SAR and CADD studies reported on PPARγ agonists, none of the molecules has made it to the clinic after the introduction of TZDs. Incomplete understanding of the dynamical nature of PPARγ-ligand interactions and translation of these interactions into physiological response could be one of the major reasons for this failure. Molecular dynamics simulation studies coupled with other experimental techniques that have been utilized by some groups to bridge these gaps are discussed briefly. Role of recently identified implications of phosphorylation of PPARγ residues and resulting nonagonistic/partial agonistic character of novel ligands is highlighted in the last section.

2. Current Treatment Options for Type 2 Diabetes

The cause of insulin resistance has been traced to defects in insulin receptor (IR) function, IR-signal transduction, glucose transport and phosphorylation, glycogen synthesis, glucose oxidation, and dysregulation of fatty acid metabolism [7]. Consequently these defects are targets of current pharmacological treatments as well as potential sites for new therapies.

Figure 1 shows the structures of currently marketed and a few withdrawn drugs which form the existing armor against Type 2 diabetes (see also Table 1). The biguanides, like metformin, reduce the hepatic glucose production and also enhance muscle insulin sensitivity. Acarbose decreases gastrointestinal absorption of carbohydrates by inhibiting α-glucosidase. The sulfonylureas bind to specific receptors on the β cells of pancreas resulting in inhibition of K^+ channels leading to depolarization of cell membrane followed by exocytosis of insulin. The dipeptidyl peptidase IV inhibitors exert their antidiabetic effects by inhibiting the metabolism of glucagon-like peptide-1 (GLP-1). GLP-1 mediates its effects through transmembrane GPC receptors leading to increased insulin secretion in response to feeding. It has also been shown to enhance the differentiation, survival, and maturation of the β cells [8]. This has encouraged the development of GLP-1 analogs, also known as incretin mimetics, like exenatide, a 39-amino acid peptide with glucoregulatory properties.

Most of the above-mentioned drug molecules act as direct or indirect insulin secretagogues of moderate to low potencies. The major cause of Type 2 diabetes, a generalized insulin resistance in the body, is actually not addressed by these lines of therapy. Thiazolidinediones (TZD) were identified in 1995 to exert their antidiabetic actions by binding to PPARγ with high affinity [9]. This is the only class of molecules that decrease generalized insulin resistance in tissues like muscle

Thiazolidinediones

Acarbose

Troglitazone (TGZ)
Withdrawn

Rosiglitazone (RGZ)

Pioglitazone (PGZ)

α-glucosidase inhibitor

Sulfonylureas

Tolbutamide

Glibenclamide

Glimepiride

Glipizide

Dipeptidyl peptidase IV inhibitors

Alogliptin
NDA submitted

Linagliptin
phase III

Saxagliptin
phase III
BMS

Vildagliptin
Approved in EU

Sitagliptin
Approved by US FDA

GLP-1 Analog

H-His-Gly-Glu-Gly-Thr-Phe-Thr-Ser-Asp-Leu-Ser-Lys-Gln-
Met-Glu-Glu-Glu-Ala-Val-Arg-Leu-Phe-Ile-Glu-Trp-Leu-Lys-
Asn-Gly-Gly-Pro-Ser-Ser-Gly-Ala-Pro-Pro-Pro-Ser-NH$_2$

Exenatide

Amylin Pharmaceuticals and Eli Lilly

Biguanides

Metformin

Phenformin
Withdrawn

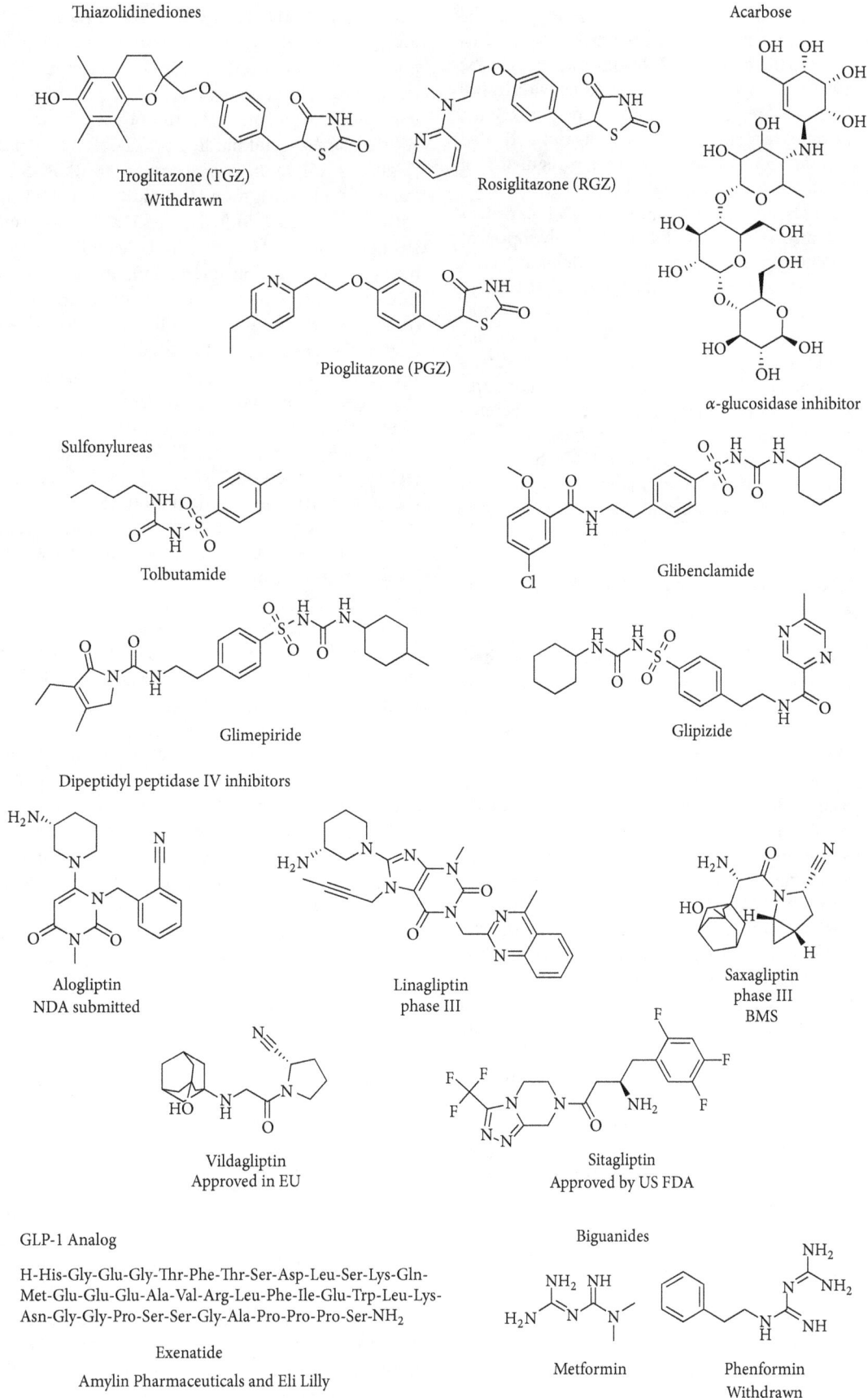

FIGURE 1: Currently marketed and a few withdrawn antidiabetic drugs.

and adipose. Rosiglitazone (RGZ, Avandia) and Pioglitazone (PGZ, Actos) are the two most widely used drugs in the treatment of diabetes. Troglitazone (TGZ, Rezulin) was also in the market since 1997, until hepatotoxicity forced its withdrawal in 2000 [10, 11]. TZDs are potent agonists of the peroxisome proliferator-activated receptor γ (PPARγ), a ligand-activated transcription factor thought to be a master regulator of adipocyte differentiation and multiple adipocyte genes. Acyl-CoA synthase/oxidase, Apolipoprotein A/C, CPTI (carnitine palmitoyl transferase I), CYP4A1/P450 IV family, lipoprotein lipase, mitochondrial 3-hydroxy-3-methylglutaryl-CoA synthase, phosphoenolpyruvate carboxykinase (PEPCK), uncoupling protein 1, and so forth are a few target proteins of PPARγ activation indicating its important role in carbohydrate and lipid metabolism. In addition to this, there is a complex feedback mechanism between the adipose tissue and insulin sensitivity. Adiponectin, a peptide hormone secreted by the adipocytes during differentiation, has been shown to decrease insulin resistance [12]. Although TZDs have been observed to increase the expression of adiponectin, it is not clear whether this is a direct result of PPAR activation or is caused by secondary effects.

3. Peroxisome Proliferator-Activated Receptor γ (PPARγ)

3.1. PPAR Location and Organization. Peroxisome proliferator-activated receptors (PPARs) belong to a super family of nuclear receptors. Phylogenetic studies suggest that the ancestral genes associated with PPAR might have appeared more than 500 million years ago during the eukaryotic evolution [13]. They are present in the cytoplasm as monomers, but upon activation by the ligand they heterodimerize with retinoid X receptor α (RXRα) and enter the nucleus to regulate transcription of a wide variety of receptors and enzymes. Three isotypes (PPARα, γ, and β/δ) have been identified, and the human-PPARγ (hPPARγ) has been located on chromosome 3 at position 3p25 close to retinoid X receptor β (RXRβ) and Thyroid hormone receptor β (TRβ) [14], while PPARα and PPARβ/δ have been assigned to chromosomes 22 and 6, respectively. For hPPARγ three isoforms have been identified (PPARγ1, PPARγ2, and PPARγ3) based on the differential use of three promoters and alternative splicing of the three $5'$-exons A1, A2, and B1 [15]. Amino acid sequences and various regions in the receptor are depicted in Figure 2.

In PPARs two main functional domains have been identified, namely, (i) DNA-binding domain (DBD) and (ii) ligand-binding domain (LBD). The DNA-binding domain is the hallmark of nuclear receptor superfamily and is formed by highly conserved two zinc finger-like motifs folded in a tertiary structure that can recognize DNA target sequences of six nucleotides. It is specific for direct repeat of two core recognition motifs, AGGTCA, spaced by one nucleotide hence called DR1. These nucleotide sequences are also known as PPAR response elements (PPREs). For CYP4A6 an extended consensus sequence for PPRE has been identified ($5'$-AACTAGGNCAAAGGTCA-$3'$). These distinguishing features of PPRE contribute to PPAR-RXR heterodimer specificity and differential regulation of transcription.

3.2. PPARγ 3D Structure. PPARγ consists of 13 α helices and four β-sheets. The overall structure is very similar to other nuclear receptors from helix H-3 to C terminus and has one extra small helix H-2$'$. Helices H-3, H-7, H-10, and H-12 along with the β-sheets arranged in antiparallel orientation constitute a large-ligand binding pocket of this nuclear receptor (Figure 3) [16]. In the crystal structure with PDB code: 2PRG, the RGZ molecule is found to straddle helix H-3 and interacts with four residues SER289, HIS323, HIS449, and TYR473 strongly. This set of interactions is generally considered as the molecular recognition interaction, and any ligand showing this set of interactions is considered as an effective agonist (though many exceptions are found). RGZ takes a U shape in this Y-shaped active site (Figure 3). Table 2 shows active site shapes and volumes of some representative cocrystal structures of important ligands with PPARγ. A search in the PDB database retrieved a large number of crystal structures (112) for PPARγ, (13) for PPARα, and (22) for PPARβ/δ (search performed on 23/11/2012). PDB codes, resolution of the crystal structures, and citation are shown in Table 3. In most of the crystal structures, agonists are bound with the LBD of PPARγ. A closer inspection and analysis of the crystal structures reveal that the active site shape and important interactions in the active site are similar for most of the agonists. The active site consists of Y-shaped binding pocket, in which the acidic head groups of the ligands interact with the H-12 helix by forming hydrogen-bonding interactions with HIS323, HIS449, and TYR473 amino acid residues.

Figure 4 shows the general pharmacophoric features present in PPARγ agonists as exemplified for RGZ. In Figure 5(a) RGZ is seen to bind in a U shape in the Y-shaped active site by forming strong hydrogen-bonding interactions with mainly polar residues (PDB code: 2PRG). The other two arms of the active site are relatively nonpolar consisting of mainly hydrophobic residues. Induced fit conformational changes in the active site shape have also been seen to accommodate larger ligands like Farglitazar leading to the formation of additional subpocket in the active site giving it an almost μ shape (PDB code: 1FM9, see Figure 5(e)). Partial agonists can bind near the H-12 helix (e.g., clofibric acid analogue, Figure 5(f)) or near the β-sheet region (e.g., BVT.13, Figure 5(g)). Endogenous ligand 15d-PGJ2 takes an almost Y shape in the active site of PPARγ (PDB code: 2ZVT, 2ZK1, and 2ZK2), thus highlighting the importance of the interactions in all the three arms of the receptor for physiological response.

Three 3D structures of DNA-RXRα-PPARγ tertiary complex were reported by Chandra et al. in 2008 [19]. The DBD and LBD of PPARγ have overall topology similar to those reported in other monomer and dimer crystal structures of PPARγ. Structures of terminal helices known to bind to the DNA were clearly seen in these heterodimer structures. Analysis of LBD of PPARγ in this heterodimer shows that it interacts with the PPRE more closely than RXRα. PPARγ resides upstream of RXRα giving a polar arrangement of these nuclear receptors on the PPRE. Helices H-7, H-9, and H-10 of each receptor form DNA-dependent contacts and

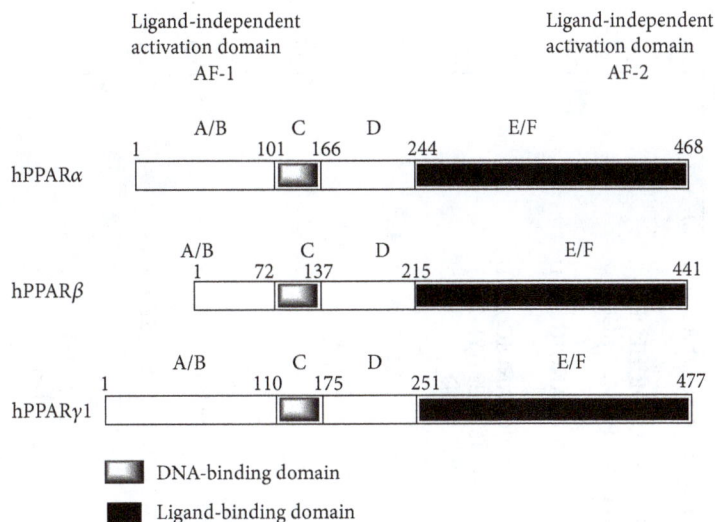

FIGURE 2: Functional domains of the PPAR family are represented schematically. Ligand-dependent activation domain (AF-1) consists of domains A/B, DNA-binding domain (C), and domain D. Ligand-dependent activation function (AF-2) consists of domains E/F and forms the ligand binding site with important molecular recognition interactions in the receptor. hPPARγ1 is the largest isoform (477 AAs). (Modified from [15]).

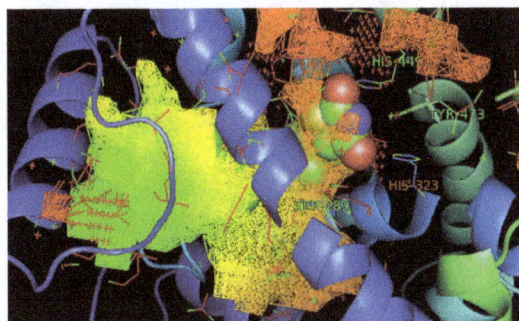

FIGURE 3: Rosiglitazone (RGZ) takes U shape in the Y-shaped active site of PPARγ (PDB code: 2PRG). The TZD ring forms hydrogen-bonding interactions with HIS323, HIS449, and TYR473 in the active site. Figure is generated using LigSite [17] and PyMol [18].

TABLE 2: Active site shape and volume for PPARγ agonists (see Figure 5).

PDB	Ligand	Active site shape	Active site volume
2PRG	RGZ (A)	Y	1703 Å^3
2PRG	PGZ (B)	Y	1703 Å^3
2PRG	Barbituric acid analogue (C)	Y	1703 Å^3
2Q59	MRL20 (D)	L	1407 Å^3
1FM9	Farglitazar (E)	μ	1815 Å^3
3CDP	Clofibric acid analogue (F)	μ	1598 Å^3
2Q5P	MRL24 (G)	L	1218 Å^3
2Q6S	BVT.13 (H)	L	1568 Å^3

lead to DBD (PPARγ)-DBD (RXRα) interaction of approximately 2,160 Å^2 solvent accessible surface area (Figure 6). The structure shows that PPARγ LBD interacts with DBD and

LBD of the RXRα and DNA. Three well understood ligands Rosiglitazone (RGZ), GW9662, and BVT.13 gave rise to a "Y-shaped" pocket. This suggests that Y-shaped ligands may fit better in the active site with higher affinity.

3.3. PPARγ Ligands

3.3.1. Natural (Endogenous) Ligands. Polyunsaturated fatty acids like linolenic acid, eicosapentaenoic acid, 9-hydroxy-10,12-octadecadienoic acid (9-HODE), 13-hydroxy-9,11-octadecadienoic acid (13-HODE), and 15-deoxy-$\Delta^{12,14}$-prostaglandin J2 (15d-PGJ2) are important endogenous ligands of PPARγ (Figure 7). They bind with lower (K_{D} ~ 2–50 μM) affinity to PPARγ. Through interaction with these fatty acids, PPARγ is thought to monitor the lipid concentrations and maintain homeostasis in the cytoplasm. The oxidized forms of prostaglandins induce adipocyte differentiation at low micromolar levels.

3.3.2. Synthetic Ligands. Since the discovery of Ciglitazone (CGZ), as effective insulin-sensitizing agent by Shoda et al., [20] many synthetic ligands of PPARγ have been identified. They have shown a wide variety of activation profiles based on receptor-binding affinity and transactivation assays. Thus, based on the dose-response curves they cac acid analogues, BVT.13 and MRL24, and so forth, (iii) dual PPARγ/α agonists, (iv) selective PPARγ modulators (SPPARMs), and the least studied (v) antagonists. A recent review has reported classification based on the agonistic activity as well as chemical group [21]. The classification based on agonistic activity is more useful for understanding the activity profiles and resulting antidiabetic effects and hence is given in the following.

Full Agonists. Full agonists like RGZ, PGZ, TGZ, and MRL20 lead to complete activation of PPARγ as shown by dose-response curves generated using transactivation assays.

TABLE 3: List of PPARγ crystal structures deposited in the PDB databank as of 23/11/2012. Resolution and primary citation for each structure are also given.

PDB ID	Resolution	Protein	Year	Ligand name	Reference
1FM9	2.10	PPARγ	2000	2-(2-BENZOYL-PHENYLAMINO)-3-(4-[2-(5-METHYL-2-PHENYL-OXAZOL-4-YL)-ETHOXY]-PHENYL)-PROPIONIC ACID	[22]
1GWX	2.50	PPARδ	1999	2-(4-(3-[1-[2-(2-CHLORO-6-FLUORO-PHENYL)-ETHYL]-3-(2,3-DICHLORO-PHENYL)-UREIDO]-PROPYL)-PHENOXY)-2-METHYL-PROPIONIC ACID	[23]
1I7G	2.20	PPARα	2001	(2S)-2-ETHOXY-3-[4-(2-(4-[(METHYLSULFONYL)OXY]PHENYL)ETHOXY)PHENYL]PROPANOIC ACID	[24]
1I7I	2.35	PPARγ	2001	(2S)-2-ETHOXY-3-[4-(2-(4-[(METHYLSULFONYL)OXY]PHENYL)ETHOXY)PHENYL]PROPANOIC ACID	[24]
1K7L	2.50	PPARα	2001	2-(1-METHYL-3-OXO-3-PHENYL-PROPYLAMINO)-3-(4-[2-(5-METHYL-2-PHENYL-OXAZOL-4-YL)-ETHOXY]-PHENYL)-PROPIONIC ACID	[25]
1KKQ	3.00	PPARα	2002	N-((2S)-2-(((1Z)-1-METHYL-3-OXO-3-[4-(TRIFLUOROMETHYL)PHENYL]PROP-1-ENYL)AMINO)-3-(4-[2-(5-METHYL-2-PHENYL-1,3-OXAZOL-4-YL)ETHOXY]PHENYL)PROPYL)PROPANAMIDE	[26]
1KNU	2.50	PPARγ	2002	(S)-3-(4-(2-CARBAZOL-9-YL-ETHOXY)-PHENYL)-2-ETHOXY-PROPIONIC ACID	[27]
1NYX	2.65	PPARγ	2003	(2S)-2-ETHOXY-3-(4-[2-(10H-PHENOXAZIN-10-YL)ETHOXY]PHENYL)PROPANOIC ACID	[28]
1PRG	2.20	PPARγ	1998		[16]
1WM0	2.90	PPARγ	2004	2-[(2,4-DICHLOROBENZOYL)AMINO]-5-(PYRIMIDIN-2-YLOXY)BENZOIC ACID	[29]
1Y0S	2.65	PPARδ	2000	(2S)-2-(4-[2-(3-[2,4-DIFLUOROPHENYL]-1-HEPTYLUREIDO)ETHYL]PHENOXY)-2-METHYLBUTYRIC ACID	[30]
1ZEO	2.50	PPARγ	2005	(2S)-(4-ISOPROPYLPHENYL)](2-METHYL-3-OXO-5,7-DIPROPYL-2,3-DIHYDRO-1,2-BENZISOXAZOL-6-YL)OXY]ACETATE	[31]
1ZGY	1.80	PPARγ	2005	2,4-THIAZOLIDINEDIONE, 5-[[4-[2-(METHYL-2-PYRIDINYLAMINO)ETHOXY]PHENYL]METHYL]-(9CL)	[32]
2ATH	2.28	PPARγ	2005	2-(5-[3-(7-PROPYL-3-TRIFLUOROMETHYLBENZO[D]ISOXAZOL-6-YLOXY)PROPOXY]INDOL-1-YL)ETHANOIC ACID	[33]
2AWH	2.00	PPARδ	2006	HEPTYL-BETA-D-GLUCOPYRANOSIDE	[34]
2B50	2.00	PPARδ	2006	HEPTYL-BETA-D-GLUCOPYRANOSIDE	[34]

TABLE 3: Continued.

PDB ID	Resolution	Protein	Year	Ligand name	Reference
2BAW	2.30	PPARδ	2006	HEPTYL-BETA-D-GLUCOPYRANOSIDE	[35]
2ENV	Solution structure	PPARδ	To be published	ZINC ION	
2F4B	2.07	PPARγ	2006	(5-(3-[(6-BENZOYL-1-PROPYL-2-NAPHTHYL)OXY]PROPOXY)-1H-INDOL-1-YL)ACETIC ACID	[36]
2FVJ	1.99	PPARγ	2006	GLYCEROL	[37]
2G0G	2.54	PPARγ	2006	3-FLUORO-N-[1-(4-FLUOROPHENYL)-3-(2-THIENYL)-1H-PYRAZOL-5-YL]BENZENESULFONAMIDE	[38]
2G0H	2.30	PPARγ	2006	N-[1-(4-FLUOROPHENYL)-3-(2-THIENYL)-1H-PYRAZOL-5-YL]-3,5-BIS(TRIFLUOROMETHYL)BENZENESULFONAMIDE	[38]
2GTK	2.10	PPARγ	2006	(2S)-3-(1-([2-(2-CHLOROPHENYL)-5-METHYL-1,3-OXAZOL-4-YL]METHYL)-1H-INDOL-5-YL)-2-ETHOXYPROPANOIC ACID	[39]
2GWX	2.30	PPARδ	1999	3-(4-METHOXYPHENYL)-N-(PHENYLSULFONYL)-1-[3-(TRIFLUOROMETHYL)BENZYL]-1H-INDOLE-2-CARBOXAMIDE	[23]
2HFP	2.00	PPARγ	2006	[1-(3-[(6-BENZOYL-1-PROPYL-2-NAPHTHYL)OXY]PROPYL)-1H-INDOL-5-YL]OXY]ACETIC ACID	[40]
2HWQ	1.97	PPARγ	2006	2-[(1-(3-[(6-BENZOYL-1-PROPYL-2-NAPHTHYL)OXY]PROPYL)-1H-INDOL-4-YL)OXY]-2-METHYLPROPANOIC ACID	[41]
2HWR	2.34	PPARγ	2006	2-[(1-(3-[(6-BENZOYL-1-PROPYL-2-NAPHTHYL)OXY]PROPYL)-1H-INDOL-4-YL)OXY]-2-METHYLPROPANOIC ACID	[41]
2I4J	2.10	PPARγ	2007	(2R)-2-(4-(2-[1,3-BENZOXAZOL-2-YL(HEPTYL)AMINO]ETHYL)PHENOXY)-2-METHYLBUTANOIC ACID	[42]
2I4P	2.10	PPARγ	2007	(2S)-2-(4-(2-[1,3-BENZOXAZOL-2-YL(HEPTYL)AMINO]ETHYL)PHENOXY)-2-METHYLBUTANOIC ACID	[42]
2I4Z	2.25	PPARγ	2007	(2S)-2-(4-(2-[1,3-BENZOXAZOL-2-YL(HEPTYL)AMINO]ETHYL)PHENOXY)-2-METHYLBUTANOIC ACID	[42]
2J14	2.80	PPARδ	2006	(3-(4-[2-(2,4-DICHLORO-PHENOXY)-ETHYLCARBAMOYL]-5-PHENYL-ISOXAZOL-3-YL)-PHENYL)-ACETIC ACID	[43]
2NPA	2.30	PPARα	2007	(2R,3E)-2-(4-[(5-METHYL-2-PHENYL-1,3-OXAZOL-4-YL)METHOXY]BENZYL)-3-(PROPOXYIMINO)BUTANOIC ACID	[44]
2OM9	2.80	PPARγ	2007	(6AR,10AR)-3-(1,1-DIMETHYLHEPTYL)-1-HYDROXY-6,6-DIMETHYL-6A,7,10,10A-TETRAHYDRO-6H-BENZO[C]CHROMENE-9-CARBOXYLIC ACID	[45]

TABLE 3: Continued.

PDB ID	Resolution	Protein	Year	Ligand name	Reference
2P4Y	2.25	PPARγ	2008	(2R)-2-(4-CHLORO-3-([3-(6-METHOXY-1,2-BENZISOXAZOL-3-YL)-2-METHYL-6-(TRIFLUOROMETHOXY)-1H-INDOL-1-YL]METHYL)PHENOXY)PROPANOIC ACID	[46]
2P54	1.79	PPARα	2007	2-METHYL-2-(4-([(4-METHYL-2-[4-(TRIFLUOROMETHYL)PHENYL]-1,3-THIAZOL-5-YL]CARBONYL)AMINO]METHYL)PHENOXY)PROPANOIC ACID	[47]
2POB	2.30	PPARγ	2007	N-[(2S)-2-[(2-BENZOYLPHENYL)AMINO]-3-(4-[2-(5-METHYL-2-PHENYL-1,3-OXAZOL-4-YL)ETHOXY]PHENYL)PROPYL]ACETAMIDE	[48]
2PRG	2.30	PPARγ	1998	2,4-THIAZOLIDINEDIONE, 5-[[4-[2-(METHYL-2-PYRIDINYLAMINO)ETHOXY]PHENYL]METHYL]-(9CL)	[16]
2Q59	2.20	PPARγ	2007	(2S)-2-(2-([1-(4-METHOXYBENZOYL)-2-METHYL-5-(TRIFLUOROMETHOXY)-1H-INDOL-3-YL]METHYL)PHENOXY)PROPANOIC ACID	[49]
2Q5G	2.70	PPARδ	2007	[(2-(3-MORPHOLIN-4-YLPROP-1-YN-1-YL)-6-([4-(TRIFLUOROMETHYL)PHENYL]ETHYNYL)PYRIDIN-4-YL]THIO)-2,3-DIHYDRO-1H-INDEN-4-YL)OXY]ACETIC ACID	[50]
2Q5P	2.30	PPARγ	2007	(2S)-2-(3-([1-(4-METHOXYBENZOYL)-2-METHYL-5-(TRIFLUOROMETHOXY)-1H-INDOL-3-YL]METHYL)PHENOXY)PROPANOIC ACID	[49]
2Q5S	2.05	PPARγ	2007	5-CHLORO-1-(4-CHLOROBENZYL)-3-(PHENYLTHIO)-1H-INDOLE-2-CARBOXYLIC ACID	[49]
2Q61	2.20	PPARγ	2007	1-BENZYL-5-CHLORO-3-(PHENYLTHIO)-1H-INDOLE-2-CARBOXYLIC ACID	[49]
2Q6R	2.41	PPARγ	2007	5-CHLORO-1-(3-METHOXYBENZYL)-3-(PHENYLTHIO)-1H-INDOLE-2-CARBOXYLIC ACID	[49]
2Q6S	2.40	PPARγ	2007		[49]
2Q8S	2.30	PPARγ	2008	(2S)-3-(4-[3-(5-METHYL-2-PHENYL-1,3-OXAZOL-4-YL)PROPYL]PHENYL)-2-(1H-PYRROL-1-YL)PROPANOIC ACID	[51]
2QMV	Solution NMR	PPARγ	To be published		
2REW	2.35	PPARα	To be published	N,N-BIS(3-D-GLUCONAMIDOPROPYL)DEOXYCHOLAMIDE	
2VSR	2.05	PPARγ	2008	(9S,10E,12Z)-9-HYDROXYOCTADECA-10,12-DIENOIC ACID	[52]

TABLE 3: Continued.

PDB ID	Resolution	Protein	Year	Ligand name	Reference
2VST	2.35	PPARγ	2008	(9Z,11E,13S)-13-HYDROXYOCTADECA-9,11-DIENOIC ACID	[52]
2VV0	2.55	PPARγ	2008	DOCOSA-4,7,10,13,16,19-HEXAENOIC ACID	[52]
2VV1	2.20	PPARγ	2008	(4S,5E,7Z,10Z,13Z,16Z,19Z)-4-HYDROXYDOCOSA-5,7,10,13,16,19-HEXAENOIC ACID	[52]
2VV2	2.75	PPARγ	2008	(5R,6E,8Z,11Z,14Z,17Z)-5-HYDROXYICOSA-6,8,11,14,17-PENTAENOIC ACID	[52]
2VV3	2.85	PPARγ	2008	(6E,10Z,13Z,16Z,19Z)-4-OXODOCOSA-6,10,13,16,19-PENTAENOIC ACID	[52]
2VV4	2.35	PPARγ	2008	(8R,9Z,12Z)-8-HYDROXY-6-OXOOCTADECA-9,12-DIENOIC ACID	[52]
2XKW	2.02	PPARγ	To be published	(5R)-5-(4-[2-(5-ETHYLPYRIDIN-2-YL)ETHOXY]BENZYL)-1,3-THIAZOLIDINE-2,4-DIONE	
2XYJ	2.30	PPARδ	2011	PENTAETHYLENE GLYCOL	[53]
2XYW	3.14	PPARδ	2011	3-CHLORO-6-FLUORO-N-[2-[4-[(5-PROPAN-2-YL-1,3,4-THIADIAZOL-2-YL)SULFAMOYL]PHENYL]ETHYL]-1-BENZOTHIOPHENE-2-CARBOXAMIDE	[53]
2XYX	2.70	PPARδ	2011	B-OCTYLGLUCOSIDE	[53]
2YFE	2.00	PPARγ	2012	AMORFRUTIN 1	[54]
2ZK0	2.36	PPARγ	2009		[55]
2ZK1	2.61	PPARγ	2009	(5E,14E)-11-OXOPROSTA-5,9,12,14-TETRAEN-1-OIC ACID	[55]
2ZK2	2.26	PPARγ	2009	GLUTATHIONE	[55]
2ZK3	2.58	PPARγ	2009	(5E,11E,14E)-8-OXOICOSA-5,9,11,14-TETRAENOIC ACID	[55]
2ZK4	2.57	PPARγ	2009	(5E,8E,11Z,13E)-15-OXOICOSA-5,8,11,13-TETRAENOIC ACID	[55]
2ZK5	2.45	PPARγ	2009	3-[5-(2-NITROPENT-1-EN-1-YL)FURAN-2-YL]BENZOIC ACID	[55]
2ZK6	2.41	PPARγ	2010	DIFLUORO(5-(2-[(5-OCTYL-1H-PYRROL-2-YL-KAPPAN)METHYLIDENE]-2H-PYRROL-5-YL-KAPPAN)PENTANOATO)BORON	[56]
2ZNN	2.01	PPARα	2009	(2S)-2-(4-PROPOXY-3-{[((4-[(3S,5S,7S)-TRICYCLO[3.3.1.1~3,7~]DEC-1-YL]PHENYL)CARBONYL)AMINO]METHYL}BENZYL)BUTANOIC ACID	[57]
2ZNO	2.40	PPARγ	2009	(2S)-2-(4-PROPOXY-3-{[((4-[(3S,5S,7S)-TRICYCLO[3.3.1.1~3,7~]DEC-1-YL]PHENYL)CARBONYL)AMINO]METHYL}BENZYL)BUTANOIC ACID	[57]
2ZNP	3.00	PPARδ	2009	HEPTYL-BETA-D-GLUCOPYRANOSIDE	[57]
2ZNQ	2.65	PPARδ	2009	(2S)-2-(3-{[(2-FLUORO-4-(TRIFLUOROMETHYL)PHENYL]CARBONYL)AMINO)METHYL]-4-METHOXYBENZYL)BUTANOIC ACID	[57]
2ZVT	1.90	PPARγ	2009	(5E,14E)-11-OXOPROSTA-5,9,12,14-TETRAEN-1-OIC ACID	[58]
3ADS	2.25	PPARγ	2010	INDOMETHACIN	[56]
3ADT	2.70	PPARγ	2010	(5-HYDROXY-1H-INDOL-3-YL)ACETIC ACID	[56]
3ADU	2.77	PPARγ	2010	(5-METHOXY-1H-INDOL-3-YL)ACETIC ACID	[56]

TABLE 3: Continued.

PDB ID	Resolution	Protein	Year	Ligand name	Reference
3ADV	2.27	PPARγ	2010	SEROTONIN	[56]
3ADW	2.07	PPARγ	2010	(5-METHOXY-1H-INDOL-3-YL)ACETIC ACID	[56]
3ADX	1.95	PPARγ	2010	INDOMETHACIN	[56]
3AN3	2.30	PPARγ	2011	(2S)-2-BENZYL-3-(4-PROPOXY-3-[[[(4-[(3S,5S,7S)-TRICYCLO[3.3.1.1~3,7~]DEC-1-YL]PHENYL]CARBONYL]AMINO]METHYL]PHENYL)PROPANOIC ACID	[59]
3AN4	2.30	PPARγ	2011	(2R)-2-BENZYL-3-(4-PROPOXY-3-[[[(4-[(3S,5S,7S)-TRICYCLO[3.3.1.1~3,7~]DEC-1-YL]PHENYL]CARBONYL]AMINO]METHYL]PHENYL)PROPANOIC ACID	[59]
3B0Q	2.10	PPARγ	To be published	(5S)-5-((6-[(2-FLUOROBENZYL)OXY]NAPHTHALEN-2-YL]METHYL)-1,3-THIAZOLIDINE-2,4-DIONE	
3B0R	2.15	PPARγ	To be published	2-CHLORO-5-NITRO-N-PHENYLBENZAMIDE	
3B1M	1.60	PPARγ	2011	(9AS)-8-ACETYL-N-[(2-ETHYLNAPHTHALEN-1-YL)METHYL]-1,7-DIHYDROXY-3-METHOXY-9A-METHYL-9-OXO-9,9A-DIHYDRODIBENZO[B,D]FURAN-4-CARBOXAMIDE	[60]
3B3K	2.60	PPARγ	2008	(2S)-2-(BIPHENYL-4-YLOXY)-3-PHENYLPROPANOIC ACID	[61]
3BC5	2.27	PPARγ	2009	(5-[3-[2-(5-METHYL-2-PHENYL-1,3-OXAZOL-4-YL)ETHOXY]BENZYL]-2-PHENYL-2H-1,2,3-TRIAZOL-4-YL)ACETIC ACID	[62]
3CDP	2.80	PPARγ	To be published	(2S)-2-(4-CHLOROPHENOXY)-3-PHENYLPROPANOIC ACID	
3CDS	2.65	PPARγ	2008	(2S)-2-(4-ETHYLPHENOXY)-3-PHENYLPROPANOIC ACID	[61]
3CS8	2.30	PPARγ	2008	2,4-THIAZOLIDINEDIONE,	[63]
3CWD	2.40	PPARγ	2008	5-[[4-[2-(METHYL-2-PYRIDINYLAMINO)ETHOXY]PHENYL]METHYL]-(9CL)	[64]
3D5F	2.20	PPARδ	To be published	(9E,12Z)-10-NITROOCTADECA-9,12-DIENOIC ACID	
3D6D	2.40	PPARγ	2008	(4-[3-(4-ACETYL-3-HYDROXY-2-PROPYLPHENOXY)PROPOXY]PHENOXY)ACETIC ACID	[61]
3DY6	2.90	PPARδ	2008	(2S)-2-(BIPHENYL-4-YLOXY)-3-PHENYLPROPANOIC ACID	[65]
3ET0	2.40	PPARγ	2009	2-((3-(3,4-DIHYDROISOQUINOLIN-2(1H)-YL]SULFONYL]PHENYL]CARBONYL]AMINO)BENZOIC ACID	[66]
3ET1	2.50	PPARα	2009	S,S-(2-HYDROXYETHYL)THIOCYSTEINE	[66]
3ET2	2.24	PPARδ	2009	3-(5-METHOXY-1-[(4-METHOXYPHENYL)SULFONYL]-1H-INDOL-3-YL)PROPANOIC ACID	[66]
				1-BUTANOL	

TABLE 3: Continued.

PDB ID	Resolution	Protein	Year	Ligand name	Reference
3ET3	1.95	PPARγ	2009	3-(5-METHOXY-1-[(4-METHOXYPHENYL)SULFONYL]-1H-INDOL-3-YL)PROPANOIC ACID	[66]
3FEI	2.40	PPARα	2009	(2S)-3-(4-([2-(4-CHLOROPHENYL)-1,3-THIAZOL-4-YL]METHOXY)-2-METHYLPHENYL)-2-ETHOXYPROPANOIC ACID	[67]
3FEJ	2.01	PPARγ	2009	(2S)-3-(4-([2-(4-CHLOROPHENYL)-1,3-THIAZOL-4-YL]METHOXY)-2-METHYLPHENYL)-2-ETHOXYPROPANOIC ACID	[67]
3FUR	2.30	PPARγ	2009	CHLORIDE ION	[68]
3G8I	2.20	PPARα	2009	(2S)-2-METHOXY-3-(4-[2-(5-METHYL-2-PHENYL-1,3-OXAZOL-4-YL)ETHOXY]-1-BENZOTHIOPHEN-7-YL)PROPANOIC ACID	[69]
3G9E	2.30	PPARγ	2009	(2S)-2-METHOXY-3-(4-[2-(5-METHYL-2-PHENYL-1,3-OXAZOL-4-YL)ETHOXY]-1-BENZOTHIOPHEN-7-YL)PROPANOIC ACID	[69]
3GBK	2.30	PPARγ	2009	2-[(1-(3-[4-(BIPHENYL-4-YLCARBONYL)-2-PROPYLPHENOXY]PROPYL)-1,2,3,4-TETRAHYDROQUINOLIN-5-YL]OXY]-2-METHYLPROPANOIC ACID	[70]
3GWX	2.40	PPARδ	1999	5,8,11,14,17-EICOSAPENTAENOIC ACID	[23]
3GZ9	2.00	PPARδ	2009	HEPTYL-BETA-D-GLUCOPYRANOSIDE	[71]
3HO0	2.60	PPARγ	2009	(2S)-2-(4-PHENETHYLPHENOXY)-3-PHENYL-PROPANOIC ACID	[72]
3HOD	2.10	PPARγ	2009	(2S)-2-(4-BENZYLPHENOXY)-3-PHENYLPROPANOIC ACID	[72]
3IA6	2.31	PPARγ	2009	(2S)-3-(4-[3-(5-METHYL-2-PHENYL-1,3-OXAZOL-4-YL)PROPYL]PHENYL)-2-(2H-1,2,3-TRIAZOL-2-YL)PROPANOIC ACID	[73]
3K8S	2.55	PPARγ	2008	2-CHLORO-N-(3-CHLORO-4-[(5-CHLORO-1,3-BENZOTHIAZOL-2-YL)SULFANYL]PHENYL)-4-(TRIFLUOROMETHYL)BENZENESULFONAMIDE	[74]
3KDT	2.70	PPARα	2010	N-(3-[(2-(4-CHLOROPHENYL)-5-METHYL-1,3-OXAZOL-4-YL]METHOXY)BENZYL)-N-(METHOXYCARBONYL)GLYCINE	[75]
3KDU	2.07	PPARα	2010	N-(3-[(2-(4-CHLOROPHENYL)-5-METHYL-1,3-OXAZOL-4-YL]METHOXY)BENZYL)-N-[(4-METHYLPHENOXY)CARBONYL]GLYCINE	[75]
3KMG	2.10	PPARγ	To be published	4'-[(2,3-DIMETHYL-5-([(1S)-1-PHENYLPROPYL]CARBAMOYL)-1H-INDOL-1-YL]METHYL]BIPHENYL-2-CARBOXYLIC ACID	
3LMP	1.90	PPARγ	2010	(9AS)-8-ACETYL-1,7-DIHYDROXY-3-METHOXY-9A-METHYL-N-(1-NAPHTHYLMETHYL)-9-OXO-9,9A-DIHYDRODIBENZO[B,D]FURAN-4-CARBOXAMIDE	[76]

TABLE 3: Continued.

PDB ID	Resolution	Protein	Year	Ligand name	Reference
3NOA	1.98	PPARγ	To be published	(5-(3-[4-(BIPHENYL-4-YLCARBONYL)-2-PROPYLPHENOXY]PROPOXY)-1H-INDOL-1-YL)ACETIC ACID	
3OSI	2.70	PPARγ	2011	S-1,2-PROPANEDIOL	[77]
3OSW	2.55	PPARγ	2011	S-1,2-PROPANEDIOL	[77]
3OZ0	3.00	PPARδ	2011	[4-(((1S)-1-[(2,4-DICHLOROPHENYL)CARBAMOYL]-1,3-DIHYDRO-2H-ISOINDOL-2-YL)METHYL]-2-METHYLPHENOXY]ACETIC ACID	[78]
3PBA	2.30	PPARγ	2011	2,6-DIBROMO-4-[2-(3,5-DIBROMO-4-HYDROXYPHENYL)PROPAN-2-YL]PHENYL HYDROGEN SULFATE	[79]
3PEQ	2.40	PPARδ	2011	[(4-(BUTYL[2-METHYL-4'-(METHYLSULFANYL)BIPHENYL-3-YL]SULFAMOYL)NAPHTHALEN-1-YL)OXY]ACETIC ACID	[80]
3PRG	2.90	PPARγ	1998	11-(4-DIMETHYLAMINO-PHENYL)-17-HYDROXY-13-METHYL-17-PROP-1-YNYL-1,2,6,7,8,11,12,13,14,15,16,17-DODEC AHYDRO-CYCLOPENTA[A]PHENANTHREN-3-ONE	[81]
3QT0	2.50	PPARγ	To be published	5,5'-DI(PROP-2-EN-1-YL)BIPHENYL-2,2'-DIOL	
3R5N	2.00	PPARγ	2011	2-ETHYL-5,7-DIMETHYL-3-((1S)-5-[2-(1H-TETRAZOL-5-YL)PHENYL]-2,3-DIHYDRO-1H-INDEN-1-YL)-3H-IMIDAZO[4,5-B]PYRIDINE	[82]
3R8A	2.41	PPARγ	2011	2-(4-(2-[1,3-BENZOXAZOL-2-YL(HEPTYL)AMINO]ETHYL)PHENOXY)-2-METHYLPROPANOIC ACID	[83]
3R8I	2.30	PPARγ	2011	(5E)-5-[(3AS,4R,5R,6AS)-5-HYDROXY-4-[(1E,3S,4R)-3-HYDROXY-4-METHYLOCT-1-EN-6-YN-1-YL]HEXAHYDROPENTALEN-2(1H)-YLIDENE]PENTANOIC ACID	[84]
3SP6	2.21	PPARα	To be published	(5E)-5-[(3AS,4R,5R,6AS)-5-HYDROXY-4-[(1E,3S,4R)-3-HYDROXY-4-METHYLOCT-1-EN-6-YN-1-YL]HEXAHYDROPENTALEN-2(1H)-YLIDENE]PENTANOIC ACID	
3SP9	2.30	PPARδ	To be published	1-(3,4-DICHLOROBENZYL)-2-METHYL-N-[(1R)-1-PHENYLPROPYL]-1H-BENZIMIDAZOLE-5-CARBOXAMIDE	
3S9S	2.55	PPARγ	2011	NONANOIC ACID	[85]
3SZI	2.30	PPARγ	2012	(5R)-5-(3-([3-(6-METHOXY-1,2-BENZOXAZOL-3-YL)-2-OXO-2,3-DIHYDRO-1H-BENZIMIDAZOL-1-YL]METHYL]PHENYL)-5-METHYL-1,3-OXAZOLIDINE-2,4-DIONE	[86]
3TY0	2.00	PPARγ	2011	(5Z)-5-(5-BROMO-2-METHOXYBENZYLIDENE)-3-(4-METHYLBENZYL)-1,3-THIAZOLIDINE-2,4-DIONE	[87]
3T03	2.10	PPARγ	2012		[88]

TABLE 3: Continued.

PDB ID	Resolution	Protein	Year	Ligand name	Reference
3U9Q	1.52	PPARγ	2012	DECANOIC ACID	[89]
3V9T	1.65	PPARγ	2012	(9AS)-8-ACETYL-N-[(3-ETHOXYNAPHTHALEN-1-YL)METHYL]-1,7-DIHYDROXY-3-METHOXY-9A-METHYL-9-OXO-9,9A-DIHYDRODIBENZO[B,D]FURAN-4-CARBOXAMIDE	[90]
3V9V	1.60	PPARγ	2011	METHYL 3-(4-[(((9AS)-8-ACETYL-1,7-DIHYDROXY-3-METHOXY-9A-METHYL-9-OXO-9,9A-DIHYDRODIBENZO[B,D]FURAN-4-YL]CARBONYL]AMINO)METHYL]NAPHTHALEN-2-YL)PROPANOATE	[90]
3VJH	2.20	PPARγ	2012	(2S)-2-[4-METHOXY-3-([[4-(TRIFLUOROMETHYL]BENZOYL]AMINO]METHYL]BENZYL]PENTANOIC ACID	[91]
3VJI	2.61	PPARγ	2012	(2S)-2-[4-BUTOXY-3-[([4-[(3S,5S,7S)-TRICYCLO[3.3.1.1~3,7~]DEC-1-YL]BENZOYL}AMINO)METHYL]BENZYL]BUTANOIC ACID	[91]
3V9Y	2.10	PPARγ	2012	4-(4-[((((9AS)-8-ACETYL-1,7-DIHYDROXY-3-METHOXY-9A-METHYL-9-OXO-9,9A-DIHYDRODIBENZO[B,D]FURAN-4-YL]CARBONYL]AMINO)METHYL]NAPHTHALEN-2-YL)BUTANOIC ACID	[90]
3VN2	2.18	PPARγ	2012	4'-[(1,7'-DIMETHYL-2'-PROPYL-1H,3'H-2,5'-BIBENZIMIDAZOL-3'-YL]METHYL]BIPHENYL-2-CARBOXYLIC ACID	[92]
4PRG	2.90	PPARγ	1999	(+/-)(2S,5S)-3-(4-CARBOXYPHENYL)BUTYL)-2-HEPTYL-4-OXO-5-THIAZOLIDINE	[93]
4A4V	2.00	PPARγ	To be published	AMORFRUTIN 2	
4A4W	2.00	PPARγ	To be published	AMORFRUTIN B	
4F9M	1.90	PPARγ	2012	(9AS)-8-ACETYL-N-[(2-ETHYL-4-FLUORONAPHTHALEN-1-YL)METHYL]-1,7-DIHYDROXY-3-METHOXY-9A-METHYL-9-OXO-9,9A-DIHYDRODIBENZO[B,D]FURAN-4-CARBOXAMIDE	

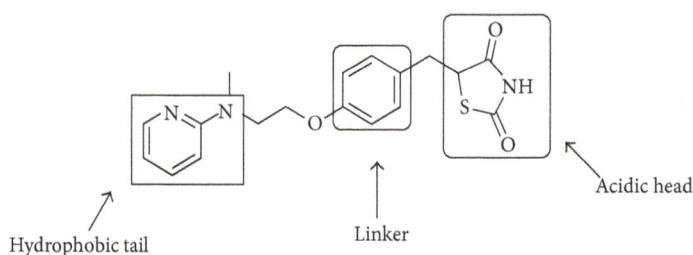

FIGURE 4: Pharmacophoric features in a PPARγ agonist Rosiglitazone (RGZ).

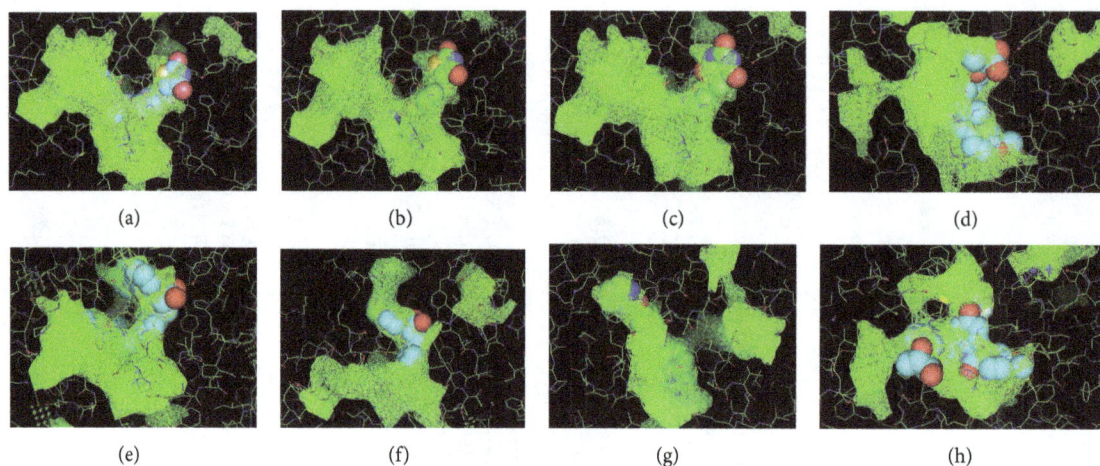

FIGURE 5: Active site shape and volumes occupied by PPARγ ligands. First row shows PPARγ full agonists: RGZ (a), PGZ (b), Barbituric acid derivative (c), and moderate agonist MRL20 (d). Second row shows PPARγ partial agonists: Farglitazar (e), clofibric acid analogue (f), BVT.13 (g), and MRL24 (h). Docked poses were used for active site analysis for PGZ and barbituric acid analogue. Calculations were performed using PocketFinder which is a modification of LigSite [17].

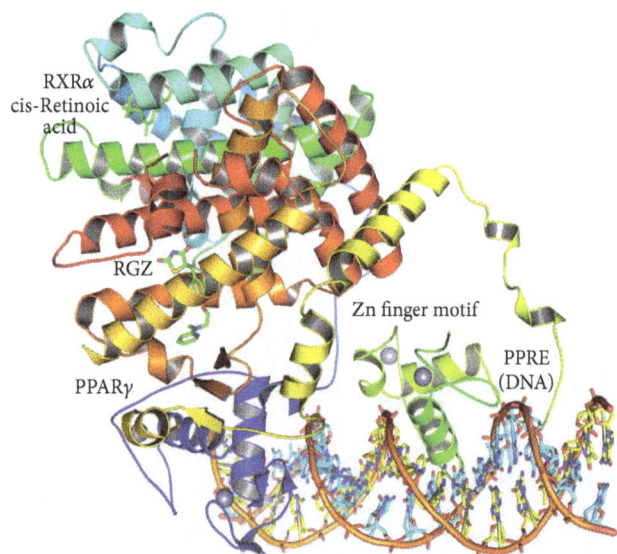

FIGURE 6: PPARγ-RXRα-DNA cocomplex crystal structure obtained with RGZ and cis-Retinoic acid bound in the active site (PDB code: 3DZY). Proximity of PPARγ LBD with RXRα LBD and PPRE (DNA) is clear. Interaction of C-terminal helices in the major grove of the DNA and Zn finger motif provides clues for graded activation of different genes by different ligands. This figure has been generated using PyMol [18].

While compounds like endogenous fatty acids and their nitrated derivatives, BVT.13, Farglitazar, MRL24, and nTZDpa do not lead to complete activation of the receptor and thus can be classified as partial agonists. Any ligand showing more than 60% of the transactivational activity shown by RGZ is classified as a full agonist. Ligands with transactivational activity near 60% are moderate agonists, but sometimes are referred as full agonists (e.g., MRL20). Partial agonists generally have less than 50% transactivational activity compared to RGZ [24, 49, 94]. Although this is a reasonably correct definition, any two ligands should be compared only when similar or identical transactivational assays have been utilized in obtaining the dose-response curves. This is due to the dependence of the observed transactivational activity on the many factors like cell type (adipose, muscle, kidney, or liver used), presence/absence of coactivators/corepressors, PPRE used, and so forth [95]. Figure 8 shows 2D structures of some full agonists. Crystallographic [16, 19] and mutation studies [46] have established the role of H-12 helix and TYR473 in the activity of full agonists.

The tyrosine amino acid residue (TYR473) present in the H-12 helix of AF-2 function forms strong hydrogen-bonding interactions with acidic head groups of full agonists as seen in Figure 3. This pocket of the active site consists of mostly polar residues (SER289, HIS323, HIS449, and TYR473), thus

Linolenic acid (**1**)

5,8,11,14,17-Icosapentaenoic acid
(eicosapentaenoic acid,**2**)

9-Hydroxy-10,12-octadecadienoic acid
(9-HODE, **3**)

13-Hydroxy-9,11-octadecadienoic acid
(13-HODE, **4**)

(Z)-7-[(1S,5E)-5-[(E)-oct-2-enylidene]-4-oxocyclopent-2-en-1-yl] hept-5-enoic acid

15-deoxy-$\Delta^{12,14}$-prostaglandin J2 (15d-PGJ2, **5**)

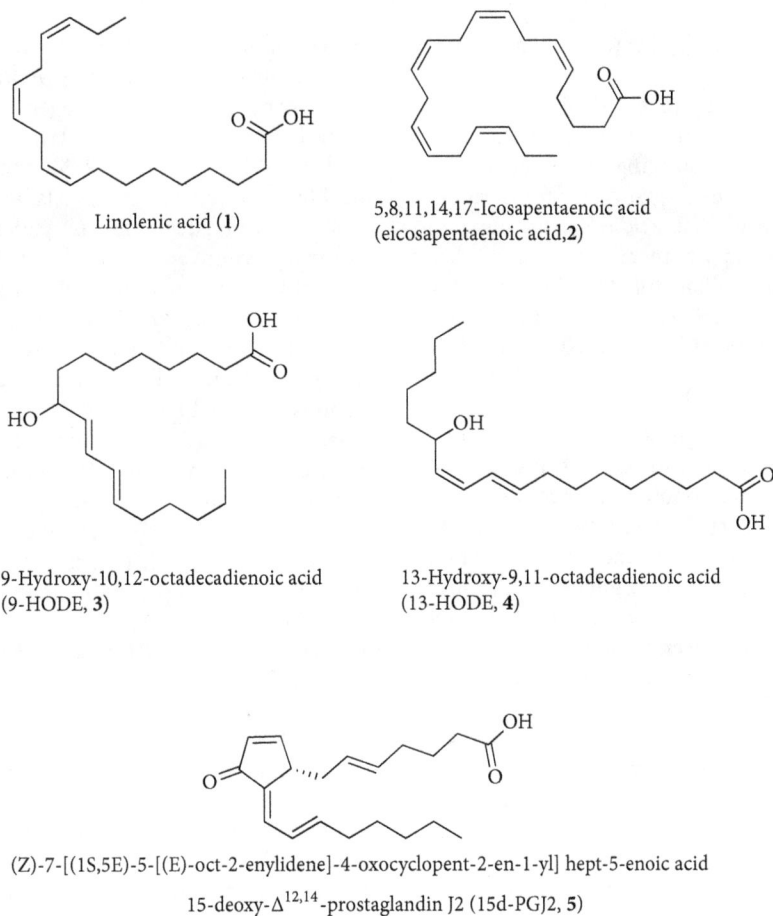

FIGURE 7: PPARγ endogenous ligands are mostly polyunsaturated fatty acids and their oxidized derivatives.

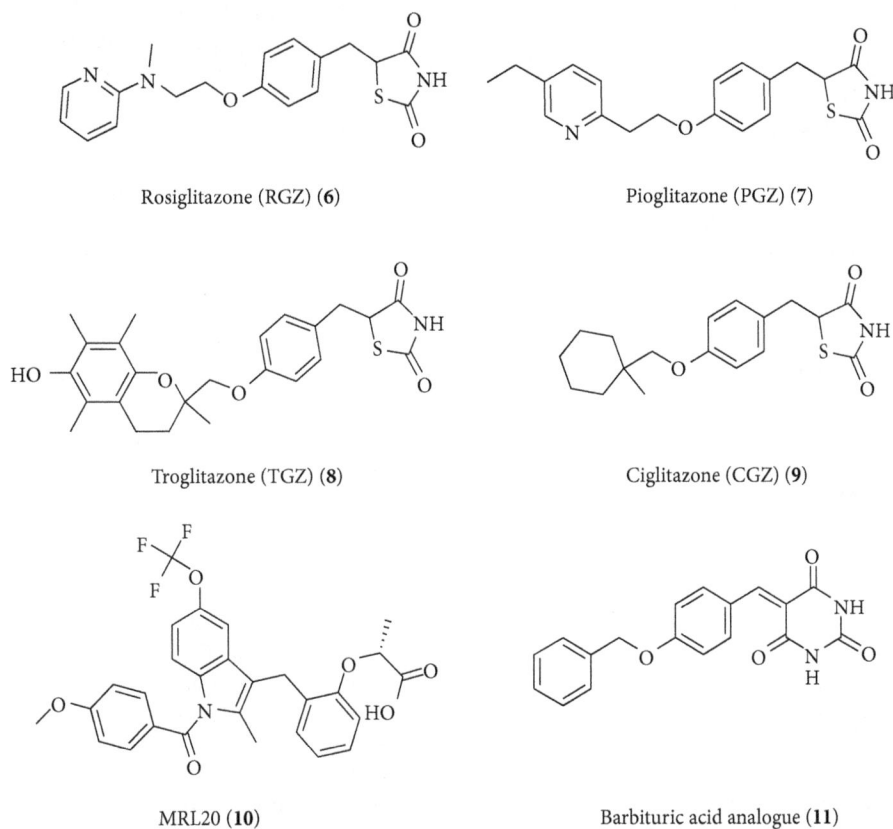

Rosiglitazone (RGZ) (**6**)

Pioglitazone (PGZ) (**7**)

Troglitazone (TGZ) (**8**)

Ciglitazone (CGZ) (**9**)

MRL20 (**10**)

Barbituric acid analogue (**11**)

FIGURE 8: PPARγ full agonists have polar acidic head groups essential for interaction with the TYR473 of H-12 helix.

interactions of full agonists with the receptor are mostly electrostatic in nature [96, 97].

Such interactions lead to significant stabilization in the fluctuations of the H-12 helix, thus stabilizing the active conformation of the receptor promoting its interaction with the coactivators and RXRα leading to gene transcription. Thus, the full agonists have polar acidic head groups and a hydrophobic tail separated by an aromatic or aliphatic linker. These three fragments constitute the pharamcophore essential for PPARγ agonistic activity (Figure 4). Endogenous ligands also have structures satisfying these pharmacophoric criteria.

Partial Agonists. Bruning et al. suggested that partial agonists (see Figure 9), in contrast to the full agonists, interact with the receptor with mostly hydrophobic interactions leading to PPAR activation that is H-12 helix independent [49]. This is evident from their radio-ligand and transactivational-binding assays. Farglitazar is known to interact with mostly hydrophobic interaction in the active site and has larger binding affinity due to the presence of extra substituent (benzophenone) that interacts in the additional subpocket near the H-12 helix.

Balaglitazone (BGZ, **12**), a partial agonist, discovered by Henriksen et al. showed lesser hemodynamic effects of fluid retention and weight gain compared to PGZ in a Phase III clinical trial [98]. PAT5A (**13**), a molecule with exocyclic double bond in the TZD ring, is a partial agonist. Treatment of PAT5A in rodents with Type 2 diabetes resulted in dose-dependent reduction in plasma glucose levels similar to RGZ along with reduced weight gain [99]. The partial agonistic character of BGZ and PAT5A points to the fact that agonistic character is not dependent on the groups present in ligands but is a function of the dynamical behavior of the H-12 helix when the ligand is bound. Thus, understanding the dynamical behavior of the AF-2 function in PPARγ is vital for future drug discovery efforts to find ligands with better pharmacological and safety profiles. Other partial agonists so far discovered generally either bind near the β-sheet region or have very weak interactions with the H-12 helix [21, 49]. These differences in the interaction features lead to recruitment of different coactivators and thus different gene expression patterns in comparison to the full agonists. For example, TZD class of compounds showed an increase in the expression of chemokine monocyte Chemoattractant protein-1 (MCP-1), whereas 15d-PGJ2 had little effect in a model of experimental glomerulonephritis (GN) in rats. TZD class of compounds also showed augmented activator protein-1 (AP-1) binding but had little effect on NF-κB, while the 15d-PGJ2 showed decrease in NF-κB without affecting AP-1 levels [95].

Dual PPARγ/α Agonists. PPARγ and PPARα show complementary effects of insulin sensitization in the adipocytes/muscles and correction of atherogenic dyslipidemia. Thus a dual agonist, combining the beneficial effects of both full and partial agonists while avoiding the side effects of weight gain, has been sought by various research groups (see Figure 10) [6, 21, 100–103]. Aleglitazar, novel α-alkoxy-β-arylpropionic acid derivative derived from SAR studies [69], has shown balanced

effects on the glucose and lipid metabolism in primate models of metabolic syndrome [104]. Acidic head group of Aleglitazar forms important hydrogen-bonding interactions with H-12 helix in both PPARγ (HIS323, HIS449, and TYR473) and PPARα (SER280, TYR314, and HIS440). It is currently in Phase III clinical trials (January 2012, NCT01042769: a study with Aleglitazar in patients with a recent acute coronary syndrome and type 2 diabetes mellitus). Aryloxy-α-methylhydrocinnamic acid derivative, LYS10929, with a thiophene tail showed insulin-sensitizing effects, decreased hyperglycemia, and improved overall lipid profiles [103]. Tesaglitazar, an α-alkoxy-propionic acid derivative, showed promise as a dual agonist [105] but was later withdrawn from a phase III clinical study due to increased serum ceratinine and decrease in glomerular filtration rates [106]. Although dual agonists demonstrated beneficial impact over selective PPAR agonists by improving both lipid and glucose homeostases, safety has been a critical issue and has led to the discontinuation of their development because of adverse toxicity profiles [101]. Molecules like Tesaglitazar and Ragaglitazar have been suspended in Phase III, and Muraglitazar has failed to get a continued FDA approval.

Selective PPARγ Modulators (SPPARMs). Selective PPARγ modulators (SPPARMs) are defined as ligands, which induce agonistic or antagonistic responses depending on the cellular context and lead to expression of specific target genes [107]. A SPPARM is different from partial agonist because the dose-response relationships for various activities are uncoupled from each other. This can be understood as resulting from tissue/organ specific responses which are not directly related to each other [21, 107]. Efforts in this direction resulted in the identification of Fmoc-L-leucine as SPPARM with most characteristics like a partial agonist [108]. Figure 11 shows 2D structures of selected SPPARMs. Metaglidasen, an enantiomer of halofenate, was found efficient at reducing glucose levels and having beneficial effects on lipid profiles. This drug candidate, a prodrug, is hydrolyzed by nonselective esterases in the plasma and converted to active metabolite. Due to uricosuric properties, this molecule was repositioned in the treatment of gout by Metabolex Inc [109]. FK-614 was found to be a structurally novel SPPARM with insulin sensitizing activities. But due to adipocyte hypertrophy its further development was halted [110]. Telmisartan, used in the treatment of hypertension, was rediscovered as a SPPARM which binds to PPARγ in a conformation different from TZDs [111]. Insulin-sensitizing effects of Telmisartan fueled its development as a combination therapy in patients with diabetes and cardiovascular complications [112]. It is currently used in the trade name MICARDIS (80 mg) for treating hypertension.

Antagonists of PPARγ. Both covalent and noncovalent antagonists of PPARγ have been identified (see Figure 12). Antagonists of PPARγ have similar insulin-sensitizing activities, but further studies are required to confirm their clinical applications. Compound GW9962 forms a covalent bond with the cysteine located on helix H-3. It has shown potent antagonistic activity against PPARγ in cell-based assays

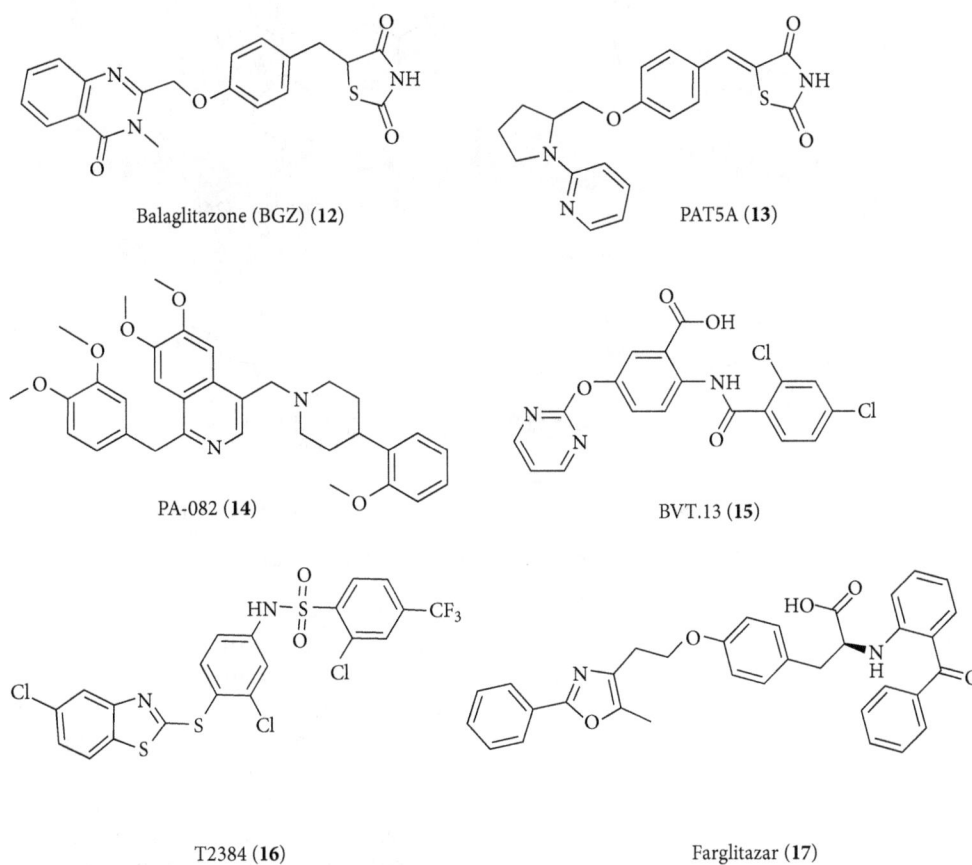

FIGURE 9: 2D structures of some representative PPARγ partial agonists, which interact with PPAR mostly by hydrophobic interactions and also have vital pharmacophoric features of PPAR agonists (Figure 4).

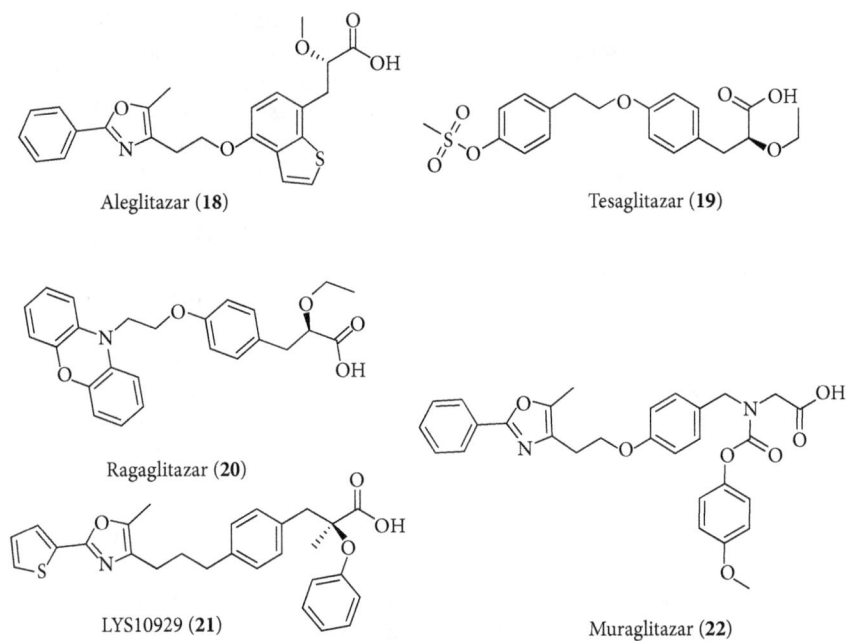

FIGURE 10: PPARα/γ dual and partial agonists.

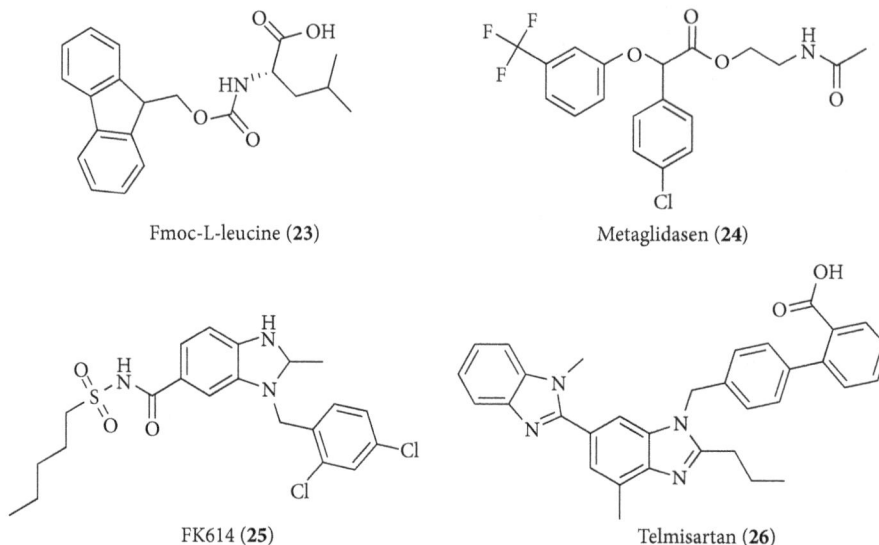

Fmoc-L-leucine (**23**)   Metaglidasen (**24**)

FK614 (**25**)   Telmisartan (**26**)

FIGURE 11: Selective PPARγ modulators (SPPARMs).

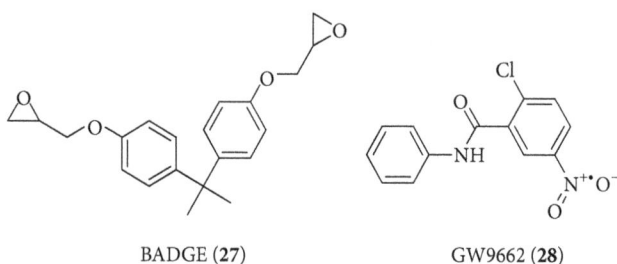

BADGE (**27**)   GW9662 (**28**)

FIGURE 12: PPARγ antagonists.

[113]. Polycarbonate-based diglycidyl ether (BADGE) is an antagonist with micromolar potency [114].

4. Structure Activity Relationship (SAR) Studies for PPARγ Ligands

With the discovery of TZDs as the potent synthetic agonists, fatty acids and their derivatives as natural ligands of PPARγ, structure activity relationship (SAR) studies were performed by many groups to understand the nature of interactions between the PPARγ and its ligands. These important SAR studies are discussed briefly in this section.

SAR between PPARγ binding affinity and antihyperglycemic effects was reported first time by Willson et al. in 1996 [115]. *In vitro* PPARγ agonistic activity correlated accurately with the *in vivo* ability of the molecules to cause antihyperglycemic effect. Difference in the *in vivo* activity profiles of compounds belonging to same chemical class having similar pharmacokinetic profiles would have most likely arisen from their differences in pharmacodynamics and thus form the intrinsic potency of the molecules. Thus results from this and similar *in vitro* analysis could logically be used to screen large libraries of molecules with confidence. This *in vitro* SAR study also established the correlation between the antidiabetic effect of TZD class of compounds and PPARγ binding affinity.

Reddy et al. reported benzyloxy derivatives of TGZ to have better euglycemic and hypolipidemic activity (see Figure 13) [116]. Introduction of ethanolamine linker and benzyl protection at the hydroxyl group of TGZ resulted in compounds with better *in vivo* glucose lowering effect in db/db mice and Wistar rats. *In vivo* analysis showed that the unsaturated analogues of TGZ are more effective in lowering the glucose levels. Transactivation assays on the other hand showed that the saturated TGZ derivatives lead to greater activation of PPARγ. Such contrasting findings in the *in vitro* and *in vivo* data were attributed to the differences in pharmacokinetic profiles and use of different salt forms of the individual drug candidates. TGZ showed toxic effects in some patients, but mechanisms of toxicity were not completely understood at that time [117]. But involvement of the hydroxyl group from the metabolic profile was becoming clear and these lead Reddy et al. to design of compounds with hydroxyl group protected by benzyl groups (**29**) [118]. In a subsequent paper Reddy et al. reported the modification of a PPARα selective agent leading to the synthesis of PPARα/γ dual agonist DRF2725 (**31**) [119]. The (-)-isomer of this compound was found to be potent in transactivation assays and showed better antidiabetic and hypolipidemic activity profile *in vivo*.

Brooks et al. reported the synthesis and dual agonistic activity of an oxazole containing phenoxypropionic acid derivative [120]. Substitution of methyl groups at α position was found to be necessary for activity. The biphenyl substitution also increased dual activation profile and gave very potent compound (**32**) as a dual PPARα/γ agonist.

Racemization in the TZD class of compounds has been well established by both experimental [121] and theoretical studies [122]. Bharatam and Khanna performed theoretical studies and proposed the importance of S-oxidation in the rapid racemization of TZD class of drugs [122]. Thus, due to this racemization administration of a pure enantiomer was not considered for this class of drugs. Haigh et al. studied

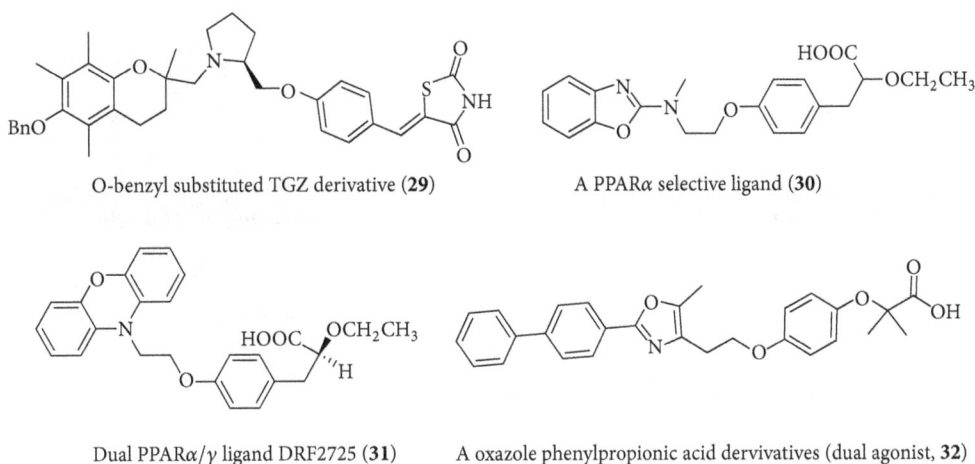

O-benzyl substituted TGZ derivative (**29**)   A PPARα selective ligand (**30**)

Dual PPARα/γ ligand DRF2725 (**31**)   A oxazole phenylpropionic acid dervivatives (dual agonist, **32**)

FIGURE 13: Benzyl protected TGZ derivatives, oxazole containing phenoxypropionic acid derivative, and DRF2725.

the effect of stereochemistry on the potency of α-methoxy-β-phenylpropanoic acids and found enzymatic racemization of R enantiomer to the S enantiomer responsible for the observed *in vivo* and *in vitro* equipotency of the two enantiomers [123].

Oguchi et al. performed molecular design, synthesis, and hypoglycemic activity studies on the imidazopyridine derivatives of TZDs [124]. In this study they developed molecules by cyclizing the N-methylaminopyridine side chain of RGZ resulting in imidazopyridine nucleus (see Figure 14). Initial design, synthesis, and biological testing in this series gave compound, 33. This compound showed potent *in vivo* hypoglycemic activity but with side effects of cardiac hypertrophy. Linkers larger than methylene showed lower activity. Substitution at the 5th-position of the imidazopyridine nucleus showed an increase in the activity with chloro, methoxy, ethoxy, benzyloxy and phenylthio groups. Especially, the methoxy substituted compound (Rivoglitazone, **34**) was found to be more potent than RGZ and showed reduced side effects compared to (**33**). Phase 3 clinical trials on Rivoglitazone were discontinued, but its applications in xerophthalmia are being considered in a Phase 2 study [21].

Yanagisawa et al., on similar lines, developed oxime containing TZD analogues (Figure 14) [125]. The biphenyl derivative (**35**) was more potent than RGZ both *in vitro* and *in vivo* assays. The authors highlighted that introduction of aromatic groups, methyl group on the oxime nitrogen, and ethylene linker are key components leading to increased activity in this series of compounds.

Novel pyrimidinone containing TZD derivatives were reported by Madhavan et al. [126]. These were derived from the modification of DRF2189 (**36**) side chain which had emerged in an earlier study by the modification of RGZ side chain [127]. PMT13 (**38**) derived from this study has shown potent antihyperglycemic activity devoid of any adverse effects in a 28-day *in vivo* study on Wistar rats (see Figure 15). The 2,4-dimethyl substituted derivative showed lower potency than PMT13. Benzyl substitution in place of the ethyl group also reduced the antihyperglycemic activity.

Analogues with 1,2,4-oxadiazolidine-3,5-dione framework in place of TZD ring were found to be less effective in producing antihyperglycemic activity.

Compound (**37**) with (2-furyl)-5-methyl substitution and 2,4-oxazolidinedione head group showed better antidiabetic effects in genetically obese and diabetic animal models (KKA[y] mice and Wistar fatty rats) [128]. Compounds with 3-arylpropyl and ethoxy spacer with *para* substitution were found to be more potent than PGZ. From this study the requirement of the spatial configuration of the three rings (oxazole, central benzene, and oxazolidinedione rings) connected with two alkyl spacers emerged (see Figure 15). Only R enantiomer of the oxazolidinedione derivatives was found to be potent activator of PPARγ. No racemization was observed under *in vivo* conditions in contrast to the TZD class of compounds; this is attributed to the oxygen atom in place of sulfur at the chiral center resulting in less stable corresponding carbanion. Asymmetric O-acetylation of the corresponding α-hydroxyvalerate with immobilized lipase was an important step in the synthesis of these compounds.

Novel 5-aryl TZD dual PPARα/γ agonists were discovered by Desai et al. in 2003 [129]. They identified that a change in the position of the substitution at the central phenyl ring converts a PPARγ selective agonist (**39**) into a dual PPARα/γ agonist (**40**).

An ethylene linker along with the *para* substitution was found to be necessary for potent PPARγ activity. Substitution of lipophilic groups on the terminal phenyl group reduced the activity, while chloro and fluoro substituents gave moderately potent dual agonists. The dual agonist, shown in Figure 16, also showed better pharmacokinetic (PK) parameters. Kim and Lee et al. reported novel pyridine and purine containing TZDs for their hypoglycemic and hypolipidemic activity in KKA[y] mice *in vivo* [130, 131]. Substitution at the 5th position of the pyridine ring resulted in compounds more potent than RGZ. Purine substituted analogues were found to be less potent than RGZ (see Figure 17).

Due to the proposed benefits, mentioned previously, with dual agonists many groups are actively developing

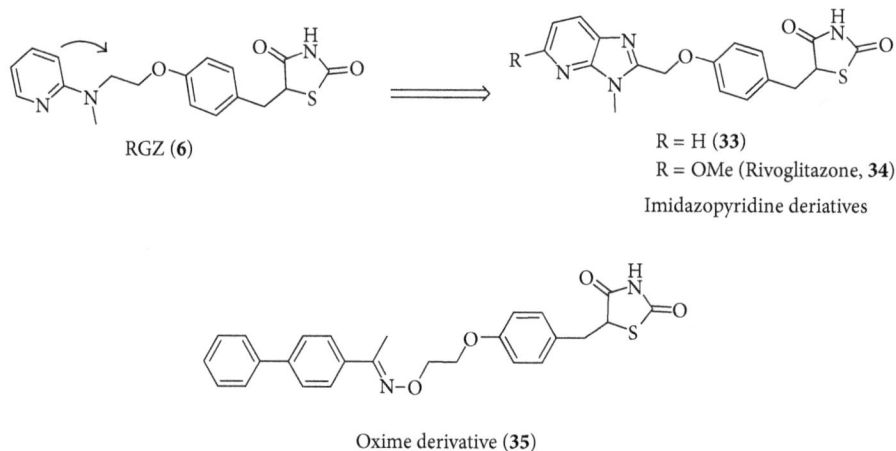

FIGURE 14: Cyclization of RGZ side chain leads to the design of imidazopyridine derivatives with hypoglycemic activity and oxime derivatives.

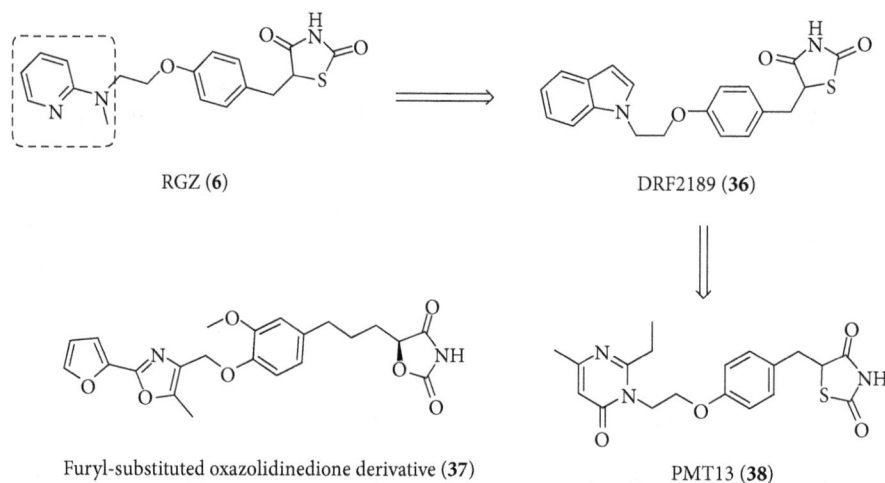

FIGURE 15: Design of pyrimidinone derivatives from RGZ and oxazolidinedione derivatives.

SAR studies for the design of dual agonists. Liu et al. combined the isobutyric acid head group of fenofibric acid (**46**), a PPARα agonist, with the lipophilic aryloxy moiety of **47** (see Figure 18) [132]. This dual ligand (**48**) was found to be more selective for PPARα and inactive at other nuclear receptors. *In vivo* the dual agonist showed significant lowering of glucose levels and had dose-dependent hypolipidemic effect. Analogues with different substitution pattern at the α position were thus prepared. Transactivation and binding studies revealed that *bis*-substitution at the aromatic ring was essential for dual activation. Extending the linker between the carboxylic acid, and the phenyl ring reduced the activity drastically. Methoxy analogue and replacement of the isoxazole ring did not significantly affect the dual activation profile.

Knowledge of the clofibric acid, aryloxyacetic acid and naphthalene containing TZDs activities leads to the design of two series of α-aryloxypropanoic acid derivatives and an β-aryl-α-oxysubstituted propanoic acid [133]. Both R and S enantiomers of the compounds were studied by transactivation assay, and only S-isomers were found to be effective in activation both PPARα and PPARγ. Substitution of the *p*-chloro substituent with more lipophilic aromatic moiety (**51**)

improved both potency and efficacy leading to compounds with full agonistic character towards PPARα and considerable activity against the PPARγ (see Figure 19). This compound was found be less effective in inducing adipocyte differentiation *in vitro* assays. Aliphatic groups lead to an increase in activity, while introduction of polar groups on the aliphatic chain reduced the activity considerably. Molecular docking analysis on the previously mentioned two compounds showed that they bind in mostly U-shaped conformation and form hydrogen bonds with key amino acids in the AF-2 function.

SAR studies on the indoleacetic acid derivatives lead to the design of dual agonists with reversed substitution pattern (see Figure 20) [41]. Initially, a PAN agonist (**52**) was converted into a PPARα selective agonist (**53**) by inverting the substitution pattern on the indoleacetic acid derivative. Adding dimethyl substitution and moving the acidic head group to the 4th or 5th position on the indole ring resulted in a PPARα/γ dual agonists (**54** and **55**). The dimethyl substitution was found to be important for PPARγ activation, as it brought the acidic head group closer to the H-12 helix leading to the formation of strong hydrogen-bonding

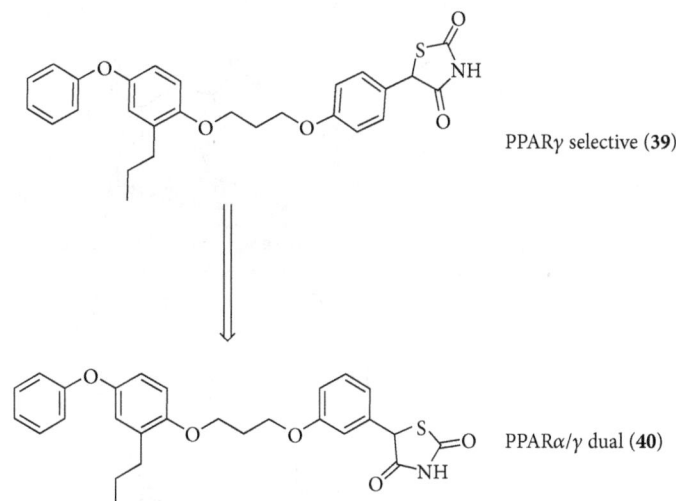

FIGURE 16: Converting a PPARγ selective ligand to PPARγ/α dual agonist.

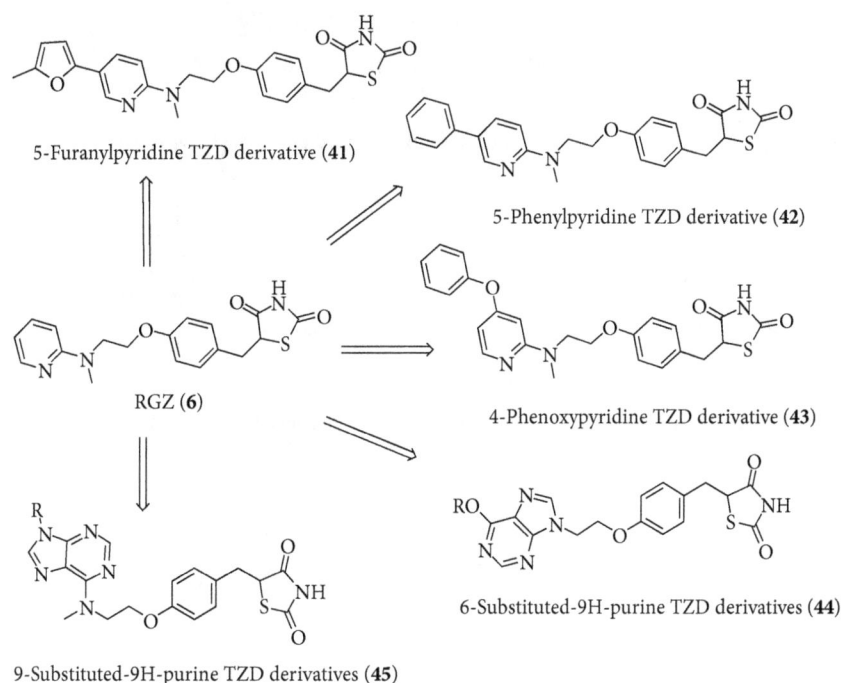

FIGURE 17: Pyridine and purine TZD derivatives derived from RGZ.

interactions with SER289, HIS323, HIS449, and TYR473 as confirmed by crystal structure analysis.

Kim et al. reported SAR studies on novel benzyl thiocarbamates as dual PPARα/γ agonists [134]. An initial study confirmed that thiocarbamates (56) are more potent than carbamates (57) (Figure 21). Aromatic terminal rings, like benzyl, gave potent compounds. Any increase or decrease in the chain length of this linker leads to decrease in activity. But bulkier substituents lead to an increase in PPARγ agonistic activity. S-isomer was found to be more active than the R-isomer towards PPARα, while both were found equally active at PPARγ. This is due to slightly larger active site volume in PPARγ in comparison to PPARα, thus both R- and S-isomers

find space inside the active site of PPARγ. But in the case of PPARα the lipophilic region in the molecule is forced to enter in hydrophilic cavity giving a lower score as confirmed by docking analysis. The presence of thiocarbamate moiety was found to be essential for dual activity as confirmed by the PPARγ selectivity of the corresponding alcohol (58).

Casimiro-Garcia et al. reported the effect of substitution at the α-position of phenylpropanoic acids on the dual PPARα/γ activation (see Figure 22) [51]. Replacement of ether moiety with acetylene, ethylene, propyl, or heteroatom-based linker lead to significant changes in the affinity and transactivation profiles. In the series with methyl group in the oxazole ring and pyrrole ring as the α-substituent, acetylene

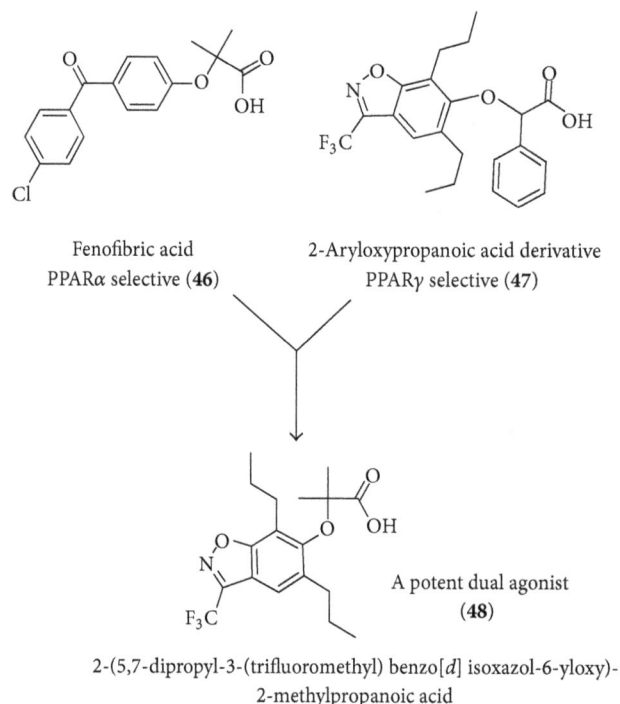

Fenofibric acid
PPARα selective (46)

2-Aryloxypropanoic acid derivative
PPARγ selective (47)

A potent dual agonist
(48)

2-(5,7-dipropyl-3-(trifluoromethyl) benzo[d] isoxazol-6-yloxy)-
2-methylpropanoic acid

FIGURE 18: Design of a dual PPARα/γ agonist from fenofibric acid and 2-aryloxypropanoic acid derivative.

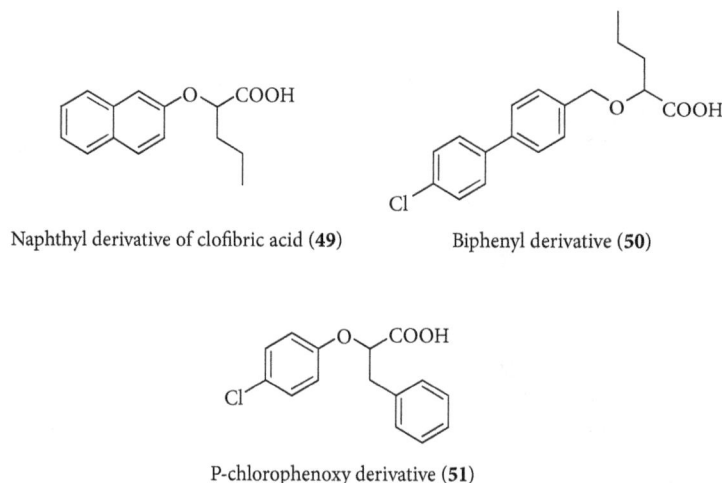

Naphthyl derivative of clofibric acid (49)

Biphenyl derivative (50)

P-chlorophenoxy derivative (51)

FIGURE 19: Dual PPARα/γ fibric acid derivatives.

linker gave nonselective ligand, while substitution with ethylene and propyl groups gave PPARγ selective compounds. These compounds showed less activation of PPARγ as compared to the pyrrole-containing compound reported earlier by GlaxoSmithKline [135]. S-isomers were found more active than the R-isomers as reported earlier for other tyrosine based compounds (59 and 60) [135, 136]. Substituents like 3-pyridinyl, 4-biphenyl, 3-biphenyl, or phenyl in place of pyrrole drastically reduced the activity at both receptors. Molecule (61) showed lower PPARα activation and was specifically selective for PPARγ. This was understood to arise due to steric interaction with TYR314 in the PPARα active site. Replacement of the ether oxygen by a nitrogen reduced PPARγ activation.

Takamura et al. have performed synthesis and biological testing on α-substituted β-phenylpropionic acid derivatives with pridin-2-ylphenyl moiety for PPAR activation and antihyperglycemic activity [137]. Oxime or amide linkers were kept in the molecules based on their earlier reported compound (37) [125]. Propyl group at α position showed potent glucose lowering activity compared to other groups like isopropyl, butyl, and phenylisopropyl (62 and 63 in Figure 23). Methylthio substitution at α position showed good dual agonistic activity. PPARγ agonistic activity could not be correlated in every molecule to its glucose lowering activity. As reported by many groups earlier, S-isomer was found to be more active in all compounds studied. The authors pointed out the fact that these compounds may be selective

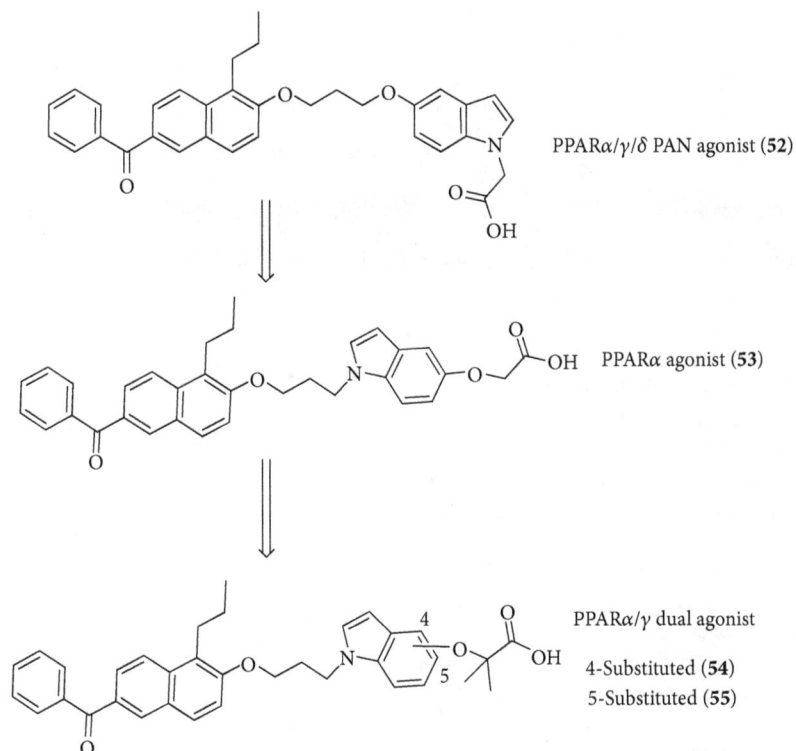

FIGURE 20: Reversal of substitution pattern in indoleacetic acid gives PPARα/γ dual agonist.

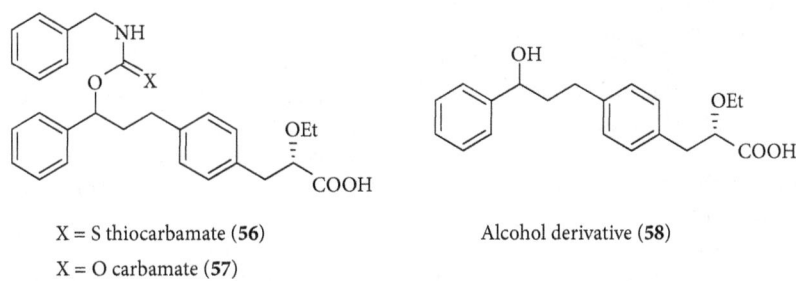

FIGURE 21: Novel benzyl thiocarbamates based Dual PPARα/γ agonists.

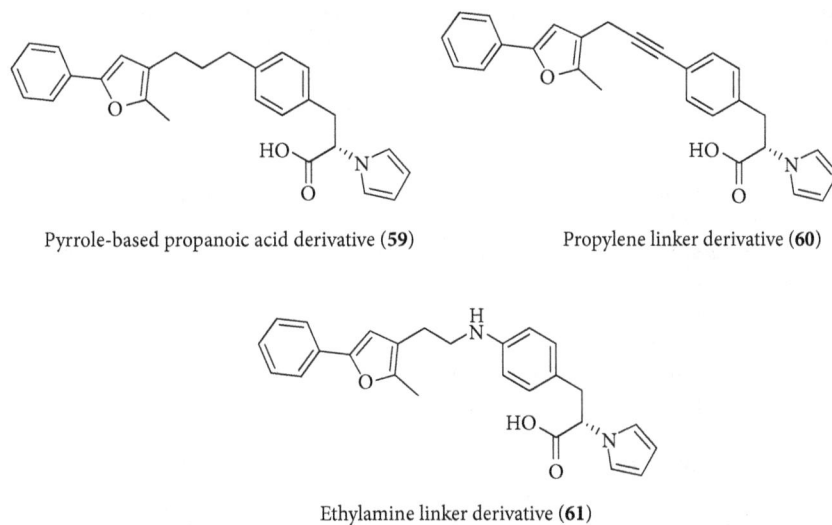

FIGURE 22: Pyrrole-based L-tyrosine derivatives with different linkers.

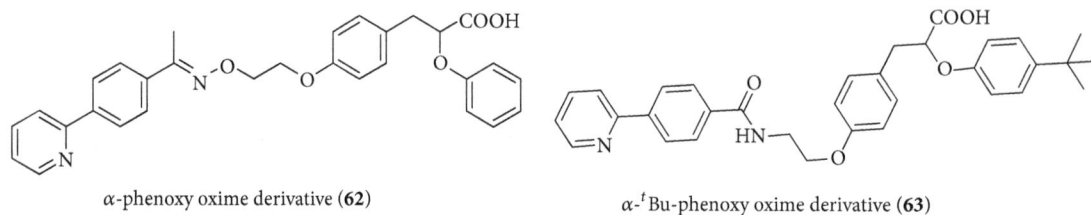

α-phenoxy oxime derivative (**62**)   α-*t*Bu-phenoxy oxime derivative (**63**)

FIGURE 23: α-substituted β-phenylpropionic acid derivatives with dual agonistic profiles.

PPARγ modulators or might activate fatty acid receptors on the pancreatic cells (GPR40/FFAR) [138]. Recently, due to the failure of PPAR agonists to reach market, the pharmaceutical industry, and academicians started looking at other targets. GPR40, a GPCR found on islet β cell membranes, is one such target known to mediate the insulin secretary effect of fatty acids [139–142].

Chromane 2-carboxylic acid derivatives were developed by Koyama et al. for discovery of novel dual PPARα/γ agonists [143]. Cyclization of fibrates was envisioned as the synthetic route leading to the compounds with chromane nucleus. Substitution at the 6th position of the chromane ring resulted in inactive compounds, while the compounds with substitution at the 7th position were found to be active dual agonists. Compounds with propyl liker were found more potent than with ethyl and methyl linkers. Propyl, hydrogen, and halogen substituents resulted in potent PPARγ activators with moderate PPARα activation. *In vitro*: binding and transactivation for affinity, *in vivo*: db/db mouse studies for antihyperglycemic, Hamster and Dog models for pharmacokinetic studies were utilized to select compound (**64**) for further studies (see Figure 24).

Parmenon et al. reported synthesis and biological evaluation of tetrahydroxyquinone derivatives for dual PPARα/γ agonistic activity [144, 145]. Di-ester- and ether-ester-based tetrahydroquinone derivatives were identified from these studies. No direct correlation between the EC_{50} (from transactivation assays) and IC_{50} values from receptor-binding studies was observed. This could be due to different binding site or interactions for the compounds under consideration and the standard (RGZ). The observed *in vitro* activity, unfortunately, did not translate into *in vivo* activity for this class of compounds.

Ohashi et al. have recently analyzed the effect of stereochemistry at the α position of the phenylpropanoic acid derivatives [146]. A reversal of enantiomeric activity was observed when a branched carbon atom is present at the β position with respect to the carbonyl group. R enantiomer was found to be more active in both phenethyl and cyclohexyl substituents, while S enantiomer was more active in the ethyl substituted compound (Figure 25). Thus authors concluded that branched or unbranched nature of the substituents determine the enantiomer selectivity. Glide docking studies were performed to support the conclusions. But further crystallographic and molecular modeling studies are required to validate these findings.

In an effort to identify CNS penetrating PPARγ agonists Virley et al. at GlaxoSmithKline have discovered

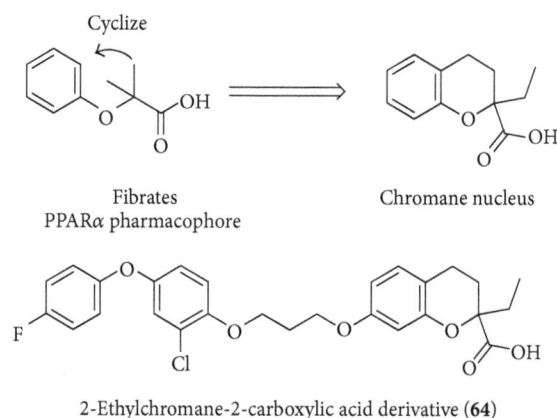

2-Ethylchromane-2-carboxylic acid derivative (**64**)

FIGURE 24: Chromane carboxylic acid derivatives developed for PPARα/γ dual activation.

GSK19971328B, a novel partial agonist. In the crystal structure benzylamide group in this molecule was found to bind in AF-2 region where TZD ring of RGZ is known to have stabilizing interactions. A series of SAR studies were performed to understand the importance of substituents on each fragment in the molecule. Thus, ethyl substituent on the benzylamide group, presence of unsubstituted C2 position in benzimidazole central ring, and fluoro substitution gave compound with most desirable pharmacological and pharmacokinetic profile.

Majority of the SAR studies discussed previously have focused on one scaffold or another while attempting to increase the potency and efficacy towards the desired receptor subtype. The activity profiles observed in the SAR studies based on *in vitro* binding studies are not always reflected as similar profiles in the *in vivo* studies due to the involvement of many factors during the absorption, distribution, and metabolism (ADME) that is the pharmacokinetics/pharmacodynamics (PK/PD) of the drug candidates. These PK/PD factors and the corresponding tissue specific (muscle and adipose) responses lead to large variability in the patient's response to the drug. The *in vitro* and *in vivo* studies provide vital information about the overall profile of the drug candidates, but they cannot provide atomic and molecular level understanding of the interactions between the drug and the macromolecular protein targets which are at the heart of the final biologically observed response. Such electronic, atomic, and molecular level information on the interaction between the drug candidate and the target macromolecule can be obtained from structure-based and computer-aided drug discovery methodologies. A review of these efforts for

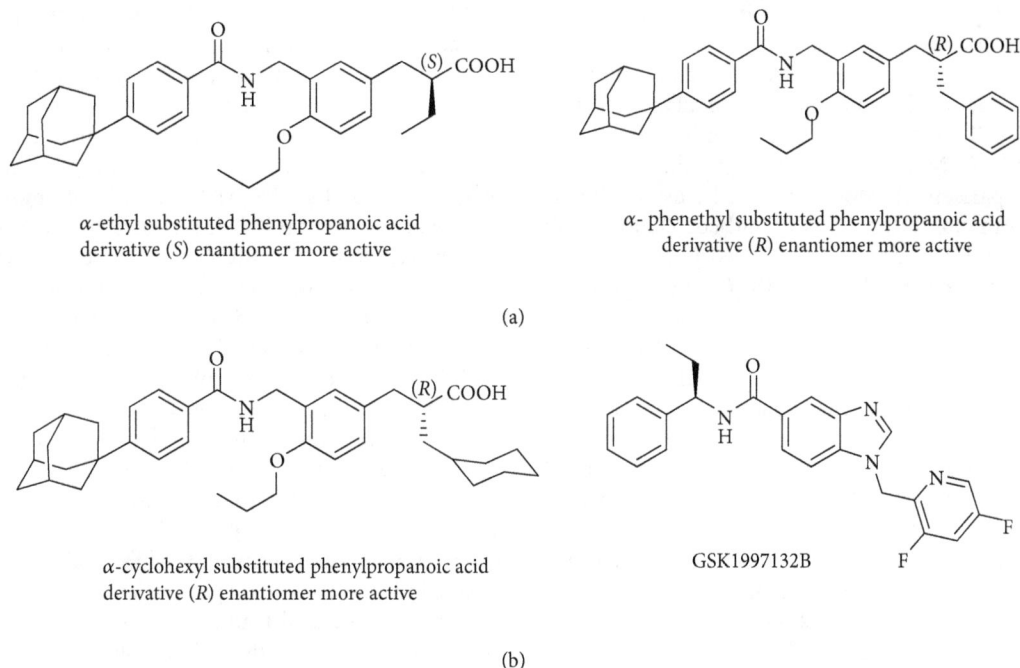

α-ethyl substituted phenylpropanoic acid
derivative (*S*) enantiomer more active

α- phenethyl substituted phenylpropanoic acid
derivative (*R*) enantiomer more active

(a)

α-cyclohexyl substituted phenylpropanoic acid
derivative (*R*) enantiomer more active

GSK1997132B

(b)

FIGURE 25: (a) Stereochemistry-activity relationship in a series of substituted phenylpropanoic acid derivatives. (b) A CNS penetrating benzimidazole derivative.

the discovery of PPARγ ligands is presented in the next section.

5. Computational Approaches for the Discovery of PPARγ Ligands

Drug discovery and development is a very time and resource demanding process in which a continuous exchange of information and knowledge takes place at the design and developmental stages. This generally involves a period of 10 to 15 years and 1.0 to 1.5 $billion (these figures tend to vary depending on the therapeutic area, but a general increase is seen with time). Thus, computational predictive tools available in the physical, chemical, and biological scientific community are extensively utilized for making quick as well as well-thought strategic decisions. In the late phases of drug discovery, for example, clinical trials, statistical tools are more often utilized to understand the hidden trends in the data. On the other end of the spectrum, where target identification, validation, molecular design, and interactions of drug candidates with targets are to be understood, computer-aided drug design (CADD) approaches are often employed [147].

CADD methods generally employ a combination of the following methodologies: (1) two-dimensional quantitative structure activity relationship (2D QSAR), (2) 3D and higher-dimensional QSAR methods, (3) pharmacophore mapping and virtual screening, (4) molecular docking in protein crystal structures (or homology models), (5) receptor-based QSAR methods, (6) receptor-based pharmacophore mapping and virtual screening, (7) *de novo* drug design, (8) molecular dynamics simulations, and (9) quantum chemical methods.

Reports making used of one or more such methodologies are described in the following.

QSAR methods based on 2D information are employed when the data set contains large variation in the chemical structures of the ligands under consideration as in the case for PPARγ [148–150]. Rücker et al. reported a 2D QSAR analysis of PPARγ ligands employing a set of molecular descriptors supplied in the program MOE. The descriptors like, atom and bond counts, connectivity indices, partial charge descriptors, pharmacophoric feature descriptors, calculated physical property descriptors and MACCS keys were used in the analysis. Data selection was based on the type of assay to derive meaningful correlation models. The receptor binding studies (pK_i) from the scintillation proximity assay and transactivation data from transient cotransfection assay were employed in the generation of models. Compounds were randomly partitioned into a training set (90%) and test set (10%). Four 2D QSAR equations were generated and thoroughly validated: (i) multiple linear regression (MLR), (ii) genetic algorithm variable selection module of MOE for receptor binding, (iii) MLR equation for gene transactivation, and (iv) activity-activity (receptor binding versus transactivation data) relationship. The authors concluded that variation in the central part of the ligand seemed to have minor importance in comparison to the other pharmacophoric features (acidic head group and hydrophobic tail). Utilizing only 2D structural features of the ligands although can allow molecules of diverse nature to be included in the analysis, it potentially leads to oversimplifications about the structure activity relationships. Thus, more robust 3D structural information about molecules can be considered while developing structure activity relationships. Efforts in this direction are presented in the following paragraphs.

QSAR methods like comparative molecular moment analysis (CoMMA) [151], comparative molecular field analysis (CoMFA) [152], molecular similarity indices in a comparative analysis (CoMSIA) [153], and adaptation of fields for molecular comparison (AFMoC) [154] make use of the 3D structural information of ligands to build correlations with biological activity. Khanna et al. have utilized a novel concept, of additivity of molecular fields using the CoMFA approach, to develop dual models for PPARα and PPARγ dual activation [100]. In this study the authors reported individual models for PPARα and PPARγ activities and a dual model by summing the *in vitro* activity data, thus generating the dual model. This dual model was shown to be superior to individual PPARα and PPARγ models in predicting the dual activation. General structure for the data set is shown in Figure 26. Individual models retained their ability to make reasonable individual activity predictions. These models were able to predict dual and selective activation for both receptors. Utility of these models in the drug design was shown by confirming the predictions of the model using molecular docking analysis and analyzing important H-bonding interactions in the active site. The authors highlighted the importance of using dual model in combination with the individual models to avoid misleading conclusions. This is because the sum of activities for two molecules can be identical in spite of having very different individual activities.

A modified, receptor-based, QSAR study on the same set of molecules was reported by Lather et al. later [155]. Volume in the active site occupied by the ligands (V_{site}) was shown as an important parameter in developing the QSAR equations. Utilizing the same dataset as used by Khanna et al. [100] they developed selective and dual models with the addition of V_{site}. Molecular descriptors like constitutional, topological (Zagreb and Balaban-type index), geometrical, electrostatic, and quantum chemical (CODESSA) were employed in this study. Balaban-type index performed better in comparison to the Zagreb index. The three models pointed out the differences in structural characteristics of PPARα and PPARγ ligands. For PPARα activity size and hydrophobicity of the ligands play a major role, while electrostatic and H-bonding interactions were found to contribute more to the PPARγ activation. The authors claimed that limitations arising from the CoMFA requirements, namely, prior alignment of 3D structures could be avoided by using their method of QSAR. The PPARγ model of Lather et al. showed that with an increase in the number of double bonds there is a decrease in the activity. This corroborates with lower activity of the endogenous PPARγ ligands which have polyunsaturated framework (Figure 26).

In the quest to find novel insulin sensitizing molecules that can avoid toxicities associated with TZD class of drugs many research groups have looked towards other chemical class with similar pharmacophoric features. A few 3D QSAR studies have been reported on such compounds. Rathi et al. have employed Apex-3D software to determine primary and secondary binding characteristics in L-tyrosine analogues necessary for PPARγ activation (Figure 26) [156].

Brown et al. have used the concept of biased chemical libraries for screening of compounds for PPAR activation [157]. A library of 480 compounds was made using a combination of three phenoxyisobutyric acid derivatives along with different amines and isocyanate derivatives to generate urea analogues. The library was screened using cell-based reporter gene assay for PPAR-GAL4 chimeric receptors. A PPARδ specific compound (GW2433, Figure 26) was identified during the screening. PPARα showed most promiscuous nature among the three receptors by binding to more than 50% of the compounds screened, while PPARγ and PPARδ showed larger selectivity profiles. The authors interpreted this result as PPARα having a special physiological role in maintaining lipid metabolism due to its presence in the liver.

A structure-based drug design strategy was employed by Kuhn et al. to identify dual PPARα/γ activators [39]. The indole-based scaffold (Figure 26) was selected from the in-house database with the hydrophobic central protein environment as a constraint while maintaining synthetic accessibility and drug-like properties. In the SAR study, effect of various structural features like position of the propionic acid chain attached to the indole scaffold, length of the linker between the indole and the oxazole ring, influence of various substituents on the activity were investigated. An increase in the size of the terminal substituents leads to an increase in the PPARα affinity, while it decreased the PPARγ affinity. These findings can be used to fine-tune the selectivity of PPAR ligands.

Scarsi et al. performed *in vitro* binding and transactivation studies on sulfonylurea class of drug molecules for potential PPARγ activation [158]. Gliquidone, Glipizide, and Nateglinide activated PPARγ at physiologically relevant concentrations. Common pharmacophoric features based on pK_a values were suggested as the basis for PPARγ activation (see Figure 27). Based on these findings and molecular docking studies the authors suggested novel molecules (e.g., **70**) by removing noninteracting nitrogen atom of the sulfonylurea group for further investigations.

Markt et al. performed pharmacophore mapping and virtual screening study on PPAR ligands [159]. Structure-based pharmacophore models (based on the active site differences) were reported for PPARα and PPARδ, while a ligand-based pharmacophore model was reported for PPARγ. Structure-based model was found less effective for PPARγ due to the small number of receptor complexes in comparison to the number of known ligands for this receptor subtype at that time. With larger number of crystal structures available now, a better receptor based pharmacophore model can be developed. Models specific for PPARα agonists, PPARγ agonists, PPARγ partial agonists, and PPARδ agonists were developed using **18**, **21**, **5**, and **7** compounds, respectively. These models were validated using a set of 357 structurally diverse sets of PPAR ligands divided into 321 actives and 36 inactives. For the PPARα and PPARδ the structure-based models were refined using the ligand-based pharmacophore models. This was done by the removal of extra hydrophobic feature form the structure based models. In the next step the authors used an in-house pharmacophore database "Inte:Ligand database" consisting of 1537 structure-based

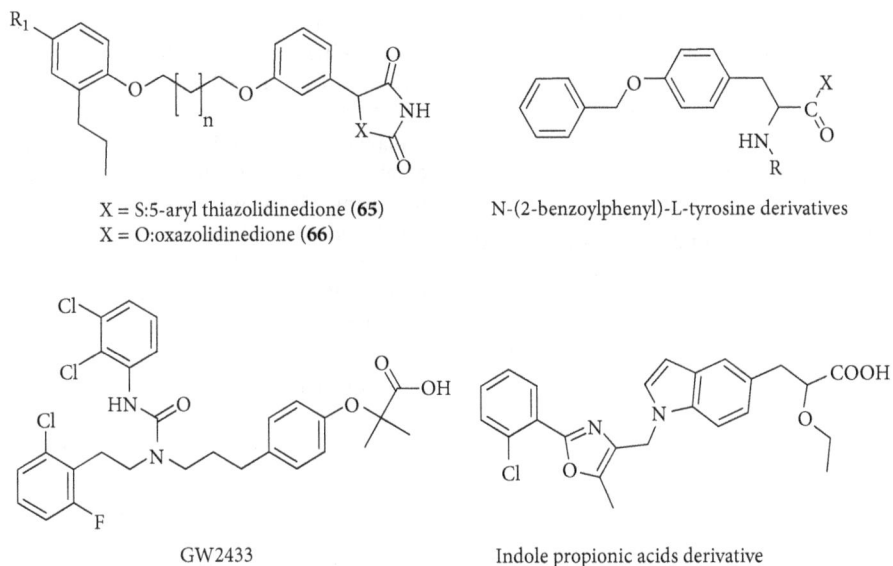

FIGURE 26: Molecules used to develop 3D CoMFA models of PPAR activity and novel PPARγ agonists discovered using QSAR and virtual screening approaches.

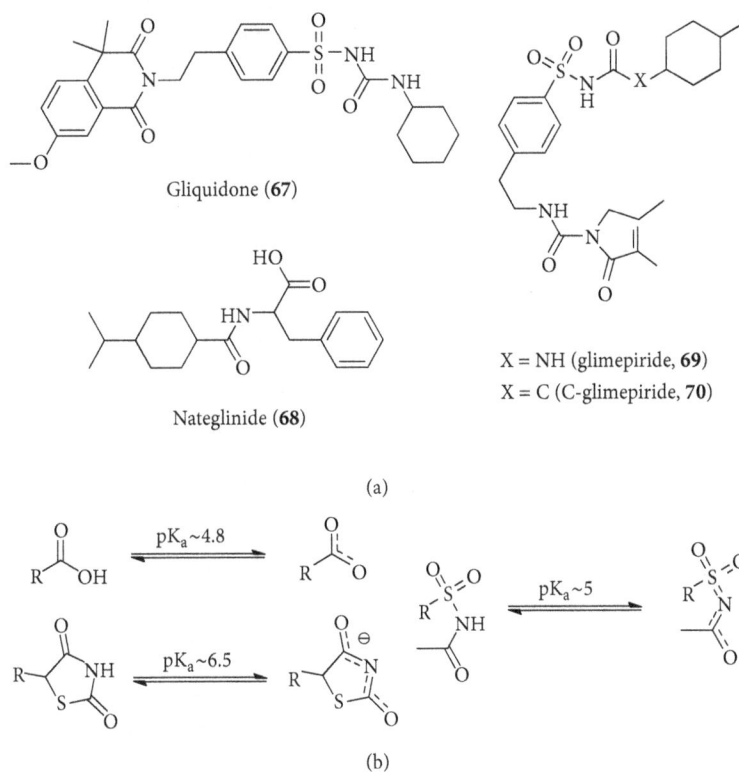

X = S:5-aryl thiazolidinedione (65)
X = O:oxazolidinedione (66)

N-(2-benzoylphenyl)-L-tyrosine derivatives

GW2433

Indole propionic acids derivative

Gliquidone (67)

Nateglinide (68)

X = NH (glimepiride, 69)
X = C (C-glimepiride, 70)

(a)

pKa~4.8

pKa~6.5

pKa~5

(b)

FIGURE 27: (a) Sulfonylureas, glinides, and N-sulfonyl carboxamides as potential PPARγ activators. (b) Pharmacophoric features common in carboxylic acids, TZDs, and sulfonamides.

models for 181 pharmacological targets for parallel screening study. Using a perl script and the target score, numbers of targets hit by the same set of ligands were identified. For one-third of the PPAR ligands PPARs were identified as the first target, while for 26% of the ligands P450 2C9 was the first target. Other protein targets identified were HRV coat protein

and only RXRβ from the rest of the nuclear receptor family. Thus, this study has proven the utility of parallel screening for determining the correct target for a set of compounds.

Giaginis et al. have analyzed correlations between lipophilic properties and the activities of PPARγ ligands [160]. A potential PPARγ ligand targeted for therapy should have,

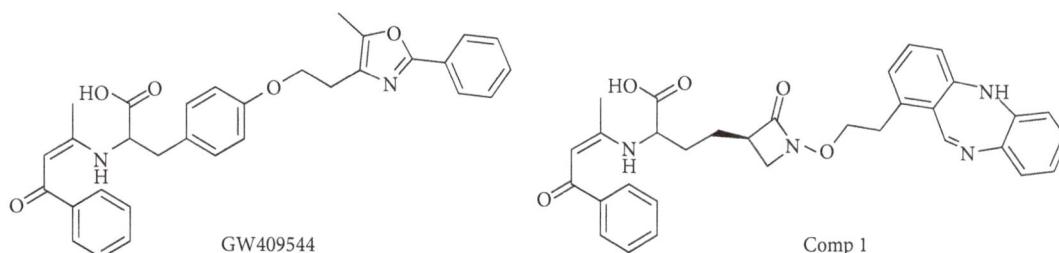

FIGURE 30: Dual agonist comp 1 identified from GW409544 using core hopping, docking, and MD approach.

both regions. These results agreed with the relative binding affinity predicted by docking.

To summarize, in the past decade a large number of structural scaffolds have been identified to show selective activation of the PPAR class of receptors. Many of the leads thus recognized have shown promising pharmacological profiles. But long-term safety and *in vivo* efficacy have remained the major challenging aspects in the development of novel molecules for the treatment of diabetes. Thus, in addition to having a deeper understanding of SAR and QSAR of novel class of molecules, focus must be equally placed on optimizing drug-like properties, pharmacodynamic/pharmacokinetic parameters of drug candidates, and clinical end points in the diabetic patients.

6. Dynamics of PPARγ and Its Relation to Activation and Antidiabetic Effects

The ligand-binding domain (LBD) of PPARγ consists of 270 amino acids, and as discussed in Section 3.2 and shown in Table 2/Figure 5, PPARγ has a large Y-shaped active site. Except the region around the AF-2 (H-12 helix) most of the interactions within the active site are hydrophobic in nature [16]. This causes the receptor to be very dynamic, and large variations in the active site volume can be seen in the crystal structures published (Tables 2 and 3). A comparison of the apo and ligand (RGZ) bound PPARγ crystal structures reveals the fact that the H-12 helix in the activation function (AF-2) can take two conformations "open" and "closed" [16]. Backbone RMS value of 1.45 Å was found between the two structures. Small RMS values for the backbone alignment suggest that the overall structural fold is maintained in the bound and unbound structures. While the RMS value for backbone atoms of the H-12 helix (residues 466–476) between the two structures was found to be 4.77 Å. Thus, significant differences are seen in the disposition of the H-12 helix in the various states accessible to the receptor. In the apo state the H-12 helix can take two positions "open" and "closed", while in the presence of agonist the closed conformation of the H-12 helix is stabilized significantly (Figure 31). This characteristic is a common feature of most of the nuclear receptors [49]. In the closed state the significant interactions of H-12 helix with the H-3 and H-10 helices are observed giving additional stability to the conformation [16, 19]. Presence of charge clamp interactions between residues in the H-12 (GLU471) and H3 (LYS301) helices with residues in the coactivators gives further stabilization in the closed conformation.

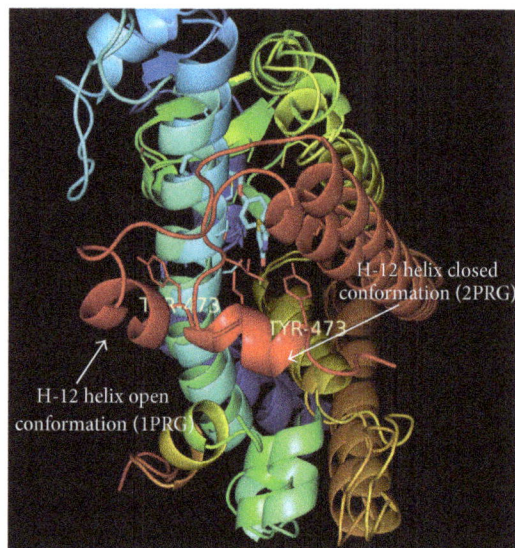

FIGURE 31: Apo (1PRG) and RGZ (2PRG) bound crystal structures of PPARγ overlaid (RMS backbone atoms = 1.45 Å). H-12 helix in the apo structure takes the open conformation, while in the RGZ bound structure (2PRG) the H-12 helix is in closed state. RMS for H-12 helix backbone atoms is 4.77 Å.

Due to these characteristic interactions full or partial agonistic behavior of various ligands was explained earlier based on H-12 helix dynamics and led to the design and synthesis of large number of structural scaffolds (Section 5) [21, 25, 42, 49, 176]. Ligands interacting with the H-12 helix and polar amino acids in the AF-2 region showed full agonistic character, while ligands with weaker or no interactions with the H-12 helix showed moderate to partial agonistic behavior. Earlier Willson et al. have correlated the binding affinity of ligands with the antihyperglycemic activity [115]. But this agonistic nature of the ligands do not always correlated with antidiabetic activity quantitatively [177, 178]. Thus the exact mechanism of activation of PPARγ and its relation to antidiabetic effects remains to be unclear.

Failure of the dual, SPPARMs and other molecules to reach the market calls for a fresh look at the molecular mechanism by which different endogenous/synthetic ligands and corepressors/coactivators of different PPAR receptors function to give a myriad of responses under different physiological conditions. It has been postulated that different ligands interact with the PPAR receptors resulting in ligand specific conformational changes. These differences translate into selective recruitment of cofactors (corepressors and coactivators) giving ligand specific gene expression patterns. Molecular dynamics (MD) simulations, which are used to follow the properties of a system as a function of time, coupled with rigid and flexible docking methods can really bridge this gap between the structurally diverse set of known ligands and a broad range of *in vitro* and *in vivo* activity profiles.

Considering the dynamic behavior of PPARγ and flexibility in its natural ligands it becomes important to find the conformational space and freedom that the natural ligands have in the active site of PPARγ. Thus, it can be suggested that any ligand, which is expected to have similar effects, should have the conformational landscape similar to these natural ligands for optimal activity. In the family of nuclear receptors role of the H-12 helix in the activation of the receptor is generally recognized. Full agonists are known to bind with the H-12 helix leading to the complete activation of the receptor. Partial agonists, on the other hand, are proposed to activate the receptor partially by binding in other end of the active site and have minimal interaction with the H-12 helix. Similar, hypotheses have been made in the literature regarding the activation of PPARγ by full and partial agonists. But the crystal structure data (see Table 3) available for PPARγ suggests that the distinction is not so simple: as many partial agonists bind to or near the H-12 helix and have important hydrogen-bonding interactions with the amino acids in/near H-12 helix. Hence, a clear understanding of the agonistic character of ligands based on the interactions within the active site is missing or obscure in the literature.

MD simulations were performed by Jyrkkarinne et al. recently to understand the agonistic and inverse agonistic behavior of constitutive androstane receptor (CAR) ligands [179]. Genest et al. have performed MD simulations on peroxisome proliferator-activated receptor γ (PPARγ), a nuclear receptor, in order to elucidate the ligand escape trajectories from the bound state [180]. They also showed that the ligands like GW0072 make use of the intrinsic flexibility in the protein structure to maneuver in the active site. Another report on ligand specificity, molecular switch, and interactions with regulators has tried to reassess the importance of various interactions of ligands (using MD studies) with PPAR and reiterated the fact that the interactions of acidic groups, although are important for efficient activity, are not the sole factor in determining the partial or full agonistic nature of the ligands [181]. Other important interactions in the Y-shaped cavity of PPARγ are hydrophobic and π-stacking interactions. Similarly, MD simulation studies by Michalik et al. have reanalyzed the role of the AF-2 region and other amino acids in the active site of PPARα [176]. In another study, MD simulations were performed with two ureidofibrate-like enantiomers and confirmed stabilization of the H-12 helix by the more active S-isomer [182]. Ji and Zhang highlighted the importance of protein polarization and electrostatic interactions in the AF-2 functional domain [97]. All these reports have substantiated the fact that full potential of the interactions in the active site have not been explored for this very important antidiabetic target and MD simulations can give useful insights into the receptor-ligand interactions and agonistic character of a ligand.

Choi et al. have alternatively suggested that the inhibition of phosphorylation of PPARγ at SER273 by cyclin-dependent kinase (Cdk5) could be mediating the beneficial antidiabetic effects of PPARγ agonists like RGZ and MRL24 [177]. SER273 (SER274 in 2PRG structure) is located in a loop between the helices H3 and H4 and occupies the surface opposite to the AF-2 region in the PPARγ active site [16, 19]. MRL24, a partial agonist, reduced the dynamic nature of the H3 helix (AAs 309–315), β-sheet region (369–379), and SER273. RGZ was found to have less effect on the dynamics of these regions but reduced the dynamics of H-12, H-11 helix, and AF-2 region significantly.

Based on these results Choi et al. have suggested the development of novel ligand with three important characteristics, namely, (1) high affinity for PPARγ, (2) blocking of Cdk5-mediated PPARγ phosphorylation, and (3) lack of classical agonism [178]. A novel indole-containing benzoic acid derivative (SR1664) was developed which stabilized the H-3 and β-sheet regions of the receptor while increasing the dynamical nature of the H-11 helix. This ligand shows minimal effect on the dynamics of H-12 helix. As expected from the dynamical nature of the H-12 helix, SR1664 did not show any classical agonistic character. Gene expression patterns of SR1664 overlapped only partially with that of RGZ, directing towards beneficial and harmful genes expression patterns. Genes like aP2, Adipsin, Cd24a, and so forth were expressed at higher level with SR1664 than with RGZ, while genes like Pdk4, Hsdl2, and so forth showed opposite expression levels. On the other hand RGZ and SR1664 showed similar effects on the expression of genes like Adiponectin, Nr1d2, Ddx17, and so forth. Further studies are thus required to fully understand the implications of these results for understanding PPAR biology and to drug discovery efforts.

Recently Amato et al. have reported, 5-(5-bromo-2-methoxy-benzylidene)-3-(4-methyl-benzyl)-thiazolidine-2,4-dione, (GQ-16) as a novel partial agonist promoting insulin sensitization without the side effects of weight gain [88]. Crystallographic studies showed that this compound binds near the β-sheet region like MRL24 and BVT.13. Inhibition of Cdk5-mediated phosphorylation of SER273 was observed and proposed as a possible explanation for its partial PPARγ activation and antidiabetic activity.

7. Conclusions and Future Directions on Developing Novel Ligands

More than a decade has passed since the introduction of TZD class of drugs in the market, but still a guided development of a novel drug with ideal balance of controlling glucose levels and simultaneously avoiding the side effects related to cardiovascular system and toxicity remains a challenging task. This is a combined effect of incomplete understanding of biology of the PPARγ, its *in vitro* and *in vivo* interactions with potential drug candidates, and correlation of these factors with clinically beneficial effects.

Nevertheless both SAR and CADD approaches have played a vital role in the identification of novel scaffolds with improved PPAR activation profiles. Glitazars, new TZD derivatives, L-tyrosine-based analogues, sulfonamide derivatives, sulfonylureas, barbituric acid derivatives, 2-hydroxynaphthoquinones, indoleacetic acid derivatives, propionic acid derivatives, oxazolidindiones, and α-substituted propanoic acid derivatives represent the remarkable success achieved so far in this area. Both ligand and receptor-based methods have contributed to this success.

Novel virtual screening techniques, pharmacophore models coupled with recent QSAR approaches, better methods of estimating binding affinities, and advances in understanding the dynamics of PPARγ-ligand interaction by employing molecular dynamics simulations have raised new hopes towards finding ligands with better pharmacological profiles.

Recently discovered alternate mechanisms of antidiabetic actions of PPARγ ligands, via inhibition of Cdk5-mediated phosphorylation, have given new impetus to efforts for the discovery of novel PPARγ ligands as antidiabetic agents. Overlap in the gene expression patterns (Section 4) of classical agonists (RGZ) and ligands (SR1664) inhibiting phosphorylation (but lacking classical agonism) suggests that partial agonists with inhibitory effects on phosphorylation could prove more effective. Thus retaining partial agonistic character with specific gene expression patterns could prove beneficial. These beneficial genes could be clustered from expression patterns of the already known ligands. A number of recent studies have begun to identify and cluster such gene sets [177, 178, 183, 184]. This suggests that ligands with following characteristic should be developed: (1) partial agonist of PPARγ, (2) potent inhibitor of Cdk-5-mediated phosphorylation at SER273 of PPARγ, and (3) high-binding affinity for PPARγ.

Abbreviations

(PPARγ):	Peroxisome proliferator-activated receptor γ
(PPARα):	Peroxisome proliferator-activated receptor α
(PPARδ):	Peroxisome proliferator-activated receptor δ
(TZD):	Thiazolidinedione
(RGZ):	Rosiglitazone
(PGZ):	Pioglitazone
(TGZ):	Troglitazone
(SPPARM):	Selective PPAR modulators
(SAR):	Structure activity relationship
(QSAR):	Quantitative structure activity relationship
(CADD):	Computer-aided drug discovery
GOLD:	(Genetic algorithm optimized ligand docking)
(ROCS):	Receiver-operating characteristic
(GLP-1):	Glucagon like peptide-1
(MCP-1):	Monocyte chemoattractant protein-1.

Conflict of Interests

Authors declare that they have no conflict of interests.

Acknowledgments

Authors are thankful to the Council of Scientific and Industrial Research (CSIR), New Delhi, India, for financial support.

References

[1] S. Wild, G. Roglic, A. Green, R. Sicree, and H. King, "Global prevalence of diabetes: estimates for the year 2000 and projections for 2030," *Diabetes Care*, vol. 27, no. 5, pp. 1047–1053, 2004.

[2] B. Pourcet, J. C. Fruchart, B. Staels, and C. Glineur, "Selective PPAR modulators, dual and pan PPAR agonists: multimodal drugs for the treatment of type 2 diabetes and atherosclerosis," *Expert Opinion on Emerging Drugs*, vol. 11, no. 3, pp. 379–401, 2006.

[3] R. H. van Huijsduijnen, W. H. B. Sauer, A. Bombrun, and D. Swinnen, "Prospects for inhibitors of protein tyrosine phosphatase 1B as antidiabetic drugs," *Journal of Medicinal Chemistry*, vol. 47, no. 17, pp. 4142–4146, 2004.

[4] D. E. Moller, "New drug targets for type 2 diabetes and the metabolic syndrome," *Nature*, vol. 414, no. 6865, pp. 821–827, 2001.

[5] C. DeSouza and V. Fonseca, "Therapeutic targets to reduce cardiovascular disease in type 2 diabetes," *Nature Reviews Drug Discovery*, vol. 8, pp. 361–367, 2009.

[6] N. Cho and Y. Momose, "Peroxisome proliferator-activated receptor γ agonists as insulin sensitizers: from the discovery to recent progress," *Current Topics in Medicinal Chemistry*, vol. 8, pp. 1483–1507, 2008.

[7] B. Panunti, A. A. Jawa, and V. A. Fonseca, "Mechanisms and therapeutic targets in type 2 diabetes mellitus," *Drug Discovery Today: Disease Mechanisms*, vol. 1, no. 2, pp. 151–157, 2004.

[8] D. K. Arulmozhi and B. Portha, "GLP-1 based therapy for type 2 diabetes," *European Journal of Pharmaceutical Sciences*, vol. 28, no. 1-2, pp. 96–108, 2006.

[9] J. M. Lehmann, L. B. Moore, T. A. Smith-Oliver, W. O. Wilkison, T. M. Willson, and S. A. Kliewer, "An antidiabetic thiazolidinedione is a high affinity ligand for peroxisome proliferator-activated receptor γ (PPARγ)," *Journal of Biological Chemistry*, vol. 270, no. 22, pp. 12953–12956, 1995.

[10] C. J. Rosen, "The rosiglitazone story—lessons from an FDA advisory committee meeting," *The New England Journal of Medicine*, vol. 357, pp. 844–846, 2007.

[11] M. T. Smith, "Mechanisms of troglitazone hepatotoxicity," *Chemical Research in Toxicology*, vol. 16, no. 6, pp. 679–687, 2003.

[12] M. Chandran, S. A. Phillips, T. Ciaraldi, and R. R. Henry, "Adiponectin: more than just another fat cell hormone?" *Diabetes Care*, vol. 26, no. 8, pp. 2442–2450, 2003.

[13] A. H. Knoll, "The early evolution of eukaryotes: a geological perspective," *Science*, vol. 256, no. 5057, pp. 622–627, 1992.

[14] M. E. Greene, B. Blumberg, O. W. McBride et al., "isolation of the human peroxisome proliferator activated receptor gamma cDNA: expression in hematopoietic cells and chromosomal mapping," *Gene Expression*, vol. 4, no. 4-5, pp. 281–299, 1995.

[15] B. Desvergne and W. Wahli, "Peroxisome proliferator-activated receptors: nuclear control of metabolism," *Endocrine Reviews*, vol. 20, no. 5, pp. 649–688, 1999.

[16] R. T. Nolte, G. B. Wisely, S. Westin et al., "Ligand binding and co-activator assembly of the peroxisome proliferator-activated receptor-γ," *Nature*, vol. 395, no. 6698, pp. 137–143, 1998.

[17] M. Hendlich, F. Rippmann, and G. Barnickel, "LIGSITE: automatic and efficient detection of potential small molecule-binding sites in proteins," *Journal of Molecular Graphics and Modelling*, vol. 15, no. 6, pp. 359–363, 1997.

[18] "The PyMOL Molecular Graphics System, Version 1.5.0.1," Schrödinger, LLC.

[19] V. Chandra, P. Huang, Y. Hamuro et al., "Structure of the intact PPAR-γ-RXR-α nuclear receptor complex on DNA," *Nature*, vol. 456, no. 7220, pp. 350–356, 2008.

[20] T. Sohda, K. Mizuno, E. Imamiya, H. Tawada, K. Meguro, and Y. Kawamatsu Yamamoto, "Studies on antidiabetic agents. III. 5-arylthiazolidine-2, 4-diones as potent aldose reductase inhibitors," *Chemical and Pharmaceutical Bulletin*, vol. 30, pp. 3601–3616, 1982.

[21] C. Pirat, A. Farce, N. Lebegue et al., "Targeting peroxisome proliferator-activated receptors (PPARs): development of modulators," *Medicinal Chemistry*, vol. 55, no. 9, pp. 4027–4061, 2012.

[22] R. T. Gampe Jr., V. G. Montana, M. H. Lambert et al., "Asymmetry in the PPARγ/RXRα crystal structure reveals the molecular basis of heterodimerization among nuclear receptors," *Molecular Cell*, vol. 5, no. 3, pp. 545–555, 2000.

[23] H. E. Xu, M. H. Lambert, V. G. Montana et al., "Molecular recognition of fatty acids by peroxisome proliferator-activated receptors," *Molecular Cell*, vol. 3, no. 3, pp. 397–403, 1999.

[24] P. Cronet, J. F. W. Petersen, R. Folmer et al., "Structure of the PPARα and -γ ligand binding domain in complex with AZ 242; ligand selectivity and agonist activation in the PPAR family," *Structure*, vol. 9, no. 8, pp. 699–706, 2001.

[25] H. E. Xu, M. H. Lambert, V. G. Montana et al., "Structural determinants of ligand binding selectivity between the peroxisome proliferator-activated receptors," *Proceedings of the National Academy of Sciences of the United States of America*, vol. 98, no. 24, pp. 13919–13924, 2001.

[26] H. E. Xu, T. B. Stanley, V. G. Montana et al., "Structural basis for antagonist-mediated recruitment of nuclear co-repressors by PPARα," *Nature*, vol. 415, no. 6873, pp. 813–817, 2002.

[27] P. Sauerberg, I. Pettersson, L. Jeppesen et al., "Novel tricyclic-α-alkyloxyphenylpropionic acids: dual PPARα/γ agonists with hypolipidemic and antidiabetic activity," *Journal of Medicinal Chemistry*, vol. 45, no. 4, pp. 789–804, 2002.

[28] S. Ebdrup, I. Pettersson, H. B. Rasmussen et al., "Synthesis and biological and structural characterization of the dual-acting peroxisome proliferator-activated receptor α/γ agonist ragaglitazar," *Journal of Medicinal Chemistry*, vol. 46, no. 8, pp. 1306–1317, 2003.

[29] T. Östberg, S. Svensson, G. Selén et al., "A new class of peroxisome proliferator-activated receptor agonists with a novel binding epitope shows antidiabetic effects," *Journal of Biological Chemistry*, vol. 279, no. 39, pp. 41124–41130, 2004.

[30] I. Takada, R. T. Yu, H. E. Xu et al., "Alteration of a single amino acid in peroxisome proliferator-activated receptor-α (PPARα) generates a PPARδ phenotype," *Molecular Endocrinology*, vol. 14, no. 5, pp. 733–740, 2000.

[31] G. Q. Shi, J. F. Dropinski, B. M. McKeever et al., "Design and synthesis of α-aryloxyphenylacetic acid derivatives: a novel class of PPARα/γ dual agonists with potent antihyperglycemic and lipid modulating activity," *Journal of Medicinal Chemistry*, vol. 48, no. 13, pp. 4457–4468, 2005.

[32] Y. Li, M. Choi, K. Suino et al., "Structural and biochemical basis for selective repression of the orphan nuclear receptor liver receptor homolog 1 by small heterodimer partner," *Proceedings*

of the National Academy of Sciences of the United States of America, vol. 102, no. 27, pp. 9505–9510, 2005.

[33] N. Mahindroo, C. F. Huang, Y. H. Peng et al., "Novel indole-based peroxisome proliferator-activated receptor agonists: design, SAR, structural biology, and biological activities," *Journal of Medicinal Chemistry*, vol. 48, no. 26, pp. 8194–8208, 2005.

[34] S. A. Fyffe, M. S. Alphey, L. Buetow et al., "Recombinant human PPAR-β/δ ligand-binding domain is locked in an activated conformation by endogenous fatty acids," *Journal of Molecular Biology*, vol. 356, no. 4, pp. 1005–1013, 2006.

[35] S. A. Fyffe, M. S. Alphey, L. Buetow et al., "Reevaluation of the PPAR-β/δ ligand binding domain model reveals why it exhibits the activated form," *Molecular Cell*, vol. 21, no. 1, pp. 1–2, 2006.

[36] N. Mahindroo, C. C. Wang, C. C. Liao et al., "Indol-1-yl acetic acids as peroxisome proliferator-activated receptor agonists: design, synthesis, structural biology, and molecular docking studies," *Journal of Medicinal Chemistry*, vol. 49, no. 3, pp. 1212–1216, 2006.

[37] E. Burgermeister, A. Schnoebelen, A. Flament et al., "A novel partial agonist of peroxisome proliferator-activated receptor-γ (PPARγ) recruits PPARγ-coactivator-1α, prevents triglyceride accumulation, and potentiates insulin signaling in vitro," *Molecular Endocrinology*, vol. 20, no. 4, pp. 809–830, 2006.

[38] I. L. Lu, C. F. Huang, Y. H. Peng et al., "Structure-based drug design of a novel family of PPARγ partial agonists: virtual screening, X-ray crystallography, and in vitro/in vivo biological activities," *Journal of Medicinal Chemistry*, vol. 49, no. 9, pp. 2703–2712, 2006.

[39] B. Kuhn, H. Hilpert, J. Benz et al., "Structure-based design of indole propionic acids as novel PPARα/γ co-agonists," *Bioorganic & Medicinal Chemistry Letters*, vol. 16, no. 15, pp. 4016–4020, 2006.

[40] C. R. Hopkins, S. V. O'Neil, M. C. Laufersweiler et al., "Design and synthesis of novel N-sulfonyl-2-indole carboxamides as potent PPAR-γ binding agents with potential application to the treatment of osteoporosis," *Bioorganic & Medicinal Chemistry Letters*, vol. 16, no. 21, pp. 5659–5663, 2006.

[41] N. Mahindroo, Y. H. Peng, C. H. Lin et al., "Structural basis for the structure-activity relationships of peroxisome proliferator-activated receptor agonists," *Journal of Medicinal Chemistry*, vol. 49, no. 21, pp. 6421–6424, 2006.

[42] G. Pochetti, C. Godio, N. Mitro et al., "Insights into the mechanism of partial agonism: crystal structures of the peroxisome proliferator-activated receptor γ ligand-binding domain in the complex with two enantiomeric ligands," *Journal of Biological Chemistry*, vol. 282, no. 23, pp. 17314–17324, 2007.

[43] R. Epple, M. Azimioara, R. Russo et al., "3,4,5-trisubstituted isoxazoles as novel PPARδ agonists. Part 2," *Bioorganic & Medicinal Chemistry Letters*, vol. 16, no. 21, pp. 5488–5492, 2006.

[44] H. Oon Han, S. H. Kim, K. H. Kim et al., "Design and synthesis of oxime ethers of α-acyl-β-phenylpropanoic acids as PPAR dual agonists," *Bioorganic & Medicinal Chemistry Letters*, vol. 17, pp. 937–941, 2007.

[45] A. L. B. Ambrosio, S. M. G. Dias, I. Polikarpov, R. B. Zurier, S. H. Burstein, and R. C. Garratt, "Ajulemic acid, a synthetic non-psychoactive cannabinoid acid, bound to the ligand binding domain of the human peroxisome proliferator-activated receptor γ," *Journal of Biological Chemistry*, vol. 282, no. 25, pp. 18625–18633, 2007.

[46] M. Einstein, T. E. Akiyama, G. A. Castriota et al., "The differential interactions of peroxisome proliferator-activated receptor γ

ligands with Tyr473 is a physical basis for their unique biological activities," *Molecular Pharmacology*, vol. 73, no. 1, pp. 62–74, 2008.

[47] M. L. Sierra, V. Beneton, A. B. Boullay et al., "Substituted 2-[(4-aminomethyl)phenoxy]-2-methylpropionic acid PPARα agonists. 1. Discovery of a novel series of potent HDLc raising agents," *Journal of Medicinal Chemistry*, vol. 50, no. 4, pp. 685–695, 2007.

[48] R. P. Trump, J. E. Cobb, B. G. Shearer et al., "Co-crystal structure guided array synthesis of PPARγ inverse agonists," *Bioorganic & Medicinal Chemistry Letters*, vol. 17, no. 14, pp. 3916–3920, 2007.

[49] J. B. Bruning, M. J. Chalmers, S. Prasad et al., "Partial agonists activate PPARγ using a helix 12 independent mechanism," *Structure*, vol. 15, no. 10, pp. 1258–1271, 2007.

[50] I. Pettersson, S. Ebdrup, M. Havranek et al., "Design of a partial PPARδ agonist," *Bioorganic & Medicinal Chemistry Letters*, vol. 17, no. 16, pp. 4625–4629, 2007.

[51] A. Casimiro-Garcia, C. F. Bigge, J. A. Davis et al., "Effects of modifications of the linker in a series of phenylpropanoic acid derivatives: synthesis, evaluation as PPARα/γ dual agonists, and X-ray crystallographic studies," *Bioorganic and Medicinal Chemistry*, vol. 16, no. 9, pp. 4883–4907, 2008.

[52] T. Itoh, L. Fairall, K. Amin et al., "Structural basis for the activation of PPARγ by oxidized fatty acids," *Nature Structural & Molecular Biology*, vol. 15, no. 9, pp. 924–931, 2008.

[53] S. Keil, H. Matter, K. Schonafinger et al., "Sulfonylthiadiazoles with an unusual binding mode as partial dual peroxisome proliferator-activated receptor (PPAR) γ/δ agonists with high potency and in vivo efficacy," *ChemMedChem*, vol. 6, pp. 633–653, 2011.

[54] C. Weidner, J. C. de Groot, A. Prasad et al., "Amorfrutins are potent antidiabetic dietary natural products," *Proceedings of the National Academy of Sciences of the United States of America*, vol. 109, pp. 7257–7262, 2012.

[55] T. Waku, T. Shiraki, T. Oyama et al., "Structural insight into PPARγ activation through covalent modification with endogenous fatty acids," *Journal of Molecular Biology*, vol. 385, no. 1, pp. 188–199, 2009.

[56] T. Waku, T. Shiraki, T. Oyama, K. Maebara, R. Nakamori, and K. Morikawa, "The nuclear receptor PPARγ individually responds to serotonin- and fatty acid-metabolites," *The EMBO Journal*, vol. 29, pp. 3395–3407, 2010.

[57] T. Oyama, K. Toyota, T. Waku et al., "Adaptability and selectivity of human peroxisome proliferator-activated receptor (PPAR) pan agonists revealed from crystal structures," *Acta Crystallographica Section D*, vol. 65, no. 8, pp. 786–795, 2009.

[58] T. Waku, T. Shiraki, T. Oyama, and K. Morikawa, "Atomic structure of mutant PPARγ LBD complexed with 15d-PGJ2: novel modulation mechanism of PPARγ/RXRα function by covalently bound ligands," *FEBS Letters*, vol. 583, no. 2, pp. 320–324, 2009.

[59] M. Ohashi, T. Oyama, I. Nakagome et al., "Design, synthesis, and structural analysis of phenylpropanoic acid-type PPARγ-selective agonists: discovery of reversed stereochemistry-activity relationship," *Journal of Medicinal Chemistry*, vol. 54, no. 1, pp. 331–341, 2011.

[60] K. Wakabayashi, S. Hayashi, Y. Matsui et al., "Pharmacology and in vitro profiling of a novel peroxisome proliferator-activated receptor γ ligand, cerco-A," *Biological & Pharmaceutical Bulletin*, vol. 34, no. 7, pp. 1094–1104, 2011.

[61] R. Montanari, F. Saccoccia, E. Scotti et al., "Crystal structure of the peroxisome proliferator-activated receptor γ (PPARγ) ligand binding domain complexed with a novel partial agonist: a new region of the hydrophobic pocket could be exploited for drug design," *Journal of Medicinal Chemistry*, vol. 51, no. 24, pp. 7768–7776, 2008.

[62] H. Zhang, D. E. Ryono, P. Devasthale et al., "Design, synthesis and structure-activity relationships of azole acids as novel, potent dual PPAR α/γ agonists," *Bioorganic & Medicinal Chemistry Letters*, vol. 19, pp. 1451–1456, 2009.

[63] Y. Li, A. Kovach, K. Suino-Powell, D. Martynowski, and H. E. Xu, "Structural and biochemical basis for the binding selectivity of peroxisome proliferator-activated receptor γ to PGC-1α," *Journal of Biological Chemistry*, vol. 283, no. 27, pp. 19132–19139, 2008.

[64] Y. Li, J. Zhang, F. J. Schopfer et al., "Molecular recognition of nitrated fatty acids by PPARγ," *Nature Structural & Molecular Biology*, vol. 15, no. 8, pp. 865–867, 2008.

[65] B. G. Shearer, H. S. Patel, A. N. Billin et al., "Discovery of a novel class of PPARδ partial agonists," *Bioorganic & Medicinal Chemistry Letters*, vol. 18, no. 18, pp. 5018–5022, 2008.

[66] D. R. Artis, J. J. Lin, C. Zhang et al., "Scaffold-based discovery of indeglitazar, a PPAR pan-active anti-diabetic agent," *Proceedings of the National Academy of Sciences of the United States of America*, vol. 106, no. 1, pp. 262–267, 2009.

[67] U. Grether, A. Bénardeau, J. Benz et al., "Design and biological evaluation of novel, balanced dual PPARα/γ agonists," *ChemMedChem*, vol. 4, no. 6, pp. 951–956, 2009.

[68] A. Motani, Z. Wang, J. Weiszmann et al., "INT131: a selective modulator of PPARγ," *Journal of Molecular Biology*, vol. 386, no. 5, pp. 1301–1311, 2009.

[69] A. Bénardeau, J. Benz, A. Binggeli et al., "Aleglitazar, a new, potent, and balanced dual PPARα/γ agonist for the treatment of type II diabetes," *Bioorganic & Medicinal Chemistry Letters*, vol. 19, no. 9, pp. 2468–2473, 2009.

[70] C. H. Lin, Y. H. Peng, M. S. Coumar et al., "Design and structural analysis of novel pharmacophores for potent and selective peroxisome proliferator-activated receptor γ agonists," *Journal of Medicinal Chemistry*, vol. 52, no. 8, pp. 2618–2622, 2009.

[71] R. V. Connors, Z. Wang, M. Harrison et al., "Identification of a PPARδ agonist with partial agonistic activity on PPARγ," *Bioorganic & Medicinal Chemistry Letters*, vol. 19, no. 13, pp. 3550–3554, 2009.

[72] G. Fracchiolla, A. Laghezza, L. Piemontese et al., "New 2-aryloxy-3-phenyl-propanoic acids as peroxisome proliferator-activated receptors α/γ dual agonists with improved potency and reduced adverse effects on skeletal muscle function," *Journal of Medicinal Chemistry*, vol. 52, no. 20, pp. 6382–6393, 2009.

[73] A. Casimiro-Garcia, C. F. Bigge, J. A. Davis et al., "Synthesis and evaluation of novel α-heteroaryl-phenylpropanoic acid derivatives as PPARα/γ dual agonists," *Bioorganic and Medicinal Chemistry*, vol. 17, no. 20, pp. 7113–7125, 2009.

[74] Y. Li, Z. Wang, N. Furukawa et al., "T2384, a novel antidiabetic agent with unique peroxisome proliferator-activated receptor γ binding properties," *Journal of Biological Chemistry*, vol. 283, no. 14, pp. 9168–9176, 2008.

[75] J. Li, L. J. Kennedy, Y. Shi et al., "Discovery of an oxybenzylglycine based peroxisome proliferator activated receptor α selective agonist 2-((3-((2-(4-chlorophenyl)-5-methyloxazol-4-yl)methoxy)benzyl)(methoxycarbonyl)amino)acetic acid

(BMS-687453)," *Journal of Medicinal Chemistry*, vol. 53, no. 7, pp. 2854–2864, 2010.

[76] A. Furukawa, T. Arita, S. Satoh et al., "Discovery of a novel selective PPARγ modulator from (-)-cercosporamide derivatives," *Bioorganic & Medicinal Chemistry Letters*, vol. 20, pp. 2095–2098, 2010.

[77] A. Riu, M. Grimaldi, A. le Maire et al., "Peroxisome proliferator-activated receptor γ is a target for halogenated analogs of bisphenol A," *Environmental Health Perspectives*, vol. 119, no. 9, pp. 1227–1232, 2011.

[78] C. A. Luckhurst, L. A. Stein, M. Furber et al., "Discovery of isoindoline and tetrahydroisoquinoline derivatives as potent, selective PPARδ agonists," *Bioorganic & Medicinal Chemistry Letters*, vol. 21, no. 1, pp. 492–496, 2011.

[79] A. Riu, A. le Maire, M. Grimaldi et al., "Characterization of novel ligands of ERα, Erβ, and PPARγ: the case of halogenated bisphenol A and their conjugated metabolites," *Toxicological Sciences*, vol. 122, pp. 372–382, 2011.

[80] K. A. Evans, B. G. Shearer, D. D. Wisnoski et al., "Phenoxyacetic acids as PPARδ partial agonists: synthesis, optimization, and in vivo efficacy," *Bioorganic & Medicinal Chemistry Letters*, vol. 21, pp. 2345–2350, 2011.

[81] J. Uppenberg, C. Svensson, M. Jaki, G. Bertilsson, L. Jendeberg, and A. Berkenstam, "Crystal structure of the ligand binding domain of the human nuclear receptor PPARγ," *Journal of Biological Chemistry*, vol. 273, no. 47, pp. 31108–31112, 1998.

[82] H. Zhang, X. Xu, L. Chen et al., "Molecular determinants of magnolol targeting both RXRα and PPARγ," *PloS ONE*, vol. 6, Article ID e28253, 2011.

[83] A. Casimiro-Garcia, G. F. Filzen, D. Flynn et al., "Discovery of a series of imidazo[4,5-b]pyridines with dual activity at angiotensin II type 1 receptor and peroxisome proliferator-activated receptor-γ," *Journal of Medicinal Chemistry*, vol. 54, no. 12, pp. 4219–4233, 2011.

[84] L. Porcelli, F. Gilardi, A. Laghezza et al., "Synthesis, characterization and biological evaluation of ureidofibrate-like derivatives endowed with peroxisome proliferator-activated receptor activity," *Journal of Medicinal Chemistry*, vol. 55, pp. 37–54, 2012.

[85] M. Sime, A. C. Allan, P. Chapman et al., "Discovery of GSK1997132B a novel centrally penetrant benzimidazole PPARγ partial agonist," *Bioorganic & Medicinal Chemistry Letters*, vol. 21, pp. 5568–5572, 2011.

[86] A. C. Puhl, A. Bernardes, R. L. Silveira et al., "Mode of peroxisome proliferator-activated receptor γ activation by luteolin," *Molecular Pharmacology*, vol. 81, no. 6, pp. 788–799, 2012.

[87] W. Liu, F. Lau, K. Liu et al., "Benzimidazolones: a new class of selective peroxisome proliferator-activated receptor γ (PPARγ) modulators," *Journal of Medicinal Chemistry*, vol. 54, pp. 8541–8554, 2011.

[88] A. A. Amato, S. Rajagopalan, J. Z. Lin et al., "GQ-16, a novel peroxisome proliferator-activated receptor γ (PPARγ) ligand, promotes insulin sensitization without weight gain," *The Journal of Biological Chemistry*, vol. 287, pp. 28169–28179, 2012.

[89] R. R. Malapaka, S. Khoo, J. Zhang et al., "Identification and mechanism of 10-carbon fatty acid as modulating ligand of peroxisome proliferator-activated receptors," *The Journal of Biological Chemistry*, vol. 287, pp. 183–195, 2012.

[90] A. Furukawa, T. Arita, T. Fukuzaki et al., "Substituents at the naphthalene C3 position of (-)-cercosporamide derivatives significantly affect the maximal efficacy as PPARγ partial agonists,"

Bioorganic & Medicinal Chemistry Letters, vol. 22, pp. 1348–1351, 2012.

[91] N. Kuwabara, T. Oyama, D. Tomioka et al., "Peroxisome proliferator-activated receptors (PPARS) have multiple binding points that accommodate ligands in various conformations: phenylpropanoic acid-type PPAR ligands bind to PPAR in different conformations, depending on the subtype," *Journal of Medicinal Chemistry*, vol. 55, pp. 893–902, 2012.

[92] Y. Amano, T. Yamaguchi, K. Ohno et al., "Structural basis for telmisartan-mediated partial activation of PPAR gamma," *Hypertension Research*, vol. 35, pp. 715–719, 2012.

[93] J. L. Oberfield, J. L. Collins, C. P. Holmes et al., "A peroxisome proliferator-activated receptor γ ligand inhibits adipocyte differentiation," *Proceedings of the National Academy of Sciences of the United States of America*, vol. 96, no. 11, pp. 6102–6106, 1999.

[94] T. S. Hughes, M. J. Chalmers, S. Novick et al., "Ligand and receptor dynamics contribute to the mechanism of graded PPARγ agonism," *Structure*, vol. 20, pp. 139–150, 2012.

[95] R. S. Chana, A. J. Lewington, and N. J. Brunskill, "Differential effects of peroxisome proliferator activated receptor-γ (PPARγ) ligands in proximal tubular cells: thiazolidinediones are partial PPARγ agonists," *Kidney International*, vol. 65, no. 6, pp. 2081–2090, 2004.

[96] K. Yamagishi, K. Yamamoto, Y. Mochizuki, T. Nakano, S. Yamada, and H. Tokiwa, "Flexible ligand recognition of peroxisome proliferator-activated receptor-γ (PPARγ)," *Bioorganic & Medicinal Chemistry Letters*, vol. 20, no. 11, pp. 3344–3347, 2010.

[97] C. G. Ji and J. Z. H. Zhang, "Protein polarization is critical to stabilizing AF-2 and helix-2' domains in ligand binding to PPAR-γ," *Journal of the American Chemical Society*, vol. 130, no. 50, pp. 17129–17133, 2008.

[98] K. Henriksen, I. Byrjalsen, P. Qvist et al., "Efficacy and safety of the PPARγ partial agonist balaglitazone compared with pioglitazone and placebo: a phase III, randomized, parallel-group study in patients with type 2 diabetes on stable insulin therapy," *Diabetes/Metabolism Research and Reviews*, vol. 27, no. 4, pp. 392–401, 2011.

[99] P. Misra, R. Chakrabarti, R. K. Vikramadithyan et al., "PAT5A: a partial agonist of peroxisome proliferator-activated receptor γ is a potent antidiabetic thiazolidinedione yet weakly adipogenic," *Journal of Pharmacology and Experimental Therapeutics*, vol. 306, no. 2, pp. 763–771, 2003.

[100] S. Khanna, M. E. Sobhia, and P. V. Bharatam, "Additivity of molecular fields: CoMFA study on dual activators of PPARα and PPARγ," *Journal of Medicinal Chemistry*, vol. 48, no. 8, pp. 3015–3025, 2005.

[101] C. Fiévet, J.-C. Fruchart, and B. Staels, "PPARα and PPARγ dual agonists for the treatment of type 2 diabetes and the metabolic syndrome," *Current Opinion in Pharmacology*, vol. 6, pp. 606–614, 2006.

[102] I. Ahmed, K. Furlong, J. Flood, V. P. Treat, and B. J. Goldstein, "Dual PPAR α/γ agonists: promises and pitfalls in type 2 diabetes," *American Journal of Therapeutics*, vol. 14, no. 1, pp. 49–62, 2007.

[103] Y. Xu, C. J. Rito, G. J. Etgen et al., "Design and synthesis of α-aryloxy-α-methylhydrocinnamic acids: a novel class of dual peroxisome proliferator-activated receptor α/γ agonists," *Journal of Medicinal Chemistry*, vol. 47, no. 10, pp. 2422–2425, 2004.

[104] B. C. Hansen, X. T. Tigno, A. Benardeau, M. Meyer, E. Sebokova, and J. Mizrahi, "Effects of aleglitazar, a balanced dual peroxisome proliferator-activated receptor α/γ agonist on glycemic and lipid parameters in a primate model of the metabolic syndrome," *Cardiovascular Diabetology*, vol. 10, p. 7, 2011.

[105] S. L. Cox, "Tesaglitazar: a promising approach in type 2 diabetes," *Drugs of Today*, vol. 42, no. 3, pp. 139–146, 2006.

[106] D. Conlon, "Goodbye glitazars?" *British Journal of Diabetes & Vascular Disease*, vol. 6, no. 3, pp. 135–137, 2006.

[107] L. S. Higgins and A. M. DePaoli, "Selective peroxisome proliferator-activated receptor γ (PPARγ) modulation as a strategy for safer therapeutic PPARγ activation," *The American Journal of Clinical Nutrition*, vol. 91, pp. 267S–272S, 2009.

[108] S. Rocchi, F. Picard, J. Vamecq et al., "A unique PPARγ ligand with potent insulin-sensitizing yet weak adipogenic activity," *Molecular Cell*, vol. 8, no. 4, pp. 737–747, 2001.

[109] T. Allen, F. Zhang, S. A. Moodie et al., "Halofenate is a selective peroxisome proliferator-activated receptorgamma modulator with antidiabetic activity," *Diabetes*, vol. 55, no. 9, pp. 2523–2533, 2006.

[110] T. Fujimura, C. Kimura, T. Oe et al., "A selective peroxisome proliferator-activated receptor γ modulator with distinct fat cell regulation properties," *Journal of Pharmacology and Experimental Therapeutics*, vol. 318, no. 2, pp. 863–871, 2006.

[111] T. Tagami, H. Yamamoto, K. Moriyama et al., "A selective peroxisome proliferator-activated receptor-γ modulator, telmisartan, binds to the receptor in a different fashion from thiazolidinediones," *Endocrinology*, vol. 150, no. 2, pp. 862–870, 2009.

[112] H. A. Pershadsingh and T. W. Kurtz, "Insulin-sensitizing effects of telmisartan: implications for treating insulin-resistant hypertension and cardiovascular disease," *Diabetes Care*, vol. 27, no. 4, p. 1015, 2004.

[113] J. Rieusset, F. Touri, L. Michalik et al., "A new selective peroxisome proliferator-activated receptor γ antagonist with antiobesity and antidiabetic activity," *Molecular Endocrinology*, vol. 16, no. 11, pp. 2628–2644, 2002.

[114] H. M. Wright, C. B. Clish, T. Mikami et al., "A synthetic antagonist for the peroxisome proliferator-activated receptor γ inhibits adipocyte differentiation," *Journal of Biological Chemistry*, vol. 275, no. 3, pp. 1873–1877, 2000.

[115] T. M. Willson, J. E. Cobb, D. J. Cowan et al., "The structure—activity relationship between peroxisome proliferator-activated receptor γ agonism and the antihyperglycemic activity of thiazolidinediones," *Journal of Medicinal Chemistry*, vol. 39, no. 3, pp. 665–668, 1996.

[116] K. A. Reddy, B. B. Lohray, V. Bhushan et al., "Novel antidiabetic and hypolipidemic agents. 5. Hydroxyl versus benzyloxy containing chroman derivatives," *Journal of Medicinal Chemistry*, vol. 42, no. 17, pp. 3265–3278, 1999.

[117] K. Matsumoto, S. Miyake, M. Yano, Y. Ueki, and Y. Tominaga, "Increase of lipoprotein (a) with troglitazone," *The Lancet*, vol. 350, no. 9093, pp. 1748–1749, 1997.

[118] K. Kawai, Y. Kawasaki-Tokui, T. Odaka et al., "Disposition and metabolism of the new oral antidiabetic drug troglitazone in rats, mice and dogs," *Arzneimittel-Forschung*, vol. 47, no. 4, pp. 356–368, 1997.

[119] B. B. Lohray, V. B. Lohray, A. C. Bajji et al., "(-)3-[4-[2-(phenoxazin-10-yl)ethoxy]phenyl]-2-ethoxypropanoic acid [(-)DRF 2725]: a dual PPAR agonist with potent antihyperglycemic and lipid modulating activity," *Journal of Medicinal Chemistry*, vol. 44, no. 16, pp. 2675–2678, 2001.

[120] D. A. Brooks, G. J. Etgen, C. J. Rito et al., "Design and synthesis of 2-methyl-2-4-[2-(5-methyl-2-aryloxazol-4-yl)ethoxy]phenoxypropionic acids: a new class of dual PPARα/γ agonists," *Journal of Medicinal Chemistry*, vol. 44, no. 13, pp. 2061–2064, 2001.

[121] T. Sohda, K. Mizuno, and Y. Kawamatsu, "Studies on antidiabetic agents. VI. Asymmetric transformation of ($\pm$)-5-[4-(1-methylcyclohexylmethoxy)benzyl]-2,4-thiazolidinedione (ciglitazone) with optically active 1-phenylethylamines," *Chemical and Pharmaceutical Bulletin*, vol. 32, no. 11, pp. 4460–4465, 1984.

[122] P. V. Bharatam and S. Khanna, "Rapid racemization in thiazolidinediones: a quantum chemical study," *Journal of Physical Chemistry A*, vol. 108, no. 17, pp. 3784–3788, 2004.

[123] D. Haigh, G. Allen, H. C. Birrell et al., "Non-thiazolidinedione antihyperglycaemic agents. Part 3: the effects of stereochemistry on the potency of α-methoxy-β-phenylpropanoic acids," *Bioorganic and Medicinal Chemistry*, vol. 7, no. 5, pp. 821–830, 1999.

[124] M. Oguchi, K. Wada, H. Honma et al., "Molecular design, synthesis, and hypoglycemic activity of a series of thiazolidine-2,4-diones," *Journal of Medicinal Chemistry*, vol. 43, no. 16, pp. 3052–3066, 2000.

[125] H. Yanagisawa, M. Takamura, E. Yamada et al., "Novel oximes having 5-benzyl-2,4-thiazolidinedione as antihyperglycemic agents: synthesis and structure-activity relationship," *Bioorganic & Medicinal Chemistry Letters*, vol. 10, no. 4, pp. 373–375, 2000.

[126] G. R. Madhavan, R. Chakrabarti, R. K. Vikramadithyan et al., "Synthesis and biological activity of novel pyrimidinone containing thiazolidinedione derivatives," *Bioorganic and Medicinal Chemistry*, vol. 10, no. 8, pp. 2671–2680, 2002.

[127] B. B. Lohray, V. Bhushan, B. P. Rao et al., "Novel euglycemic and hypolipidemic agents," *Journal of Medicinal Chemistry*, vol. 41, no. 10, pp. 1619–1630, 1998.

[128] Y. Momose, T. Maekawa, T. Yamano et al., "Novel 5-substituted 2,4-thiazolidinedione and 2,4-oxazolidinedione derivatives as insulin sensitizers with antidiabetic activities," *Journal of Medicinal Chemistry*, vol. 45, no. 7, pp. 1518–1534, 2002.

[129] R. C. Desai, W. Han, E. J. Metzger et al., "5-Aryl thiazolidine-2,4-diones: discovery of PPAR dual α/γ agonists as antidiabetic agents," *Bioorganic & Medicinal Chemistry Letters*, vol. 13, no. 16, pp. 2795–2798, 2003.

[130] B. Y. Kim, J. B. Ahn, H. W. Lee et al., "Synthesis and antihyperglycemic activity of erythrose, ribose and substituted pyrrolidine containing thiazolidinedione derivatives," *Chemical and Pharmaceutical Bulletin*, vol. 51, no. 3, pp. 276–285, 2003.

[131] H. W. Lee, Y. K. Bok, B. A. Joong et al., "Molecular design, synthesis, and hypoglycemic and hypolipidemic activities of novel pyrimidine derivatives having thiazolidinedione," *European Journal of Medicinal Chemistry*, vol. 40, no. 9, pp. 862–874, 2005.

[132] K. Liu, L. Xu, J. P. Berger et al., "Discovery of a novel series of peroxisome proliferator-activated receptor α/γ dual agonists for the treatment of type 2 diabetes and dyslipidemia," *Journal of Medicinal Chemistry*, vol. 48, no. 7, pp. 2262–2265, 2005.

[133] A. Pinelli, C. Godio, A. Laghezza et al., "Synthesis, biological evaluation, and molecular modeling investigation of new chiral fibrates with PPARα and PPARγ agonist activity," *Journal of Medicinal Chemistry*, vol. 48, no. 17, pp. 5509–5519, 2005.

[134] N. J. Kim, K. O. Lee, B. W. Koo et al., "Design, synthesis, and structure-activity relationship of carbamate-tethered aryl propanoic acids as novel PPARα/γ dual agonists," *Bioorganic & Medicinal Chemistry Letters*, vol. 17, no. 13, pp. 3595–3598, 2007.

[135] K. G. Liu, M. H. Lambert, A. H. Ayscue et al., "Synthesis and biological activity of L-tyrosine-based PPARγ agonists with

reduced molecular weight," *Bioorganic & Medicinal Chemistry Letters*, vol. 11, no. 24, pp. 3111–3113, 2001.

[136] B. R. Henke, S. G. Blanchard, M. F. Brackeen et al., "N-(2-benzoylphenyl)-L-tyrosine PPARγ agonists. 1. Discovery of a novel series of potent antihyperglycemic and antihyperlipidemic agents," *Journal of Medicinal Chemistry*, vol. 41, no. 25, pp. 5020–5036, 1998.

[137] M. Takamura, M. Sakurai, E. Yamada et al., "Synthesis and biological activity of novel α-substituted β-phenylpropionic acids having pyridin-2-ylphenyl moiety as antihyperglycemic agents," *Bioorganic and Medicinal Chemistry*, vol. 12, no. 9, pp. 2419–2439, 2004.

[138] Y. Itoh, Y. Kawamata, M. Harada et al., "Free fatty acids regulate insulin secretion from pancreatic β cells through GPR40," *Nature*, vol. 422, pp. 173–176, 2003.

[139] E. Christiansen, C. Urban, N. Merten et al., "Discovery of potent and selective agonists for the free fatty acid receptor 1 (FFA1/GPR40), a potential target for the treatment of type II diabetes," *Journal of Medicinal Chemistry*, vol. 51, pp. 7061–7064, 2008.

[140] E. Christiansen, M. E. Due-Hansen, and T. Ulven, "A rapid and efficient Sonogashira protocol and improved synthesis of free fatty acid 1 (FFA1) receptor agonists," *Journal of Organic Chemistry*, vol. 75, no. 4, pp. 1301–1304, 2010.

[141] S. B. Bharate, K. V. Nemmani, and R. A. Vishwakarma, "Progress in the discovery and development of small-molecule modulators of G-protein-coupled receptor 40 (GPR40/FFA1/FFAR1): an emerging target for type 2 diabetes," *Expert Opinion on Therapeutic Patents*, vol. 19, pp. 237–264, 2009.

[142] S. Y. Lu, Y. J. Jiang, J. Lv, T. X. Wu, Q. S. Yu, and W. L. Zhu J, "Molecular docking and molecular dynamics simulation studies of GPR40 receptor-agonist interactions," *Journal of Molecular Graphics and Modelling*, vol. 28, no. 8, pp. 766–774, 2010.

[143] H. Koyama, D. J. Miller, J. K. Boueres et al., "(2R)-2-ethylchromane-2-carboxylic acids: discovery of novel PPARα/γ dual agonists as antihyperglycemic and hypolipidemic agents," *Journal of Medicinal Chemistry*, vol. 47, no. 12, pp. 3255–3263, 2004.

[144] C. Parmenon, J. Guillard, D. H. Caignard et al., "4,4-dimethyl-1,2,3,4-tetrahydroquinoline-based PPARα/γ agonists. Part. II: synthesis and pharmacological evaluation of oxime and acidic head group structural variations," *Bioorganic & Medicinal Chemistry Letters*, vol. 19, no. 10, pp. 2683–2687, 2009.

[145] C. Parmenon, J. Guillard, D. H. Caignard et al., "4,4-Dimethyl-1,2,3,4-tetrahydroquinoline-based PPARα/γ agonists. Part I: synthesis and pharmacological evaluation," *Bioorganic & Medicinal Chemistry Letters*, vol. 18, no. 5, pp. 1617–1622, 2008.

[146] M. Ohashi, I. Nakagome, J.-i. Kasuga et al., "Design, synthesis and in vitro evaluation of a series of α-substituted phenylpropanoic acid PPARγ agonists to further investigate the stereochemistry—activity relationship," *Bioorganic & Medicinal Chemistry*, vol. 20, no. 21, pp. 6375–6383, 2012.

[147] I. M. Kapetanovic, "Computer-aided drug discovery and development (CADDD): *in silico*-chemico-biological approach," *Chemico-Biological Interactions*, vol. 171, no. 2, pp. 165–176, 2008.

[148] C. Hansch, D. Hoekman, A. Leo, D. Weininger, and C. D. Selassie, "Chem-bioinformatics: comparative QSAR at the interface between chemistry and biology," *Chemical Reviews*, vol. 102, no. 3, pp. 783–812, 2002.

[149] C. Hansch, D. Hoekman, and H. Gao, "Comparative QSAR: toward a deeper understanding of chemicobiological interactions," *Chemical Reviews*, vol. 96, no. 3, pp. 1045–1075, 1996.

[150] S. P. Gupta, "QSAR studies on enzyme inhibitors," *Chemical Reviews*, vol. 87, no. 5, pp. 1183–1253, 1987.

[151] B. D. Silverman and D. E. Platt, "Comparative molecular moment analysis (coMMA): 3D-QSAR without molecular superposition," *Journal of Medicinal Chemistry*, vol. 39, no. 11, pp. 2129–2140, 1996.

[152] R. D. Cramer, D. E. Patterson, and J. D. Bunce, "Comparative molecular field analysis (CoMFA). 1. Effect of shape on binding of steroids to carrier proteins," *Journal of the American Chemical Society*, vol. 110, no. 18, pp. 5959–5967, 1988.

[153] G. Klebe, U. Abraham, and T. Mietzner, "Molecular similarity indices in a comparative analysis (CoMSIA) of drug molecules to correlate and predict their biological activity," *Journal of Medicinal Chemistry*, vol. 37, no. 24, pp. 4130–4146, 1994.

[154] H. Gohlke and G. Klebe, "Drugscore meets CoMFA: adaptation of fields for molecular comparison (AFMoC) or how to tailor knowledge-based pair-potentials to a particular protein," *Journal of Medicinal Chemistry*, vol. 45, no. 19, pp. 4153–4170, 2002.

[155] V. Lather, V. Kairys, and M. X. Fernandes, "Quantitative structure-activity relationship models with receptor-dependent descriptors for predicting peroxisome proliferator-activated receptor activities of thiazolidinedione and oxazolidinedione derivatives," *Chemical Biology and Drug Design*, vol. 73, no. 4, pp. 428–441, 2009.

[156] L. Rathi, S. K. Kashaw, A. Dixit, G. Pandey, and A. K. Saxena, "Pharmacophore identification and 3D-QSAR studies in *N*-(2-benzoyl phenyl)-L-tyrosines as PPARγ agonists," *Bioorganic and Medicinal Chemistry*, vol. 12, no. 1, pp. 63–69, 2004.

[157] P. J. Brown, T. A. Smith-Oliver, P. S. Charifson et al., "Identification of peroxisome proliferator-activated receptor ligands from a biased chemical library," *Chemistry and Biology*, vol. 4, no. 12, pp. 909–918, 1997.

[158] M. Scarsi, M. Podvinec, A. Roth et al., "Sulfonylureas and glinides exhibit peroxisome proliferator-activated receptor γ activity: a combined virtual screening and biological assay approach," *Molecular Pharmacology*, vol. 71, no. 2, pp. 398–406, 2007.

[159] P. Markt, D. Schuster, J. Kirchmair, C. Laggner, and T. Langer, "Pharmacophore modeling and parallel screening for PPAR ligands," *Journal of Computer-Aided Molecular Design*, vol. 21, no. 10-11, pp. 575–590, 2007.

[160] C. Giaginis, S. Theocharis, and A. Tsantili-Kakoulidou, "A consideration of PPAR-γ ligands with respect to lipophilicity: current trends and perspectives," *Expert Opinion on Investigational Drugs*, vol. 16, no. 4, pp. 413–417, 2007.

[161] N. K. Salam, T. H. Huang, B. P. Kota, M. S. Kim, Y. Li, and D. E. Hibbs, "Novel PPAR-gamma agonists identified from a natural product library: a virtual screening, induced-fit docking and biological assay study," *Chemical Biology & Drug Design*, vol. 71, no. 1, pp. 57–70, 2008.

[162] Y. Tanrikulu, O. Rau, O. Schwarz et al., "Structure-based pharmacophore screening for natural-product-derived PPARγ agonists," *ChemBioChem*, vol. 10, no. 1, pp. 75–78, 2009.

[163] Y. Tanrikulu, M. Nietert, U. Scheffer et al., "Scaffold hopping by "fuzzy" pharmacophores and its application to RNA targets," *ChemBioChem*, vol. 8, no. 16, pp. 1932–1936, 2007.

[164] B. O. Al-Najjar, H. A. Wahab, T. S. Tengku, A. C. Shu-Chien, N. A. Ahmad, and M. O. Taha, "Discovery of new nanomolar peroxisome proliferator-activated receptor γ activators via elaborate ligand-based modeling," *European Journal of Medicinal Chemistry*, vol. 46, no. 6, pp. 2513–2529, 2011.

[165] D. Barnum, J. Greene, A. Smellie, and P. Sprague, "Identification of common functional configurations among molecules," *Journal of Chemical Information and Computer Sciences*, vol. 36, no. 3, pp. 563–571, 1996.

[166] S. Sundriyal, B. Viswanad, P. Ramarao, A. K. Chakraborti, and P. V. Bharatam, "New PPARγ ligands based on barbituric acid: virtual screening, synthesis and receptor binding studies," *Bioorganic & Medicinal Chemistry Letters*, vol. 18, no. 18, pp. 4959–4962, 2008.

[167] H. Zheng, S. Li, L. Ma et al., "A novel agonist of PPAR-γ based on barbituric acid alleviates the development of non-alcoholic fatty liver disease by regulating adipocytokine expression and preventing insulin resistance," *European Journal of Pharmacology*, vol. 659, no. 2-3, pp. 244–251, 2011.

[168] S. Sundriyal, B. Viswanad, E. Bharathy, P. Ramarao, A. K. Chakraborti, and P. V. Bharatam, "New PPARγ ligands based on 2-hydroxy-1,4-naphthoquinone: computer-aided design, synthesis, and receptor-binding studies," *Bioorganic & Medicinal Chemistry Letters*, vol. 18, pp. 3192–3195, 2008.

[169] S. Sundriyal and P. V. Bharatam, "Important pharmacophoric features of pan PPAR agonists: common chemical feature analysis and virtual screening," *European Journal of Medicinal Chemistry*, vol. 44, no. 9, pp. 3488–3495, 2009.

[170] S. Sundriyal and P. V. Bharatam, "'Sum of activities' as dependent parameter: a new CoMFA-based approach for the design of pan PPAR agonists," *European Journal of Medicinal Chemistry*, vol. 44, no. 1, pp. 42–53, 2009.

[171] J. Choi, Y. Park, H. S. Lee, Y. Yang, and S. Yoon, "1,3-diphenyl-1H-pyrazole derivatives as a new series of potent PPARγ partial agonists," *Bioorganic and Medicinal Chemistry*, vol. 18, no. 23, pp. 8315–8323, 2010.

[172] Z. L. Wei, P. A. Petukhov, F. Bizik et al., "Isoxazolyl-serine-based agonists of peroxisome proliferator-activated receptor: design, synthesis, and effects on cardiomyocyte differentiation," *Journal of the American Chemical Society*, vol. 126, no. 51, pp. 16714–16715, 2004.

[173] T. Kaya, S. C. Mohr, D. J. Waxman, and S. Vajda, "Computational screening of phthalate monoesters for binding to PPARγ," *Chemical Research in Toxicology*, vol. 19, no. 8, pp. 999–1009, 2006.

[174] V. G. Maltarollo and K. M. Honorio, "Molecular properties of fatty acids related to PPAR binding and metabolic diseases," *Medicinal Chemistry Research*, pp. 1–8, 2012.

[175] Y. Ma, S.-Q. Wang, W.-R. Xu, R.-L. Wang, and K.-C. Chou, "Design novel dual agonists for treating type-2 diabetes by targeting peroxisome proliferator-activated receptors with core hopping approach," *PloS ONE*, vol. 7, no. 6, Article ID e38546, 2012.

[176] L. Michalik, V. Zoete, G. Krey et al., "Combined simulation and mutagenesis analyses reveal the involvement of key residues for peroxisome proliferator-activated receptor α helix 12 dynamic behavior," *Journal of Biological Chemistry*, vol. 282, no. 13, pp. 9666–9677, 2007.

[177] J. H. Choi, A. S. Banks, J. L. Estall et al., "Anti-diabetic drugs inhibit obesity-linked phosphorylation of PPARγ 3 by Cdk5," *Nature*, vol. 466, no. 7305, pp. 451–456, 2010.

[178] J. H. Choi, A. S. Banks, T. M. Kamenecka et al., "Antidiabetic actions of a non-agonist PPARγ ligand blocking Cdk5-mediated phosphorylation," *Nature*, vol. 477, pp. 477–481, 2011.

[179] J. Jyrkkarinne, J. Kablbeck, J. Pulkkinen et al., "Molecular dynamics simulations for human CAR inverse agonists," *Journal of Chemical Information and Modeling*, vol. 52, pp. 457–464, 2012.

[180] D. Genest, N. Garnier, A. Arrault, C. Marot, L. Morin-Allory, and M. Genest, "Ligand-escape pathways from the ligand-binding domain of PPARγ receptor as probed by molecular dynamics simulations," *European Biophysics Journal*, vol. 37, no. 4, pp. 369–379, 2008.

[181] V. Zoete, A. Grosdidier, and O. Michielin, "Peroxisome proliferator-activated receptor structures: ligand specificity, molecular switch and interactions with regulators," *Biochimica et Biophysica Acta*, vol. 1771, no. 8, pp. 915–925, 2007.

[182] G. Pochetti, N. Mitro, A. Lavecchia et al., "Structural insight into peroxisome proliferator-activated receptor γ binding of two ureidofibrate-like enantiomers by molecular dynamics, cofactor interaction analysis, and site-directed mutagenesis," *Journal of Medicinal Chemistry*, vol. 53, no. 11, pp. 4354–4366, 2010.

[183] A. Rogue, C. Spire, M. Brun, N. Claude, and A. Guillouzo, "Gene expression changes induced by PPAR gamma agonists in animal and human liver," *PPAR Research*, vol. 2010, Article ID 325183, 16 pages, 2010.

[184] A. Rogue, M. P. Renaud, N. Claude, A. Guillouzo, and C. Spire, "Comparative gene expression profiles induced by PPARγ and PPARα/γ agonists in rat hepatocytes," *Toxicology and Applied Pharmacology*, vol. 254, no. 1, pp. 18–31, 2011.

21

Computational Simulation of Tumor Surgical Resection Coupled with the Immune System Response to Neoplastic Cells

J. Jesús Naveja,[1] Flavio F. Contreras-Torres,[1,2]
Andrés Rodríguez-Galván,[1] and Erick Martínez-Lorán[1]

[1] Technology and Consultancy, CTDAT, 04360 Mexico City, Mexico
[2] Universidad de Investigación de Tecnología Experimental Yachay, 100119 Urcuqui, Ecuador

Correspondence should be addressed to J. Jesús Naveja; naveja.jesus@ctdat.com

Academic Editor: Gabriela M. Wilson

Numerous mathematical and computational models have arisen to study and predict the effects of diverse therapies against cancer (e.g., chemotherapy, immunotherapy, and even therapies under research with oncolytic viruses) but, unfortunately, few efforts have been directed towards development of tumor resection models, the first therapy against cancer. The model hereby presented was stated upon fundamental assumptions to produce a predictor of the clinical outcomes of patients undergoing a tumor resection. It uses ordinary differential equations validated for predicting the immune system response and the tumor growth in oncologic patients. This model could be further extended to a personalized prognosis predictor and tools for improving therapeutic strategies.

1. Introduction

The most recent mathematical models are relegating Gompertzian growth curves out of tumor growth modeling. Gompertzian growth strongly depends on time [1], and it can be demonstrated that this leads to artifacts in tumor growth models working with external perturbations, that is, any given therapy. Thus, ordinary differential equations (ODEs) that resemble more the behavior of perturbed tumors [2–4] also share more similarities with the ODEs from the Lotka-Volterra predator-prey model and with the logistic curve described by Verhulst. These ODEs are less time-dependent and focus on interactions among different populations and the carrying capacity of the system [5]. Other approaches for modeling tumor growth use complexity models [6, 7] or physically based models [8, 9], although they have been applied less on therapeutic models than ODEs.

Metastasis, the spread of the malignant cells through the body, causes the degeneration of different body functions, depending on the systems affected. Some of the computational models for metastasis are (a) those belonging to the field of complexity—where discrete models based on single cell interactions have been developed [10]—and (b) models

with ODEs [11, 12]. These models are useful for predicting outcomes for patients under antimetastatic drugs therapies.

Another important factor affecting the dynamics of the tumor is the immune system. De Pillis et al. developed a model that includes as input some features of natural killer cells (NK) and T CD8+ cells (TCD8), as well as the tumor growth rate. NK and TCD8 cells mediate most of the immune response against tumor growth. This model was incorporated into another one that was able to predict clinical outcomes in patients receiving immunotherapy. Interestingly, this model neglects metastasis but obtains clinically significant data [13].

Tumor resection, although a traditional treatment for cancer that is still applied as a treatment for some types of cancer, is a therapy whose mathematical modeling has not been fully developed. Remarkably, a biophysical model correlates histopathology findings with nutrient diffusion of tumor cells, thus permitting a prediction of the required tumor surgical resection for enhancing the probability of total remission [14]. Also, some studies in the field of probability predict the necessity of radiotherapy in postsurgical oncologic patients [15]. However, there are no models with ODEs or in the field of complexity, even though much clinical data have been recollected about tumor resection. It is well known that many tumor surgeries lead to recurrence, and the most accepted mechanism for this is that resections are not always complete, so that negative surgical margins are critical for ensuring a better resection [16]. Also, deliberated partial resections are common, particularly when the tumor is located in organs whose function's maintenance is necessary (e.g., kidney, brain) [16, 17].

In this study, De Pillis et al. ordinary differential equations were coupled with a computational model of tumor resection to observe if the response of the immune system could be modified by a resection of a massive percentage of the tumor. This is a novel study using ODEs for modeling the immune system and tumor partial resection as perturbations on a tumor.

2. Methodology

Using Python 2.7 a program was developed to integrate the ODEs describing the immune system, the tumor, and their interactions. From De Pillis et al.,

$$\frac{dT}{dt} = aT(1 - bT) - cNT - D,$$

$$\frac{dN}{dt} = \sigma - fN + \frac{gT^2}{h + T^2}N - pNT, \quad (1)$$

$$\frac{dL}{dt} = -mL + \frac{jD^2}{k + D^2}L - qLT + rNT,$$

where

$$D = d\frac{(L/T)^\lambda}{s + (L/T)^\lambda}T, \quad (2)$$

where t is time, T is the number of tumor cells, N is the number of NK cells, L is the number of TCD8 cells, and D is the fractional cell kill. The other terms are constants describing the characteristics of the immune system and tumor cells and are better defined in the article from the group of De Pillis, although a brief description of them is given in Table 1.

The parameters that predict whether the immune systems response is either competent (i.e., an immune system capable of defeating a malignant tumor) or incompetent (i.e., the opposite, an immune system whose response is not sufficient and would be overwhelmed by a malignant tumor) against the tumor growth were extracted from the same reference and are given in Table 1.

The incompetent immune system was perturbed during tumor growth with a sudden removal of tumor cells at an arbitrary time. It was then observed whether the immune response remained insufficient against the tumor. The time of the surgery and its extent were deliberately changed in different simulations. Thus, the surgery is evidently an algorithm, not an ODE in this model.

3. Results

The data from De Pillis et al. for competent and incompetent immune system responses against tumors were reproduced.

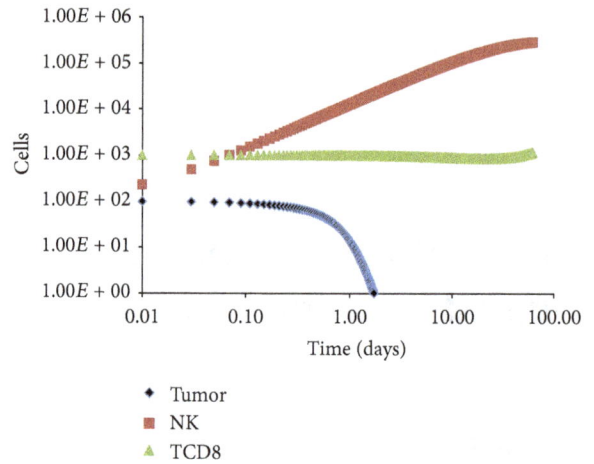

FIGURE 1: Competent immune system versus tumor. NK cell number increase of about 3 orders of magnitude. TCD8 cell increment is less marked, but necessary for an efficient response.

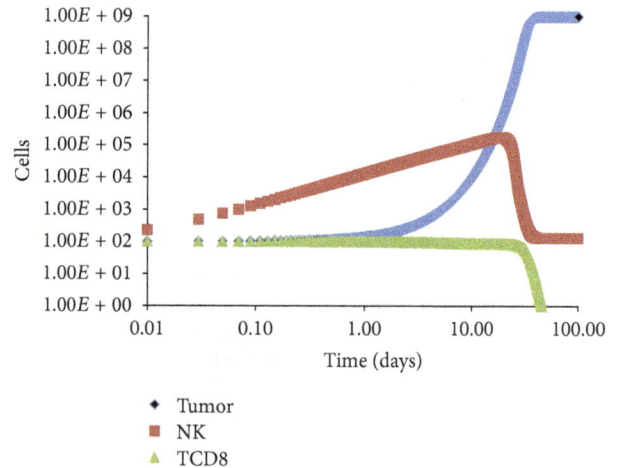

FIGURE 2: Incompetent immune system overwhelmed by a tumor.

The parameters used for the simulations are described in Table 1. When the immune system is overwhelmed by the tumor, a marked decrement of its response is observed, an effect that does not happen in competent immune systems, as shown in Figures 1 and 2. In Figure 1, NK cells exhibit a rapid growth that leads to tumor extinction; interestingly, TCD8 cells number is not modified at a large extent. Nonetheless, TCD8 cell stability is essential for attacking the tumor, as may be seen in Figure 2, where tumor growth elicits a rapid response, at first primarily dependent on NK cells, but with entire collapse of the immune system occurring at around day 20.

Remarkably, when the incompetent immune system is perturbed with a partial but important surgery, an inflection in the remaining tumor cells is observed with practically the same immune response, which does not modify (Figure 3). However, the immune system collapse observed in Figure 2 is not reproduced when the surgery is performed. The key

TABLE 1: Parameters defining a competent and an incompetent immune system for a given tumor (modified from [13]).

Parameter	Units	Meaning	Competent	Incompetent
a	Day^{-1}	Tumor growth rate	5.14×10^{-1}	5.14×10^{-1}
b	Cell^{-1}	$1/b$ is tumor carrying capacity	1.02×10^{-9}	1.02×10^{-9}
c	Cell^{-1} day^{-1}	Fractional tumor cell kill by NK cells	3.23×10^{-7}	3.23×10^{-7}
d	Day^{-1}	Saturation level of fractional tumor cell kill by TCD8 cells	5.8	5.8
λ	None	Exponent of fractional tumor cell kill by TCD8 cells	1.36	1.36
s	None	Steepness coefficient of the tumor-TCD8 cells competition	2.5	2.5
σ	Cells day^{-1}	Constant source of NK cells	1.3×10^{4}	1.3×10^{4}
f	Day^{-1}	Death rate of NK cells	4.12×10^{-2}	4.12×10^{-2}
g	Day^{-1}	Maximum NK cell recruitment rate by tumor cells	2.5×10^{-2}	2.5×10^{-2}
h	Cell^{2}	Steepness coefficient of the NK cell recruitment curve	2.02×10^{7}	2.02×10^{7}
p	Cell^{-1} day^{-1}	NK cell inactivation rate by tumor cells	1.0×10^{-7}	1.0×10^{-7}
m	Day^{-1}	Death rate of TCD8 cells	2.0×10^{-2}	2.0×10^{-2}
j	Day^{-1}	Maximum TCD8 cell recruitment rate	3.75×10^{-2}	3.75×10^{-2}
k	Cell^{2}	Steepness coefficient of the TCD8 cell recruitment curve	2.0×10^{7}	2.0×10^{7}
q	Cell^{-1} day^{-1}	TCD8 cell inactivation rate by tumor cells	3.42×10^{-10}	3.42×10^{-10}
r	Cell^{-1} day^{-1}	Rate at which tumor-specific TCD8 cells are stimulated to be produced as a result of tumor cells killed by NK cells	1.1×10^{-7}	1.1×10^{-7}
$T(0)$	Cells	Initial number of tumor cells	100	100
$N(0)$	Cells	Initial number of NK cells	200	200
$L(0)$	Cells	Initial number of TCD8 cells	1000	100

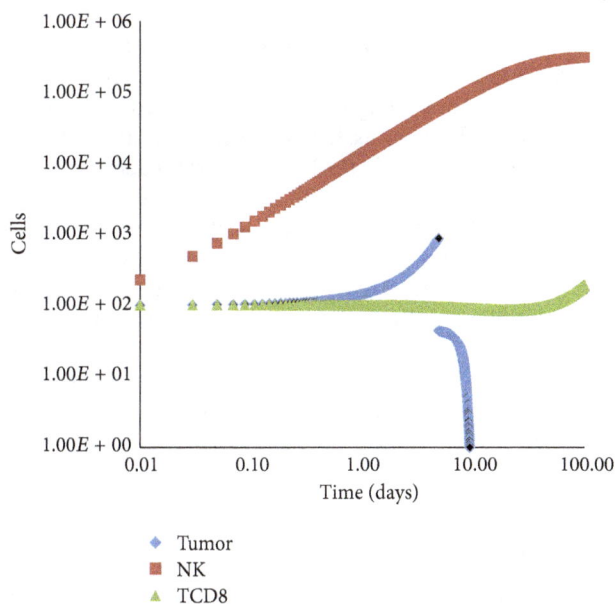

FIGURE 3: The same incompetent immune system depicted in Figure 2, plus a 95 percent resection at day 5; an inflection in the tumor growth curve is seen after the surgery.

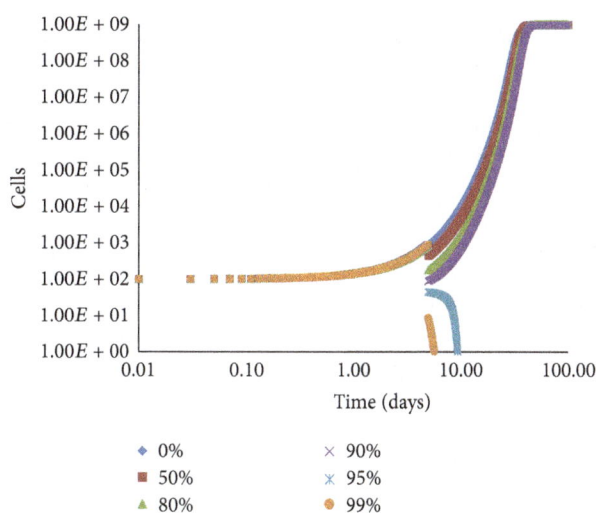

FIGURE 4: Tumor growth resulting from different percentages of tumor resection: 0, 50, 80, 90, 95, and 99% of the tumor, but with the same immune system as in Figure 2 and all of them at day 5.

finding is that this more vulnerable system is capable of reducing the remaining tumor cells.

In order to recognize the extent and the time of the surgery as important variables when a tumor surgical resection is performed, different percentages of tumor removal and times for surgery were tested (Figures 4 and 5, resp.). At day 5, and for the same immune system response seen in Figure 2, only surgeries that remove 95% or more of the tumor would cure the patient (assuming that no other intervention is performed) (Figure 4). On the other hand, a 95% resection would only cure the patient if it is performed earlier than day 10 (Figure 5).

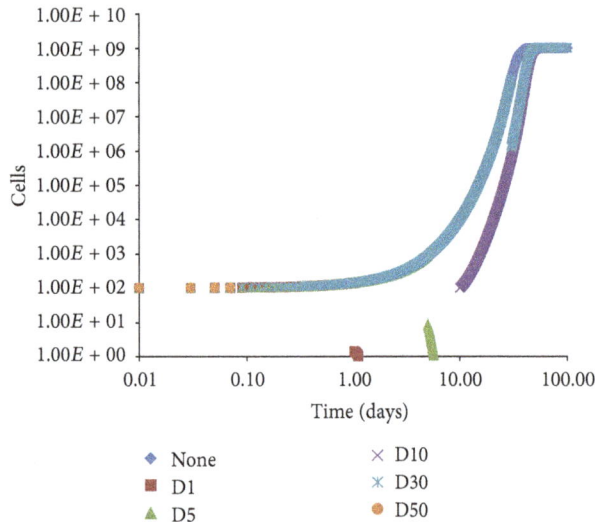

FIGURE 5: Tumor growth for resections at days 1, 5, 10, 30, and 50; the extent of the surgery was set at 95% and the immune system is the same as that shown in Figure 2.

4. Discussion

A decline in tumor growth could not be elicited by the immune system in every case. In Figure 1, a sufficient immune response performed by a competent immune system leads to the inhibition of the tumor. However, a partial but sufficient surgery may reverse the overwhelming of the immune system response when otherwise it would be incompetent (e.g., Figures 2 and 3). When the surgery was implemented, the most important variables turned out to be (a) the tumor size at the time of the surgery, which is a variable dependent on the time of the surgery, as can be seen in Figure 5, where only resections performed before tumor growth reaches a significant inflexion point are curative; (b) the extent of the surgery: Figure 4 shows how resections reducing the number of tumor cells below a critical number (50 cells for this particular tumor interacting with this particular immune system) may lead to total remission; and (c) the immune system response at the time of the surgery, which was found to be equivalent to the number of cells in the immune system, which only defines a higher or lower critical tumor mass (data not shown). Interestingly, clinical data from a study with resection of different percentages of the tumor highly resembled this data: only resections spanning 90% or more of the tumor volume were likely to lead to a total remission of abdominal Burkitt's lymphoma; this can be seen in Figure 4 [18]. It must be noted that in the simulation depicted in Figure 5 the critical number of cells (a threshold that, if trespassed, will lead to a massive growth of the tumor) is consistent with that in Figure 4. This effect shows that the time of resection is not by itself a prognostic factor.

The assumptions taken by this model define its limitations. It does not take into account metastasis, adjuvant chemotherapy, or tumor angiogenesis. Nonetheless, studying a single variable in this case would be more reliable. Thus, this model would work better for predicting the behavior of tumors in which angiogenesis and metastasis may be neglected. This is an evident limitation when predicting outcomes distant in time. Hence, this model would work better for predicting clinical events foreseen to occur soon when considering tumors that metastasize, since the possibility of distant metastasis increases with time. Although the timing of the interventions in this model is early, it must be taken into account that the patients from [13] had an advanced disease. This does not diminish the reliability of the model, as it may be personalized to every patient. On the other hand, it could be difficult to estimate the proportion of the tumor extracted. This problem may be avoided since a correlation exists between the volume of the tumor and the number of cells in the tumor, and computed tomography can estimate tumor volume accurately [19]. Diffusion-tensor magnetic resonance may even estimate brain tumor cellularity precisely [20].

This study was performed on a validated model of immune system against tumor growth and could be further developed to consider metastasis, chemotherapy, and any other therapy for every individual case. This will bring a more personalized health care and prognosis depending on more than population statistic variables, as in the prevalent prognosis calculation [21]. Besides this, it would be highly beneficial if surgeons could be aided with computer programs for improving the patients' follow-up and scheduling subsequent surgeries based on evidence.

5. Conclusion

A novel computational model is hereby proposed, which predicts the interaction of tumors and immune system response and their behavior after a partial surgical resection using ordinary differential equations. It was shown that a partial but sufficient surgery could help the immune system defeat a tumor *in silico*. Otherwise, the immune system explored would have collapsed and been incapable of eradicating the neoplasm.

Further research is needed in order to improve prognostic tools and therapeutic strategies using computational models predicting clinical outcomes of patients with cancer. This computational model requires clinical validation, although it is based on a model of immune system that correlated well with the outcomes of patients with cancer. Moreover, ODEs should be tested, for example, against stochastic differential equations, in order to assess their reliability.

Conflict of Interests

The authors declare that there is no conflict of interests regarding the publication of this paper.

Acknowledgments

The authors thank Ricardo Espinosa-González for his contribution revising the paper and for his pertinent annotations. J. Jesús Naveja acknowledges PECEM M.D./Ph.D. program from the Faculty of Medicine of UNAM for the organization of the fellowship. Flavio F. Contreras-Torres thanks Yachay Tech University for supporting his academic stay.

References

[1] A. K. Laird, "Dynamics of tumor growth," *British Journal of Cancer*, vol. 18, no. 3, pp. 490–502, 1964.

[2] N. L. Komarova and D. Wodarz, "ODE models for oncolytic virus dynamics," *Journal of Theoretical Biology*, vol. 263, no. 4, pp. 530–543, 2010.

[3] R. K. Sachs, L. R. Hlatky, and P. Hahnfeldt, "Simple ODE models of tumor growth and anti-angiogenic or radiation treatment," *Mathematical and Computer Modelling*, vol. 33, no. 12-13, pp. 1297–1305, 2001.

[4] E. Comen, P. G. Morris, and L. Norton, "Translating mathematical modeling of tumor growth patterns into novel therapeutic approaches for breast cancer," *Journal of Mammary Gland Biology and Neoplasia*, vol. 17, no. 3-4, pp. 241–249, 2012.

[5] A. A. Berryman, "The origins and evolution of predator-prey theory," *Ecology*, vol. 73, no. 5, pp. 1530–1535, 1992.

[6] C. F. Lo, "Stochastic Gompertz model of tumour cell growth," *Journal of Theoretical Biology*, vol. 248, no. 2, pp. 317–321, 2007.

[7] A. R. Kansal, S. Torquato, G. R. Harsh IV, E. A. Chiocca, and T. S. Deisboeck, "Simulated brain tumor growth dynamics using a three-dimensional cellular automaton," *Journal of Theoretical Biology*, vol. 203, no. 4, pp. 367–382, 2000.

[8] T. Yamano, "Statistical ensemble theory of Gompertz growth model," *Entropy*, vol. 11, no. 4, pp. 807–819, 2009.

[9] P. Castorina and D. Zappalà, "Tumor Gompertzian growth by cellular energetic balance," *Physica Acta*, vol. 365, no. 2, pp. 473–480, 2006.

[10] L. A. Liotta, G. M. Saidel, and J. Kleinerman, "Stochastic model of metastases formation," *Biometrics. Journal of the Biometric Society*, vol. 32, no. 3, pp. 535–550, 1976.

[11] V. Haustein and U. Schumacher, "A dynamic model for tumour growth and metastasis formation," *Journal of Clinical Bioinformatics*, vol. 2, no. 1, article 11, 2012.

[12] A. R. A. Anderson, M. A. J. Chaplain, E. L. Newman, R. J. C. Steele, and A. M. Thompson, "Mathematical modelling of tumour invasion and metastasis," *Journal of Theoretical Medicine*, vol. 2, no. 2, pp. 129–154, 2000.

[13] L. G. De Pillis, A. E. Radunskaya, and C. L. Wiseman, "A validated mathematical model of cell-mediated immune response to tumor growth," *Cancer Research*, vol. 65, no. 17, pp. 7950–7958, 2005.

[14] M. E. Edgerton, Y.-L. Chuang, P. MacKlin, W. Yang, E. L. Bearer, and V. Cristini, "A novel, patient-specific mathematical pathology approach for assessment of surgical volume: application to ductal carcinoma in situ of the breast," *Analytical Cellular Pathology*, vol. 34, no. 5, pp. 247–263, 2011.

[15] F. M. O. Al-Dweri, D. Guirado, A. M. Lallena, and V. Pedraza, "Effect on tumour control of time interval between surgery and postoperative radiotherapy: An empirical approach using Monte Carlo simulation," *Physics in Medicine and Biology*, vol. 49, no. 13, pp. 2827–2839, 2004.

[16] S. E. Sutherland, M. I. Resnick, G. T. Maclennan, and H. B. Goldman, "Does the size of the surgical margin in partial nephrectomy for renal cell cancer really matter?" *The Journal of Urology*, vol. 167, no. 1, pp. 61–64, 2002.

[17] I. Ciric, M. Ammirati, N. Vick, and M. Mikhael, "Supratentorial gliomas: surgical considerations and immediate postoperative results. Gross total resection versus partial resection," *Neurosurgery*, vol. 21, no. 1, pp. 21–26, 1987.

[18] I. T. Magrath, S. Lwanga, W. Carswell, and N. Harrison, "Surgical reduction of tumour bulk in management of abdominal Burkitt's lymphoma," *British Medical Journal*, vol. 2, no. 914, pp. 308–312, 1974.

[19] C. R. Johnson, H. D. Thames, D. T. Huang, and R. K. Schmidt-Ullrich, "The tumor volume and clonogen number relationship: tumor control predictions based upon tumor volume estimates derived from computed tomography," *International Journal of Radiation Oncology, Biology, Physics*, vol. 33, no. 2, pp. 281–287, 1995.

[20] K. M. Gauvain, R. C. McKinstry, P. Mukherjee et al., "Evaluating pediatric brain tumor cellularity with diffusion-tensor imaging," *American Journal of Roentgenology*, vol. 177, no. 2, pp. 449–454, 2001.

[21] B. Gwilliam, V. Keeley, C. Todd et al., "Development of prognosis in palliative care study (PiPS) predictor models to improve prognostication in advanced cancer: prospective cohort study," *British Medical Journal*, vol. 343, no. 7821, Article ID d4920, 2011.

22

2D-QSAR Study of Indolylpyrimidines Derivative as Antibacterial against *Pseudomonas aeruginosa* and *Staphylococcus aureus*: A Comparative Approach

Prasanna A. Datar

Department of Pharmaceutical Chemistry, Sinhgad Institute of Pharmacy, Narhe, Pune 411041, India

Correspondence should be addressed to Prasanna A. Datar; d_pras_anna@rediffmail.com

Academic Editor: Gabriela Mustata Wilson

A set of 15 indolylpyrimidine derivatives with their antibacterial activities in terms of minimum inhibitory concentration against the gram-negative bacteria *Pseudomonas aeruginosa* and gram-positive *Staphylococcus aureus* were selected for 2D quantitative structure activity relationship (QSAR) analysis. QSAR was performed using a combination of various descriptors such as steric, electronic and topological. Stepwise regression method was used to derive the most significant QSAR equation for predicting the inhibitory activity of this class of molecules. The best QSAR model was further validated by a leave one out technique as well as by the random trials. A high correlation between experimental and predicted inhibitory values was observed. A comparative picture of behavior of indolylpyrimidines against both of the microorganisms is discussed.

1. Introduction

Pseudomonas aeruginosa (PA), a gram-negative pathogen, has been known as a major cause of hospital acquired infection and antimicrobial resistance [1, 2]. *Pseudomonas aeruginosa* is responsible for various infectious cases such as nosocomial pneumonia urinary tract infections, surgical wound infections, and bloodstream infections [3]. Structural differences exist between cell walls of gram-positive and gram-negative bacteria. Gram-positive bacteria have more peptidoglycan layers as compared to gram-negative bacteria. Therefore the cell wall of gram-positive bacteria is thicker than the cell wall of gram-negative bacteria.

Gram-negative bacterial cell wall is different from gram-positive bacterial cell wall by having an outer membrane of lipoproteins that covers the peptidoglycan layer. The outer membrane of gram-negative bacteria is made up of phospholipids, lipoproteins, and lipopolysaccharides. The outer membrane is negatively charged and helps prevent the bacteria from being phagocytosed by macrophages. The outer membrane provides protection from effects of antibiotics, digestive enzymes, and heavy metals.

Many chemical entities work as antibacterial agents by inhibiting the DNA synthesis of cell wall by blocking the enzymes such as DNA gyrase and dihydrofolate reductase and even inhibiting enzymes processing the development of peptidoglycan layer [4, 5].

Approach of antibacterial drug is initially a surface phenomenon. The wall of gram-positive and gram-negative bacteria will resist the surface interaction. Therefore there is a difference in antibacterial activity of chemical entity towards gram-positive and gram-negative bacteria. In the present work, we have made an attempt to differentiate the behavior of chemical entities towards gram-positive and gram-negative bacteria using QSAR molecular descriptors which explains surface phenomenon. This would have been possible to express in terms of Hammett parameters and pKa values of the compounds as descriptors, but our approach gives emphasis on calculated surface parameter to express the antibacterial activity. There are many equations in the literature expressing antibacterial activity using Hammett and pKa values but these equations are insignificant in virtual screening of molecular databases for finding significant antibacterial hits.

The objective of the present investigation was to study the usefulness of QSAR in the prediction of the antibacterial activity of indolylpyrimidine derivatives against *Pseudomonas aeruginosa* (PA) and *Staphylococcus aureus* (SA) and understand how multiple linear regression (MLR) equations can explain the structural key points correlating to differential behavior in activity against both gram-positive and gram-negative strains.

The pharmaceutical importance of pyrimidine compounds lies in the fact that they can be effectively used as analgesic, anti-inflammatory, anticonvulsant, insecticidal, herbicidal, antitubercular, anticancer and antidiabetic agents. The indole ring is known to exhibit anti-inflammatory, antimicrobial and antifungal activities [6–10]. The fused ring system of substituted indolylpyrimidines is remarkably effective as antitumor and antibacterial activity [11, 12]. The QSAR method requires data collection from the same laboratory experiment, molecular descriptor selection, QSAR model development and finally model validation. A QSAR study has predictive ability and even provides clues for mechanism of drug receptor interactions [13, 14].

2. Biological Activity

Very few research articles are available from the same laboratory on indolylpyrimidines as antibacterial agents. Indolylpyrimidines tested were obtained from the studies reported by Panda and Chowdhary [15] where *in vitro* antibacterial activity against *Pseudomonas aeruginosa* and *Staphylococcus aureus* was carried out at uniform concentration of 100 μg/mL and zone of inhibition is reported in distance unit, that is, millimeters (mm). The values are directly proportional since the more the distance in mm for zone of inhibition is, the more the potency would be. The distance in mm is used as dependent variable in QSAR study. Zone of inhibition against *Pseudomonas aeruginosa* (PAantibact) varies from 10 mm to 24 mm while, for *Staphylococcus aureus*, it varies from 13 mm to 31 mm (SAantibact). Figures 1 and 2 give the activity distribution plot for antibacterial activity against *Pseudomonas aeruginosa* and *Staphylococcus aureus*, respectively. The plot shows blue columns representing training set while brown columns represent test set distribution.

3. Data Sets

Due to constraints of data selection based on the same laboratory experimental studies, study with exact numerical values was selected for QSAR study. According to the variation in substituents at various positions in a set of indolylpyrimidine derivatives, molecules were divided into the training set and test set using sphere exclusion method. The training set comprised 15 derivatives (4a, 4c, 4e, 4g, 4i, 5c, 5f, 5g, 5h, 5j, 6a, 6b, 6d, 6i, and 6j) while the and test set comprised 9 derivatives (4d, 4f, 4h, 4j, 5a, 5d, 6c, 6e, 6f, and 6g) of indolylpyrimidines published by Panda and Chowdary [15], which have been shown to possess antibacterial activity against *Pseudomonas aeruginosa*.

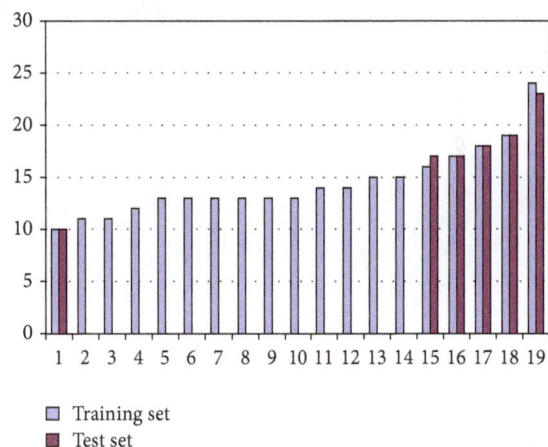

FIGURE 1: Activity distribution plot for antibacterial activity against PA.

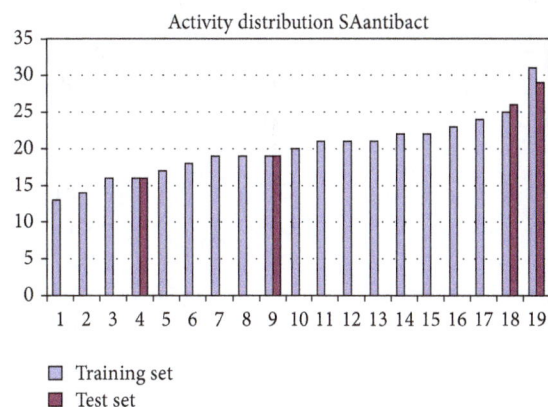

FIGURE 2: Activity distribution plot for antibacterial activity against SA.

The case of QSAR model studied for activity against *Staphylococcus aureus* has a training set comprising 14 molecules (4a, 4c, 4d, 4f, 5a, 5b, 5d, 5g, 5h, 6b, 6c, 6f, 6i, 6j) and test set comprising 6 molecules (4b, 5c, 5f, 6a, 6d, 6h). The test compounds were selected manually considering the activity distribution and structural diversity as compared to the training set. Chemical structures of indolylpyrimidines and corresponding biological data are shown in Table 1.

4. Molecular Modeling

All molecular modeling studies were performed by using Schrodinger software running on windows platform. Ligprep module was used to draw the 3D structures. The 3D structures were further cleaned up and subjected to energy minimization using conjugate gradient method using MMFF force field. The minimization was performed until the RMS gradient value reaches a value smaller than 0.1 kcal/mol°A. Optimization was further performed using BFGS method until the RMS gradient attains a value smaller than 0.0001 kcal/mol°A. The lowest energy structure of each molecule was subjected to calculate molecular descriptors.

TABLE 1: Structures of indolylpyrimidines and their antibacterial activity used for the QSAR studies.

Compound number	R_1	R_2	Zone of inhibition against *Pseudomonas aeruginosa* in mm (PAantibact)	Zone of inhibition against *Staphylococcus aureus* in mm (SAantibact)
4a	OH	H	13	16
4b	OH	p-NH$_2$	24	26
4c	OH	p-Br	19	20
4d	OH	p-Cl	18	19
4e	OH	o,p-OH	14	14
4f	OH	p-F	17	18
4g	OH	p-CH$_3$	13	10
4h	OH	p-OCH$_3$	17	21
4i	OH	p-OH	11	16
4j	OH	p-NO$_2$	23	22
5a	SH	H	12	13
5b	SH	p-NH$_2$	18	19
5c	SH	p-Br	15	16
5d	SH	p-Cl	16	17
5f	SH	p-F	14	19
5g	SH	p-CH$_3$	10	21
5h	SH	p-OCH$_3$	13	25
5j	SH	p-NO$_2$	19	16
6a	NH$_2$	H	11	10
6b	NH$_2$	p-NH$_2$	10	24
6c	NH$_2$	p-Br	17	23
6d	NH$_2$	p-Cl	15	19
6e	NH$_2$	o,p-OH	13	16
6f	NH$_2$	p-F	23	22
6g	NH$_2$	p-CH$_3$	13	14
6h	NH$_2$	p-OCH$_3$	25	29
6i	NH$_2$	p-OH	13	21
6j	NH$_2$	p-NO$_2$	24	31

5. Descriptor Generation

The numerical descriptors are responsible for encoding information of important features of the molecular structure and can be categorized into different properties such as electronic, geometric, hydrophobic and topological. Various molecular descriptors were calculated such as molecular weight, dipole moment and partition coefficient (ClogP), surface area descriptors, H-bond donor count, H-bond acceptor count, ionization potential and electron affinity. Among the set of equations, generated descriptors that explain surface phenomenon were retained as shown in Table 2. Biological activity and descriptor values were scaled to unit variance as shown in Table 3.

Pearson's correlation matrix was used to select the suitable descriptors for MLR analysis. Pearson's correlation matrix

TABLE 2: Description of descriptors used in QSAR study.

Descriptor name	Description
mol_MW	Molecular weight of the molecule.
dipole	Computed dipole moment of the molecule.
EA (eV)	PM3 calculated electron affinity.
donorHB	Estimated number of hydrogen bonds that would be donated by the solute to water molecules in an aqueous solution. Values are averages taken over a number of configurations, so they can be noninteger.
PSA	Van der Waals surface area of polar nitrogen and oxygen atoms.
SASA	Total solvent accessible surface area (SASA) in square angstroms using a probe with a 1.4 Å radius.
PISA	π (carbon and attached hydrogen) component of the SASA.
WPSA	Weakly polar component of the SASA (halogens, P and S).
FISA	Hydrophilic component of the SASA (SASA on N, O, and H on heteroatoms).
FOSA	Hydrophobic component of the SASA (saturated carbon and attached hydrogen).

TABLE 3: Descriptors used in 2D QSAR studies.

Compound number	mol_MW	dipole	FOSA	FISA	PISA	WPSA	donorHB	EA (eV)	PSA
4a	287.3	5.2	0	109.3	423.9	0	2	0.631	57.9
4b	302.3	3.4	0	170.7	377.8	0	3.5	0.394	83.9
4c	366.2	6.9	0	109.1	375.9	77.9	2	0.747	57.9
4d	321.7	7.3	0	109.3	376.3	72.5	2	0.784	57.9
4e	319.3	4.3	0	201.0	354.2	0	4	0.428	98.5
4f	305.3	7.4	0	109.3	386.7	47.2	2	0.804	57.9
4g	301.3	5.0	89.4	109.3	368.1	0	2	0.608	57.9
4h	317.3	5.9	93.0	111.3	365.1	0	2	0.693	67.8
4i	303.3	5.1	0	164.7	382.2	0	3	0.605	80.6
4j	332.3	14.3	0	207.5	365.3	0	2	1.852	103.0
5a	303.3	4.2	0	47.1	420.0	81.2	1.8	0.721	35.2
5b	318.3	3.2	0	108.6	373.9	81.2	3.3	0.47	61.2
5c	382.2	5.7	0	46.9	371.9	159.2	1.8	0.836	35.2
5d	337.8	6.1	0	47.2	372.3	153.8	1.8	0.874	35.2
5e	335.3	3.6	0	139.3	350.5	79.9	3.8	0.507	75.8
5f	321.3	6.3	0	47.1	382.7	128.5	1.8	0.894	35.2
5g	317.4	3.9	89.4	47.2	364.2	81.2	1.8	0.696	35.2
5h	333.4	4.9	93.0	47.1	361.2	81.2	1.8	0.721	44.1
5i	319.3	4.0	0	102.6	378.2	81.2	2.8	0.692	57.9
5j	348.3	13.1	0	145.3	361.4	81.2	1.8	1.903	80.4
6a	286.3	4.3	0	113.8	422.3	0	3	0.388	60.7
6b	301.3	1.8	0	175.3	376.1	0	4.5	0.166	86.7
6c	365.2	6.3	0	113.6	374.2	77.9	3	0.511	60.7
6d	320.7	6.7	0	113.8	374.6	72.5	3	0.555	60.7
6e	318.3	5.4	0	205.3	352.7	0	5	0.204	101.3
6f	304.3	6.7	0	113.8	385.0	47.2	3	0.572	60.7
6g	300.3	3.9	89.4	113.9	366.4	0	3	0.369	60.7
6h	317.3	5.9	93.0	111.3	365.1	0	2	0.693	67.8
6i	302.3	5.4	0	169.3	380.5	0	4	0.365	83.4
6j	331.3	13.7	0	212.0	363.7	0	3	1.716	105.8

was performed on all descriptors by using "BuildQSAR" module available in Schrodinger software. Tables 4 and 5 show correlation matrix for the descriptors used in the resulting models for *Pseudomonas aeruginosa* and *Staphylococcus aureus*, respectively. The descriptors correlated above 0.5 were eliminated from the QSAR study. The correlated descriptor that duplicates the meaning of other descriptors was eliminated. ClogP was found to be correlated to FISA by 0.94 and to FOSA by 0.46, respectively. Correlation matrix shows that ClogP correlates well with FISA and PSA (Tables 4 and 5).

TABLE 4: Pearson's correlation matrix for descriptors in QSAR model of *Pseudomonas aeruginosa*.

	PAantibact	Dipole	mol_MW	donorHB	FISA	PSA	ClogP
PAantibact	1.0	—	—	—	—	—	—
Dipole	0.803	1.0	—	—	—	—	—
mol_MW	0.321	0.170	1.0	—	—	—	—
donorHB	0.037	0.075	0.186	1.0	—	—	—
FISA	0.090	0.076	0.080	0.581	1.0	—	—
PSA	0.122	0.115	0.053	0.536	0.979	1.0	—
ClogP	−0.013	0.013	0.510	−0.898	−0.93	−0.914	1.0

TABLE 5: Pearson's correlation matrix for descriptors in QSAR model of *Staphylococcus aureus*.

	SAantibact	Dipole	EA (eV)	PSA	PISA	WPSA	FOSA	ClogP
SAantibact	1.0	—	—	—	—	—	—	—
Dipole	0.200	1.0	—	—	—	—	—	—
EA (eV)	0.175	0.016	1.0	—	—	—	—	—
PSA	0.328	0.810	0.087	1.0	—	—	—	—
PISA	0.618	0.065	0.084	0.038	1.0	—	—	—
WPSA	0.055	0.065	0.001	0.506	0.080	1.0	—	—
FOSA	0.182	0.032	0.001	0.072	0.212	0.001	1.0	—
ClogP	−0.488	−0.159	0.113	−0.933	0.010	0.855	0.468	1.0

Since ClogP is unable to express charge of a molecule, therefore descriptors based on solvent accessible surface area such as FISA and FOSA were used to overcome this limitation [16, 17].

Linear QSAR equations were developed by a stepwise addition of terms. Each descriptor was chosen as input for variable selection method such as stepwise addition method. The method selects the descriptor that contributes to the antibacterial activity of indolylpyrimidine derivatives. To reduce the variation in the biological data, stepwise equations were generated using autoscaling of the dataset.

MLR method only can be used when a relatively small number of molecular descriptors are used. The ratio of descriptor to number of molecules in a QSAR equation generated was kept as $1 : 5$. Thus for training set of 15 molecules, 3 descriptors were optimal. However, PCR and PLS would also be used which allow using more descriptors, but too many descriptors may cause difficulties in model interpretability. Besides, using several factors (principal components or latent variables) can make model interpretation tedious. Validation is a crucial aspect of any QSAR analysis [18, 19]. Predictive power of selected MLR equation is validated by the live one out (LOO) technique. The QSAR equations were validated by the calculation of the following statistical parameters: CV $r^2(q^2)$, r^2, ran_r^2, and std_error (Tables 6a and 6b).

Randomization was performed by randomly shuffling the dependent parameter and then generating the equation using MLR method for the same set of descriptors and training set molecule. The resulting r^2 is denoted by ran_r^2. If ran_r^2 is consistent and equivalent to r^2 value of the QSAR model, then the QSAR equation is spurious. Consider

$$\text{CV } r^2 = \frac{1 - \text{Press}}{\text{SSY}}, \quad (1)$$

where,

$$\text{Press} = \sum \left(Y_{\text{obs}} - Y_{\text{calc}}\right)^2, \quad (2)$$

$$\text{SSY} = \sum \left(Y_{\text{obs}} - Y_{\text{mean}}\right)^2, \quad (3)$$

where Y_{obs}, Y_{calc}, and Y_{mean} are observed, calculated, and mean values, respectively, "n" is the number of compounds, and "p" is the number of independent parameters. The value PRESS is indicated by prediction sum of squares. The PRESS value can be used to calculate CV $r^2(q^2)$, called cross-validated r^2, which represents the prediction ability of the QSAR equation. This is a good way to validate the prediction of a regression equation. The CV $r^2(q^2)$ value ranges from zero to one. To calculate PRESS, each observation is individually omitted once. The remaining $n - 1$ observations are used to calculate a regression equation and value of the omitted observation is estimated. This is done "n" times, once for each observation. The difference between the actual Y value (Y_{obs}) and the predicted Y value (Y_{calc}) is called the prediction error. The sum of the squared prediction errors is indicated as PRESS value.

A compound is said to be outlier whose activity cannot be predicted by generated QSAR equation. The structural diversity of these molecules is responsible for their nonpredictability. Equation 1 in Table 6(a) gives outliers, which can be identified by Z score value [20]. Z score value is calculated by the following formula:

$$Z \text{ score} = \frac{(x - x\_\text{mean})}{s}, \quad (4)$$

where initially the mean is subtracted from every value and then the mean-shifted values are divided by the standard

TABLE 6: Best MLR models for the prediction of antibacterial activity.

(a) Stepwise regression result for antibacterial activity against PA

Eq. number	Equation	N	r^2	CV r^2 (q^2)	Std_error (s)	Pred. r^2	Ran_r^2	Z score r^2
1	PAantibact = (0.8455) dipole + (0.0464) mol_MW + (0.0135) FISA − 7.5189	15	0.879	0.709	0.499	0.399	0.264	4.938
1.1	PAantibact = (1.0249) dipole + (0.0538) mol_MW − (0.0555) SASA + 21.7974	15	0.878	0.673	1.504	0.518	0.391	1.876

(b) Stepwise regression result for antibacterial activity against SA

Eq. number	Equation	N	r^2	CV r^2 (q^2)	Std_error (s)	Pred. r^2	Ran_r^2	Z score r^2
2	SAantibact = −0.2246 PISA − 0.0595 WPSA + 2.9410 EA (eV) + 107.5483	15	0.874	0.767	0.222	1.469	0.356	3.938
2.1	SAantibact = −(0.1343) PISA + (0.1660) PSA + (0.0494) FOSA + 61.1447	15	0.876	0.743	2.210	1.544	0.288	3.461

deviation (s). Z score is a value that estimates in terms of the number of standard deviations the value above or below the mean of a data set.

6. Results

In QSAR equation development for *Pseudomonas aeruginosa*, the regression equation indicated dipole moment as the most significant in contribution to inhibitory activity (Equation 1, Table 6(a)) since it has the highest correlation with the activity. Molecular weight (mol_MW) is an additional parameter to dipole, which significantly increases the correlation coefficient from 0.7910 to 0.8587. The selection of variable was such that it minimizes the mean squared error of prediction. Similarly, the addition of a third parameter, FISA, also increased the correlation coefficient from 0.8587 to 0.8793. Other regression equations were also obtained just by altering third parameter FISA with donorHB or PSA and so forth. Tables 6(a) and 6(b) give the best equations (1 and 2) selected in comparison to 1.1 and 2.1, respectively, since the latter ones are having high standard error (s) value and therefore are insignificant.

In Table 6(a), Equation 1, all the descriptors are directly proportional to the activity and it is highly correlated to dipole more than molecular weight. Similarly, in case of QSAR equation developed for activity against *Staphylococcus aureus* is shown in Table 6(b), PISA is a prominent parameter. Successive addition of WPSA or PSA and the third parameter EA (eV) enhanced QSAR equation significantly. N is the number of molecules in training set, r^2 is squared correlation coefficient and F-test is a variance-related statistical value that compares two models differing by one or more variable. The QSAR equation is supposed to be good if the F-test is above a threshold value. The statistical quality of the resulting models, as depicted in Table 6(a), is determined by r, standard error (std_error), and randomization test (ran_r^2) [21, 22].

A data point was considered to be an outlier if its residual value exceeded two times the value of standard error of estimate of the model. It is noteworthy that all these equations were derived using the entire data set of compounds ($n = 28$) and the outliers were identified for both of the QSAR equations. For QSAR equation of *Pseudomonas aeruginosa*, outliers were obtained as 5b, 6h with Z score value of 4.938. While QSAR equation of activity against *Staphylococcus aureus* had outliers as 4e, 4g, 5j, 6e, 6g with Z score value of 3.938. The reason for the molecules being found as outliers was investigated. It was found that the descriptor value for these molecules was away from the range of descriptor values of the training set molecules [23]. Removal of these outliers has improved the statistics of the equations.

The best measure of reliability of a 2D-QSAR model is a high q^2, not just a high r^2 that could be a result of overfitting to data. More often, a value of $q^2 > 0.5$ is considered acceptable [24–26]. Self-consistency of the derived models was verified using the leave one out (LOO) process and the predictability of each model was assessed using cross-validated r^2, called q^2.

Figures 3 and 4 shows plots of predicted versus experimentally observed inhibitory activity for training set and test set of indolylpyrimidines against PA respectively. While Figures 5 and 6 shows plots of predicted versus experimentally observed inhibitory activity for training set and test set of indolylpyrimidines against SA respectively. The plots for QSAR models of PA and SA show a very good fit in the range of $r^2 = 0.87$ to 0.80. It indicates that these models can be successfully applied to predict the antibacterial activity of this class of molecules. Randomization studies show ran_r^2 of 0.2 and 0.3 for Equation 1 (Table 6(a)) and 2 (Table 6(b)), respectively; thus the equations are not chance correlations. Moreover, it was possible to use the reported QSAR models to predict the activity of analogous molecules for antibacterial activity against PA and SA. The

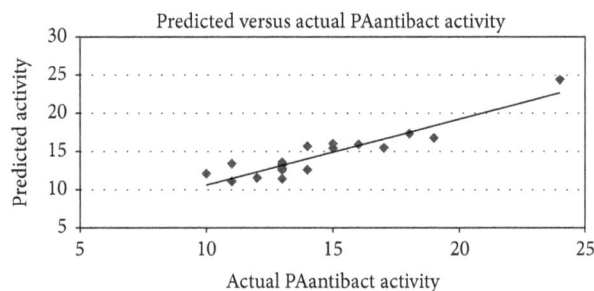

FIGURE 3: Plots of predicted versus experimentally observed inhibitory activity for training set of indolylpyrimidines against PA.

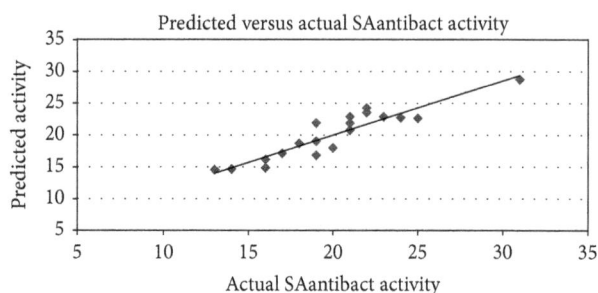

FIGURE 5: Plot of predicted versus experimentally observed inhibitory activity for training set of indolylpyrimidines against SA.

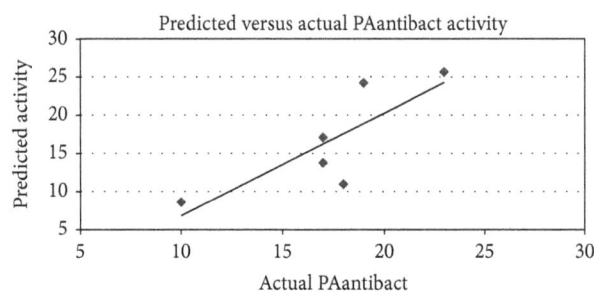

FIGURE 4: Plot of predicted versus experimentally observed inhibitory activity for test set of indolylpyrimidines against PA.

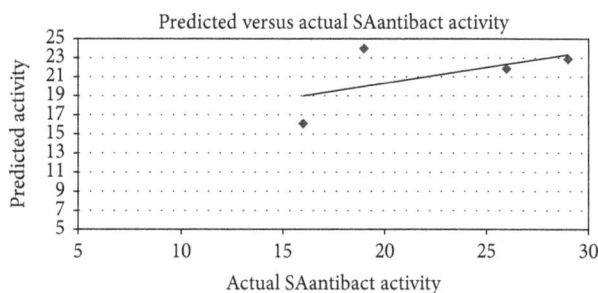

FIGURE 6: Plot of predicted versus experimentally observed inhibitory activity for test set of indolylpyrimidines against SA.

applicability domain of the derived QSAR models is restricted to substituted indolylpyrimidine derivatives.

7. Discussion

It clearly showed that QSAR Equation 1 in Table 6(a) obtained for antibacterial activity against PA includes dipole, mol_MW, and third descriptor FISA. Thus the equation is a combination of size of molecule, polar nature, and hydrophilicity of molecule as shown in Table 6(a). While QSAR equation obtained for antibacterial activity against SA includes PISA, PSA, and third descriptor FOSA. Thus QSAR Equation 2 in Table 6(b) shows combination of hydrophobicity and electron density centers and weakly polar groups (halogens P and S).

Since both of the activities were conducted in the same laboratory and at the same concentration of drug, that is, 100 μg/mL, the comparisons with respect to activity were possible.

Equation 1 in Table 6(a) gives descriptors for PA activity such as dipole, molecular weight, and FISA. In QSAR Equation 1 of Table 6(a), all the descriptors are directly proportional to the activity. Dipole is highly correlated with the activity followed by molecular weight. It is observed that the higher the dipole and the higher the PA activity, the higher the FISA activity and the higher the PA activity and molecular weight to be in the range of 320 to 332. Overall, this equation gives the relationship of polarity of a molecule as the essential characteristics required for the antibacterial activity against PA.

In QSAR Equation 2 which is developed for SA activity, as shown in Table 6(b), PISA is a prominent parameter. Successive addition of WPSA and the third parameter EA (eV) enhanced the model significantly. In interpretation of SA activity, the following descriptors were found to have general observations. PISA is a π (carbon and attached hydrogen) component of the SASA. The lower the PISA value the higher the SA activity. The lower value of PISA is due to presence of electronegative groups the higher SA activity is. Higher value of PISA is due to presence of protons connected to C, N, and O and has more influence at the R_2 position. WPSA is a weakly polar component of the SASA (halogens P and S). Sulfhydryl group and halogens are not essential but impart moderate activity. Among halogens, activity diminishes at R_2 as Br > F in the presence of S. Electron acceptor is an atom that has a more positive value of electron affinity and the electron donor atom has less positive electron affinity. Electron affinity follows the trend of electronegativity. Fluorine (F) has a higher electron affinity than oxygen and chlorine most strongly attracts extra electrons. Atoms whose anions are stabler than neutral atoms have a greater electron affinity. Electron withdrawing group at R_2 is having more electron affinity and electron donating groups have moderate electron affinity which seems to be responsible for high to moderate activity, respectively. The activity would be higher for a combination of anion and proton donor at R_1 or R_2 position or vice versa, respectively. Overall, this equation gives the relationship of hydrophobicity of a molecule as essential characteristics required for the antibacterial activity against SA. Compounds 4b, 4j, 6f, 6h, and 6j were active at both the gram-positive and gram-negative bacterial strains.

This can be explained by using both of the QSAR equations. The compounds have high electron affinity and high dipole along with high values of FISA for activity against PA. The molecules have sufficient PISA contribution and low values of WPSA. Any extension to substituted phenyl by bulky groups would be favorable for activity against SA.

Polar surface area (PSA) descriptor represents drug transport properties such as intestinal absorption and blood-brain barrier penetration [27]. It is the sum of the contributions to the molecular (usually van der Waals) surface area of polar atoms such as oxygen, nitrogen, and their attached hydrogens. The polarity and polarizability of a molecule have been well known to be important for description of various physicochemical properties and chemical reactivity of molecule. Molecular polarity accounts for chromatographic retention on a polar stationary phase [28]. Most often, dipole moment is used which reflects only global polarity of molecule. Local polarities can be represented by atomic charges in the localized regions of the molecule.

8. Conclusions

The 2D-QSAR study on a series of indolylpyrimidine compounds showed that the presence of functional groups that balance the dipole and hydrophobicity would lead to increase in the activity of indolylpyrimidines against both PA and SA. The regression equation indicates that presence of polar components weighs more than hydrophobicity in the R_2 position of indolylpyrimidines for activity against *Pseudomonas aeruginosa*, while absence of protonated electronegative bulky groups at R_2 is suitable for antibacterial activity against *Staphylococcus aureus*.

Abbreviations

PA: *Pseudomonas aeruginosa*
SA: *Staphylococcus aureus*
MLR: Multiple linear regression
QSAR: Quantitative structure activity relationship
MMFF: Merck molecular force field
RMS: Root mean square
LOO: Leave one out

Conflict of Interests

The author declares no competing financial interests regarding the publication of this paper.

Acknowledgments

The author thanks his father, Mr. Anand Datar, and his guide, Dr. E. C. Coutinho, for providing facilities as well as continuous encouragement during this work.

References

[1] L. Nicoll, "*Pseudomonas aeruginosa*: infections and treatment," *New England Journal of Medicine*, vol. 332, pp. 616–617, 1995.

[2] J. Vila and T. Pal, "Update on antibacterial resistance in low-income countries: factors favoring the emergence of resistance," *Open Infectious Diseases Journal*, vol. 4, no. 1, pp. 38–54, 2010.

[3] C. Van Delden and B. H. Iglewski, "Cell-to-cell signaling and *Pseudomonas aeruginosa* infections," *Emerging Infectious Diseases*, vol. 4, no. 4, pp. 551–560, 1998.

[4] P. S. Charifson, T. H. Grossman, and P. Mueller, "The use of structure-guided design to discover new anti-microbial agents: focus on antibacterial resistance," *Anti-Infective Agents in Medicinal Chemistry*, vol. 8, no. 1, pp. 73–86, 2009.

[5] J. Vila, J. Sánchez-Céspedes, and E. Giralt, "Old and new strategies for the discovery of antibacterial agents," *Current Medicinal Chemistry: Anti-Infective Agents*, vol. 4, no. 4, pp. 337–353, 2005.

[6] H. D. Patel, B. D. Mistry, and K. R. Desai, "Synthesis and antimicrobial activity of pyrazolo [3,4-d] pyrimidines," *Indian Journal of Heterocyclic Chemistry*, vol. 13, no. 2, pp. 179–180, 2003.

[7] A. Kreutzberger and M. Sellheim, "Antimycotic agents. XIX. [1,2]. 4,6-disubstituted 2-(cyanamino)pyrimidine derivatives," *Journal of Heterocyclic Chemistry*, vol. 22, no. 3, pp. 721–723, 1985.

[8] V. Lather and P. V. Chowdary, "Synthesis and antimicrobial activity of N1-(arylidine hydrazidomethyl)-indoles, 2-(substituted aryl)-3-(N1-indolyl acetamidyl)-4-oxo-thiazolidines and 5-benzylidine derivatives of thiazolidinones," *Indian Journal of Pharmaceutical Sciences*, vol. 65, no. 6, pp. 576–579, 2003.

[9] G. S. Gadaginamath, A. S. Shyadligeri, and R. R. Kavali, "Chemoselectivity of indole-dicarboxylates towards hydrazine hydrate: part III-synthesis and antimicrobial activity of novel 4- thiazolidinonylindoles," *Indian Journal of Chemistry B: Organic and Medicinal Chemistry*, vol. 38, no. 2, pp. 156–159, 1999.

[10] P. Renukadevi and J. S. Biradar, "Synthesis and antimicrobial activity of 3,5-disubstituted-2-[1′-phenyl-5′-thioalkyl-s-triazol-2′-yl] indoles and 3,5-disubstituted-2-[1′-substituted aminomethyl-4′-phenyl-5′ (4′h)-thione-s-triazol-3-yl] indoles," *Indian Journal of Heterocyclic Chemistry*, vol. 9, no. 2, pp. 107–112, 1999.

[11] B. Jiang, C. Yang, W. Xiong, and J. Wang, "Synthesis and cytotoxicity evaluation of novel indolylpyrimidines and indolylpyrazines as potential antitumor agents," *Bioorganic and Medicinal Chemistry*, vol. 9, no. 5, pp. 1149–1154, 2001.

[12] M. A. A. Radwan and M. El-Sherbiny, "Synthesis and antitumor activity of indolylpyrimidines: marine natural product meridianin D analogues," *Bioorganic and Medicinal Chemistry*, vol. 15, no. 3, pp. 1206–1211, 2007.

[13] C. Hansch, A. Leo, and D. H. Hoekman, *Exploring QSAR, Hydrophobic, Electronic and Steric Constants*, American Chemical Society, Washington, DC, USA, 1995.

[14] C. Hansch, A. Leo, and D. H. Hoekman, *Exploring QSAR, Fundamentals and Application in Chemistry and Biology*, American Chemical Society, Washington, DC, USA, 1995.

[15] S. Panda and P. V. R. Chowdary, "Synthesis of novel indolylpyrimidine antiinflammatory, antioxidant and antibacterial agents," *Indian Journal of Pharmaceutical Sciences*, vol. 70, no. 2, pp. 208–215, 2008.

[16] D. F. Veber, S. R. Johnson, H. Cheng, B. R. Smith, K. W. Ward, and K. D. Kopple, "Molecular properties that influence the oral bioavailability of drug candidates," *Journal of Medicinal Chemistry*, vol. 45, no. 12, pp. 2615–2623, 2002.

[17] T. Masuda, T. Jikihara, K. Nakamura, A. Kimura, T. Takagi, and H. Fujiwara, "Introduction of solvent-accessible surface area in

the calculation of the hydrophobicity parameter log P from an atomistic approach," *Journal of Pharmaceutical Sciences*, vol. 86, no. 1, pp. 57–63, 1997.

[18] Guidance Document on the Validation of (Quantitative) Structure-Activity Relationship [(Q)SAR] Models. OECD Environment Health and Safety Publications Series on Testing and Assessment No. 69. OECD: Paris, 2007, http://www.oecd.org/dataoecd/55/35/38130292.pdf.

[19] J. G. Topliss and R. P. Edwards, "Chance factors in studies of quantitative structure-activity relationships," *Journal of Medicinal Chemistry*, vol. 22, no. 10, pp. 1238–1244, 1979.

[20] R. D. Cramer III, D. E. Patterson, and J. D. Bunce, "Comparative molecular field analysis (CoMFA). 1. Effect of shape on binding of steroids to carrier proteins," *Journal of the American Chemical Society*, vol. 110, no. 18, pp. 5959–5967, 1988.

[21] G. W. Snedecor and W. G. Cochran, *Statistical Methods*, Oxford and IBH, New Delhi, India, 1967.

[22] S. Chaltterjee, A. S. Hadi, and B. Price, *Regression Analysis by Examples*, Wiley VCH, New York, NY, USA, 2000.

[23] M. V. Diudea, *QSPR/QSAR Studies for Molecular Descriptors*, Nova Science, Huntingdon, NY, USA, 2000.

[24] A. M. Doweyko, "3D-QSAR illusions," *Journal of Computer-Aided Molecular Design*, vol. 18, no. 7–9, pp. 587–596, 2004.

[25] Y. Marrero Ponce, J. A. Castillo Garit, F. Torrens, V. Romero Zaldivar, and E. A. Castro, "Atom, atom-type, and total linear indices of the "molecular pseudograph's atom adjacency matrix": application to QSPR/QSAR studies of organic compounds," *Molecules*, vol. 9, no. 12, pp. 1100–1123, 2004.

[26] A. Golbraikh and A. Tropsha, "Beware of q^2!," *Journal of Molecular Graphics and Modelling*, vol. 20, no. 4, pp. 269–276, 2002.

[27] N. Strazielle and J. Ghersi-Egea, "Factors affecting delivery of antiviral drugs to the brain," *Reviews in Medical Virology*, vol. 15, no. 2, pp. 105–133, 2005.

[28] L. Buydens, D. L. Massart, and P. Geerlings, "Prediction of gas chromatographic retention indexes with topological, physicochemical, and quantum chemical parameters," *Analytical Chemistry*, vol. 55, no. 4, pp. 738–744, 1983.

23

Context-Based Separation of Cell Clusters for the Automatic Biocompatibility Testing of Implant Materials

S. Buhl, B. Neumann, and S. C. Schäfer

Institute for Computer Science, Vision and Computational Intelligence, South Westphalia University of Applied Sciences, Frauenstuhlweg 31, 58644 Iserlohn, Germany

Correspondence should be addressed to S. Buhl; sven.buhl@web.de

Academic Editor: Daniel Kendoff

This paper presents a new method to separate cells on microscopic surfaces joined together in cell clusters into individual cells. Important features of this method are that the remaining object geometry is preserved and few contour points are required for finding joints between neighboring cells. There are alternative methods such as morphological operations or the watershed transformation based on the inverse distance transformation but they have certain disadvantages compared to the method presented in this paper. The discussed method contains knowledge-based components in form of a decision function and exchangeable rules to avoid unwanted separations.

1. Introduction

In the process of testing implant materials for biocompatibility, it is important to evaluate whether a material is suitable for use in human bodies. An important aspect of biocompatibility is the determination of the exact number of cells which are in contact with the surface of the material being tested. For the specimen preparation process, a suspension with a defined cell concentration reacts for a certain time with the substrate under test and allows the cells to settle on the contact surface. Afterwards, the cells are stained using the May-Grünwald suspension [1] to be easily identifiable amongst each other. Microscopic images (Figure 1) are used to evaluate the results. A major challenge is the separation of single cells in a cluster due to their very variable morphology. The examination of many samples shows that L929 cells often exhibit cell clusters at various positions. This paper is based on providing a method of identifying individual cells within these cell clusters.

Several papers deal with different image processing methods for cell segmentation [2–7]. Depending on the image quality or the dyeing process, different segmentation methods may be the appropriate choice. If, for example, a noisy image has to be analyzed, the use of active contours could be advisable [3, 5–7].

The separation of connected cells is still a great challenge. Several papers provide different approaches to separate cells of a specific type [8–11]. Due to the often simple morphology of the analyzed cell types, a separation of clusters with simple rules is possible.

An iterative erosion method may create a separation of cells or objects at joining points between cells. After each iteration, it has to be checked whether separated objects have been created. The algorithm is not able to separate the cells without altering the cell contours. Therefore, a reconstruction of the cell area is required. A big disadvantage of this method is that it also removes or separates cell extensions, which is not acceptable in our case. An improved method for separating cells is described in [12] that leaves the cell contour unchanged. This method is known as opening by reconstruction. Compared to the method presented in the next section, this approach partially results in unwanted separation processes and requires about five times more computing time. If the local joining regions are considered to be objects which are being traced, the use of a hit-and-miss transformation [13] or a model-based method [14] is potential solution. But the morphological variation of the cells also leads to a variation of the joining shapes. Thus, a method is required which considers these circumstances.

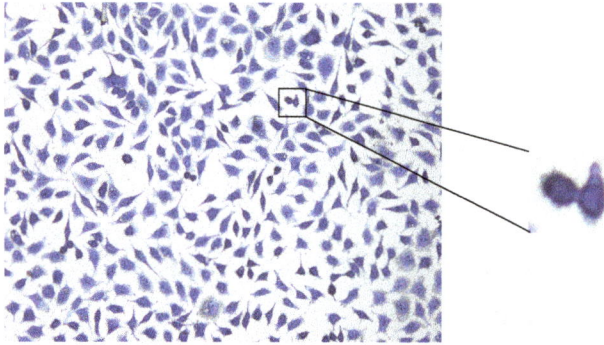

FIGURE 1: L929 cells on the substrate steel. Right: a biological cell division process, two joint cells which have a sand glass appearance.

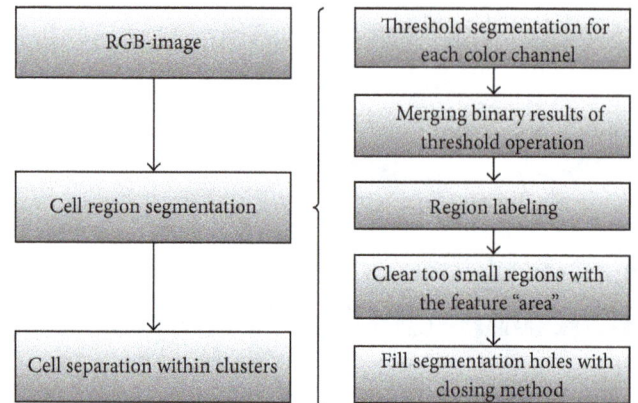

FIGURE 2: Cell segmentation process. The steps within the brackets are carried out for the cell region segmentation (Section 2.1). The subsequent separation of clusters is described in Section 2.2.

Another common procedure to separate connected cells is the watershed transformation based on the inverse distance transformation [15]. The method works well for cell types with a simple morphology, for example, peripheral blood and bone marrow samples. For biocompatibility testing, often cells of type L929 are used (Figure 1) but they are characterized by a strong varying morphology. Some cells are also creating cell extensions which are not allowed to be separated. These aspects have a negative impact on the segmentation result using the watershed transformation (Figure 12(e)).

The method for the separation of connected cells described in [16] turns out to be suitable. This algorithm first detects the nuclei with the Histogram Backprojection method [17]; then the shortest paths between the nuclei are calculated by means of the A^* algorithm [18]. The contact points of connected cells usually have local joints between cells, which are determined by calculating the so-called dominant contour points (DCPs) [19]. With the help of these DCPs, the separation of the cells can be carried out. The disadvantage of the method described in [16] is the high computing time for the separation process due to the high complexity of the algorithm (Table 3). A further disadvantage of the above-mentioned algorithm is the inability to separate cells which are in a biological cell division process (Figure 1) since they contain no visible nucleus regions. The method presented in this paper increases the separation performance and reduces significantly the computing time for the process in [16]. The method is not restricted to cell structures; it can also be applied to general objects which have to be separated.

2. Materials and Methods

2.1. Cell Segmentation. The images were created by the Olympus XC10 camera, which is installed on an Olympus Bx51 M microscope with 100x magnification. The size of the images is 1376×1032 pixel. The segmentation of the cell areas is carried out by a standard threshold procedure for all three color channels. The thresholds depend on the used staining method. In the case of the present May-Grünwald staining, the thresholds $T_R = 128$, $T_G = 150$, and $T_B = 150$ are used. To determine suitable thresholds, an expert draws the contours of 20 different cells in the image. The same cells are also automatically segmented by using the default threshold

values $T_R = T_G = T_B = 128$. With the help of the Jaccard coefficient, the similarity of the automatically generated cell areas compared to the reference areas can be measured. The automatic cell segmentation with subsequent calculation of the Jaccard coefficient is now iteratively performed with different threshold values. Finally the parameter set with the maximum Jaccard coefficient is used for cell segmentation. Due to a reliable staining process, the chosen parameters are robust for different images of one or more test samples.

The resulting three binary images B_R, B_G, and B_B are then merged into one image $B_{\text{Ges}} = B_R \cup B_G \cup B_B$ and a region labeling is performed. Only those segmented regions with a minimum area A_{Min} which depends on the used cell type are further analyzed. To determine the minimum cell area for cells of type L929, the cells in 50 images were automatically segmented and had their respective cell areas calculated. Afterwards, a manual check by an expert was done to determine whether the segmented object is a cell or merely an artifact on the substrate surface. The smallest segmented cell was determined to have an area of $C_{\text{MIN}} = 276$ pixel and the biggest segmented artifact was found to have an area of $E_{\text{Max}} = 102$ pixel. A_{Min} is defined as the average of the smallest cell area and the biggest artifact area:

$$A_{\text{Min}} = \frac{(C_{\text{Min}} + E_{\text{Max}})}{2} = 189 \text{ pixel}. \tag{1}$$

Finally small holes within the regions produced by the segmentation process are filled by the closing algorithm. The complete cell segmentation process is visualized in Figure 2.

Figure 2 shows the process of the presented method to segment the cell regions (Section 2.1) and then separating the clusters with help of the context-based separation method (Section 2.2).

2.2. Context-Based Separation. The new method presented in this paper is called the context-based separation (CBS). This method performs splitting operations on cells or other objects. This splitting is restricted to narrow joints between cells or objects. In an image m clusters $R_{C_1}, R_{C_2}, \ldots, R_{C_m}$ are contained. Each cluster consists of several cells which have

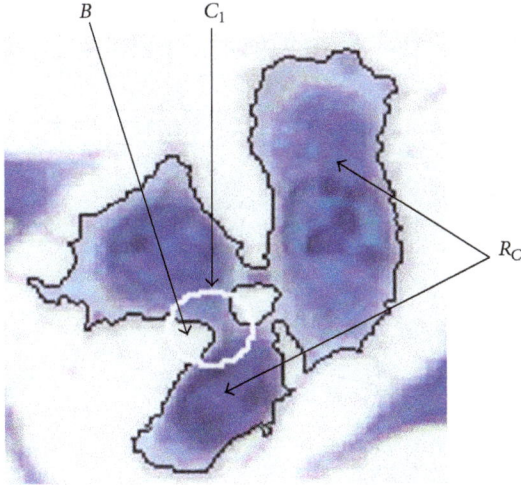

FIGURE 3: The contour of the object R_C is sampled by a circular structural element C_1.

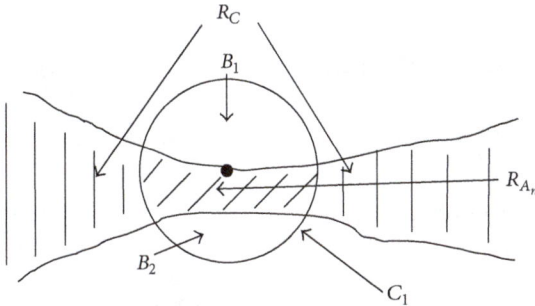

FIGURE 4: The background B within C_1 is separated by R_A in two subsets B_1 and B_2.

TABLE 1: Average relative deviation of the automatic cell count (2376 cells) to the reference cell count compiled by an expert is determined.

	$a = 1.25$	$a = 1.5$	$a = 2.0$	$a = 2.5$	$a = 3.0$
Relative deviation	8.6%	4.6%	2.7%	3.1%	5.4%

TABLE 2: Average relative deviation of the automatic cell count (2376 cells) to the reference cell count compiled by an expert.

	$x = 1.25$	$x = 1.5$	$x = 2.0$	$x = 2.5$	$x = 3.0$
Relative deviation	5.8%	2.7%	2.9%	3.8%	7.4%

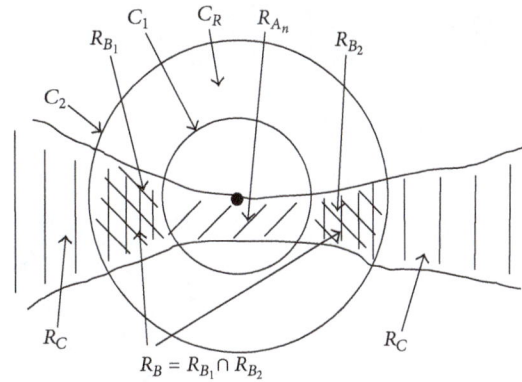

FIGURE 5: With help of C_1 and C_R it is checked whether a narrowing is present.

to be separated for further analysis. The approach of this method is shown by one cluster R_C. For purposes of clarity, R_C is defined as a representative of a cluster. Therefore, the cluster index can be ignored. This method is performed only at narrow joints R_{A_n} with $n = 1, 2, \ldots, x$ (Figure 5) where a separation process is carried out. For this purpose, the contour of the object R_C is sampled with a circular structural element C_1 with radius r_1 (Figure 3).

For each nth (step width) contour point it is checked whether the background area B enclosed by C_1 consists of two separated subsets B_1 and B_2. B_1 and B_2 must be separated by the cell area enclosed by C_1 with $R_{A_n} = C_1 \cap R_C$ (Figure 4). This is a necessary condition for a local joining of the object. A join is characterized by a dilatation at the ends. This is determined by creating a circular mask C_2 with radius $r_2 = a \cdot r_1$ which is generated concentrically around C_1. The parameter a is adjusted to this cell type. In our case $a = 2$ is suitable. If values smaller than 1.5 are chosen, not all local joints are found. In contrast, if the value of a is set higher than 2.75, the circular mask gets much bigger than most of the local joints and the failure rate increases (Table 1).

With the help of C_1 and C_2, the circular ring mask C_R is calculated with $C_R = C_2 \setminus C_1$ and in the further course of the algorithm $R_B = C_R \cap R_C$ is determined (Figure 5). A join

should be present when the decision function $f_1(x)$ assumes the value is true. For the case shown in Figure 5, where the point set R_B consists of 2 nonoverlapping or adjacent point sets R_{B_1} and R_{B_2}, the decision function is defined as

$$f_1(x) = \left(\left| R_{B_1} \right| \geq \left| R_{A_n} \right| \cdot x \right) \wedge \left(\left| R_{B_2} \right| \geq \left| R_{A_n} \right| \cdot x \right). \quad (2)$$

The set R_B can also comprise q nonoverlapping or adjacent sets of points (Table 4). The decision function $f_1(x)$ is then given by

$$f_1(x) = \left(\left| R_{B_1} \right| \geq \left| R_{A_n} \right| \cdot x \right) \wedge \left(\left| R_{B_2} \right| \geq \left| R_{A_n} \right| \cdot x \right)$$
$$\wedge \cdots \left(\left| R_{B_q} \right| \geq \left| R_{A_n} \right| \cdot x \right). \quad (3)$$

The symbol $|\cdots|$ denotes the number of pixels of a set. In our case the parameter x is set to $x = 1.5$. If the chosen value of x is too high, some local joints are not found. On the other hand if the value of x is a too small, the algorithm provides too many local joints (Table 2).

If $f_1(x)$ returns the value true, the object separation is done with the assignment

$$R_C' = R_C \setminus R_{A_n},$$
$$R_C := R_C'. \quad (4)$$

The cell region R_C is overridden to prevent multiple separations of neighboring contour points. R_{A_n} is added as an element of the set R_{A_Ges}. The mentioned separation process is carried out at the n narrowing joints of the cluster.

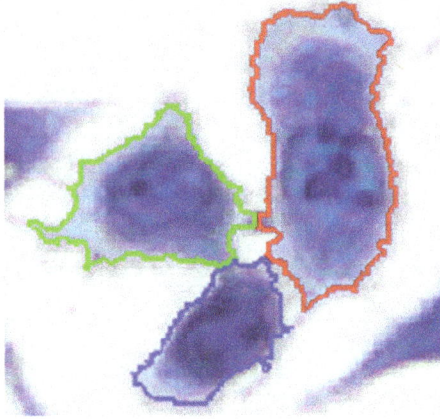

FIGURE 6: The result of the cell separation process. Three new cells R_{S_1}, R_{S_2}, and R_{S_3} are created.

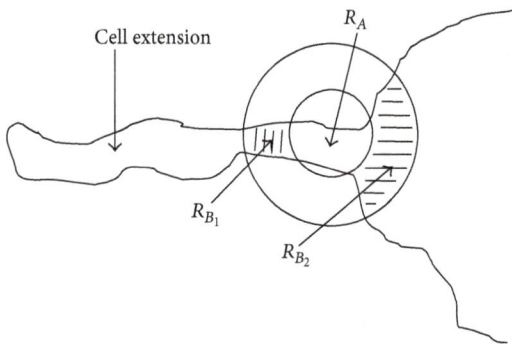

FIGURE 7: Incorrect separation of a cell extension from its cell.

TABLE 3: Average relative deviation of the automatic cell count (2376 cells) to the reference cell count compiled by an expert.

	$y = 1.5$	$y = 2$	$y = 3$	$y = 4$	$y = 5$
Relative deviation	26.7%	5.3%	2.7%	4.2%	8.1%

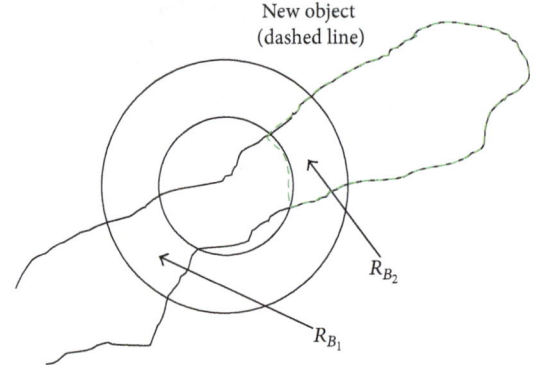

FIGURE 8: Incorrect splitting of a cell extension.

The extended decision function is $f(x, y) = f_1(x) \wedge f_2(y)$ with

$$f_2(y) = \left(\left| R_{B_1} \right| \leq y \cdot \left| R_{B_2} \right| \right) \vee \left(\left| R_{B_2} \right| \leq y \cdot \left| R_{B_1} \right| \right). \tag{5}$$

Figure 7 illustrates the case $|R_{B_2}| > 3|R_{B_1}|$. Thus $f_2(3) =$ false and therefore $f(1.5, 3) =$ false. A separation must not be carried out, because a cell extension which belongs to the cell was recognized. In some cases, the width of an elongated cell extension varies so much that $f(1.5, 3)$ has the value true (Figure 8). Again, this is obviously an incorrect decision and must be prevented with additional optional conditions.

Condition 1. All object regions in R_n, generated by the separation process, must have a minimum size $A_{\min}$; otherwise they are not separated.

Condition 2. The compactness of all object regions in R_n must be $K \leq a$ up to a maximum object size $A_{\max}$, with $a = 10$ in our case.

Generally in image processing the compactness is defined as

$$K = \left(\frac{L^2}{4A \cdot \pi} \right). \tag{6}$$

L is the contour length of the object and A is the object surface. If an element of R_n has an area $> A_{\max}$, it is a narrow elongated single cell and a separation is correct.

Figure 9 shows a simple flow-diagram of the CBS.

The agglomerate R_C has n different narrowing joints $R_{A_1}, R_{A_2}, \ldots, R_{A_n}$. These are processed sequentially in a loop with the CBS, shown with a thick border in Figure 9. The separation process of R_C results in r new object regions $R_{S_1}, R_{S_2}, \ldots, R_{S_r}$ from R_C, which are stored as elements of O_{List}. The mentioned procedure is valid for every segmented cluster. The detailed CBS algorithm is presented in the flow-diagram in Figure 10.

Applying the region labeling after the separation process of the cluster shown in Figure 6 results in 3 cells R_{S_1}, R_{S_2}, and R_{S_3}. In the context of the 3 separation processes R_{A_1}, R_{A_2}, and R_{A_3} are subtracted from R_C and the results are reassigned to R_C afterwards. The object regions stored in R_{A_Ges} are subsets of the original object region R_{C_Copy} and have to be assigned to the neighboring regions. For this purpose, each region R_{A_n} is separated into two regions using erosion. Each of the two separated regions is then assigned to the closest neighboring cell. Afterwards the assigned regions are enlarged to their original sizes using dilation. The dilation process stops if the two regions collide.

There may be situations in which object separations do not make sense, for example, at contact points between cell extensions and cell body, even though $f_1(x)$ delivers true. For this reason, the decision function $f_1(x)$ has to be expanded for a cell separation. The experience shows that a division should be avoided if one of the two regions R_{B_1} or R_{B_2} (Figure 7) is y-times greater than the other region. As in the earlier cases, y is a parameter adjusted to the situation. In our case $y = 3$ is chosen. If the parameter y is set too high, then cell extensions are partially separated from the cell. For the case that the value of y is set too small, the algorithm partially prevents the separation of connected cells (Table 3).

Start

Actual cluster R_C has n narrow joints $R_{A_1}, R_{A_2}, \ldots, R_{A_n}$

A copy R_{C_Copy} is made of the current object

Context-based separation of the current object R_C at the n narrow joints if $f(x, y)$ is true and the conditions 1 and 2 are fulfilled

Number of separated regions $r > 1$?

No — The copy R_{C_Copy} of the original object is appended to O_{List}

Stop

Yes — R_C is separated into r new objects $R_{S_1}, R_{S_2}, \ldots, R_{S_r}$ which are appended in O_{List}

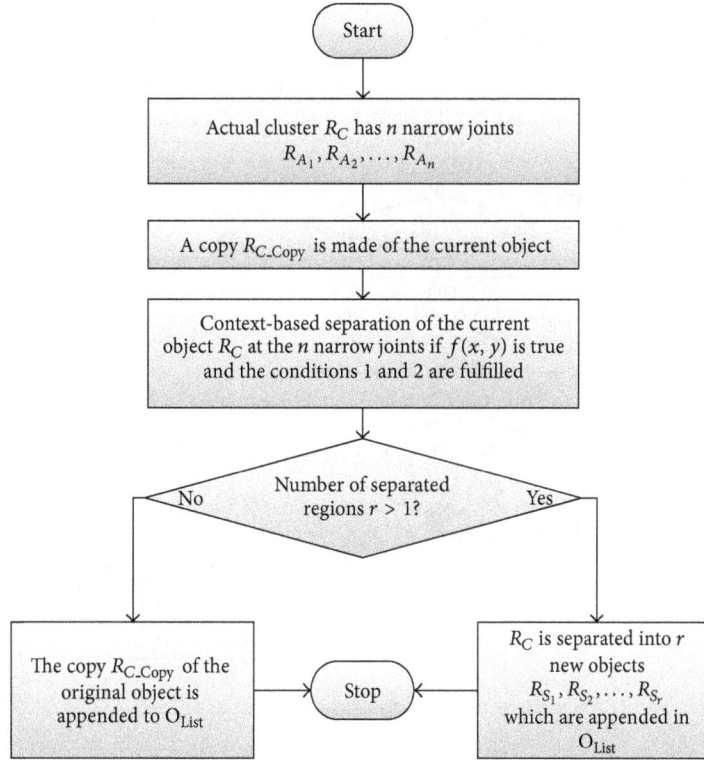

FIGURE 9: Simple flow-diagram of separating objects at the narrow joints.

Figure 10 shows a decision-based structure of the algorithm, with which the possible geometric variations of the objects are processed.

After calculation of $R_{A_n} = C_1 \cap R_C$ with subsequent region labeling R_{A_n} consists of k sets. For the case $k > 1$, only the set is addressed, which includes the center of C_1. If R_A consists only of one set, the calculation of $R_B = C_R \cap R_C$ follows. R_B is region labeled, so l subsets $R_{B_1}, R_{B_2}, \ldots, R_{B_l}$ are created, which form a coherent set when combined with R_{A_n}. If $l = 2$, the decision function $f(x, y)$ checks whether the two subsets R_{B_1} and R_{B_2} represent a join. In the case $l > 2$ it is checked whether all subsets fulfill

$$\left(\left| R_{B_p} \right| \geq x \cdot \left| R_{A_n} \right| \right) \wedge \left(\left| R_{B_p} \right| \geq \frac{\left| R_{B_p} \right|_{max}}{y} \right) \quad (7)$$

with $p = 1, 2, \ldots, l$; $x = 1.5$; $y = 3$

at which $\left| R_{B_p} \right|_{max}$ matches the biggest subset from $\{R_{B_1}, R_{B_2}, \ldots, R_{B_l}\}$.

If $R_{B_1}, R_{B_2}, \ldots, R_{B_l}$ contain at least two sets, which fulfill the previously mentioned conditions, the separation process is initiated. If q sets exist in $\{R_{B_1}, R_{B_2}, \ldots, R_{B_l}\}$ which do not fulfill the conditions, they are added as elements in R_{BD}, $R_{BD} = \{R_{BD_1}, R_{BD_2}, \ldots, R_{BD_q}\}$. After the object separation, the undesirably separated object regions are determined with the help of the elements in R_{BD}. A separated object region R_{S_j} with $j = 1, 2, \ldots, i$ is considered to be undesirable if $R_{U_{j,t}} = R_{S_j} \cap R_{BD_t}$ (with $t = 1, 2, \ldots, q$) results in $\left| R_{U_{j,t}} \right| > 0$. An undesired object region R_{S_j} is assigned randomly to one of the remaining objects. In this way, an object separation can be done even in cases where several object regions come together but not all of them must be separated (Table 4, case 5). The possible cases that can occur in context of a separation process are listed in Table 4. Figure 11 is used as a legend for Table 4.

The number of cell areas within C_1 and C_R can vary but this was not considered in Table 4 for reasons of clarity. Mixed forms of the illustrated cases are also possible, although this would not cause a problem for the algorithm.

3. Results and Discussion

In the context of biocompatibility testing of implant materials, the determination of the proliferation rate (cell count) and the evaluation of the cell morphology are important features. Therefore, an accurate determination of the cell borders within the clusters is necessary. The cytotoxicity of an implant material is classified in 4 levels depending on the proliferation rate (Table 5).

Table 5 shows that the minimum classification interval of the proliferation rate is 10% (Low cytotoxicity (80%–71%) and Moderate cytotoxicity (70%–61%)). If the automated cell count was to deviate by more than 10% from the reference cell

Start

Calculation of the contour points of the current cell cluster results in p contour points.

$j := 1$

$j \leq p$	No	Yes

A region labeling is carried out to R_C. The result contains i objects $R_{S_1}, R_{S_2}, \ldots, R_{S_i}$

Generate circular element C_1 with radius r_1 and midpoint at the position of the current contour point

$C_1 \cap B$ consists of at least 2 separated regions?	Yes	No

$R_A = C_1 \cap R_C$ R_A contains k separated sets $R_{A_1}, R_{A_2}, \ldots, R_{A_k}$	$k > 1$	$k = 1$

$i > 1$	Yes	No

$j := j +$ step width

Define $R_A = R_{A_k}$ with R_{A_k} containing the midpoint of C_1

Generate circular element C_2 with radius $r_2 = 2 \cdot r_1$ and circular ring $C_R = C_2 \backslash C_1$ $R_B = C_R \cap R_C$

Assign the object regions stored in R_{A_Ges} to the newly created neighbouring cells

$l < 2$

$l = 2$

All sets in R_B which are not connected to R_A are deleted. R_B now contains l separated sets $R_{B_1}, R_{B_2}, \ldots, R_{B_l}$

$l > 2$

If sets $R_{BD_1}, R_{BD_2}, \ldots, R_{BD_t}$ are stored in R_{BD}, the undesirable separated object regions are determined as follows. If $R_{U_{j,t}} = R_{S_j} \cap R_{BD_t}$ results in $|R_{U_{j,t}}| > 0$, then R_{S_j} is an undesired region and is assigned to one of the remaining objects; finally the result is r separated objects $R_{S_1}, R_{S_2}, \ldots, R_{S_r}$

Check the 2 sets R_{B_1}, R_{B_2}: Returns $f(x, y)$ true and constraints 1 and 2 are fulfilled?	No	Yes

Determine the biggest set $|R_{B_i}|_{max}$ in R_B

Check all sets R_{B_i} in R_B: $\left(|R_{B_i}| \geq x \cdot R_{A_n}|\right) \wedge \left(|R_{B_i}| \geq \dfrac{|R_{B_i}|_{max}}{y}\right)$ R_B contains s sets which fulfill the constraints and q sets which do not fulfill the constraints

$s \geq 2$	$s < 2$

Subtract R_{A_n} from R_C and combine R_{A_n} with R_{A_Ges}. $R_C := R_C \backslash R_{A_n}$ $R_{A\_Ges} := R_{A\_Ges} \cup R_{A_n}$ $n := n + 1$

Add the q sets $R_{BD_1}, R_{BD_2}, \ldots, R_{BD_t}$ with $t = 1, 2, \ldots, q$ in R_{BD}

$r > 1$	No	Yes

The original object R_{C_Copy} is added as an element to O_{List}

Save the r new objects $R_{S_1}, R_{S_2}, \ldots, R_{S_r}$ as elements of O_{List}

Stop

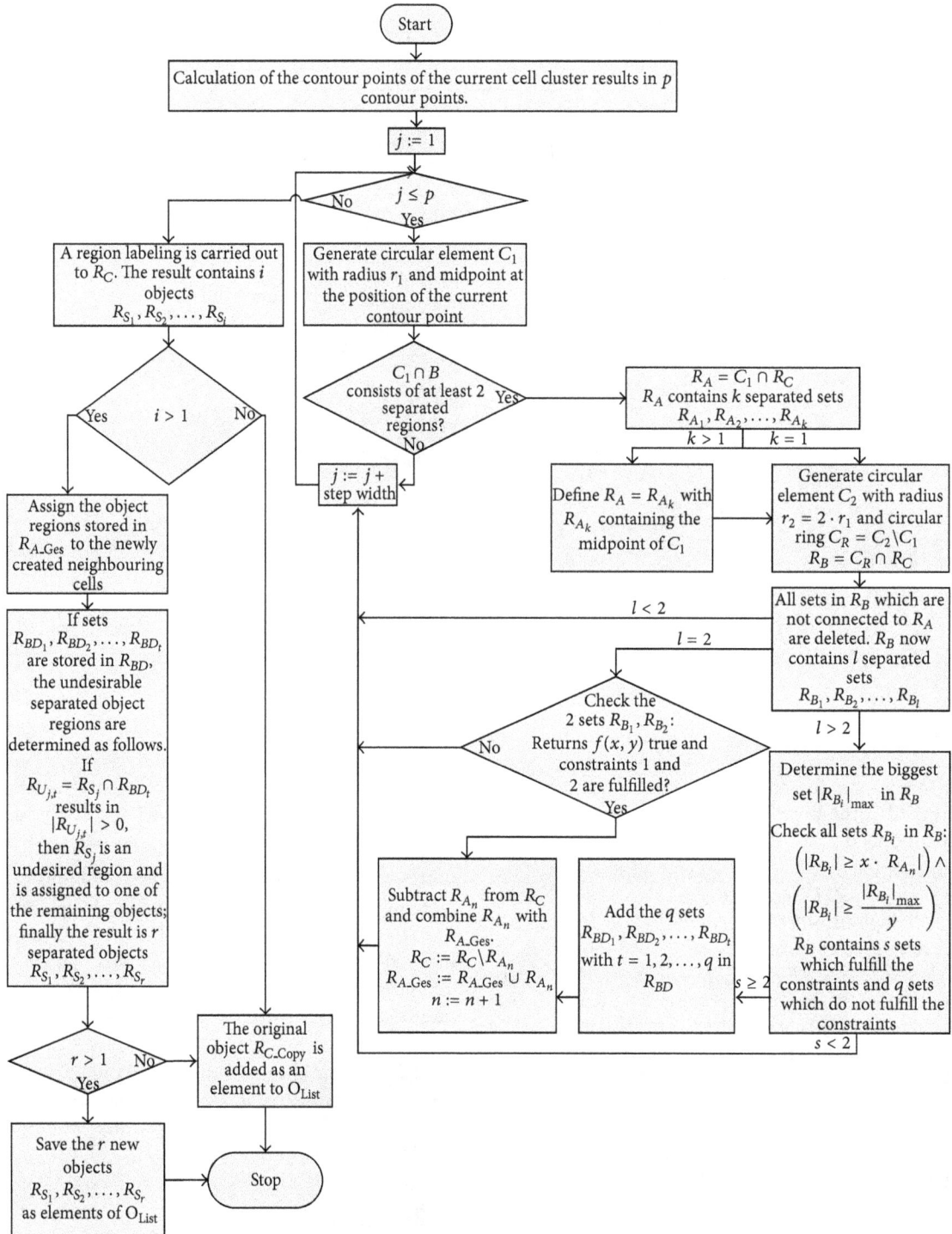

Figure 10: Activity diagram of the CBS.

count, it would not be possible to reliably classify the cytotoxicity level of implant materials. Therefore, the automated counting of cells in the field of biocompatibility is only feasible if a counting accuracy of more than 95% is attainable.

To evaluate the efficiency of the presented method, first the number of cells for 10 samples (2409 cells) of the cell type L929 on the substrates steel as well as titanium is determined and compared to the number of cells specified by an expert (reference cell count). The part of L929 cells which are connected to clusters is in average 23.3%. Table 6 shows the cell counting for the method presented in this paper compared to two other separation methods [15, 20]. The algorithm in [20] is old but cell separation with the help of morphological operations is still a common procedure. The method

TABLE 4: Schematic illustration of possible object shapes at a cell contact point.

	Schema	Description
Case 1		The circular ring C_1 includes the cell region R_{A_n} that separates the background pixels in two separate sets B_1 and B_2 (Figure 5). The circular ring C_R includes two noncontiguous sets R_{B_1} and R_{B_2}. To allow object separating, $f(x, y)$ has to return the value true for R_{B_1} and R_{B_2} and the additional conditions 1 and 2 must be met.
Case 2		There are two separated cell regions within C_1. For further processing only the cell area is selected which contains the center of C_1 in its point set. As a result of this processing, this case is case type 3 from now on.
Case 3		There is a separated cell area within C_R which does not enter the region of C_1. This cell region will be ignored for further processing. As a result the case is type 1 from this point forward.
Case 4		C_R contains a separated cell area, which is connected to R_{A_n}, but not with other object areas. For all three subsets contained in R_B, it is checked whether $f(x, y)$ returns true and the conditions 1 and 2 are fulfilled. If at least two subsets remain in R_B which fulfill the above-mentioned criteria; the separation takes place at this point. All subsets in R_B, which do not satisfy the above-mentioned criteria, will be added as elements in R_{BD} so that the cell regions separated in error can be reunited with the neighboring object.
Case 5		Compared to case 4, there are one or more separate cell areas located within C_R, which are connected to R_{A_n} and other parts of R_C in this case. It is determined for all subsets in R_B whether $f(x, y)$ returns true and conditions 1 and 2 are met. If at least two subsets in R_B remain which fulfill the above-mentioned criteria, the separation takes place at this point. All subsets in R_B which do not satisfy the above-mentioned criteria are stored as elements in R_{BD} similarly to Case 4 so that the cell regions separated in error can be reunited with the neighboring object.

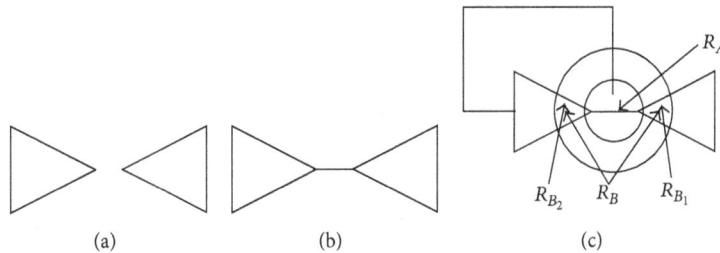

FIGURE 11: (a) 2 cells; (b) two connected cells; (c) two connected cells where a left cells region extends into C_1.

TABLE 5: Assignment of the cell proliferation rate to the four levels of cytotoxicity.

Cytotoxicity level	Proliferation rate (%)	Interpretation
0	100–81	Not cytotoxic
1	80–71	Low cytotoxicity
2	70–61	Moderate cytotoxicity
3	60–0	Strong cytotoxicity

introduced in [15] is based on the watershed transformation applied to the inverse distance transformation of the segmented cell areas. This is a state-of-the-art procedure to separate connected nuclei or cells in microscopic images.

Separating the cells with the CBS method results in a mean cell count error of 2.7%. In comparison, using the methods described in [15, 20], an average cell count error of 9.3% and 5.1% results. Table 6 shows that the algorithms described in [15, 20] have a high false positive detection rate (10.3% and 5.7%). The main reason is that that these methods are not able to detect the cell extensions as part of the cell and therefore separate them incorrectly. On the other hand, these methods provide a very small false negative detection rate (1.0% and 0.6%) yet due to the high false positive detection rate the overall error is higher in comparison to the CBS algorithm. Thus, the method described in this paper is more suitable for the determination of the L929 cell number as the methods described in [15, 20]. Figure 12 shows the cell separation results for the investigated methods.

TABLE 6: Comparison of cell counting using the CBS and the methods presented in [20] and [15].

Sample	ACC	FP	FN	PC	REF	RFP (%)	RFP (%)	ERR (%)
				CBS Algorithm				
1	234	4	2	230	232	1.7	0.9	0.9
2	350	3	22	347	369	0.8	6.0	5.1
3	240	2	12	238	250	0.8	4.8	4.0
4	193	3	9	190	199	1.5	4.5	3.0
5	232	4	12	228	240	1.7	5.0	3.3
6	205	9	3	196	199	4.5	1.5	3.0
7	217	3	1	214	215	1.4	0.5	0.9
8	208	5	7	203	210	2.4	3.3	1.0
9	220	6	1	214	215	2.8	0.5	2.3
10	270	6	16	264	280	2.1	5.7	3.6
					Ø Err	**2.0**	**3.3**	**2.7**
				Method described in [20]				
1	255	24	1	231	232	10.3	0.4	9.9
2	380	16	5	364	369	4.3	1.4	3.0
3	269	21	2	248	250	8.4	0.8	7.6
4	223	25	1	198	199	12.6	0.5	12.1
5	260	23	3	237	240	9.6	1.3	8.3
6	222	25	2	197	199	12.6	1.0	11.6
7	247	36	4	211	215	16.7	1.9	14.9
8	231	23	2	208	210	11.0	1.0	10.0
9	236	22	1	214	215	10.2	0.5	9.8
10	296	20	4	276	280	7.1	1.4	5.7
					Ø Err	**10.3**	**1.0**	**9.3**
				Method described in [15]				
1	245	14	1	231	232	6.0	0.4	5.6
2	391	25	3	366	369	6.8	0.8	6.0
3	258	8	0	250	250	3.2	0.0	3.2
4	211	14	2	197	199	7.0	1.0	6.0
5	252	13	1	239	240	5.4	0.4	5.0
6	208	10	1	198	199	5.0	0.5	4.5
7	226	13	2	213	215	6.0	0.9	5.1
8	219	10	1	209	210	4.8	0.5	4.3
9	230	16	1	214	215	7.4	0.5	7.0
10	292	14	2	278	280	5.0	0.7	4.3
					Ø Err	**5.7**	**0.6**	**5.1**

ACC: automatic cell count; FP: false positive detection; FN: false negative (missed) detection; PC: positive correct detection (ACC − FP); REF: reference cell count; RFP: relative false positive detection (FP/REF ∗ 100); RFN: relative false negative detection (FN/REF ∗ 100); ERR: relative error (((REF − ACC)/REF) ∗ 100).

The used algorithms described in [15, 20] lead to a partial splitting of one cell or cell extensions indicated by the arrows in Figures 12(c) and 12(e). However, these cell extensions are part of the cell and thus they are not allowed to be separated from the rest of the cell area.

As mentioned the CBS can be used independently of other procedures or it can be combined with other methods, for example, the algorithm described in [16], to decrease the calculation time (Table 7) and to improve the cell count quality.

By using the CBS a speed-up factor of about 8 may be achieved, compared to the cell count algorithm without the use of CBS (Table 7). The calculation time is varying since the number of clusters is changing from image to image.

In comparison, the method described in [9] results in 3.9% deviation from the reference cell count for leukocyte cells. In contrast to type L929, the leukocyte cells morphology does not vary so much. Therefore, it can be assumed that the deviation gets worse for cells with stronger varying morphology than the leucocyte cells.

The evaluation of the cell morphology is an important aspect in the context of biocompatibility testing. Therefore, an accurate segmentation of the cell boundaries within the clusters is important in order to obtain a reliable result. To evaluate the methods precision concerning the cell area segmentation, 100 automatically segmented cell regions within clusters were compared with the cell regions evaluated manually by an expert. The Jaccard coefficient is a suitable method to

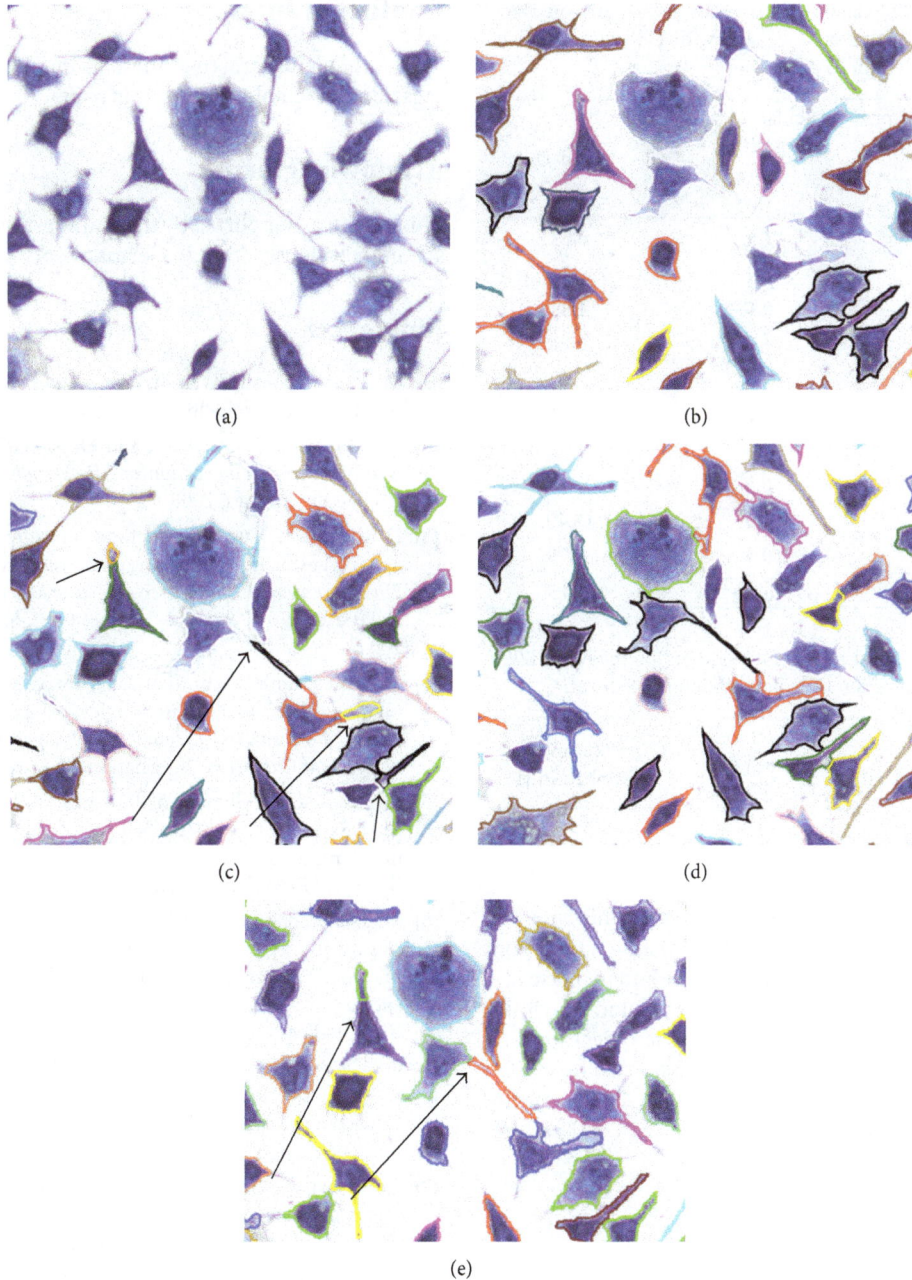

FIGURE 12: (a) Cells of type L929. (b) Cell segmentation result before the separation process. Some cells are connected to each other. (c) Cell separation with the method described in [20]. The arrows indicate wrong separation results. (d) Cell separation with the CBS method. (e) Cell separation with the method described in [15]. The arrows indicate wrong separation results.

determine the quality of the separation. If two objects are equal in shape and area, the Jaccard coefficient is 1. Table 8 shows the Jaccard coefficient of the CBS and four other separation algorithms.

Table 8 shows a Jaccard Coefficent of 0.84 for the CBS. In comparison, the other methods [15, 16, 20] provide with 0.76, 0.75 and 0.8 poorer results.

The methods [15, 20] partially split cellular extensions or even holes cells (Figures 12(c) and 12(e)). However, with the presented method and the algorithm introduced in [16], no cell extensions are separated and most cells are cut at

reasonable places from a biological point of view. The method described in [16] is, in contrast to the CBS, not suitable for the separation of cells which are in a biological division process. Therefore, the Jaccard coefficient is slightly worse in comparison to the presented procedure.

The required parameters for the decision function $f(x, y)$ for the cell type L929 were adjusted experimentally. With $f(1.5, 3)$, the smallest deviation of the automated cell count compared to the reference value is obtained. The cell-specific rules such as object size and compactness were set up specifically for this application and can, if necessary, be replaced

TABLE 7: Comparison of calculation time for the separation algorithm described in [16] without CBS and with CBS on a 3.2 GHz Intel Core i7 CPU with parallel processing.

Sample	Calculation time Algorithm excluding CBS (s)	Calculation time Algorithm including CBS (s)	Speed-Up
1	12.4	**1.9**	6.53
2	5.8	**2.1**	2.76
3	4.4	**0.9**	4.89
4	11.8	**1.9**	6.21
5	2.1	**0.6**	3.50
6	4.1	**1.1**	3.73
7	1.1	**0.4**	2.75
8	2.0	**0.5**	4.00
9	6.2	**0.5**	12.40
10	15.1	**0.4**	37.75
		Ø Speed-up	**8.45**

TABLE 8: Calculated Jaccard coefficient based on 100 reference L929 cells within clusters for different cell separation procedures.

CBS	Method described in [16]	Method described in [20]	Method described in [15]
0.84	0.80	0.75	0.76

by other rules without changing the method. In this case the method is used as a supplement to the existing separation algorithm [16] to reduce the calculation time and increase the accuracy of cell counting and cell area segmentation within the clusters. It is possible to apply the CBS to object joining situations independently of other algorithms. By doing so, the calculation time needed is milliseconds. The CBS algorithm can also be applied to other types of objects and is therefore suitable for other similar types of problems.

4. Conclusion

In this paper, a method for segmenting and separating cells in clusters is presented. The algorithm first segments histological stained cell regions in microscopic images with a standard threshold method applied to each color channel. The separation of connected cells at narrow joints is carried out by sampling the cluster contour with a circular structural element. Within the circular element, the cell geometry is analyzed and the result of a decision function indicates whether a local narrowing exists or not. An extension of the decision function with two exchangeable conditions avoids unwanted separation processes and improves the cell area segmentation. The method can be used to separate any segmented objects which have narrow joints at their contact areas. It has a very fast execution speed since not all contour points have to be processed. The procedure can be combined very well with other separation methods. This leads to better results and reduces the overall calculation time.

Conflict of Interests

The authors declare that there is no conflict of interests regarding the publication of this paper.

Acknowledgment

This work was supported by the "Bundesministerium für Forschung und Entwicklung," Germany (no. 17033X10).

References

[1] M. Mulisch and U. Welsch, *Mikroskopische Technik*, Spektrum Akademischer, Heidelberg, Germany, 2010.

[2] S. Colantonio, I. Gurevich, and O. Salvetti, *Automatic Fuzzy-Neural Based Segmentation of Microscopic Cell Images*, Inderscience Enterprises, 2008.

[3] D. Murashov, "Two-level method for segmentation of cytological images using active contour model," in *Proceedings of the 7th International Conference on Pattern Recognition and Image Analysis (PRIA-7 '04)*, vol. 3, pp. 814–817, St Petersburg, Russia, 2004.

[4] G. Ramella and G. Sanniti di Baja, "Image segmentation by nontopological erosion and topological expansion," in *Advances in Mass Data Analysis of Signals and Images in Medicine Biotechnology and Chemistry*, International Converences MDA, 2007.

[5] F. Sadeghian, Z. Seman, A. R. Ramli, B. H. Abdul Kahar, and M.-I. Saripan, "A framework for white blood cell segmentation in microscopic blood images using digital image processing," *Biological Procedures Online*, vol. 11, no. 1, pp. 196–206, 2009.

[6] M. Tscherepanow, F. Zöllner, M. Hillebrand, and F. Kummert, "Automatic segmentation of unstained living cells in bright-field microscope images," in *Proceedings of the International Conference on Mass-Data Analysis of Images and Signals in Medicine, Biotechnology, Chemistry and Food Industry (MDA)*, vol. 5108, pp. 158–172, Springer, Heidelberg, Germany, 2008.

[7] F. A. Velasco and J. L. Marroquín, "Robust parametric active contours: the Sandwich Snakes," *Machine Vision and Applications*, vol. 12, no. 5, pp. 238–242, 2001.

[8] S. Kothari, Q. Chaudry, and M. D. Wang, "Automated cell counting and cluster segmentation using concavity detection and ellipse fitting techniques," in *Proceedings of the IEEE International Symposium on Biomedical Imaging: From Nano to Macro (ISBI '09)*, pp. 795–798, Boston, Mass, USA, July 2009.

[9] B. Nilsson and A. Heyden, "Segmentation of complex cell clusters in microscopic images: application to bone marrow samples," *Cytometry Part A*, vol. 66, no. 1, pp. 24–31, 2005.

[10] A. Sheehy, G. Martinez, J.-G. Frerichs, and T. Scheper, "Region and contour based cell cluster segmentation algorithm for insitu microscopy," in *Proceedings of the 5th International Conference on Electrical Engineering, Computing Science and Automatic Control (CCE '08)*, pp. 168–172, Mexico City, Mexico, November 2008.

[11] W. Weixing and S. Hao, "Cell cluster image segmentation on form analysis," in *Proceedings of the 3rd International Conference on Natural Computation (ICNC '07)*, pp. 833–836, Haikou, China, August 2007.

[12] L. Vincent, "Morphological grayscale reconstruction in image analysis: applications and efficient algorithms," *IEEE Transactions on Image Processing*, vol. 2, no. 2, pp. 176–201, 1993.

[13] R. Haralick and L. Shapiro, *Computer and Robot Vision*, vol. 1, Addison-Wesley, 1992.

[14] K.-M. Lee and W. N. Street, "Model-based detection, segmentation, and classification for image analysis using on-line shape learning," *Machine Vision and Applications*, vol. 13, no. 4, pp. 222–233, 2001.

[15] J. Cheng and J. C. Rajapakse, "Segmentation of clustered nuclei with shape markers and marking function," *IEEE Transactions on Biomedical Engineering*, vol. 56, no. 3, pp. 741–748, 2009.

[16] S. Buhl, B. Neumann, and E. Eisenbarth, "Segmentation of cytological stained cell areas and generation of cell boundaries," in *Complex Shaded Cell Clusters*, 55. IWK—International Scientific Colloquium, pp. 511–514, Isle Publisher, Ilmenau, Germany, 2010.

[17] M. J. Swain and D. H. Ballard, "Indexing via color histograms," in *Proceedings of the 3rd International Conference on Computer Vision*, pp. 390–393, December 1990.

[18] P. E. Hart, N. J. Nilsson, B. Raphael et al., "Correction to a formal basis for the heuristic determination of minimum cost paths," *SIGART Newsletter*, vol. 37, pp. 28–29, 1972.

[19] U. Pal, K. Rodenacker, and B. B. Chaudhuri, "Automatic cell segmentation in cyto- and histometry using dominant contour feature points," *Analytical Cellular Pathology*, vol. 17, no. 4, pp. 243–250, 1998.

[20] V. Metzler, H. Bienert, T. Lehmann, K. Mottaghy, and K. Spitzer, "A novel method for quantifying shape deformation applied to biocompatibility testing," *ASAIO Journal*, vol. 45, no. 4, pp. 264–271, 1999.

Permissions

The contributors of this book come from diverse backgrounds, making this book a truly international effort. This book will bring forth new frontiers with its revolutionizing research information and detailed analysis of the nascent developments around the world.

We would like to thank all the contributing authors for lending their expertise to make the book truly unique. They have played a crucial role in the development of this book. Without their invaluable contributions this book wouldn't have been possible. They have made vital efforts to compile up to date information on the varied aspects of this subject to make this book a valuable addition to the collection of many professionals and students.

This book was conceptualized with the vision of imparting up-to-date information and advanced data in this field. To ensure the same, a matchless editorial board was set up. Every individual on the board went through rigorous rounds of assessment to prove their worth. After which they invested a large part of their time researching and compiling the most relevant data for our readers.

The editorial board has been involved in producing this book since its inception. They have spent rigorous hours researching and exploring the diverse topics which have resulted in the successful publishing of this book. They have passed on their knowledge of decades through this book. To expedite this challenging task, the publisher supported the team at every step. A small team of assistant editors was also appointed to further simplify the editing procedure and attain best results for the readers.

Apart from the editorial board, the designing team has also invested a significant amount of their time in understanding the subject and creating the most relevant covers. They scrutinized every image to scout for the most suitable representation of the subject and create an appropriate cover for the book.

The publishing team has been an ardent support to the editorial, designing and production team. Their endless efforts to recruit the best for this project, has resulted in the accomplishment of this book. They are a veteran in the field of academics and their pool of knowledge is as vast as their experience in printing. Their expertise and guidance has proved useful at every step. Their uncompromising quality standards have made this book an exceptional effort. Their encouragement from time to time has been an inspiration for everyone.

The publisher and the editorial board hope that this book will prove to be a valuable piece of knowledge for researchers, students, practitioners and scholars across the globe.

List of Contributors

R. A. Thuraisingham
1A, Russell Street, Eastwood, NSW 2122, Australia

Steady Mushayabasa
Department of Mathematics, University of Zimbabwe, P.O. Box MP 167, Harare, Zimbabwe

Sean Ekins
Collaborations in Chemistry, 5616 Hilltop Need more Road, Fuquay-Varina, NC 27526, USA

Antony J. Williams
Royal Society of Chemistry, 904 Tamaras Circle, Wake Forest, NC 27587, USA

Michael-R. Goldsmith
National Exposure Research Laboratory, US-Environmental Protection Agency, 109 TW Alexander Drive, Research Triangle Park, NC 27711, USA

Aniko Simon, Zsolt Zsoldos and Orr Ravitz
SimBioSys, Inc., 135 Queen's Plate Drive, Suite 520, Toronto, ON, Canada M9W6V1

Ghasem Ghasemi, Shahab Shariati and Zinab Rastgoo
Department of Chemistry, Rasht Branch, Islamic Azad University, Rasht, Iran

Sattar Arshadi
Department of Chemistry, Payame Noor University, Behshahr Branch, Behshahr, Iran

Nemati Rashtehroodi
Department of Chemistry, Payame Noor University, Sari Branch, Sari, Iran

Alireza Mahyar Nirouei
Department of Electrical Engineering, Lahijan Branch, Islamic Azad University, Lahijan, Iran

S. R. Ghodsi
VFE Research Institute, University of Tehran (Campus 2), College of Engineering, 4th Floor of Institute of Petroleum Engineering Building, North Kargar Avenue, Tehran 14399-56191, Iran

V. Esfahanian
School of Mechanical Engineering, University of Tehran, Tehran 14399-56191, Iran

S. M. Ghodsi
Sina Trauma Research Center, Tehran University of Medical Science, Tehran 14399-56191, Iran

Shalini Singh and Pradeep Srivastava
School of Biochemical Engineering, Indian Institute of Technology (Banaras Hindu University), Varanasi 221005, India

Kirsi Varpa, Kati Iltanen and Martti Juhola
Computer Science, School of Information Sciences, University of Tampere, 33014 Tampere, Finland

Maria A. Ivanchuk
Department of Biological Physics and Medical Informatics, Bukovinian State Medical University, Kobyljanska Street 42, Chernivtsi 58000, Ukraine

Vitalij V. Maksimyuk
Department of Surgery, Bukovinian State Medical University, Golovna Street 137, Chernivtsi 58000, Ukraine

Igor V. Malyk
Department of the System Analysis and Insurance and Financial Mathematics, Chernivtsi National University of Yuriy Fedkovich, Unversitetska Street 12, Chernivtsi 58012, Ukraine

Adnan Khan, Sultan Sial and Mudassar Imran
Department of Mathematics, Lahore University of Management Sciences, Lahore 54792, Pakistan

Rahul P. Gangwal, Gaurao V. Dhoke, Mangesh V. Damre, Kanchan Khandelwal and Abhay T. Sangamwar
Department of Pharmacoinformatics, National Institute of Pharmaceutical Education and Research (NIPER), Sector 67, S.A.S. Nagar, Punjab 160 062, India

Donghua Liao and Jingbo Zhao
GIOME Academia, Institute of Clinical Medicine, Aarhus University Hospital, 8200 Aarhus, Denmark
Mech-Sense, Department of Gastroenterology and Surgery, Aalborg University Hospital, 9000 Aalborg, Denmark

Peng Wang
Department of Mechanical and Manufacturing Engineering, Aalborg University, 9220 Aalborg, Denmark

Hans Gregersen
College of Bioengineering, Chongqing University, Chongqing 400050, China The GIOME Institute, Dubai, UAE

Edward T. Dougherty
Mathematics Department, Rowan University, Glassboro, NJ 08028, USA

James C. Turner
Mathematics Department, Virginia Polytechnic Institute and State University, Blacksburg, VA 24061, USA

Tien Tuan Dao and Philippe Pouletaut
Sorbonne Universités, Université de Technologie de Compiégne, CNRS, UMR 7338 Biomécanique et Bioingénierie, Centre de Recherche Royallieu, CS 60 319,60 203 Compiégne, France

Tien Tuan Dao
Sorbonne Universités, Université de Technologie de Compiégne, CNRS, UMR 7338, Biomécanique et Bioingénierie, Centre de Recherche Royallieu, CS 60 319, 60 203 Compiégne, France

Tien Tuan Dao
Sorbonne Universités, Université de Technologie de Compiégne, CNRS, UMR 7338, Biomécanique et Bioingénierie, Centre de Recherche Royallieu, CS 60 319, 60 203 Compiégne, France

Ambreen Hafeez, Afshan Naz and Naheed Akhtar
Biophysics Research Unit, Department of Biochemistry, University of Karachi, Karachi 75270, Pakistan

Zafar Saied Saify
International Center for Biological and Chemical Sciences, HEJ Research Institute of Chemistry, University of Karachi, Karachi 75270, Pakistan

Farzana Yasmin
Biomedical Engineering Department, NED University of Engineering and Technology, Karachi 75270, Pakistan

Durjoy Majumder and Sayan Mukherjee
Department of Physiology, West Bengal State University, Berunanpukuria, P.O. Malikapur, Barasat, North 24 Parganas, Kolkata 700126, India

Anup K. Paul and Rupak K. Banerjee
School of Dynamic Systems, Mechanical Engineering Program, University of Cincinnati, Cincinnati, OH 45221, USA

Arumugam Narayanan, Mohamed A. Effat and Jason J. Paquin
Division of Cardiovascular Diseases, University of Cincinnati, Cincinnati, OH 45221, USA

Julia Vianna Gallinaro, Fernando Mendes de Azevedo and Daniela Ota Hisayasu Suzuki
Instituto de Engenharia Biomédica, Departamento de Engenharia Elétrica, CTC, Universidade Federal de Santa Catarina, 88040-900 Florianópolis, SC, Brazil

Claudia Mirian de Godoy Marques
Centro de Ciências da Saúde e do Esporte, Universidade do Estado de Santa Catarina, 88080-350 Florianópolis, SC, Brazil

Vaibhav A. Dixit and Prasad V. Bharatam
Department of Medicinal Chemistry, National Institute of Pharmaceutical Education and Research (NIPER), S. A. S. Nagar, Punjab 160062, India

J. Jesús Naveja, Andrés Rodríguez-Galván and Erick Martínez-Lorán
Technology and Consultancy, CTDAT, 04360 Mexico City, Mexico

Flavio F. Contreras-Torres
Technology and Consultancy, CTDAT, 04360 Mexico City, Mexico
Universidad de Investigación de Tecnología Experimental Yachay, 100119 Urcuqui, Ecuador

Prasanna A. Datar
Department of Pharmaceutical Chemistry, Sinhgad Institute of Pharmacy, Narhe, Pune 411041, India

S. Buhl, B. Neumann and S. C. Schäfer
Institute for Computer Science, Vision and Computational Intelligence, South Westphalia University of Applied Sciences, Frauenstuhlweg 31, 58644 Iserlohn, Germany

www.ingramcontent.com/pod-product-compliance
Lightning Source LLC
Chambersburg PA
CBHW080517200326
41458CB00012B/4237